Access Videos, Podcasts, and More!

Self-Study Companion Website resources included with any new book.

Access to MyHealthLab, including assignments and eText, sold separately.

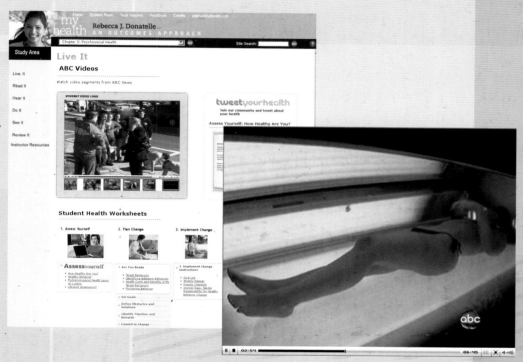

REGISTER NOW!

Registration will let you:

— See It! with *ABC News* videos.

— See It! with New Student "Video Blogs (vlogs)" which show real students' attempts at behavior change throughout a semester, showing their triumphs and failures, and allowing for assignments and learning experiences.

Registration also gives you access to multiple practice quizzes, mobile apps, web links, critical thinking exercises, and more.

www.pearsonhighered.com/donatelle

TO REGISTER

1. Go to www.pearsonhighered.com/donatelle
2. Click on your book cover.
3. Select any chapter from the drop-down menu and click "Go."
4. Click on "See It" and then one of the video options.
5. Click "Register."
6. Follow the on-screen instructions to create your login name and password.

Your Access Code is:

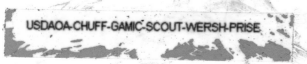

USDAOA-CHUFF-GAMIC-SCOUT-WERSH-PRISE

Note: If there is no silver foil covering the access code, it may already have been redeemed, and therefore may no longer be valid. In that case, you can purchase access online using a major credit card or PayPal account. To do so, go to www.pearsonhighered.com/donatelle click on "Buy Access," and follow the on-screen instructions.

TO LOG IN

1. Go to www.pearsonhighered.com/donatelle
2. Click on your book cover.
3. Select any chapter from the drop-down menu and click "Go."
4. Click on "See It" and then one of the video options.
5. Enter your login name and password.

Hint:
Remember to bookmark the site after you log in.

Technical Support:
http://247pearsoned.custhelp.com

BEHAVIOR CHANGE CONTRACT

Complete the Assess Yourself questionnaire. After reviewing your results and considering the various factors that influence your decisions, choose a health behavior that you would like to change, starting this quarter or semester. Sign the contract at the bottom to affirm your commitment to making a healthy change and ask a friend to witness it.

My behavior change will be:

_____

My long-term goal for this behavior change is:

_____

These are three obstacles to change (things that I am currently doing or situations that contribute to this behavior or make it harder to change):

1. _____
2. _____
3. _____

The strategies I will use to overcome these obstacles are:

1. _____
2. _____
3. _____

Resources I will use to help me change this behavior include:

a friend/partner/relative: _____

a school-based resource: _____

a community-based resource: _____

a book or reputable website: _____

In order to make my goal more attainable, I have devised these short-term goals:

short-term goal	target date	reward
short-term goal	target date	reward
short-term goal	target date	reward

When I make the long-term behavior change described above, my reward will be:

_____ target date: _____

I intend to make the behavior change described above. I will use the strategies and rewards to achieve the goals that will contribute to a healthy behavior change.

Signed: _____   Witness: _____

Your colleagues agree that *My Health: An Outcomes Approach* will help students succeed—in this course and in the future.

I love ALL of the tables and figures presented in the book. I would use them in my class today. The chapters are student-friendly, colorful, informative, and relevant to today's college students. I love your book! —Marshina Baker, Bowie State University

I already like this textbook better than the one I currently use. The topics are more up-to-date and the information is very useful. . . . I don't even require the current textbook, but I would require this textbook based on what I have seen and read so far. —Kimberli Stassen, Ball State University

This manuscript is better than my current text. It gets right to the point. It isn't wordy or preachy. The learning outcomes direct the student and the summary questions help to reinforce that. —Karla Rues, Ozarks Technical Community College

I think that the material in this chapter is presented more clearly than in the textbook that I currently use. I would assign the edge to your textbook because it is clear in its design and presentation of the material discussed in the chapter. —Elaine Bryan, Georgia Perimeter College

Overall, the student learning outcomes are clearly stated and presented. As good SLOs should be, these are simply stated and easy for both instructor and learner to comprehend.—James Forkum, Ph.D., Santa Rosa Junior College

The Learning Outcomes accurately reflect the material and provide a solid basis to the students as to what they should learn from each module. . . . I really like the Check Yourself questions and I believe they all go hand in hand with the Learning Outcomes. —Cody Trefethen, Palomar College

A textbook designed for easier studying now and healthier lifelong behavior choices

Each concept is covered in a **one- or two-page spread,** allowing students to pace their learning. The text flows smoothly from outcomes to questions without being interrupted by feature boxes or other distractions.

Learning Outcomes give students clear and specific goals for what they should be able to accomplish after completing the module

3.7 Internal Causes of Stress

learning outcomes

- **Discuss and classify internal causes of stress.**

Although stress can come from the environment and other external sources, it can result from internal factors as well. Internal stressors such as negative appraisal, low self-esteem, and low self-efficacy can cause unsettling thoughts or feelings, and can ultimately affect your health.[52] It is important to address and manage these internal stressors.

Appraisal and Stress Throughout life, we encounter many different demands and potential stressors—some biological, some psychological, and others sociological. In any case, it is our **appraisal** of these demands, rather than the demands themselves, that results in our experiencing stress. Appraisal is defined as the interpretation and evaluation of information provided to the brain by the senses. Appraisal is not a conscious activity, but rather a natural process that the brain constantly performs. As new information becomes available, appraisal helps us recognize stressors, evaluate them on the basis of past experiences and emotions, and decide how to cope with them. When you perceive that your coping resources are sufficient to meet life's demands, you experience little or no stress. By contrast, when you perceive that life's demands exceed your coping resources, you are likely to feel strain and distress.

Self-Esteem and Self-Efficacy *Self-esteem* refers to how you feel about yourself. Self-esteem varies; it can and does continually change.[53] When you feel good about yourself, you are less likely to respond to or interpret an event as stressful. Conversely, if you place little or no value on yourself and believe you have inadequate coping skills, you become susceptible to stress and strain.[54] Of particular concern, research with high school and college students has found that low self-esteem and stressful life events significantly predict **suicidal ideation**, a desire to die and thoughts about suicide. On a more positive note, research has also indicated that it is possible to increase an individual's ability to cope with stress by increasing self-esteem.[55]

Self-efficacy is another important factor in the ability to cope with life's challenges. Self-efficacy refers to belief or confidence in one's skills and performance abilities.[56] Self-efficacy is considered one of the most important personality traits that influences psychological and physiological stress responses and has been found to predict a number of health behaviors in college students.[57]

Developing self-efficacy is also vital to coping with and overcoming academic pressures and worries. For example, by learning to handle anxiety around testing situations, you improve your chances of performing well; the more you feel yourself capable of handling testing situations, the greater will be your sense of academic self-efficacy.

Type A and Type B Personalities It should come as no surprise to you that personality can have an impact on whether you are happy and socially well adjusted or sad and socially isolated. However, your personality may affect more than just your social interactions: It may be a critical factor in your stress level, as well as in your risk for CVD, cancer, and other chronic and infectious diseases.

In 1974, physicians Meyer Friedman and Ray Rosenman published a book indicating that Type A individuals had a greatly increased risk of heart disease.[58] *Type A* personalities are defined as hard-driving, competitive, time-driven perfectionists. In contrast, *Type B* personalities are described as being relaxed, noncompetitive, and more tolerant of others.

Today, most researchers recognize that none of us will be wholly Type A or Type B all of the time. We might exhibit either type as we respond to the various challenges of our daily lives. In addition, recent research indicates that not all Type A people experience negative health consequences; in fact, some hard-driving

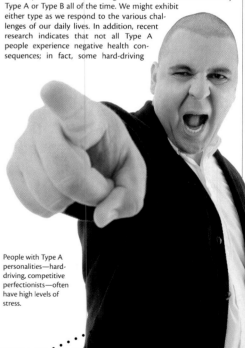

People with Type A personalities—hard-driving, competitive perfectionists—often have high levels of stress.

56

Striking photos and graphics capture student attention

individuals seem to thrive on their supercharged lifestyles. Only those Type A individuals who exhibit a "toxic core"—who have disproportionate amounts of anger; are distrustful of others; and have a cynical, glass-half-empty approach to life, in total, a set of characteristics referred to as **hostility**—are at increased risk for heart disease.[59]

Type C and Type D Personalities In addition to CVD risks, personality types have been linked to increased risk for a variety of illnesses ranging from asthma to cancer. *Type C* personality is one such type. Typically, Type C people are stoic and tend to deny feelings. They have a tendency to conform to the wishes of others (or to be "pleasers"), a lack of assertiveness, and an inclination toward feelings of helplessness or hopelessness. Possibly as a result of these characteristics, research indicates they are more susceptible to illnesses such as asthma, multiple sclerosis, autoimmune disorders, and cancer.[60] These are the "nice" guys and gals who really do finish last when it comes to their health.

A more recently identified personality type is *Type D* (distressed), characterized by a tendency toward excessive negative worry, irritability, gloom, and social inhibition. Several recent studies have shown that Type D people may be up to eight times more likely to die of a heart attack or sudden cardiac death.[61]

Psychological Hardiness According to psychologist Susanne Kobasa, **psychological hardiness** may negate self-imposed stress associated with Type A behavior. Psychologically hardy people are characterized by control, commitment, and willingness to embrace challenge.[62] People with a sense of control are able to accept responsibility for their behaviors and change those that they discover to be debilitating. People with a sense of commitment have good self-esteem and understand their purpose in life. Those who embrace challenge see change as a stimulating opportunity for personal growth. The concept of hardiness has been studied extensively, and many researchers believe it is the foundation of an individual's ability to cope with stress and remain healthy.[63]

Patterns of Thinking People fall into patterns and ways of thinking that can cause stress and increase their levels of anxiety. The fact is, your thought patterns can be your own worst enemy. If you can become aware of the internal messages you are giving yourself, you can recognize them and work to change them. Some strategies for doing this include:

- **Reframe a distressing event from a positive perspective.** Reframing is a stress-management technique that helps you change your perspective on a situation to a more positive vantage point. For example, if you feel perpetually frustrated that you can't be the best in every class, reframe the issue to highlight your strengths.
- **Break the worry habit.** If you are preoccupied with "what if's" and worst case scenarios, doubts and fears can sap your strength and send your stress levels soaring. The following suggestions can help slow the worry drain:
  - If you must worry, create a "worry period"—a 20 minute time period each day when you can journal or talk about it. After that, move on.

- Try to focus on the many things that are going right, rather than the one thing that might go wrong.
- Learn to accept what you cannot change. Chronic worriers want to be in control, but each of us must learn to live with some uncertainty.
- **Look at life as being fluid.** If you accept that change is a natural part of living and growing, the jolt of changes will become less stressful.
- **Moderate your expectations.** Aim high, but be realistic about your circumstances and motivation.
- **Weed out trivia.** Cardiologist Robert Eliot offers two rules for coping with life's challenges: "Don't sweat the small stuff," and remember, "It's all small stuff."
- **Tolerate mistakes by yourself and others.** Rather than getting angry or frustrated by mishaps, evaluate what happened and learn from it.

Skills for Behavior Change

OVERCOMING TEST-TAKING ANXIETY

Here's an example of how to increase self-efficacy in a familiar situation—an academic exam. Try these helpful hints when approaching your next exam, and you might just reduce your stress levels as well as improve your grade.

Before the Exam
- Manage your study time. Start studying a week before your test to reduce anxiety. Do a limited review the night before, get a good night's sleep, and arrive for the exam early.
- Build your test-taking self-esteem. On an index card, write down three reasons you will pass the exam. Keep the card with you and review it whenever you study. When you get the test, write your three reasons on the test or on a piece of scrap paper.
- Eat a balanced meal before the exam. Avoid sugar and rich or heavy foods, as well as foods that might upset your stomach. You want to feel your best.
- If you feel that you are a slow reader and need more time, discuss this in advance with your teacher or test administrator.

During the Test
- Manage your time during the test. Decide how much time you need to take the test, review your answers, and go back over questions you might be stuck on. Hold to this schedule.
- Slow down and pay attention. When you open your test book, always write "RTFQ" (Read the Full Question) at the top. Make sure you understand the question before answering.
- Stay on track. If you begin to get anxious, reread your three reasons for success.

check yourself

- **What are five causes of internal stress?**
- **Which internal causes of stress do you experience most frequently?**

Skills for Behavior Change tips give students the tools they need to make immediate changes for healthier lifestyles

Check Yourself questions give students immediate feedback on their mastery of the content of the module

1, 2, 3 . . . We give you the tools you need to teach with *My Health* now!

1. Teaching Tool Box

Save hours of valuable planning time with one comprehensive course planning kit. The Teaching Tool Box provides all of the prepping and lecture tools you need:

- For instructors: an Instructor Resource DVD (which includes PowerPoint lecture outlines, *ABC News* videos, and the Computerized Test Bank); the printed Instructor Resource and Support Manual and the Test Bank; the User's Quick Guide for using the book's media resources; the new *Teaching with Student Learning Outcomes* and *Teaching with Web 2.0* publications; and more.
- For students: the new *Behavior Change Log Book; Eat Right!; Live Right!;* and the *Take Charge of Your Health* worksheets.

Each learning resource that you may choose to use in your course has been thoroughly correlated with the text's learning outcomes. PowerPoint lecture slides, Test Bank questions, and instructor resources are tied to the relevant learning outcomes for each topic.

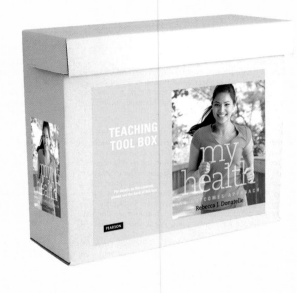

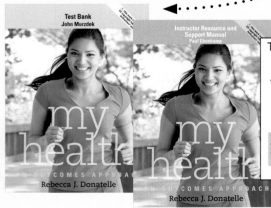

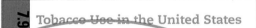

Tobacco Use in the United States: Module 7.9

- Approximately 70 million Americans report using tobacco products (cigarettes, cigars, smokeless tobacco, and pipe tobacco) at least once in the past month.

Module 7.9 Learning Outcomes:

- Discuss advertising tactics used by the tobacco industry.
- Examine reasons that people start smoking.
- List factors that contribute to tobacco use by college students.

7.9 Tobacco Use in the United States

learning outcomes

- Discuss advertising tactics used by the tobacco industry.
- Examine reasons that people start smoking.
- List factors that contribute to tobacco use by college students.

Approximately 70 million Americans report using tobacco products (cigarettes, cigars, smokeless tobacco, and pipe tobacco) at least once in the past month. In 2009, 25.3 percent of men and 21.4 percent of women were current cigarette smokers. Every day approximately 1,100 people under 18 and 1,900 people over 18 become daily smokers.[65]

Education is closely linked to cigarette use: Adults with a bachelor's degree or higher education are three times *less* likely to smoke than are those with less than a high school education. Cigarette smoking also varies by ethnicity and gender, with the highest rates of smoking found among non-Hispanic black men and American Indian and Alaska Native men.[66]

More than 20 percent of Americans are former smokers; about 60 percent have never smoked. The most commonly used tobacco product is cigarettes, followed by cigars and smokeless tobacco. Approximately 6 percent of Americans smoke cigars, and 7 percent of men and less than 1 percent of women use smokeless tobacco.[67]

Why Do People Use Tobacco?

Nicotine Addiction Beginning smokers usually feel the effects of nicotine with their first puff. These symptoms, called **nicotine poisoning**, can include dizziness, lightheadedness, rapid and erratic pulse, clammy skin, nausea, vomiting, and diarrhea. Symptoms cease as tolerance develops, which happens as quickly as the second or third cigarette. Many regular smokers experience no "buzz," but continue to smoke because stopping is too difficult.

Two studies on twins found genetic factors to be more influential than environmental factors in smoking initiation and nicotine dependence.[68] Two specific genes may influence smoking behavior by affecting the action of the brain chemical dopamine.[69] Understanding the influence of genetics on nicotine addiction could be crucial to developing more effective treatments for smoking cessation.[70]

Behavioral Dependence People who smoke are not just physically but also psychologically dependent. Nicotine "tricks" the brain into creating pleasurable associations with sensory stimuli or environmental cues that may trigger the urge for a cigarette.[71] Some former smokers remain vulnerable to sensory and environmental cues for many years after they quit.

Weight Control Nicotine is an appetite suppressant and slightly increases basal metabolic rate. After smoking a cigarette, one's metabolism quickly increases then returns to normal; heavy smokers have such surges throughout the day. When a smoker quits, the metabolic rate slows down and appetite returns. People tend to eat more, particularly sweets. Fear of gaining weight is one of the biggest reasons smokers are reluctant to quit. To avoid weight gain after quitting smoking, avoid crash diets, keep low-calorie treats handy, and drink plenty of water.

Advertising The tobacco industry spends an estimated $36 million per day on advertising and promotion.[72] Because children and teenagers constitute 90 percent of all new smokers, much of the advertising has been directed toward them. Evidence of product recognition among underage smokers is clear: 86 percent prefer one of the three most heavily advertised brands—

Figure 7.8 Reasons for Smoking among College Student Smokers

Source: Adapted from *Wasting the Best and the Brightest: Substance Abuse at America's Colleges and Universities* (New York: National Center on Addiction and Substance Abuse at Columbia University, March 2007), 48. Copyright © 2007. Used with permission.

2. Teaching with Student Learning Outcomes

This exciting publication contains essays from 11 instructors who are using student learning outcomes in their courses. They share their goals in using outcomes, the processes that they follow to develop and refine the outcomes, and many useful suggestions and examples for successfully incorporating outcomes into a personal health course.

Recent attendees at the Pearson Student Learning Outcomes webinar said:

My college is beginning an extensive assessment process for our SLOs and I will be representing HED so it was great to hear what other professors are doing. —Kathleen Smyth, College of Marin

Great interaction with other educators about SLOs and how they incorporate them in their courses. —Steve Hartman, Citrus College

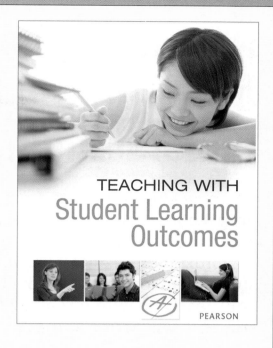

TEACHING WITH
Student Learning Outcomes

PEARSON

3. Health & Wellness Teaching Community Website

www.pearsonhighered.com/healthcommunity

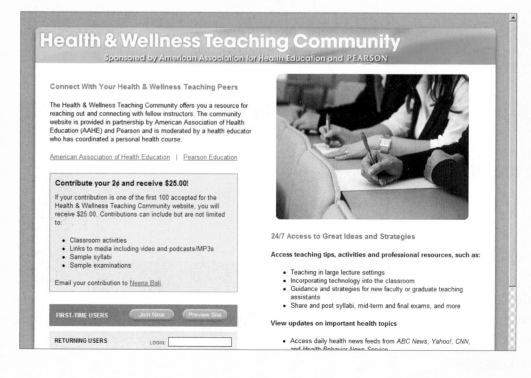

Connect with other health instructors to share teaching tips and ideas, talk about health-related issues, and more. Post a question, provide a solution, interact with your colleagues!

A newly redesigned MyHealthLab® helps create the moment of understanding

The new MyHealthLab® from Pearson has been designed and refined with a single purpose in mind: To help educators create that moment of understanding with their students. The MyHealthLab system helps instructors maximize class time with customizable, easy-to-assign, and automatically graded assignments that motivate students to learn outside of class and arrive prepared for lecture. By complementing your teaching with our engaging technology and content, you can be confident your students will arrive at that moment—the moment of true understanding.

Engaging Experiences

MyHealthLab provides a one-stop spot for accessing a wealth of preloaded content and tools, while giving you the ability to customize your course as much (or as little) as you'd like.

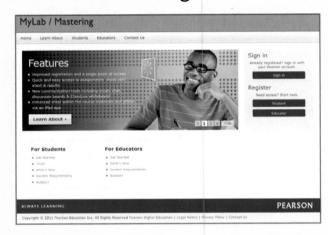

Fresh, clean, and easily customizable design layout is pleasing to both new and experienced users of technology.

Over 150 Pre-Built, Publisher-Created Assignments

Assignments are easily assignable and gradable and include:

- student learning outcomes pre- and post-course exam
- pre-reading chapter tests
- post-reading chapter tests
- ABC News videos multiple choice quiz questions
- MP3 case studies assignable quizzes
- entire content from the Test Bank categorized by Bloom's Taxonomy and by student learning outcome
- gradable discussion board questions

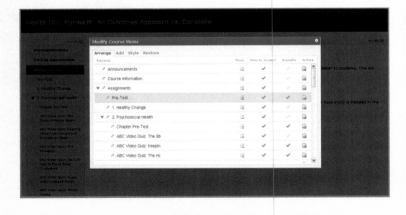

A New Gradebook Helps Instructors Track Their Course

- The gradebook provides instructors with a quick entry page for assignments, so they can tab rapidly through the assignments for each student, updating grades efficiently.
- The gradebook automatically calculates students' grades to date and lets instructors see detailed views of that assignment and receive an accurate student reflection of what's been assigned.
- Student names and grades are fixed in the left hand screen, allowing for easy navigation at any point in the semester and with any number of students.
- Student discussion responses appear in the gradebook for easy grading.

Health 101

Gradebook - Gradebook

Announcements
Course Information
eText
Study Area
Assignments
Course Tools

Name	Grade to Date	Students Learning Outcomes Pre-Course Exam out of 25	Chapter 4 Test out of 25	Chapter 4 Pre-Reading Quiz out of 25	ABC Video Quiz out of 25	MP3 Quiz out of 25
Eighteen, Student	60.67%	20	22	23	23	19
Eleven, Student	59.67%	17	24	21	24	17
Fifteen, Student	54.33%	13	19	24	21	19
Fifty, Student	62%	25	24	20	23	16
Five, Student	67.67%	24	25	21	24	25
Forty, Student	54.67%	19	18	19	17	18
Forty-Eight, Student	57.67%	17	20	23	22	19
Forty-Five, Student	80%	16	21	21	20	24
Forty-Four, Student	78%	17	19	24	19	25
Forty-Nine, Student	67.33%	21	14	22	19	25

Proven Results

MyHealthLab has a consistently positive impact on the quality of learning in higher education personal health instruction. MyHealthLab can be successfully implemented in any environment—lab-based, hybrid, fully online, traditional—and demonstrates the quantifiable difference that integrated usage of these products has on student retention, subsequent success, and overall achievement.

A Trusted Partner

MyHealthLab delivers engaging, dynamic learning opportunities—focused on instructor learning objectives and responsive to each student's progress—with improved registration and instructor support.

- Quick Start Videos demonstrate MyHealthLab basics for instructors, giving you help right when you need it.
- Dedicated instructor and student support via internet chat at http://247pearsoned.custhelp.com/ or dedicated customer service line at 800-677-6337.

Flexible options help you make the right choice for your students!

The Pearson eText gives students access to the text whenever and wherever they can access the Internet. The eText pages look exactly like the printed text, and include powerful interactive and customization functions. Students can create notes, highlight text, create bookmarks, zoom in and out, click hyperlinked words and phrases to view definitions. Students and instructors using MyHealthLab gain access to the eText for the iPad via the Pearson App at no additional charge. Contact your local Pearson sales representative for more information.

CourseSmart eTextbooks are an exciting new choice for students looking to save money. As an alternative to purchasing the print textbook, students can subscribe to the same content online and save 40% off the suggested list price of the print text. Access the CourseSmart eText at www.coursesmart.com.

Book à la Carte offers the exact same content as *My Health: An Outcomes Approach* in a convenient, three-hole punched, loose-leaf version. Books à la Carte offers a great value for your students—this format costs 35% less than a new textbook!

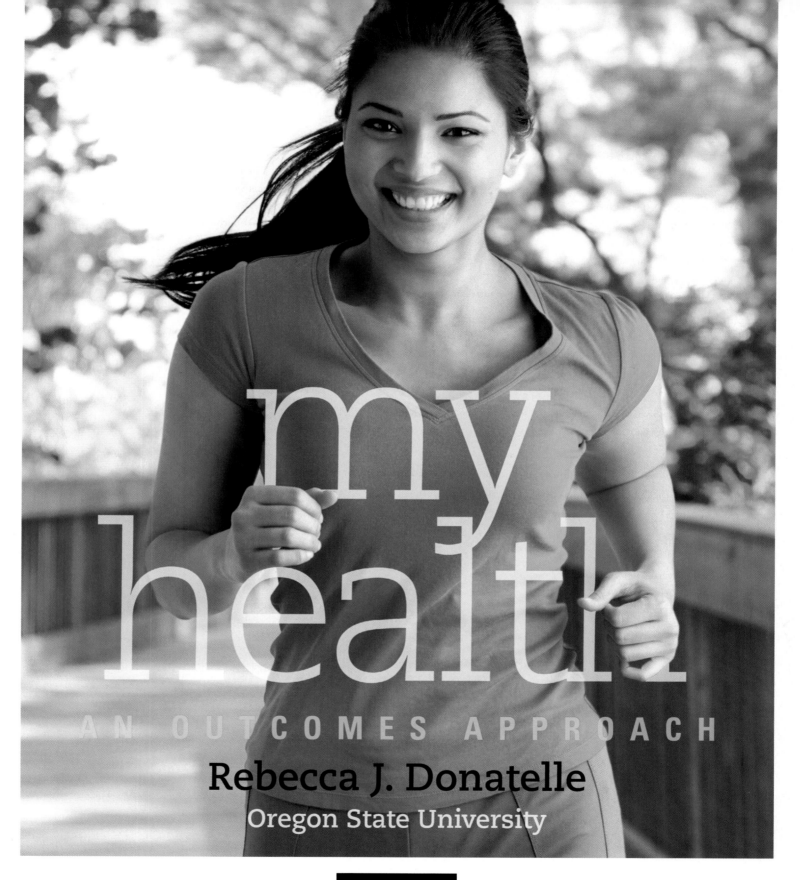

my health

AN OUTCOMES APPROACH

Rebecca J. Donatelle

Oregon State University

PEARSON

Boston Columbus Indianapolis New York San Francisco Upper Saddle River
Amsterdam Cape Town Dubai London Madrid Milan Munich Paris Montréal Toronto
Delhi Mexico City São Paulo Sydney Hong Kong Seoul Singapore Taipei Tokyo

Executive Editor: Sandra Lindelof
Editorial Manager: Susan Malloy
Development Manager: Barbara Yien
Development Editor: Lisa Gluskin Stonestreet
Assistant Editor: Meghan Zolnay
Editorial Assistant: Briana Verdugo
Executive Media Producer: Liz Winer
Assistant Media Producer: Annie Wang
Senior Managing Editor: Deborah Cogan
Assistant Managing Editor: Nancy Tabor

Design Director/Cover and Interior Designer:
    Mark Ong
Art Development Editor: Kelly Murphy
Production Management: Thistle Hill Publishing Services
Composition: Nesbitt Graphics, Inc.
Illustration: Precision Graphics
Photo Researcher: Bill Smith Group, Laura Murray
Senior Manufacturing Buyer: Stacey Weinberger
Executive Marketing Manager: Neena Bali
Senior Market Development Manager: Brooke Suchomel

Cover Photo Credit: Blend Images/Alamy

Credits and acknowledgments borrowed from other sources and reproduced, with permission, in this textbook appear on page C-1.

Library of Congress Cataloging-in-Publication Data

Donatelle, Rebecca J., 1950–
 My health : an outcomes approach / Rebecca J. Donatelle.
    p. cm.
 Includes bibliographical references and index.
 ISBN 978-0-321-75123-2 — ISBN 0-321-75123-X
1. Health. 2. Health behavior. 3. Diseases—Prevention. I. Title.
RA776.D6635 2011
613—dc23
                              2011041247

ISBN 10: 0-321-75123-X; ISBN 13: 978-0-321-75123-2 (Student Edition)
ISBN 10: 0-321-80379-5; ISBN 13: 978-0-321-80379-5 (Instructor's Review Copy)

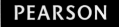

About the Author

Rebecca J. Donatelle, Ph.D.

Associate Professor Emeritus, Oregon State University

Rebecca Donatelle has served as a faculty member in the Department of Public Health, College of Health and Human Sciences, at Oregon State University for the last two decades. In that role, she has chaired the department and been Program Coordinator for the Health Promotion and Health Behavior programs (Bachelor's Degree, Master of Public Health, and Ph.D. degree programs), as well as serving on over 50 national, state, regional, and university committees focused on improving the public's health. Most importantly to her, she has also taught and mentored thousands of undergraduate and graduate students, and she is proud of the many outstanding accomplishments of her students! Many of these students gained community-based intervention and research skills while working on Dr. Donatelle's national, state, and locally funded research projects. These projects often focused on behaviorally based interventions designed to promote health and reduce risks for chronic diseases, particularly for those at risk for cardiovascular disease and diabetes.

Dr. Donatelle has a Ph.D. in Community Health/Health Education with specializations in health behaviors, aging, and chronic disease prevention from the University of Oregon, a Master of Science Degree in Health Education from the University of Wisconsin, La Crosse, and a Bachelor of Science degree from the University of Wisconsin, La Crosse, with majors in Health/Physical Education and English.

In recent years, Dr. Donatelle has received several awards for leadership, teaching, and service within the university and for her work on the Oregon Masters of Public Health degree program, a joint collaborative degree program with Portland State University and Oregon Health and Science University. She also has received a Robert Wood Johnson Foundation Presidential Award for Promising New Research in the Smoke-Free Families National Initiative.

Her primary research and scholarship areas have focused on the use of incentives, social and community supports, and risk communication strategies in motivating diverse populations to change their risk behaviors. She has worked with pregnant women who smoke in an effort to motivate them to quit smoking, obese women of all ages who are at risk for cardiovascular disease and diabetes, pre-diabetic women at risk for progression to type 2 diabetes, and a wide range of other health issues and problems. Earlier research projects have focused on decision making and factors influencing the use of alternative and traditional health care providers for treatment of low back pain, illness and sick role behaviors, occupational stress and stress claims, and worksite health promotion.

From her earliest years of college instruction, Dr. Donatelle was convinced that there was a better way of providing health education material to students that wouldn't lecture *at* them, but would serve to involve and motivate them to search for the best information and to make informed choices after considering all of their options. Writing a text such as this one has helped keep her current in her teaching and research and has allowed her to provide the very best resources to assist students in their learning experience. In addition, it is in keeping with her philosophy of working hard to continually improve the pedagogical and overall educational experience of her students, to use technology where possible, and to encourage student engagement in the classroom. As part of the process, she has trained and supervised teaching assistants and worked with them to help them have the tools and resources necessary to make their teaching experiences positive ones.

Brief Contents

Contents

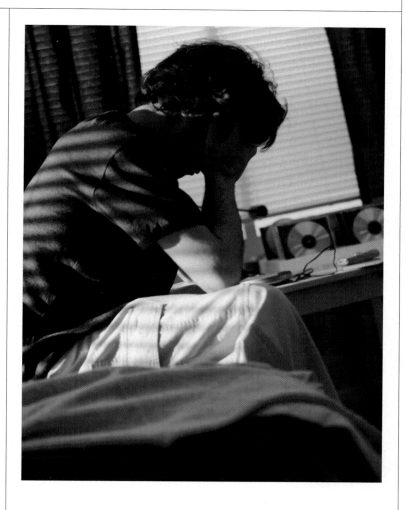

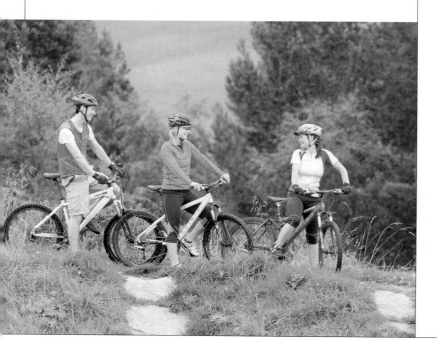

3 Stress 45

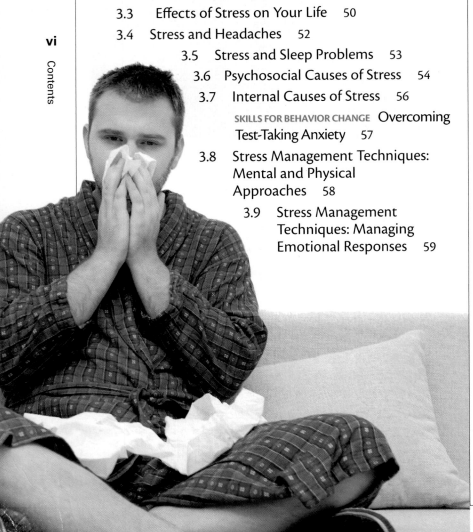

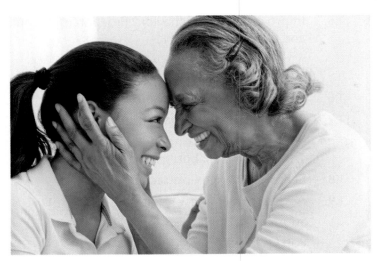

4 Relationships and Sexuality 67

5 Reproductive Choices 93

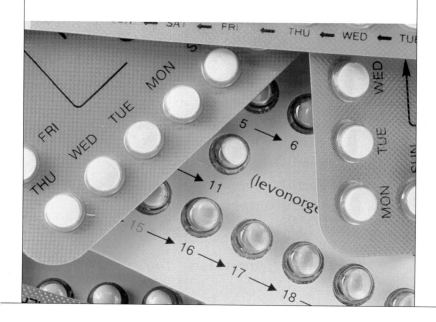

6 Addiction and Drug Abuse 121

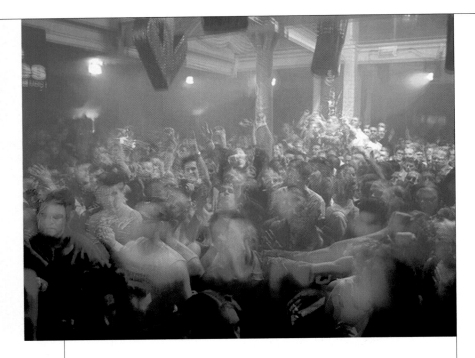

viii

Contents

7 Alcohol and Tobacco 145

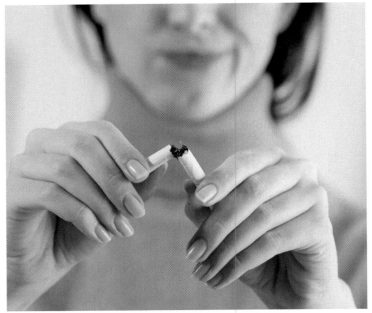

8 Nutrition 171

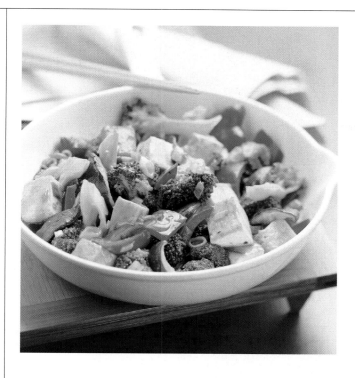

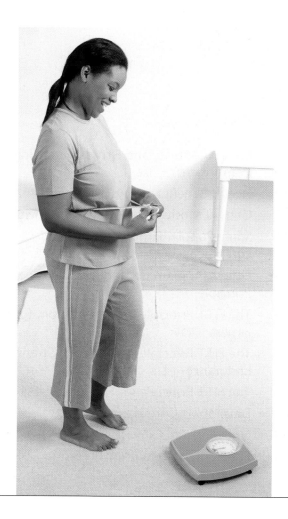

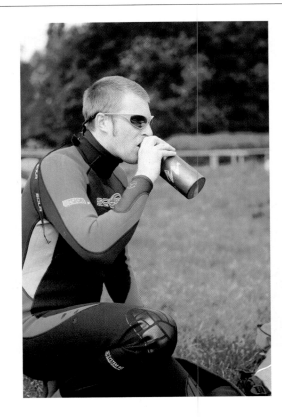

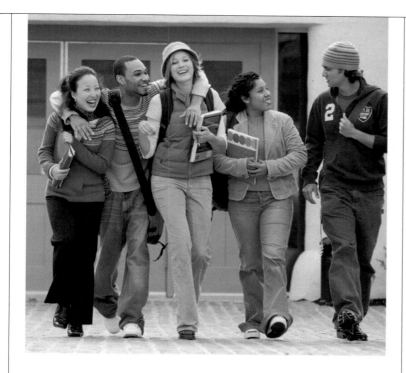

12 Infectious Conditions   289

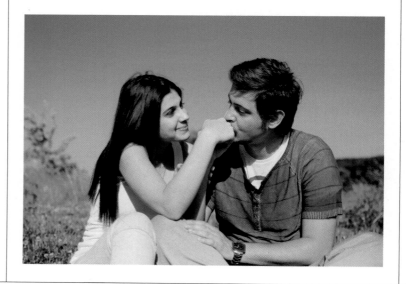

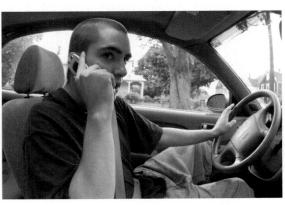

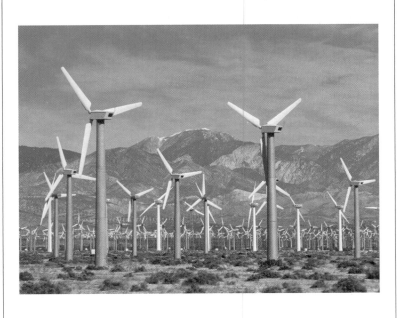

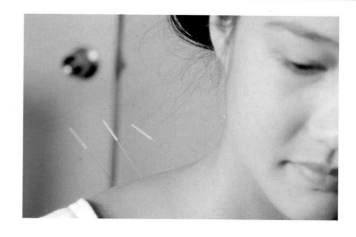

15 Consumerism and Complementary and Alternative Medicine 359

Preface

For students today, health is headline news. Whether it's the latest cases of deadly *E. coli* infections from eating infected produce, a new environmental catastrophe, or increasing rates of obesity and diabetes, the issues often seem big and far-reaching. At the same time, health is personal and individual: How can I reduce my stress? What can I do to improve my diet? When can I find time to study? As I have taught personal health courses over the past two decades, I have seen changes in students and in their learning styles and I came to realize that a new way of providing critical health information to students was needed. Students today want their information to be organized and concise. They want to know what they should be learning and be able to test themselves to confirm that they understand the material. What's more, both they and their instructors want to be able to prove that they know more about health—and how to improve it—at the end of the course than they did at the beginning. For these reasons and more, I decided to write *My Health: An Outcomes Approach*.

Key Features of This Text

This book is the result of a great deal of thought about students and how they learn. Among the features that we have developed are:

- **The modular organization,** which presents information in one- and two-page spreads, helping students to pace their learning.
- **Student learning outcomes,** which give instructors and students measurable goals for each module.
- **Check Yourself questions** to help students confirm that they have mastered the content of each module.
- **Assess Yourself modules,** which provide opportunities for students to assess their current behaviors, with at least one Assess Yourself at the end of every chapter.
- **Skills for Behavior Change boxes,** which are featured in many modules, so that students attain the skills to apply what they have learned.
- **Striking figures and photos** on every page to engage students and encourage learning.
- **A streamlined approach,** with feature-box material integrated into the text, so that students can follow the narrative without interruptions.

Student learning outcomes were a critical part of the development of this book. Learning outcomes are a powerful tool to set clear expectations for our students and then to measure their achievement. The outcomes for this book were written based on the standard personal health course content, then revised and edited based on feedback from colleagues from around the country (their names are listed later in the Acknowledgments section). As students turn to each module, the outcomes for that module are clearly specified. Students understand the key points of the module and know where to focus their attention.

At the end of each module, students are challenged by Check Yourself questions. If students can answer these questions, then they have understood the key concepts of the module and are ready to move on to the next module. If they cannot, then they can stop and read the material again, before adding onto it with yet more information.

We know that students are often pressed for time and may only be able to read through a few pages of this book at one time. With the outcomes and the Check Yourself questions, even if students can only complete part of a reading assignment, they can learn the material in one or two modules, test themselves, and know that they have accomplished a measurable portion of their reading goal.

In addition to the modular organization and the outcomes and questions, you will notice Skills for Behavior Change boxes throughout the chapters. Using the skills learned from these boxes, students can make concrete changes in their behaviors that will contribute to improved health. You will also see that these are the only feature boxes in the text. In order to keep the book streamlined and focused on main points, the type of information that traditionally has been relegated to a feature box has been included in the text, where it is important for student understanding, or omitted. I hope that you will agree that this provides students with a clear, concise presentation of the most important health information.

Supplementary Materials

Available with *My Health: An Outcomes Approach* is a comprehensive set of ancillary materials designed to enhance learning and to facilitate teaching.

Student Supplements

- **MyHealthLab** (www.pearsonhighered.com/myhealthlab). MyHealthLab is organized by learning areas. *Read It* houses the Pearson eText, with which users can create notes, highlight text in different colors, create bookmarks, zoom, click hyperlinked words for definitions, and change the page view. The Pearson eText also links to associated media files and can be accessed via the Pearson App on the iPad at no additional charge. *See It* includes more than 70 *ABC News* videos on important health topics and the key concepts of each chapter presented in PowerPoint® lecture outline form. *Hear It* contains MP3 files of the big-picture concepts for the text and audio case studies. *Do It* contains critical-thinking questions, case studies, and weblinks. *Review It* contains four types of study quizzes for each chapter. *Live It* is a newly redesigned electronic tool kit that will help jumpstart students' behavior-change projects; students can fill out a Behavior Change Contract, journal and log behaviors, and prepare a reflection piece.

- **Companion Website** (www.pearsonhighered.com/donatelle). This website is organized by learning areas. Students can study chapter objectives (Read It), listen to MP3 clips of main concepts and case studies (Hear It), learn hands-on with critical-thinking questions (Do It), take practice quizzes (Review It), and access a brand new electronic behavior-change tool kit (Live It).
- **Take Charge of Your Health! Worksheets.** This pad of 50 self-assessment activities allows students to further explore their health behaviors.
- *Behavior Change Log Book and Wellness Journal.* This assessment tool helps students track daily exercise and nutritional intake and create a long-term nutrition and fitness prescription plan. It includes Behavior Change Contracts and topics for journal-based activities.
- *Eat Right! Healthy Eating in College and Beyond.* This booklet provides students with practical nutrition guidelines, shopper's guides, and recipes.
- *Live Right! Beating Stress in College and Beyond.* This booklet gives students useful tips for coping with stressful life challenges both during college and for the rest of their lives.
- **TweetYourHealth,** a powerful, easy-to-use, Twitter-based application allows students to track and keep an online journal of everyday health behaviors (such as what you eat, how often you exercise, and how much sleep you get) via any mobile device with text messaging capabilities, or directly from a computer.
- **Digital 5-Step Pedometer.** Take strides to better health with this pedometer, which measures steps, distance (miles), activity time, and calories, and provides a clock.
- **MyDietAnalysis** (www.mydietanalysis.com). Powered by ESHA Research, Inc., MyDietAnalysis features a database of nearly 20,000 foods and multiple reports. It allows students to track their diet and activity using up to three profiles and to generate and submit reports electronically.

Instructor Supplements

A full resource package accompanies *My Health: An Outcomes Approach* to assist the instructor with classroom preparation and presentation.

- **MyHealthLab** (www.pearsonhighered.com/myhealthlab). This tool provides a one-stop spot for accessing a wealth of preloaded content and makes paper-free assigning and grading easier than ever. Pre-loaded assignments include pre- and post-course exams, pre- and post-reading chapter tests, *ABC News* video quiz questions, and Test Bank questions categorized by Bloom's Taxonomy and by student learning outcome. MyHealthLab contains the Pearson eText, which allows for instructor annotation to be shared with the class; includes over 70 *ABC News* videos; and provides robust electronic behavior-change tools.
- *ABC News* **Health and Wellness Lecture Launcher Videos.** Seventy videos, each 5 to 10 minutes long, help instructors stimulate critical discussion in the classroom. Videos are provided already linked within PowerPoint® lectures and are available separately in large-screen format with optional closed captioning on the Instructor Resource DVD and through MyHealthLab.

- **Instructor Resource DVD.** The Instructor Resource DVD includes 30 *ABC News* Lecture Launcher videos, clicker questions, Quiz Show questions, PowerPoint® lecture outlines, all illustrations and tables from the text, selected photos, Transparency Masters, as well as Microsoft Word® files for the Instructor Resource and Support Manual and the Test Bank. The DVD also holds the Computerized Test Bank.
- **Teaching Tool Box.** This kit offers all the tools necessary to guide an instructor through the course: *Teaching with Student Learning Outcomes; Teaching with Web 2.0;* Instructor Resource and Support Manual; Test Bank; Instructor Resource DVD with *ABC News* Lecture Launcher videos and Computerized Test Bank; Course-at-a-Glance grid; MyHealthLab Instructor Access Kit; *Great Ideas! Active Ways to Teach Health and Wellness; Behavior Change Logbook and Wellness Journal; Eat Right!, Live Right!,* and *Take Charge of Your Health* worksheets.
- *Teaching with Student Learning Outcomes.* This new publication contains essays from 11 instructors who are teaching using student learning outcomes. They share their goals in using outcomes and the processes that they follow to develop and refine the outcomes. They offer many useful suggestions and examples for successfully incorporating outcomes into a personal health course.
- *Teaching with Web 2.0.* From Facebook to Twitter to blogs, students are using and interacting with Web 2.0 technologies. This handbook provides an introduction to these popular online tools and offers ideas for incorporating them into your personal health course. Written by personal health and health education instructors, each chapter examines the basics about a technology and ways to make it work for you and your students.
- *User's Quick Guide.* Newly redesigned to be even more useful, this valuable supplement gives you the information you need to quickly access all of the media and print supplements. Included is a step-by-step illustrated guide to transferring resources from the Instructor Resource DVD to your computer desktop and an overview of the features of the MyHealthLab course management system.
- **Instructor Resource and Support Manual.** This teaching tool provides chapter summaries and outlines and a step-by-step visual walkthrough of all the resources available to instructors. It includes information on available PowerPoint® lectures with the accompanying figures and art, integrated *ABC News* Lecture Launcher video discussion questions, tips and strategies for managing large classrooms, ideas for in-class activities, and suggestions for integrating MyHealthLab and MyDietAnalysis into your classroom activities and homework assignments.
- **Test Bank.** The Test Bank is organized around Bloom's Taxonomy, or the Higher Order of Learning, to help instructors create exams that encourage students to think analytically and critically. The learning outcome being tested is listed for each test bank item.
- *Great Ideas! Active Ways to Teach Health & Wellness.* This manual provides ideas for classroom activities related to specific health and wellness topics, as well as suggestions for activities that can be adapted to various topics and class sizes.

- **Community Website** (www.pearsonhighered.com/ healthcommunity). The new Health & Wellness Teaching Community website serves instructors by offering teaching tips and ideas and a forum for peers to discuss health-related issues, how to incorporate student learning outcomes into the course, and more.

Flexible Options

My Health: An Outcomes Approach is available in two electronic versions:

- The **Pearson eText** gives students access to the text whenever and wherever they can access the Internet. The eText pages look exactly like the printed text and include powerful interactive and customization functions. Students can create notes, highlight text, create bookmarks, zoom in and out, click hyperlinked words and phrases to view definitions, and search quickly and easily for specific content. (Note: Not available in MyLabs.) Students and instructors using MyHealthLab gain access to the eText for the iPad via the Pearson App at no additional charge. Contact your local Pearson sales representative for more information.

- **CourseSmart eTextbooks** are an exciting new choice for students looking to save money. As an alternative to purchasing the print textbook, students can subscribe to the same content online and save 40% off the suggested list price of the print text. Access the CourseSmart eText at www.coursesmart.com.

Additional print versions available include Books a la Carte and the Pearson Custom Library:

- **Books a la Carte** offers the exact same content as *My Health: An Outcomes Approach* in a convenient, three-hole punched, loose-leaf version. Books a la Carte offers a great value for your students—this format costs 35% less than a new textbook!

- Creating a customized version of the book from the **Pearson Custom Library,** with only the chapters that you select, is also possible. Contact your Pearson sales representative for more details.

Acknowledgments

Writing and developing a textbook is truly a team effort. Each step along the way in planning, developing, and translating critical health information to students and instructors requires a tremendous amount of work from many dedicated professionals, and I cannot help but think how fortunate I have been to work with the gifted publishing professionals at Pearson. Through time constraints, decision making, and computer meltdowns, this group handled every detail, every obstacle with patience, professionalism, and painstaking attention to detail. From this author's perspective, the personnel personify key aspects of what it takes to be successful in the publishing world: (1) drive and motivation; (2) commitment to excellence; (3) a vibrant, youthful, forward-thinking and enthusiastic approach; and (4) personalities that motivate an author to continually strive to produce market-leading texts. I have been amazed at the way that this team continually strives to be well ahead of the curve in terms of cutting-edge information. Asking "what do students need to know" and "what will help instructors and students thrive" in today's high-pressure academic settings was a foundation of our efforts. I am deeply indebted to everyone who has played a role in making this book come alive for students.

In particular, credit goes to my project editor for this edition, Susan Malloy, who drafted outlines and made recommendations for organization and coverage for every module. Further praise and thanks go to the highly skilled and hardworking, creative, and charismatic Executive Editor Sandra Lindelof, who has catapulted this book into a competitive twenty-first century. Sandy searches out and procures cutting-edge technology to meet the demands of an increasingly savvy student and keeps her finger on the pulse of what instructors and students need in their classrooms today. In addition, I would like to acknowledge the wonderful contributions of Development Editor Lisa Gluskin Stonestreet. Lisa did an extraordinary job of streamlining and revising material to fit within the constraints of the modular outline, while retaining accuracy and readability. Without her, this book would not exist—thank you!

Although these women were key contributors to the finished work, there were many other people who worked on *My Health: An Outcomes Approach*. In particular, I would like to thank Assistant Managing Editor Nancy Tabor who created a unique production process to accommodate the peculiar demands of this book and then kept the book moving along with grace and good humor. Thanks also to Angela Urquhart at Thistle Hill Publishing Services who reliably kept us on track with flexibility and dedication. Design director Mark Ong was almost a second author on this book. He painstakingly laid out every page, making constant adjustments to accommodate editorial needs while always keeping the visual impact of the design for students and instructors in mind. We could not have created this book without his creativity and dedication. Mark also created the remarkable cover, which we feel perfectly conveys the unique qualities of the text. Assistant Editor Meghan Zolnay gets major kudos for overseeing the print supplements package, including the new resource *Teaching with Student Learning Outcomes*. Liz Winer, Executive Media Producer, put together an innovative and comprehensive media supplements package. Additional thanks go to the rest of the team at Pearson, especially Editorial Assistant Briana Verdugo, Production Supervisor Meghan Power, Managing Editor Deborah Cogan, and Development Manager Barbara Yien.

The editorial and production teams are critical to a book's success, but I would be remiss without thanking another key group who ultimately help determine a book's success: the textbook sales group and Executive Marketing Manager Neena Bali. With Neena's support, the Pearson sales representatives traverse the country, promoting the book, making sure that instructors know how it compares to the competition, and providing support to customers. From directing an outstanding marketing campaign to the everyday tasks of being responsive to instructor needs, Neena does a superb job of making sure that *My Health: An Outcomes Approach* gets into instructors' hands and that adopters receive the service they deserve. Brooke Suchomel, Senior Market Development Manager, spearheaded class testing of the book as well as invaluable focus groups. In keeping with my overall experiences with Pearson, the marketing and sales staff are among the best of the best. I am very lucky to have them working with me on this project and want to extend a special thanks to all of them!

This book was developed in part from material from my other textbooks, *Access to Health* and *Health: The Basics*. I would like to thank the contributors to those books, particularly Dr. Patricia Ketcham (Oregon State University), Dr. Peggy Pederson (Western Oregon State University), Dr. Angela Thompson (St. Francis Xavier University), Dr. Kathy Munoz (Humboldt State University), Dr. Karen Elliot (Oregon State University), and Dr. Jennifer Jabson (Boston University). A special thanks to Niloofar Bavarian (Oregon State University), who drafted the original student learning outcomes on which the book is based. Thanks also to the talented people who contributed to the supplements package: Paul Ebenkamp, who authored the Instructor Resource and Support Manual; John Murzdek, who wrote the Test Bank; John Kowalczyk (University of Minnesota-Duluth), who provided the Bloom's taxonomy for the Test Bank; Melanie Healey (University of Washington-La Crosse) and Cody Trefethen (Palomar College), who wrote the PowerPoint lecture slides; and Jane House (Wake Technical Community College), who created the PowerPoint quiz show slides.

Reviewers

This book is the result not only of my efforts, but also the invaluable contributions of the many reviewers. From the initial idea to the fine-tuning of each and every learning outcome, the thoughtful comments from reviewers shaped this book in many ways. I am extremely grateful for your feedback.

Many thanks to all!
Rebecca J. Donatelle, PhD

Chapter Reviewers

Doug Athey
Xavier University of Louisiana

Marshina Baker
Bowie State University

Kristy Ballard
St. Edward's University

Katharine Bloom
Salem State University

Elaine D. Bryan
Georgia Perimeter College

Annette Carrington
North Carolina Central University

Lisa Chaudhari
Northern Arizona University

Dusty Childress
Ozarks Technical Community College

Jeanne M. Clerc
Western Illinois University

Brent Damron
Bakersfield College

Teresa Dolan
Lincoln University

Maqsood M. Faquir
Palm Beach State College

Ari Fisher
Louisiana State University

James Forkum
Santa Rosa Junior College

Anna Stiles Hanlon
Orange Coast College

Charlene G. Harkins
University of Minnesota Duluth

Chris T. Harman
California University of Pennsylvania

Guoyuan Huang
University of Southern Indiana

Mary E. Iten
University of Nebraska at Kearney

Jacqueline V. Jackson
Jackson State University

John Janowiak
Reich College of Education

Cheryl Kerns-Campbell
Grossmont College

Dr. John Kowalczyk
University of Minnesota Duluth

Ellen Larson
Northern Arizona University

James Ledrick
Grand Valley State University

Debbie Lynch
Rose State College

Jamie Mansell
Lincoln University

Donna McGill-Cameron
Woodland Community College

Bridget Melton
Georgia Southern University

Kristin Moline
Lourdes University

Brenda Moore
Georgia Perimeter College

Maria Okeke
Florida A&M University

Toni A. Pannell
Tarrant County College, Northwest Campus

Grace Pokorny
Long Beach City College

Natasha Romeo
Wake Forest University

Pamela Rost
Erie Community College—South Campus

Karla Rues
Ozarks Technical Community College

Andrea Salis
Queensborough Community College

Kelly Fisher Shobe
Georgia Perimeter College

Kathleen Smyth
College of Marin

Kim Stassen
Ball State University

Natalie Stickney
Georgia Perimeter College

Nancy Storey
Georgia Perimeter College

Jeremy Termini
Finger Lakes Community College

Cody Trefethen
Palomar College

Hilda C. Whitmire
Georgia Perimeter College

Carl Wilson
Lincoln University

Bonnie J. Young
Georgia Perimeter College

Lana Zinger
Queensborough Community College

Student Learning Outcomes Reviewers

Carol Allen
Lane Community College

Angela Backus
Kent State University

Dusty Childress
Ozarks Technical Community College

Daniel Czech
Georgia Southern University

Kelly Falcone
Palomar College

Chris T. Harman
California University of Pennsylvania

Steve Hartman
Citrus College

Leslie Hickcox
Portland Community College

Emogene Johnson-Vaughn
Norfolk State University

Patricia Kearney
Bridgewater College

Dr. John Kowalczyk
University of Minnesota Duluth

Dale Landenberger
University of Akron

Ellen Larson
Northern Arizona University

Dean Lofgren
El Camino College

Debbie Lynch
Rose State College

Jamie Mansell
Lincoln University

Rich Morris
Rollins College

Jennifer Musick
Long Beach City College

Lindy Pickard
Palm Beach State College

Grace Pokorny
Long Beach City College

Andrea Salis
Queensborough Community College

Cody Trefethen
Palomar College

Debra Trigoboff
Palm Beach State College

Glenda Warren
University of the Cumberlands

Hilda C. Whitmire
Georgia Perimeter College

Sharon Woodard
Wake Forest University

Barbara Wright
Virginia Western Community College

Personal Health Forum and Focus Group Participants

Kathleen Allison
Lockhaven University

Fay Cook
Lockhaven University

Steven Dion
Salem State University

David V. Harackiewicz
Central Connecticut State University

Andrew Kanu
Virginia State University

Ellen Larson
Northern Arizona University

Ayanna Lyles
California University of Pennsylvania

Mitch Mathis
Arkansas State University

Holly Moses
University of Florida

Cody Trefethen
Palomar College

MyHealthLab Reviewers

Christine Bouffard
Waubonsee Community College

Steve Hartman
Citrus College

William Huber
County College of Morris

Kris Jankovitz
California Polytechnic State University

Dee Jones
Bucks County Community College

Carol Kennedy-Armbruster
Indiana University

Dean Lofgren
El Camino College

Jennifer Musick
Long Beach Community College

Cynthia Smith
Central Piedmont Community College

Debra Smith
Ohio University

Jenny Vannoy
Oregon State University

Healthy Change

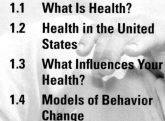

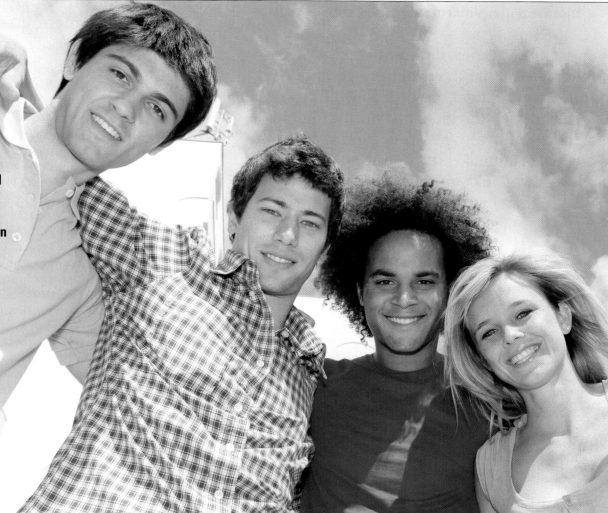

1

Got health? That may sound like a simple question, but it isn't; health is a process, not something we just "get." People who are healthy in their forties, fifties, sixties, and beyond aren't just lucky or the beneficiaries of hardy genes. In most cases, those who are healthy and thriving in their later years have set the stage for good health by making it a priority in their early years. You've probably heard others say that your college years will be the best years of your life; the canvas is hung upon which you will paint the story of your life. Whether your story is filled with good health, happiness, and fulfillment of your life goals is largely dependent on the health choices you make—beginning right now.

We aspire to be fit; we want to be more environmentally conscious; we search for relationships that are meaningful, loving, and lasting; and we want to live to a healthy, happy old age. How does what you do today influence you and those around you?

What Is Health?

- **Discuss definitions of *health* used throughout history.**
- **Discuss dimensions of health and wellness.**

Over the centuries, different ideals—or models—of human **health** have dominated. Our current model has broadened from a focus on the individual body to an understanding of health as a reflection of not only ourselves but also our communities. The choices we make about our health affect our lives in many ways. For instance, did you

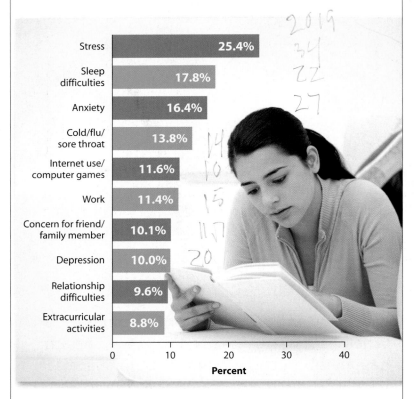

Figure 1.1 Top 10 Reported Impediments to Academic Performance—Past 12 Months

In a recent survey by the National College Health Association, students indicated that stress, poor sleep, recurrent minor illnesses, and anxiety, among other things, had prevented them from performing at their academic best.

Source: Data are from American College Health Association, *American College Health Association—National College Health Assessment II (ACHA-NCHA II) Reference Group Data Report, Fall 2010,* Available at www.acha-ncha.org.

know that the amount of sleep that you get each night could affect your body weight, your ability to ward off colds, your mood, and your driving? What's more, inadequate sleep is one of the most commonly reported impediments to academic success (Figure 1.1).

Models of Health

Before the twentieth century, if you made it to your fiftieth birthday, you were regarded as lucky. Survivors were believed to be of healthy stock—having what we might refer to today as "good genes." During this time, perceptions of health were dominated by the **medical model**, in which health status focused primarily on the individual and his or her tissues and organs. The way to bring about improved health was to cure the individual's disease, either with medication to treat the disease-causing agent or through surgery to remove the diseased body part. Government resources focused on initiatives that led to disease treatment rather than prevention.

In the early 1900s, researchers begin to see entire populations of poor people, particularly those living in certain locations, as victims of environmental factors—such as polluted water, air, and food—over which they often had little control. Experts then began to realize that disease and health are related to more than just physical factors. A field of study examining interactions between the social and physical environment evolved, leading to a more comprehensive **ecological** or **public health model**.

Recognition of the public health model enabled health officials to control contaminants in water, for example, by building adequate sewers, and to control burning and other forms of air pollution. Over time, public health officials began to recognize and address other forces affecting human health, including hazardous work conditions; negative influences in the home and social environment; stress; unsafe behavior; diet; and sedentary lifestyle.

By the 1940s, progressive thinkers began calling for policies, programs, and services to improve individual health and that of the population as a whole. Their focus shifted from treatment of individual illness to **disease prevention**, reducing or eliminating the factors that cause illness and injury. For example, childhood vaccination programs reduced the incidence and severity of infectious disease, and laws governing occupational safety reduced worker injuries and deaths. In 1947 at an international conference focusing on global health issues, the World Health Organization (WHO) proposed a new definition of health that rejected the old medical model: "Health is the state of complete physical, mental, and social well-being, not just the absence of disease or infirmity."[1]

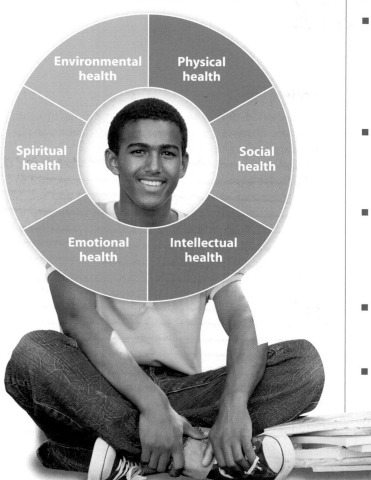

Figure 1.2 The Dimensions of Health
When all dimensions of health are in balance and well developed, they can support your active and thriving lifestyle.

Alongside prevention, the public health model emphasized **health promotion**—policies and programs promoting behaviors known to support health. Such programs identify people engaging in **risk behaviors** (behaviors increasing susceptibility to negative health outcomes) and motivate them to change their actions by changing the larger environment..

Wellness and the Dimensions of Health

In 1968, René Dubos proposed an even broader definition of health. In his book, *So Human an Animal*, Dubos defined *health* as "a quality of life, involving social, emotional, mental, spiritual, and biological fitness on the part of the individual, which results from adaptations to the environment."[2] This concept of adaptability became a key element in our overall understanding of health.

Eventually the word **wellness** entered the popular vocabulary, further enlarging Dubos's definition of health by recognizing levels—or gradations—of health within each category. Today, the words *health* and *wellness* are often used interchangeably to mean the dynamic, ever-changing process of trying to achieve one's potential in each of six interrelated dimensions (Figure 1.2):

- **Physical health.** This includes characteristics such as body size and shape, sensory acuity and responsiveness, susceptibility to disease and disorders, body functioning, physical fitness, and recuperative abilities. Newer definitions of physical health include our ability to perform normal *activities of daily living (ADLs)*, or those tasks necessary to normal existence in society, such as getting up from a chair, bending to tie your shoes, or writing a check.
- **Social health.** The ability to have satisfying interpersonal relationships with friends, family members, and partners is a key part of overall wellness. This implies being able to give and receive love, be nurturing and supportive in social interactions, and to interact and communicate with others.
- **Intellectual health.** The ability to think clearly, reason objectively, analyze critically, and use brainpower effectively to meet life's challenges. This includes learning from successes and mistakes; making sound, responsible decisions that consider all aspects of a situation; and having a healthy curiosity about life and an interest in learning new things.
- **Emotional health.** Being able to express emotions when appropriate, and to control them when not. Self-esteem, self-confidence, self-efficacy, trust, and love are all part of emotional health.
- **Spiritual health.** Having a sense of meaning and purpose in your life. This may involve belief in a supreme being or a specified way of living prescribed by a particular religion. It may also include the ability to understand and express one's purpose in life; to feel part of a greater spectrum of existence; to experience peace, contentment, and wonder over life's experiences; and to care about and respect all living things.
- **Environmental health.** Understanding how the health of the environments in which you live, work, and play can affect you; protecting yourself from hazards in your own environment; and working to protect and improve environmental conditions for everyone.

Achieving wellness means attaining the optimal level of well-being for your unique limitations and strengths. For example, a physically disabled person may function at his or her optimal level of performance; enjoy satisfying interpersonal relationships; work to maintain emotional, spiritual, and intellectual health; and have a strong interest in environmental concerns. In contrast, those who spend hours lifting weights to perfect each muscle but pay little attention to social or emotional health may look healthy but may not maintain a balance in all dimensions.

Although we often consider physical attractiveness and athletic performance key measures of health, these external trappings reveal very little about a person's overall health. The perspective we need is *holistic*, emphasizing balanced integration of mind, body, and spirit.

check yourself

- **How have definitions of health changed over time?**
- **What are the dimensions of health? Explain the differences among them.**

HEALTHY CHANGE

Health in the United States

learning **outcomes**

- **Specify major present-day health issues affecting the United States population.**
- **Explain the overall goals of *Healthy People 2020*.**

Our health choices are not only personal; they affect the lives of others in many ways. For example, overeating and inadequate physical activity contribute to individual obesity. But obesity also burdens the U.S. health care system and economy. *Direct* medical costs, including the costs of diagnosis and treatment, recently reached $147 billion.[3] And obesity costs the public *indirectly*, via, for example, increased disability payments and health insurance rates. Similarly, smoking, excessive consumption of alcohol, and use of illegal drugs place an economic burden on our communities and our society as a whole—not to mention social and emotional burdens on families and caregivers.

How Healthy Are We?

According to current **mortality** statistics—which reflect the proportion of deaths within a population—average life expectancy at birth in the United States is projected to be 78.8 years for a child born in 2010.[4] In other words, we can expect American infants born today to live to an average age of over 78, much longer than the 47-year life expectancy for people born in the early 1900s.

In the last century, with the development of vaccines, antibiotics, and other public health successes, as well as advances in medications, diagnostic technologies, surgery, and cancer treatments, life expec-

tancy increased dramatically.[5] The leading cause of death shifted to **chronic diseases**, such as heart disease, cerebrovascular disease (which leads to strokes), cancer, and diabetes.

Unfortunately, some researchers question whether this trend of increasing life expectancy will continue. One contributor to possible future reductions in life expectancy is obesity and sedentary lifestyle. A study from the Harvard School of Public Health and the University of Washington indicates that smoking, high blood pressure, elevated blood glucose, and overweight/obesity currently reduce life expectancy in the United States by 4.9 years in men and 4.1 years in women.[6] As Table 1.1 shows, today's four leading causes of death—heart disease, cancer, chronic respiratory disease, and stroke[7]—are strongly linked to lifestyle. The four leading causes of chronic disease are all under our individual control as well (Figure 1.3).

Clearly, healthful choices increase **life expectancy**. But they also increase **healthy life expectancy**—the years of full health a person enjoys without disability, chronic pain, or significant illness. For example, if we could delay the onset of diabetes until age 60 rather than 30, there would be a 30-year increase in that individual's healthy life expectancy. The prevalence of health issues affecting the U.S. population highlights the need to focus on healthy life expectancy as a cornerstone of public health.

Healthy People 2020: Setting Health Objectives

The Surgeon General's health promotion plan, *Healthy People*, has been published every 10 years since 1990 with the goal of improving quality of life and years of life for all Americans.[8] Each plan consists of a series of long-term objectives for the decade to come, with two broad goals for the health of the U.S. population: (1) increase both life spans and quality of life and (2) reduce and ultimately eliminate health disparities—major factors that can affect an individual's ability to attain optimal health.

In recognition of the changing demographics of the U.S. population and vast differences in health status based on racial or ethnic background, *Healthy People 2020* included strong language about the importance of reducing these disparities.[9]

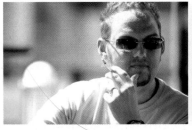 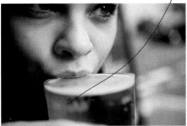 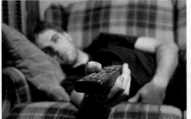 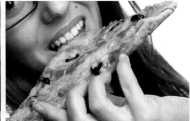

Figure 1.3 Four Leading Causes of Chronic Disease in the United States
Tobacco use, excessive alcohol consumption, lack of physical activity, and poor nutrition—all modifiable health determinants—are the four most significant factors leading to chronic disease among Americans today.

TABLE 1.1 Leading Causes of Death in the United States, 2009, Overall and by Age Group

All Ages	Number of Deaths
Diseases of the heart	598,607
Malignant neoplasms (cancer)	568,668
Chronic lower respiratory diseases	137,082
Cerebrovascular diseases	128,603
Accidents (unintentional injuries)	117,176
AGED 15–24	
Accidents (unintentional injuries)	12,351
Assault (homicide)	4,820
Self-harm (suicide)	4,341
Malignant neoplasms	1,659
Diseases of the heart	1,010
AGED 25–44	
Accidents (unintentional injuries)	28,844
Malignant neoplasms (cancer)	16,236
Diseases of the heart	14,053
Self-harm (suicide)	11,871
Assault (homicide)	6,883

Source: Data from K. D. Kochanek, et al., "Deaths: Preliminary Data for 2009," *National Vital Statistics Reports* 59, no. 4 (2011).

At the root of *Healthy People 2020* are four "foundation health measures" designed to "monitor progress toward promoting health, preventing disease and disability, eliminating disparities, and improving quality of life":[10]

- Measures of *general health status*, including life expectancy, healthy life expectancy, and chronic disease prevalence
- Measures of *health-related quality of life and well-being*, including physical, mental, and social factors and participation in common activities
- *Determinants of health*, which are the personal, social, economic, and environmental factors that influence health status
- Measures of *disparities* and inequity, including differences in health status based on race/ethnicity, gender, physical and mental ability, and geography

At the heart of *Healthy People 2020* are 39 topic areas, each representing a public health priority, such as diabetes, physical activity, or substance abuse.[11] Under each area is an overview describing health issues within its scope, objectives for the nation to achieve during the decade to come, and resources for communities and individuals. For instance, objectives for the nutrition topic include "Increase the proportion of schools that offer nutritious foods and beverages outside of school meals" and "Increase the proportion of physician office visits that include counseling or education related to nutrition or weight." For each objective, in turn, the report lists baseline statistics and a target goal for the year 2020.

Perhaps one of the most revealing aspects of the report are the 13 topic areas newly added for this decade, which reflect concern over health disparities, the relationship of lifestyle and wellness, and

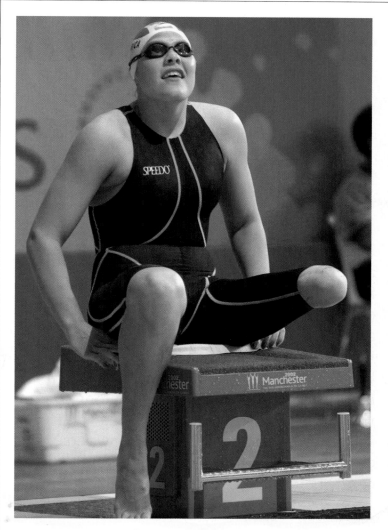

How are *health* and *quality of life* related?

Health-related quality of life refers to perceived physical and mental health over time. Just because a person has an illness or disability doesn't mean his or her quality of life is necessarily low. Swimmer Natalie du Toit lost her leg at age 14, but that hasn't prevented her from achieving her goals and a high quality of life. In 2008, she became the first amputee to qualify for and compete in the Olympic Games.

issues affecting the young and the very old.[12] These include adolescent health; global health; lesbian, gay, bisexual, and transgender health; older adults; sleep health, and health-related quality of life and well-being. Health is viewed as a comprehensive system encompassing the individual and the society, with influences both intensely personal and broadly global in scope.

check yourself

- **What are four key health issues in the United States?**
- **How are national health objectives used to improve health among Americans?**

What Influences Your Health?

- **Describe the major factors affecting an individual's ability to attain optimal health.**
- **Examine the connection between lifestyle and health outcomes.**

If you're lucky, aspects of your world promote health: Your family is active and fit; there are fresh apples on sale at the neighborhood farmer's market; and a new walking trail opens along the river. If you're not so lucky, aspects of your world discourage health: Your family eats a high-fat diet; cigarettes, alcohol, and junk food dominate the corner market; and you wouldn't dare walk along the river for fear of being mugged. This variety of influences explains why seemingly personal choices aren't totally within an individual's control.

Public health experts refer to the factors that influence health as **determinants of health**, a term the U.S. Surgeon General defines as "the array of critical influences that determine the health of individuals and communities" (Figure 1.4).[13]

Biology and Genetics

In the domain of health determinants, *biology* refers to an individual's genetics, ethnicity, age, and gender. Biology also includes family history; for example, if your parents developed diabetes in their forties, that's a biological determinant for you. Your history of illness and injury factors in, too; a serious injury might influence your ability to participate in physical activity. Biological determinants—what health experts refer to as *nonmodifiable determinants*—are things you can't change or modify.

Also included in this category are physiological differences between men and women that can extend into health behaviors and disease risk:

The effects of family on health can be both biological and environmental. Genetics determine some of your health status, but the actions and values of your family also have a strong influence on health.

- The size, structure, and function of the brain differ in women and men, particularly in areas that affect mood and behavior and in areas used to perform tasks.
- Bone mass in women peaks in the twenties; in men, it increases gradually until 30. After menopause, women lose bone at an accelerated rate.
- Women's immune systems are stronger than men's, though women are more prone to autoimmune diseases.
- When consuming the same amount of alcohol, women have a higher blood alcohol content than men, even allowing for size differences.
- Men smoke more than women, but women who smoke have higher rates of lung disease.
- Women are twice as likely than men to contract a sexually transmitted infection and 10 times more likely to contract HIV via unprotected intercourse.
- Depression is two to three times more common in women than in men, and women are more likely to attempt suicide; however, men are more likely to succeed at suicide.

Individual Behavior

In contrast to biological factors, *behaviors* are responses to internal and external conditions. By definition, behaviors are changeable; health experts refer to them as *modifiable determinants*. They significantly influence your risk for chronic disease, which is responsible for 7 out of 10 deaths in the United States.[14] Just four modifiable determinants are responsible for most illness and early death related to chronic diseases:[15]

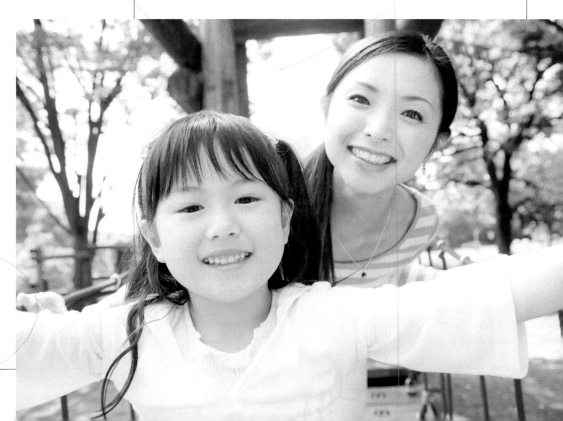

- **Lack of physical activity.** Physical inactivity and overweight/obesity are each responsible for nearly 1 in 10 deaths in U.S. adults.
- **Poor nutrition.** High salt, low omega-3 fatty acids, and high *trans* fatty acids are the dietary risks with the largest mortality effects.
- **Excessive alcohol consumption.** Alcohol causes 90,000 deaths in adults annually, through cardiovascular disease, other medical conditions, traffic accidents, and violence.
- **Tobacco use.** Tobacco smoking and the high blood pressure it causes are responsible for about 1 in 5 deaths in American adults.

Social and Physical Environment

Social determinants of health refer to the social factors and physical conditions in the environment in which people are born or live. Your social environment includes interactions with family, friends, and others in your community. It encompasses social institutions such as your campus, place of worship, and worksite, as well as services such as law enforcement and transportation. Cultural customs and languages are also aspects of the social environment, as is the level of violence in a community.[16]

Among the most powerful determinants of health in the social environment are economic factors; even in affluent nations such as the United States, people in lower socioeconomic brackets have substantially shorter life expectancies and more illnesses.[17] Economic disadvantages exert their effects on health in areas such as access to quality education, safe housing, nourishing food, warm clothes, medication, and transportation.

The physical environment is anything—from skyscrapers to snowfall—that you can perceive with your senses. It also includes less tangible things such as radiation and air pollution.

The built environment includes anything created or modified by human beings, from buildings to transportation to electrical lines. Changes to the built environment can improve the health of community members.[18] For example, Walter Willett of the Harvard School of Public Health proposes that sidewalks and bike lanes be part of every federally funded road project; when sidewalks are built in neighborhoods and downtowns, people are more apt to start walking and slim down.[19]

Individuals and communities exposed to toxins, radiation, irritants, and infectious agents can suffer significant harm. And the effects go beyond the local; the pollutants one region produces, or the diseases it harbors, can affect people worldwide. Examples include the burning of the South American rainforest contributing to global warming and the swift transmission of strains of severe influenza across populations.

Health Services and Health Disparities

The health of individuals and communities is also determined by access to quality health care, not only provider services but also accurate information and products such as eyeglasses, medical supplies, and medications. This determinant is related to both economics and public policy. **Health disparities** can arise from a variety of factors, including:[20]

- **Race and ethnicity.** Research indicates dramatic health disparities across racial and ethnic backgrounds. Socioeconomic dif-

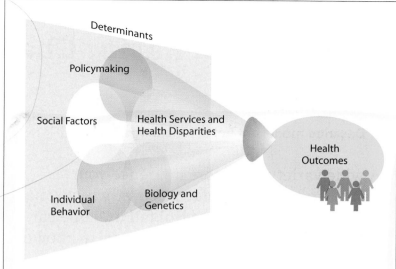

Figure 1.4 *Healthy People 2020* Determinants of Health
The determinants of health often overlap one another. Collectively, they impact the health of individuals and communities.

ferences, stigma based on "minority status," poor access to care, cultural barriers and beliefs, discrimination, and limited education and employment opportunities can all affect health.
- **Inadequate health insurance.** A large and growing number of the *uninsured* or *underinsured* face high copayments, high deductibles, or limited care in their area.
- **Sex and gender.** At all stages of life, men and women experience differences in rates of disease and disability.
- **Economics.** Poverty may make it difficult to afford healthy food, preventive medical visits, or medication. Economics also influences access to safe, affordable exercise.
- **Geographic location.** Whether you live in an urban or rural area and have access to public transportation or your own vehicle can have a huge impact on what you eat, your physical activity, and your ability to visit the doctor or dentist.
- **Sexual orientation.** Gay, lesbian, bisexual, or transgender individuals may lack social support, are often denied health benefits due to unrecognized marital status, and face unusually high stress levels and stigmatization by other groups.
- **Disability.** Disproportionate numbers of disabled individuals lack access to health care services, social support, and community resources.

Policymaking

Public policies and interventions can have a powerful effect on the health of individuals and communities. Examples include campaigns to prevent smoking, laws mandating seatbelt use, vaccination programs, and public funding for mental health services.[21]

check yourself

- **What are the determinants that affect health identified in this section?**
- **Give three examples of the connection between lifestyle and health outcomes.**

Models of Behavior Change

learning **outcomes**

■ **Describe models of behavior change.**

A wide variety of factors influence your health status. But the factors over which you have by far the most control fall into one category: individual behaviors (otherwise known as *modifiable determinants*). Clearly, change is not always easy. But your chances of successfully changing negative habits improve when you first identify a behavior that you want to change, then develop a plan for gradual transformation—one that allows you time to unlearn negative patterns and substitute positive ones. Many experts advocate breaking any health behavior you want to change into small parts, then working on them one at a time in "baby steps."

In other words, to successfully change a behavior, you need to see change not as a singular *event* but instead as a *process*—one that requires preparation, consists of several stages, and takes time to succeed.

Over the years, social scientists and public health researchers have developed a variety of models to reflect the multifaceted process of behavior change. We explore three such models here.

The Health Belief Model

Many people see changing health behaviors as a straightforward process: When rational people realize that their behaviors put them at risk, they will change those behaviors and reduce that risk. But, for many (even most) of us, it's more complicated than that. Consider the number of health professionals who smoke, consume junk food, and act in other unhealthy ways. They surely know better, but "knowing" is disconnected from "doing." One classic model of behavior change proposes that our beliefs may help to explain why this occurs.

A **belief** is an appraisal of the relationship between some object, action, or idea (e.g., smoking) and some attribute of that object, action, or idea (e.g., "Smoking is expensive, dirty, and causes cancer"— or "Smoking is sociable and relaxing"). Psychologists studying the relationship between beliefs and health behaviors have determined that although beliefs may subtly influence behavior, they may or may not cause people to actually behave differently. In 1966, psychologist I. Rosenstock developed a classic theory, the **health belief model (HBM)**, to show when beliefs about health affect behavior change.[22] The HBM holds that, before change is likely to happen, our beliefs must reflect the following:

■ **Perceived seriousness of the health problem.** How severe would the medical and social consequences be if the health problem were to develop or be left untreated? The more serious the perceived effects, the more likely that action will be taken.
■ **Perceived susceptibility to the health problem.** What is the likelihood of developing the health problem? People who perceive themselves at high risk are more likely to take preventive action.
■ **Cues to action.** A person who is reminded or alerted about a potential health problem is more likely to take action.

People follow the HBM many times every day. Take, for example, smokers. Older smokers are likely to know other smokers who have developed serious heart or lung problems. They are thus more likely to perceive tobacco as a threat to their health than are teenagers who have just begun smoking. The greater the perceived threat of health problems caused by smoking, the greater the chance a person will quit.

But many chronic smokers know the risks, yet continue to smoke. Why do they miss these cues to action? According to Rosenstock, some people do not believe that they, personally, are susceptible to a severe problem, and so act as though they are immune to it. Such people are unlikely to change their behavior.

35% of people who make New Year's resolutions break them before the end of January.

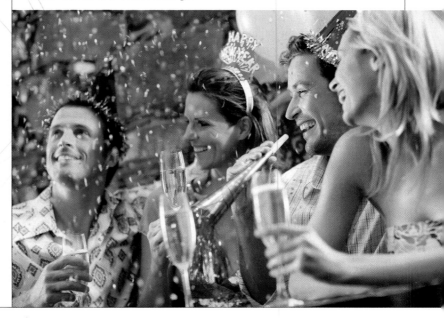

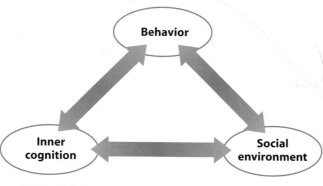

Figure 1.5 Social Cognitive Model
We are constantly changing our behavior in response to factors in our social environment and our inner world (our thoughts and feelings). But in return, our behaviors also change our environments as well as our thoughts and feelings—including our sense of our ability to make positive change.

The Social Cognitive Model

The **social cognitive model** developed from the work of multiple researchers over the past several decades, though it is most closely associated with the work of psychologist Albert Bandura. Fundamentally, the model proposes that three factors interact in a reciprocal fashion to promote and motivate change. These are the social environment in which we live, our thoughts or cognition (including our values, perceptions, beliefs, expectations, and sense of self-efficacy), and our behaviors (Figure 1.5). We change our behavior, in part, by observing models in our environments—from childhood to the present moment—reflecting on our observations, and regulating ourselves accordingly.

For instance, if as a child you observed your mother successfully quitting smoking, you may be more apt to believe that you can quit, too. In addition, when we succeed in changing ourselves, we change our thoughts about ourselves. This in turn may promote further behavior change: After you've successfully quit smoking, you may feel empowered to increase your level of physical activity. Moreover, as we change ourselves, we change our world; in this case, you become a model of successful smoking cessation for others to observe. In this model, we are not just products of our environments, but also producers of it.

The Transtheoretical Model

Why do so many New Year's resolutions fail before Valentine's Day? According to Drs. James Prochaska and Carlos DiClemente, it's because we are going about things in the wrong way; fewer than 20 percent of us are really prepared to take action on our resolutions. After considerable research, Prochaska and DiClemente have concluded that behavior changes that start with the change itself usually do not succeed; instead, we must go through a series of stages to adequately prepare ourselves for an eventual change.[23] According to Prochaska and DiClemente's **transtheoretical model** of behavior

is the number of times most people will attempt to change an unhealthy behavior before succeeding.

change (also called the *stages of change model*), our chances of keeping those New Year's resolutions will be greatly enhanced if we have proper reinforcement and help during each of the following stages:

1. **Precontemplation.** People in the precontemplation stage have no current intention of changing. They may have tried to change a behavior before and given up, or they may be in denial and unaware of any problem.
2. **Contemplation.** In this phase, people recognize that they have a problem and begin to contemplate the need to change. Despite this acknowledgment, people can languish in this stage for years, realizing a problem but lacking the time or energy to make the change.
3. **Preparation.** Most people at this point are close to taking action. They've thought about what they might do and may even have come up with a specific plan.
4. **Action.** In this stage, people begin to follow their action plans. Those who have prepared for change appropriately and made a plan of action are more ready for action than those who have given it little thought.
5. **Maintenance.** During the maintenance stage, a person continues the actions begun in the action stage and works toward making them a permanent part of his or her life. In this stage, it is important to be aware of the potential for relapses and to develop strategies for dealing with such challenges.
6. **Termination.** By this point, the change in behavior is so ingrained that constant vigilance may be unnecessary. The new behavior has become an essential part of daily living.

We don't necessarily go through these stages sequentially. They may overlap, or we may shuttle back and forth from one to another—say, contemplation to preparation, then back to contemplation—for a while before we become truly committed to making the change. Still, it's useful to recognize "where we're at" with a change, so we can consider the appropriate strategies to move us forward.

check yourself

- **Compare and contrast models of behavior change.**
- **Which model of behavior change reflects most accurately your experiences? Why?**

Improving Health Behaviors: Precontemplation and Contemplation

- **Identify strategies to employ prior to engaging in behavior change.**
- **Identify common behavior change strategies.**
- **Examine the factors that influence behavior and behavior change decisions.**

Step One: Increase Your Awareness

Before you can decide what you want to change, you'll need to learn about both the behaviors that affect your health and the health determinants in your life. What aspects of your biology, behavior, and social and physical environment support your health, and which are obstacles to overcome?

Step Two: Contemplate Change

Examine Your Health Habits and Patterns Do you routinely stop at Dunkin' Donuts for breakfast? Smoke when you're stressed? Party too much? Get to bed way past 2 AM? When considering habits, ask yourself the following:

- How long has this been going on?
- How often does it happen?
- How serious are its consequences?
- What are your reasons for the behavior?
- What situations trigger it?
- Are others involved? How?

Health behaviors involve personal choice, but are also influenced by determinants that make them more or less likely. Some are *predisposing factors*—for instance, if your parents smoke, you're 90 percent more likely to start smoking than a child of nonsmokers. Some are *enabling factors*—if your peers smoke, you're 80 percent more likely to smoke.

Reinforcing factors can also contribute to habits. If you decide to stop smoking but your friends all smoke, you may lose your resolve.

In such cases, it can be helpful to employ the social cognitive model and deliberately change your environment—spending more time with nonsmoking friends who model behavior you want to emulate.

Identify a Target Behavior Ask yourself these questions:

- **What do I want?** What is your ultimate goal? To lose weight? Exercise more? Reduce stress? Have a lasting relationship? Get a clear picture of your outcome.
- **Which change is my priority now?** Suppose you're gaining unwanted weight. Rather than saying, "I need to eat less and exercise," identify one specific behavior that contributes to your problem; tackle that first.
- **Why is this important to me?** Do you want to change for your health? To improve academic performance? To look better? To win someone's approval? It's best to target a behavior because it's right for you rather than because it will please others.

Learn about the Target Behavior Get solid information from reliable sources (see **Do Your Research**, below). Look at the behavior, its effects. and aspects of your world that could hinder your success. Let's say you want to meditate daily. You need to learn what meditation is, how it's practiced, and its benefits. What else might pose an obstacle? Do you think of yourself as hyper? Do you live in a noisy dorm? Are you afraid your friends might find meditating weird? To prepare for change, learn everything you can about your target behavior now.

Assess Your Motivation and Readiness To change, you need not just desire but **motivation**—a social and cognitive force that directs your behavior. To understand motivation, think about the health belief model (HBM) and the social cognitive model (SCM). According to the HBM, beliefs affect ability to change.

Find reliable health information at your fingertips!

Smokers may think, "I'll stop tomorrow" or "They'll have a cure for lung cancer before I get it." These beliefs allow them to continue smoking—they dampen motivation. Ask yourself the following:

- Do you believe your current pattern could lead to a serious problem? The more severe the consequences, the more motivation for change. For example, smoking can cause deadly diseases. But what if cancer and emphysema were just words to you? To increase your motivation, you could study these disorders and the suffering they cause.
- Do you see yourself as personally likely to experience the consequences of your behavior? Losing a loved one to lung cancer could motivate you to stop smoking.

If you're struggling to perceive a behavior as serious or its consequences as personal, use the SCM. You could interview people struggling with the consequences of the behavior and ask if when they were engaging in the behavior they believed it would harm them. And don't ignore the motivating potential of positive role models. Do you know people who have successfully lost weight, stopped drinking, or quit smoking? Hang out with them!

Motivation is powerful, but it must be combined with common sense, commitment, and a realistic understanding of how to move from A to B. *Readiness* precedes behavior change. People who are ready to change possess the knowledge, skills, and external and internal resources that make change possible.[24]

Develop Self-Efficacy **Self-efficacy**—a belief that one is capable of achieving certain goals or of influencing events in life—is one of the greatest influences on health. People who exhibit high self-efficacy are confident that they can succeed and approach challenges positively. They may therefore be more likely to succeed. Conversely, someone with low self-efficacy may give up easily, or never try to change. Such people tend to avoid challenges and are more likely to revert to old patterns. If you suspect your have low self-efficacy, a technique of cognitive-behavioral therapy called *cognitive restructuring* can help; find out more by visiting your campus counseling services.

Cultivate an Internal Locus of Control The conviction that you have the power and ability to change is a powerful motivator. Individuals with an *external* **locus of control** feel that they have limited control over their lives; they often find it difficult to initiate positive changes.[25] In contrast, people with an *internal* locus of control believe that they have power over their own actions. They are more likely to state their opinions and be true to their beliefs.

Do Your Research The Internet is a wonderful resource for finding answers to your questions, but it can also be a source of *misinformation*. If you're not careful, you could end up frazzled, confused, and worst, misinformed. To ensure that the sites you visit are trustworthy, follow these tips:

- Look for websites sponsored by government agencies (identified by .gov extensions—e.g., the National Institute of Mental Health at www.nimh.nih.gov), universities or colleges (.edu extensions—e.g., Johns Hopkins University at www.jhu.edu), or hospitals/medical centers (often .org—e.g., the Mayo Clinic at www.mayoclinic

.org). Major philanthropic foundations (such as the Robert Wood Johnson Foundation and the Kellogg Foundation) and national nonprofit organizations (such as the American Heart Association and the American Cancer Society) are good, authoritative sources. Most foundation and nonprofit sites have *.org* extensions.
- Search for peer-reviewed journals such as the *New England Journal of Medicine* (http://content.nejm.org) and *Journal of the American Medical Association* (JAMA; http://jama.ama-assn.org). Though some of these sites require an access fee, many colleges give students free access to them.
- Other reliable sites include the Centers for Disease Control and Prevention (www.cdc.gov), the World Health Organization (www.who.int/en), FamilyDoctor.org (http://familydoctor.org), MedlinePlus (www.nlm.nih.gov/medlineplus), Go Ask Alice! (www.goaskalice.columbia.edu), and WebMD (http://my.webmd.com).
- Don't believe everything you read. Cross-check information against reliable sources. Be wary of websites selling you something. When in doubt, check with your health care provider or health professor.

Skills for Behavior Change

MAINTAIN YOUR MOTIVATION

- **Pick one specific behavior you want to change.** Trying to change many things at once can be overwhelming and can cause you to lose motivation.
- **Assess the behavior you wish to change.** Why is it important to change? If you can't find a compelling reason to motivate you, you probably shouldn't address this behavior right now.
- **Set achievable and incremental goals.** Developing short- and long-term goals, and taking small steps to meet them, improves your chances of staying motivated.
- **Reward yourself.** Create a list of things you find rewarding; link each to a specific goal. Having something to look forward to can help you stay focused and motivated.
- **Avoid or anticipate barriers and temptations.** Control or eliminate the environmental cues that provoke the behavior you want to change.
- **Remind yourself why you're trying to change.** List the benefits you'll get from this change, both now and down the road, as well as the risks of doing nothing.
- **Enlist the support of others.** They can serve as role models, a cheering squad, or partners in change. Let the people you care about know your plans, and ask for help.
- **Don't be discouraged.** Everyone, no matter how committed, experiences setbacks. A brief lapse doesn't mean the cause is lost. Look for new strategies, set new short-term goals, and then get back on the horse.

check yourself

- **What are some activities you should do before undertaking a behavior change?**
- **What are five common behavior change strategies?**
- **What are important factors that influence behavior and behavior change decisions?**

HEALTHY CHANGE

Improving Health Behaviors: Preparation

- **Set a behavior change goal.**
- **Identify obstacles to behavior change.**

Prepare for Change

You've contemplated change for long enough—now it's time to set a realistic goal, anticipate barriers, reach out to others, and commit.

Set a Realistic Goal A realistic goal is one that you truly can achieve—not someday, when things in your life change, but within the circumstances of your life right now. Knowing that your goal is attainable increases your motivation. This, in turn, leads to a better chance of success and to a greater sense of self-efficacy—which can in turn motivate you to succeed even more. To set realistic goals, do the following:

Use the SMART System Unsuccessful goals are vague and open-ended—for instance, "Get into shape by exercising more." In contrast, successful goals are SMART:

- **S**pecific. "Attend the Tuesday/Thursday aerobics class at the YMCA."
- **M**easurable. "Reduce my alcohol intake on Saturday nights from three drinks to two."
- **A**ction-oriented. "Volunteer at the animal shelter on Friday afternoons."
- **R**ealistic. "Increase my daily walk from 15 to 20 minutes."
- **T**ime-oriented. "Stay in my strength-training class for the full 10-week session, then reassess."

Use Shaping **Shaping** is a process of making a series of small changes. Suppose you want to start jogging 3 miles every other day, but right now you get tired and winded after half a mile. Shaping would dictate a process of slow, progressive steps, perhaps beginning with walking 1 hour every other day at a slow, relaxed pace for the first week; walking for an hour every other day but at a faster pace that covers more distance the second week; and speeding up to a slow run the third week.

Regardless of the change you plan, remember that your current habits didn't develop overnight; they won't change overnight, either. Prepare your goals and your plan of action with these shaping points in mind:

- Start slowly to avoid hurting yourself or causing undue stress.
- Keep the steps of your program small and achievable.
- Be flexible and ready to change your original plan if it proves uncomfortable.
- Master one step before moving on to the next.

Anticipate Barriers to Change Anticipating *barriers to change*, or possible stumbling blocks, will help you prepare fully and adequately for change. For example, if you want to lose weight, you may face several barriers to change, including social determinants (your family members and friends are overweight), aspects of the built environment (the only food vendors on or near your campus are convenience stores and fast-food outlets), or lack of adequate health care (you have an inexpensive health insurance policy that doesn't cover treatment for weight loss). In addition to negative determinants, the following are a few general barriers to change that you may need to overcome:

- **Overambitious goals.** Remember the advice to set realistic goals? Even with the strongest motivation, overambitious goals can derail change. Most people cannot lose weight, stop smoking, and begin running 3 miles a day all at the same time. Wanting to achieve dramatic change within unrealistically short time frames—for example, aiming to lose 20 pounds in 1 month—tends to be equally unsuccessful. Habits are best changed one small step at a time.
- **Self-defeating beliefs and attitudes.** As the health belief model explains, believing you're too young or fit or lucky to have to worry about the consequences of your behavior can keep you from making a solid commitment to change. Likewise, seeing yourself as helpless to change your eating, smoking, or other habits can undermine your efforts. Greater self-efficacy and more positive expectations may help.
- **Failing to accurately assess your current state of wellness.** You might assume that you will be able to walk the 2 miles to campus each morning, for example, only to find yourself aching and winded after only a mile. Failing to make sure that the planned change is realistic for *you* can leave you with weakened motivation and commitment.
- **Lack of support and guidance.** If you want to cut down on your drinking, peers who drink heavily may be powerful barriers to that change. To succeed, you will need to recognize the people in your life who can't support, or might even actively oppose, your decision to change, then limit your interactions with them.
- **Emotions that sabotage your efforts and sap your will.** Some-

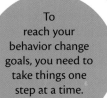

To reach your behavior change goals, you need to take things one step at a time.

times the best laid plans go awry because you're having a bad day or are fighting with someone you care about. While emotional reactions to life's challenges aren't inherently bad, they can sabotage your efforts to change by distracting you and draining your reserves. Seek help for more severe psychological problems, and recognize that you may need to focus on those before you can effect significant change in other aspects of your health.

Enlist Others as Change Agents The social cognitive model recognizes the importance of our social contacts in successful change. Most of us are highly influenced by the approval or disapproval (real or imagined) of close friends, family members, and the social and cultural group to which we belong. In addition, watching others successfully change their behavior can give you ideas and encouragement for your own change. This **modeling**, or learning from role models, is a key component of the social cognitive model of change. Observing a friend who is a good conversationalist, for example, can help you improve your communication skills. Or find someone to share your plan for change! For instance, get your roommate to commit to taking a daily walk or run with you or sign a contract with a friend stipulating that you will never let each other drink and drive.

Family Members From the time of your birth, your parents and other family members have given you strong cues about which actions are and are not socially acceptable. Your family has also influenced your food choices, your religious beliefs, your political beliefs, and many of your other values and actions. Strong and positive family units provide care, trust, and protection; are dedicated to the healthful development of all family members; and work to reduce problems.

When a loving family unit does not exist or when it does not provide for basic human needs, a child can find it difficult to learn positive health behaviors. Healthy families provide the foundation for a clear and necessary understanding of what is right and wrong, what is positive and negative. Without this fundamental grounding, many young people have great difficulties.

Friends Just as your family influences your actions during your childhood, your friends and significant others influence your behaviors as you grow older. Most of us desire to fit the "norm" and avoid hassles in our daily interactions with others. If you deviate from the actions expected in your hometown or among your friends, you may suffer ostracism, strange looks, and other negative social consequences. But if your friends offer encouragement, or even express interest in joining you in a behavior change, you are more likely to remain motivated. Cultivating and maintaining close friends who share your personal values can greatly affect your behaviors and improve your chances of success.

Professionals Sometimes the change you seek requires more than the help of well-meaning family members and friends. Depending on the type and severity of the problem, you may want to enlist support from professionals such as your health instructor, PE instructor, coach, health care provider, academic adviser, or minister. As appropriate, consider counseling services offered on

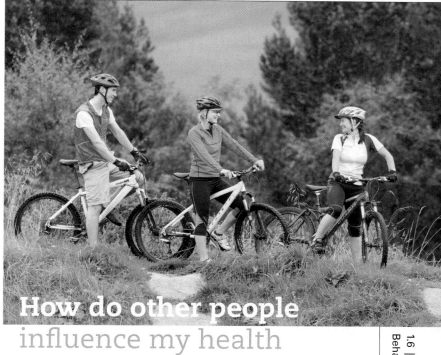

How do other people influence my health behaviors?

The people in your life—including family, friends, neighbors, coworkers, and society in general—can play a huge role—both positive and negative—in the health choices you make. The behaviors of those around you can predispose you to certain health habits, at the same time enabling and reinforcing them. Seeking out the support and encouragement of friends who have similar goals and interests will strengthen your commitment to develop and maintain positive health behaviors.

campus, as well as community services such as smoking cessation programs, Alcoholics Anonymous support groups, and your local YMCA.

Sign a Contract It's time to get it in writing! A formal *behavior change contract* serves many powerful purposes. It functions as a promise to yourself, a public declaration of intent, an organized plan that lays out start and end dates and daily actions, a list of barriers you may encounter, a place to brainstorm strategies to overcome barriers, a list of sources of support, and a reminder of the benefits of sticking with the program.

Writing a behavior change contract will help you clarify your goals and make a commitment to change. In the next module, you will see a completed behavior change contract and later in the chapter, a blank behavior change contract. Use this to put your behavior change plan in writing.

check yourself

- **What is your behavior change goal? Does it fit the SMART system?**

- **What are some obstacles to change that you expect to face? What strategies will you employ to overcome them?**

Improving Health Behaviors: Action

- **Employ behavior change strategies to make a behavior change.**

Take Action to Change

It's time to put your plan into action! Behavior change strategies include visualization, countering, controlling the situation, changing your self-talk, rewarding yourself, and journaling. The options don't stop here, but these are a good place to start.

Visualize New Behavior Mental practice can transform unhealthy behaviors into healthy ones. Using **imagined rehearsal** to visualize an action ahead of time can help you be prepared. Careful mental and verbal rehearsal of how you intend to act will help you anticipate problems, and greatly improve the likelihood of success.

Learn to "Counter" Substituting a desired behavior for an undesirable one is called **countering**. You may want to stop eating junk food, but going "cold turkey" isn't realistic. Instead, compile a list of substitute foods and where to get them—and have it ready before your mouth starts to water at the smell of a burger and fries.

Control the Situation Sometimes, the right setting or the right group of people will positively influence your behaviors. Any behavior has both antecedents and consequences. *Antecedents* are aspects of a situation that come beforehand, cueing or stimulating a person to act in certain ways. *Consequences*—the results of behavior—affect whether a person repeats an action. Both antecedents and consequences can be events, thoughts, emotions, or the actions of others. Try using a diary noting your undesirable behaviors, and the settings in which they occur, to help determine their antecedents and consequences. Then use **situational inducement** to improve your chances for change—consider which settings help and which hurt your effort to change. Identifying substitute antecedents that support a more positive result helps you control the situation further.

Change Your Self-Talk The way you think to yourself—**self-talk**—can reflect your feelings of *self-efficacy*. When we feel we have little control, it's tempting to engage in negative self-talk, which can sabotage our best intentions.

Use Rational, Positive Statements Rational-emotive cognitive therapy, or self-directed behavior change, is based on the premise that there is a close connection between what people say to themselves and how they feel. According to psychologist Albert Ellis, most emotional problems and related behaviors stem from irrational statements that people make to themselves when events in their lives are different from what they would like them to be.[26]

Suppose you say to yourself, "I can't believe I flunked that exam. I'm so stupid." Changing such irrational, "catastrophic" self-talk into rational, positive statements about what is really going on can increase the likelihood of positive change: "I didn't study enough for

Behavior Change Contract

My behavior change will be:
To snack less on junk food and more on healthy foods.

My long-term goal for this behavior change is:
Eat junk food snacks no more than once a week.

These are three obstacles to change (things that I am currently doing or situations that contribute to this behavior or make it harder to change):
1. The grocery store is closed by the time I come home from school.
2. I get hungry between classes, and the vending machines only carry candy bars.
3. It's easier to order pizza or other snacks than to make a snack at home.

The strategies I will use to overcome these obstacles are:
1. I'll leave early for school once a week so I can stock up on healthy snacks in the morning.
2. I'll bring a piece of fruit or other healthy snack to eat between classes.
3. I'll learn some easy recipes for snacks to make at home.

Resources I will use to help me change this behavior include:
a friend/partner/relative: my roommates: I'll ask them to buy healthier snacks instead of chips when they do the shopping.
a school-based resource: The dining hall: I'll ask the manager to provide healthy foods we can take to eat between classes.
a community-based resource: The library: I'll check out some cookbooks to find easy snack ideas.
a book or reputable website: The USDA nutrient database at www.nal.usda.gov/fnic I'll use this site to make sure the foods I select are healthy choices.

In order to make my goal more attainable, I have devised these short-term goals:
short-term goal Eat a healthy snack 3 times per week   target date September 15   reward new CD
short-term goal Learn to make a healthy snack   target date October 15   reward concert tickets
short-term goal Eat a healthy snack 5 times per week   target date November 15   reward new shoes

When I make the long-term behavior change described above, my reward will be:
ski lift tickets for winter break   target date: December 15

I intend to make the behavior change described above. I will use the strategies and rewards to achieve the goals that will contribute to a healthy behavior change.

Signed: Elizabeth King   Witness: **Susan Bauer**

Figure 1.6 Example of a Completed Behavior Change Contract

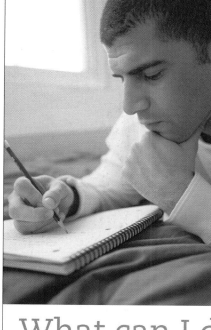

One of the best tools for helping you change your habits is journaling. Keeping track of your goals, behaviors, feelings, accomplishments, and setbacks can reinforce the healthy changes you are trying to make and provide motivation to continue. Other useful tools include shaping, enlisting supports, visualization, countering, controlling the situation, changing your self-talk, and rewarding yourself.

What can I do to change an unhealthy habit?

that exam. I'm not stupid; I just need to prepare better for the next test." Positive self-talk can help you recover from disappointment and take steps to correct problems.

Practice Blocking and Stopping Blocking or stopping negative thoughts can help you concentrate on positive steps toward behavior change. Suppose you're preoccupied with your ex-partner, who left you for someone else. By refusing to dwell on negative images and forcing yourself to focus elsewhere, you can avoid wasting energy, time, and emotional resources and move on to positive change.

Reward Yourself Promote positive behavior change with **positive reinforcement**. Each of us is motivated by different positive reinforcers. Most of these fall into one of the following categories:

- *Consumable reinforcers* are edible items such as a favorite fruit or snack mix.
- *Activity reinforcers* are opportunities to do something enjoyable, such as going on a hike or taking a trip.
- *Manipulative reinforcers* are incentives such as reduced rent in exchange for mowing the lawn or the promise of a better grade for doing an extra-credit project.
- *Possessional reinforcers* are tangible rewards such as a new gadget or car.
- *Social reinforcers* are signs of appreciation, approval, or love such as hugs or praise.

Successful positive reinforcement often lies in choosing successful incentives. Your reinforcers may initially come from others (extrinsic

rewards), but as you see positive changes in yourself you will begin to reward and reinforce yourself (intrinsic rewards). Reinforcers should immediately follow a behavior, but beware of overkill; if you reward yourself with a movie every time you go jogging, the reinforcer will soon lose its power. It would be better to give yourself such a reward after, say, a full week of adherence to your jogging program.

Journal Journaling, or writing down personal experiences, interpretations, and results, is an important skill for behavior change. You can log your daily activities, monitor your progress, record your feelings, and note ideas for improvement.

Let's Get Started

Once you have the skills to support successful behavior change, you can apply them to your target behavior. Create a behavior change contract incorporating the goals and skills discussed here, and place it where you'll see it every day, as a reminder that change doesn't "just happen." (See Figure 1.6 for an example.) Reviewing your contract helps you stay alert to potential problems, be aware of your alternatives, maintain a firm sense of your values, and stick to your goals under pressure.

Skills for Behavior Change

CHALLENGE THE THOUGHTS THAT SABOTAGE CHANGE

Are thought patterns and beliefs holding you back? Try these strategies:

- **"I don't have enough time!"** Chart your activities for 1 day. What are your highest priorities? What can you eliminate or reduce? Plan to make some time for a healthy change next week.
- **"I'm too stressed!"** Assess your major stressors right now. List those you can control and those you can change or avoid. Then identify two things you enjoy that can help you reduce stress now.
- **"I worry what others may think."** How much do others influence your decisions about drinking, sex, eating habits, and the like? What is most important to you? What actions can you take to act in line with your values?
- **"I don't think I can."** Just because you haven't done something before doesn't mean you can't do it now. To develop confidence, take baby steps and break tasks into small chunks of time.
- **"I can't break this habit!"** Habits are difficult to break, but not impossible. What triggers your behavior? List ways you can avoid triggers. Ask for support from friends and family.

check yourself

- **Describe the behavior change strategies that you used. What were the benefits and disadvantages of each strategy?**

Behavior Change Contract

■ **Complete a behavior change contract.**

Complete the Assess Yourself questionnaire. After reviewing your results and considering the various factors that influence your decisions, choose a health behavior that you would like to change, starting this quarter or semester. Sign the contract at the bottom to affirm your commitment to making a healthy change and ask a friend to witness it.

My behavior change will be:

_____

My long-term goal for this behavior change is:

_____

These are three obstacles to change (things that I am currently doing or situations that contribute to this behavior or make it harder to change):

1.   _____
2.   _____
3.   _____

The strategies I will use to overcome these obstacles are:

1.   _____
2.   _____
3.   _____

Resources I will use to help me change this behavior include:

  a friend/partner/relative: _____

  a school-based resource: _____

  a community-based resource: _____

  a book or reputable website: _____

In order to make my goal more attainable, I have devised these short-term goals:

_____   _____   _____
short-term goal   target date   reward

_____   _____   _____
short-term goal   target date   reward

_____   _____   _____
short-term goal   target date   reward

When I make the long-term behavior change described above, my reward will be:

_____   target date: _____

I intend to make the behavior change described above. I will use the strategies and rewards to achieve the goals that will contribute to a healthy behavior change.

Signed: _____   Witness: _____

■ **Do you think that completing the contract will make it more likely that you will succeed in your behavior change? Why or why not?**

Assessyourself

How Healthy Are You?

Although we all recognize the importance of being healthy, it can be a challenge to sort out which behaviors are most likely to cause problems or which ones pose the greatest risk. *Before* you decide where to start, it is important to look at your current health status.

By completing the following assessment, you will have a clearer picture of health areas in which you excel and those that could use some work. Taking this assessment will also help you to reflect on components of health that you may not have thought about.

Answer each question, then total your score for each section and fill it in on the Personal Checklist at the end of the assessment for a general sense of your health profile. Think about the behaviors that influenced your score in each category. Would you like to change any of them? Choose the area that you'd like to improve, and then complete the Behavior Change Contract on the previous page. Use the contract to think through and implement a behavior change over the course of this class.

Each of the categories in this questionnaire is an important aspect of the total dimensions of health, but this is not a substitute for the advice of a qualified health care provider. Consider scheduling a thorough physical examination by a licensed physician or setting up an appointment with a mental health counselor at your school if you need help making a behavior change.

For each of the following, indicate how often you think the statements describe you.

1 Physical Health

	Never	Rarely	Some of the time	Usually or Always
1. I am happy with my body size and weight.	1	2	3	4
2. I engage in vigorous exercises such as brisk walking, jogging, swimming, or running for at least 30 minutes per day, three to four times per week.	1	2	3	4
3. I get at least 7 to 8 hours of sleep each night.	1	2	3	4
4. My immune system is strong, and my body heals itself quickly when I get sick or injured.	1	2	3	4
5. I listen to my body; when there is something wrong, I try to make adjustments to heal it or seek professional advice.	1	2	3	4

Total score for this section: _____

2 Social Health

	Never	Rarely	Some of the time	Usually or Always
1. I am open, honest, and get along well with others.	1	2	3	4
2. I participate in a wide variety of social activities and enjoy being with people who are different from me.	1	2	3	4
3. I try to be a "better person" and decrease behaviors that have caused problems in my interactions with others.	1	2	3	4
4. I am open and accessible to a loving and responsible relationship.	1	2	3	4
5. I try to see the good in my friends and do whatever I can to support them and help them feel good about themselves.	1	2	3	4

Total score for this section: _____

3 Emotional Health

	Never	Rarely	Some of the time	Usually or Always
1. I find it easy to laugh, cry, and show emotions like love, fear, and anger, and try to express these in positive, constructive ways.	1	2	3	4
2. I avoid using alcohol or other drugs as a means of helping me forget my problems.	1	2	3	4
3. I recognize when I am stressed and take steps to relax through exercise, quiet time, or other calming activities.	1	2	3	4
4. I try not to be too critical or judgmental of others and try to understand differences or quirks that I note in others.	1	2	3	4
5. I am flexible and adapt or adjust to change in a positive way.	1	2	3	4

Total score for this section: _____

4 Environmental Health

	Never	Rarely	Some of the time	Usually or Always

1. I buy recycled paper and purchase biodegradable detergents and cleaning agents, or make my own cleaning products, whenever possible. — 1 2 3 4

2. I recycle paper, plastic, and metals; purchase refillable containers when possible; and try to minimize the amount of paper and plastics that I use. — 1 2 3 4

3. I try to wear my clothes for longer periods between washing to reduce water consumption and the amount of detergents in our water sources. — 1 2 3 4

4. I vote for pro-environment candidates in elections. — 1 2 3 4

5. I minimize the amount of time that I run the faucet when I brush my teeth, shave, or shower. — 1 2 3 4

Total score for this section: _____

5 Spiritual Health

1. I take time alone to think about what's important in life—who I am, what I value, where I fit in, and where I'm going. — 1 2 3 4

2. I have faith in a greater power, be it a supreme being, nature, or the connectedness of all living things. — 1 2 3 4

3. I engage in acts of caring and goodwill without expecting something in return. — 1 2 3 4

4. I sympathize and empathize with those who are suffering and try to help them through difficult times. — 1 2 3 4

5. I go for the gusto and experience life to the fullest. — 1 2 3 4

Total score for this section: _____

6 Intellectual Health

1. I carefully consider my options and possible consequences as I make choices in life. — 1 2 3 4

2. I learn from my mistakes and try to act differently the next time. — 1 2 3 4

3. I have at least one hobby, learning activity, or personal growth activity that I make time for each week, something that improves me as a person. — 1 2 3 4

	Never	Rarely	Some of the time	Usually or Always

4. I manage my time well rather than let time manage me. — 1 2 3 4

5. My friends and family trust my judgment. — 1 2 3 4

Total score for this section: _____

Although each of these six aspects of health is important, there are some factors that don't readily fit in one category. As college students, you face some unique risks that others may not have. For this reason, we have added a section to this self-assessment that focuses on personal health promotion and disease prevention. Answer these questions and add your results to the Personal Checklist in the following section.

7 Personal Health Promotion/Disease Prevention

1. If I were to be sexually active, I would use protection such as latex condoms, dental dams, and other means of reducing my risk of sexually transmitted infections. — 1 2 3 4

2. I can have a good time at parties or during happy hours without binge drinking. — 1 2 3 4

3. I have eaten too much in the last month and have forced myself to vomit to avoid gaining weight. — 4 3 2 1

4. If I were to get a tattoo or piercing, I would go to a reputable person who follows strict standards of sterilization and precautions against bloodborne disease transmission. — 1 2 3 4

5. I engage in extreme sports and find that I enjoy the highs that come with risking bodily harm through physical performance. — 4 3 2 1

Total score for this section: _____

Personal Checklist

Now, total your scores for each section on the next page and compare them to what would be considered optimal scores. Are you surprised by your scores in any areas? Which areas do you need to work on?

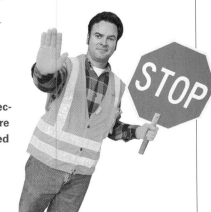

1.9

	Ideal Score	Your Score
Physical health	20	_____
Social health	20	_____
Emotional health	20	_____
Environmental health	20	_____
Spiritual health	20	_____
Intellectual health	20	_____
Personal health promotion/ disease prevention	20	_____

What Your Scores in Each Category Mean

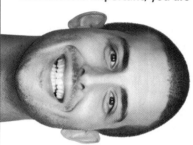

Scores of 15–20: Outstanding! Your answers show that you are aware of the importance of these behaviors in your overall health. More important, you are putting your knowledge to work by practicing good health habits that should reduce your overall risks. Although you received a very high score on this part of the test, you may want to consider areas in which your scores could be improved.

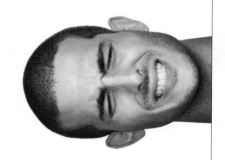

Scores of 10–14: Your health risks are showing! Find information about the risks you are facing and why it is important to change these behaviors. Perhaps you need help in deciding how to make the changes you desire. Assistance is available from this book, your professor, and student health services at your school.

Scores below 10: You may be taking unnecessary risks with your health. Perhaps you are not aware of the risks and what to do about them. Identify each risk area and make a mental note as you read the associated chapter in the book. Whenever possible, seek additional resources, either on your campus or through your local community health resources, and make a serious commitment to behavior change. If any area is causing you to be less than functional in your class work or personal life, seek professional help. In this book you will find the information you need to help you improve your scores and your health. Remember that these scores are only indicators, not diagnostic tools.

Your Plan for Change

The Assess Yourself activity gave you the chance to look at the status of your health in several dimensions. Now that you have considered these results, you can take steps toward changing certain behaviors that may be detrimental to your health.

Today, you can:

○ Evaluate your behavior and identify patterns and specific things you are doing.

○ Select one pattern of behavior that you want to change.

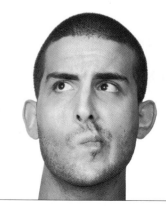

○ Fill out the Behavior Change Contract in this chapter. Be sure to include your long- and short-term goals for change, the rewards you'll give yourself for reaching these goals, the potential obstacles along the way, and your strategies for overcoming these obstacles. For each goal, list the small steps and specific actions that you will take.

Within the next 2 weeks, you can:

○ Start a journal and begin charting your progress toward your behavior change goal.

○ Tell a friend or family member about your behavior change goal, and ask him or her to support you along the way.

○ Reward yourself for reaching your short-term goals, and reevaluate your plan if you find that they are too ambitious.

By the end of the semester, you can:

○ Review your journal entries and consider how successful you have been in following your plan. What helped you be successful? What made change more difficult? What will you do differently next week?

○ Revise your plan as needed: Are the goals attainable? Are the rewards satisfying? Do you have enough support and motivation?

Summary

- Choosing good health has immediate benefits, such as reducing the risk of injury and illness; long-term rewards, such as disease prevention and improved quality of life; and societal and global benefits, such as reducing the global disease burden.
- For the U.S. population as a whole, the leading causes of death are heart disease, cancer, and stroke.
- The definition of *health* has changed over time. The medical model focused on treating disease; the current public health model focuses on factors contributing to health, disease prevention, and health promotion.
- Health is the process of fulfilling one's potential in physical, social, emotional, spiritual, intellectual, and environmental dimensions of life. Wellness means achieving the best health possible in several dimensions.
- Health is influenced by *determinants*, which the Surgeon General's health promotion plan, *Healthy People*, classifies as individual biology and behavior, the social environment, the physical environment, policies and interventions, and access to quality health care. Disparities in health among groups contribute to increased risks.
- Models of behavior change include health belief, the social cognitive, and transtheoretical (stages of change) models. You can increase the chance of changing a behavior by viewing change as a process.
- When contemplating change, examine current habits, learn about a target behavior, and assess readiness. When preparing to change, set incremental goals, anticipate barriers to change, enlist support, and sign a behavior change contract. When taking action, visualize new behavior, practice countering, control the situation, change self-talk, reward yourself, and keep a log or journal.

Pop Quiz

1. Our ability to perform everyday tasks, such as walking up the stairs or tying shoes, is an example of
   a. improved quality of life.
   b. physical health.
   c. health promotion.
   d. activities of daily living.

2. Janice displays both high self-esteem and high self-efficacy. The dimension of health this relates to is the
   a. social dimension.
   b. emotional dimension.
   c. spiritual dimension.
   d. intellectual dimension.

3. Cody has decided that he needs to improve his diet. He observes his roommates' healthy meal choices and decides to adopt some of their eating habits. This is an example of which model of behavior change?
   a. social cognitive
   b. health belief
   c. transtheoretical
   d. stages of change

4. Because Craig's parents smoked, he is 90 percent more likely to start smoking than someone whose parents didn't. This is an example of what factor influencing behavior change?
   a. Circumstantial factor
   b. Enabling factor
   c. Reinforcing factor
   d. Predisposing factor

5. Suppose you want to lose 20 pounds. To reach your goal, you start by counting calories. After 2 weeks, you begin an exercise program and gradually build up to your desired fitness level. What behavior change strategy are you using?
   a. Shaping
   b. Visualization
   c. Modeling
   d. Reinforcement

6. After Kirk and Tammy pay their bills, they reward themselves by watching TV together. The type of positive reinforcement is a(n)
   a. activity reinforcer.
   b. consumable reinforcer.
   c. manipulative reinforcer.
   d. possessional reinforcer.

7. Jake is exhibiting *self-efficacy* when he
   a. claims he will never be able to bench-press 125 pounds.
   b. doubts he'll ever bench-press the weight he hopes for.
   c. believes that he can and will be able to bench-press 125 pounds in his specified time frame.
   d. does not believe he possesses personal control over this situation.

8. Aspects of a situation that cue or stimulate a person to act in certain ways are called
   a. reinforcers.
   b. antecedents.
   c. consequences.
   d. cues to action.

9. What strategy is advised for an individual in the preparation stage of change?
   a. Seeking recommended readings
   b. Finding ways to maintain positive behaviors
   c. Setting realistic goals
   d. Publicly stating the desire for change

10. *Healthy People 2020* is:
    a. a blueprint for actions designed to improve U.S. health.
    b. a projection for life expectancy rates in the United States in the year 2020.
    c. an international plan for achieving global health priorities for the environment by the year 2020.
    d. a set of specific goals that states must achieve in order to receive federal funding for health.

    Answers to these questions can be found on page A-1.

Web Links

1. **CDC Wonder.** A clearinghouse for information from the Centers for Disease Control and Prevention. http://wonder.cdc.gov
2. **Mayo Clinic.** A reputable resource for information about health topics, diseases, and treatment options. www.mayoclinic.com
3. **National Center for Health Statistics.** Information about health status in the United States, including key reports and national survey information. www.cdc.gov/nchs

Psychological Health

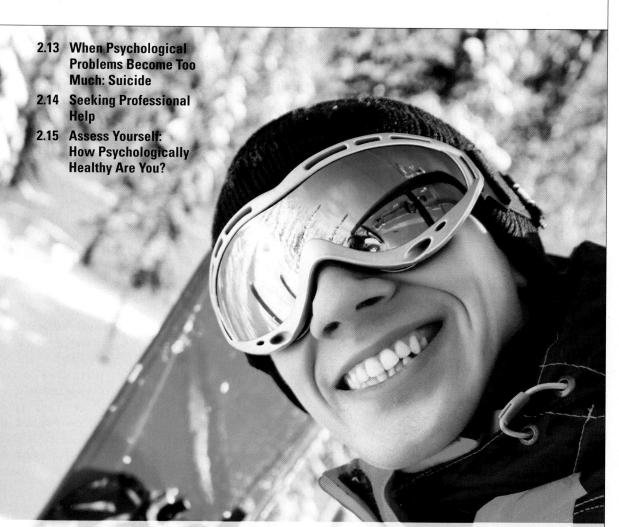

Although the vast majority of college students describe their college years as among the best of their lives, many find the pressures of grades, financial concerns, relationship problems, and the struggle to find themselves to be extraordinarily difficult. Psychological distress caused by relationship issues, family issues, academic competition, and adjusting to life as a college student is rampant on college campuses today. Many experts believe that the often anxiety-inducing campus environment is a major contributor to poor health decisions, such as high levels of alcohol consumption, and, in turn, to health problems that ultimately affect academic success and success in life.

Fortunately, even though we often face seemingly insurmountable pressures, human beings possess a resiliency that can enable us to cope, adapt, and even thrive in the face of life's challenges. How we feel and think about ourselves, those around us, and our environment can tell us a lot about our psychological health and whether we are healthy emotionally, socially, spiritually, and mentally.

What Is Psychological Health?

■ **Identify basic characteristics shared by psychologically healthy people.**

■ **Identify each level in Maslow's hierarchy of needs.**

Psychological health is the sum of how we think, feel, relate, and exist in our day-to-day lives. Our thoughts, perceptions, emotions, motivations, interpersonal relationships, and behaviors are the product of a combination of our experiences and the skills we have developed along the way to meet life's challenges. Most experts identify several basic elements shared by psychologically healthy people:

■ **They feel good about themselves.** They are not typically overwhelmed by fear, love, anger, jealousy, guilt, or worry. They know who they are, have a realistic sense of their capabilities, and respect themselves even though they realize that they aren't perfect.

■ **They feel comfortable with other people, and express respect and compassion toward others.** They enjoy satisfying and lasting personal relationships, and do not take advantage of others or allow others to take advantage of them. They recognize that there are others whose needs are greater than their own and take responsibility for their

fellow human beings. They can give love, consider others' interests, take time to help others, and respect personal differences.

■ **They control tension and anxiety.** They recognize the underlying causes and symptoms of stress and anxiety in their lives and consciously avoid irrational thoughts, hostility, excessive excuse making, and blaming others for their problems. They use resources and learn skills to control their reactions to stressful situations.

■ **They meet the demands of life.** Psychologically healthy people try to solve problems as they arise, accept responsibility, and plan ahead. They set realistic goals, think for themselves, and make independent decisions. Acknowledging that change is inevitable, they welcome new experiences.

■ **They curb hate and guilt.** They acknowledge and combat tendencies to respond with anger, thoughtlessness, selfishness, vengefulness, or feelings of inadequacy. They do not try to knock others aside to get ahead, but rather reach out to help others.

■ **They maintain a positive outlook.** They approach each day with a presumption that things will go well. They look to the future with enthusiasm rather than dread. Having fun and making time for themselves are integral parts of their lives.

■ **They value diversity.** Psychologically healthy people do not feel threatened by those of a different race, gender, religion, sexual orientation, ethnicity, or political party. They are nonjudgmental and do not force their beliefs and values on others.

■ **They appreciate and respect nature.** They take time to enjoy their surroundings, are conscious of their place in the universe, and act responsibly to preserve their environment.

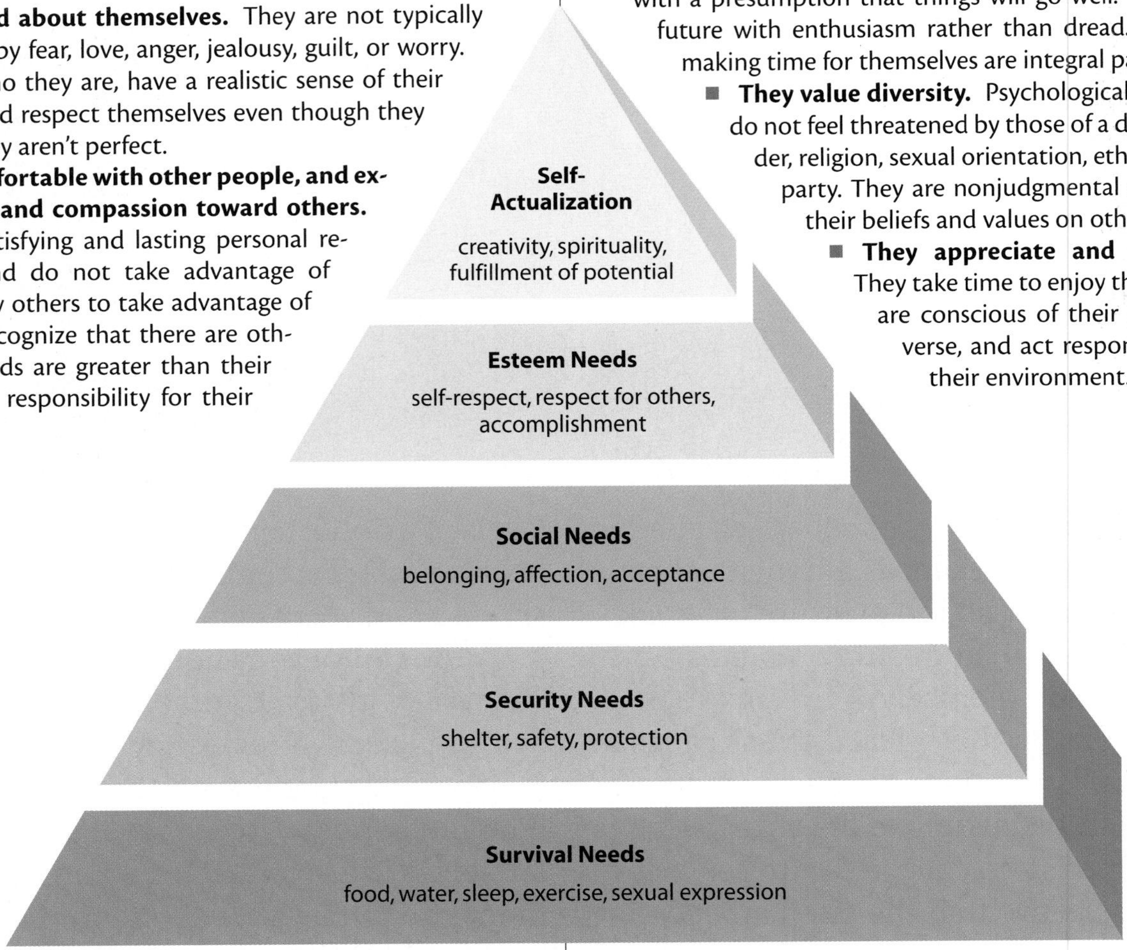

Self-Actualization
creativity, spirituality, fulfillment of potential

Esteem Needs
self-respect, respect for others, accomplishment

Social Needs
belonging, affection, acceptance

Security Needs
shelter, safety, protection

Survival Needs
food, water, sleep, exercise, sexual expression

Figure 2.1 Maslow's Hierarchy of Needs

Psychologically unhealthy ←→ **Psychologically healthy**

No zest for life; pessimistic/cynical most of the time; spiritually down

Laughs, but usually at others, has little fun

Has serious bouts of depression, "down" and tired much of time; has suicidal thoughts

A "challenge" to be around, socially isolated

Experiences many illnesses, headaches, aches/pains, gets colds/infections easily

Shows poorer coping than most, often overwhelmed by circumstances

Has regular relationship problems, finds that others often disappoint

Tends to be cynical/critical of others; tends to have negative/critical friends

Lacks focus much of the time, hard to keep intellectual acuity sharp

Quick to anger, sense of humor and fun evident less often

Works to improve in all areas, recognizes strengths and weaknesses

Healthy relationships with family and friends, capable of giving and receiving love and affection

Has strong social support, may need to work on improving social skills but usually no major problems

Has occasional emotional "dips" but overall good mental/emotional adaptors

Possesses zest for life; spiritually healthy and intellectually thriving

High energy, resilient, enjoys challenges, focused

Realistic sense of self and others, sound coping skills, open minded

Adapts to change easily, sensitive to others and environment

Has strong social support and healthy relationships with family and friends

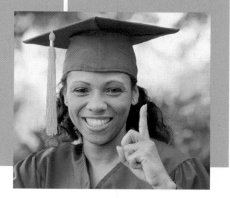

Figure 2.2 Characteristics of Psychologically Healthy and Unhealthy People
Where do you fall on this continuum?

Psychologists have long argued that before we can achieve any of the above characteristics of psychologically healthy people, we must have certain basic needs met in our lives. In the 1960s, psychologist Abraham Maslow developed a *hierarchy of needs* to describe this idea (**Figure 2.1**). At the bottom of his hierarchy are basic *survival needs*, such as food, sleep, and water; at the next level are *security needs*, such as shelter and safety; at the third level—*social needs*—is a sense of belonging and affection; at the fourth level are *esteem needs*, self-respect and respect for others; and at the top are needs for *self-actualization* and self-transcendence.

According to Maslow's theory, a person's needs must be met at each of these levels before that person can ever truly be healthy. Failure to meet any of the lower levels of needs will interfere with a person's ability to address upper-level needs. For example, someone who is homeless or worried about threats of violence will be unable to focus on fulfilling social, esteem, or actualization needs. Maslow believed that people are more likely to behave badly if they are frustrated by a lack of need fulfillment.[1]

In sum, psychologically healthy people are emotionally, mentally, socially, and spiritually resilient. They most often respond to challenges and frustrations in appropriate ways, despite occasional slips (see **Figure 2.2**). When they do slip, they recognize that fact and take action to rectify the situation.

Attaining psychological well-being involves many complex processes. This chapter will help you understand not only what it means to be psychologically well, but also why we may run into problems in our psychological health. Learning how to assess your own health and take action to help yourself are important aspects of psychological health.

check yourself

- **What are the basic characteristics shared by psychologically healthy people?**
- **At which level of Maslow's hierarchy of needs do you face the most challenges?**

Dimensions of Psychological Health

- **List and define each dimension of psychological health.**

Psychological health includes mental, emotional, social, and spiritual dimensions (see Figure 2.3).

Mental Health

The term **mental health** is used to describe the "thinking" or "rational" dimension of our health. A mentally healthy person perceives life in realistic ways, can adapt to change, can develop rational strategies to solve problems, and can carry out personal and professional responsibilities. In addition, a mentally healthy person has the intellectual ability to sort through information, messages, and life events; attach meaning to these events; and respond appropriately. This latter capacity is often referred to as *intellectual health*, a subset of mental health.[2]

Emotional Health

The term **emotional health** refers to the feeling, or subjective, side of psychological health. **Emotions** are intensified feelings or complex patterns of feelings that we experience on a regular basis—for example, love, hate, frustration, anxiety, and joy. Typically, emotions are described as the interplay of four components: physiological arousal, feelings, cognitive (thought) processes, and behavioral reactions. As rational beings, we are responsible for evaluating our individual emotional responses, the environment that is causing them, and the appropriateness of our actions.

Emotionally healthy people usually respond appropriately to upsetting events. Rather than reacting in an extreme fashion or behaving inconsistently or offensively, they can express their feelings, communicate with others, and show emotions in appropriate ways. Emotionally unhealthy people are much more likely to let their feelings overpower them. They may be highly volatile and prone to unpredictable emotional responses, which may be followed by inappropriate communication or actions.

Emotional health also affects social and intellectual health. A person who is feeling hostile, withdrawn, or moody may become socially isolated.[3] Because such people are not much fun to be around, friends may avoid them at the very time they are most in need of emotional support. For students, a more immediate concern is the impact of emotional trauma on academic performance. Have you ever tried to study for an exam after a fight with a close friend or family member? Emotional turmoil may seriously affect your ability to think, reason, and act rationally.

Social Health

Social health includes a person's interactions with others on an individual and group basis, the ability to use social resources and support in times of need, and the ability to adapt to a variety of social situations. Socially healthy individuals enjoy a wide range of interactions with family, friends, and acquaintances and are able to have healthy interactions with an intimate partner. Typically, socially healthy individuals can listen, express themselves, form healthy attachments, act in socially acceptable and responsible ways, and find the best fit for themselves in society. Numerous studies have documented the importance of positive relationships with family

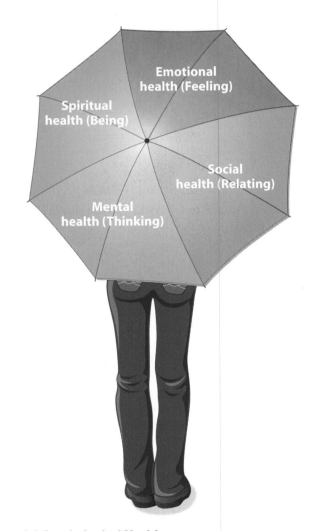

Figure 2.3 Psychological Health
Psychological health is a complex interaction of the mental, emotional, social, and spiritual dimensions of health. Possessing strength and resiliency in these dimensions can maintain your overall well-being and help you weather the storms of life.

How can I increase the social support in my life?

Fostering a solid social support group can be as simple as spending time playing a game, such as soccer, with friends. Physical health affects mental health, so doing something active with others is doubly beneficial.

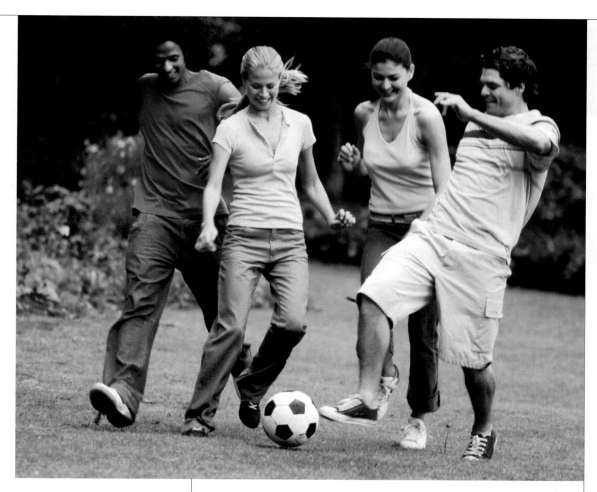

members, friends, and significant others in overall well-being and longevity.[4]

Social bonds, which reflect the level of closeness and attachment that we develop with other individuals, are the very foundation of human life. They provide intimacy, feelings of belonging, opportunities for giving and receiving nurturance, reassurance of one's worth, assistance and guidance, and advice. You may have many friends; those you share your deepest thoughts with, those you seek out when you are in trouble, and those you miss the most when they are away are those with whom you are most closely bonded. Social bonds take multiple forms, the most common of which are social support and community engagements.

The concept of **social support** is more complex than many people realize. In general, it refers to the networks of people and services with whom and which we interact and share social connections. These ties can provide *tangible support*, such as babysitting services or money to help pay the bills, or *intangible support*, such as encouraging you to share intimate thoughts. Sometimes, support can be felt as perceiving that someone would be there for us in a crisis. Generally, the closer and the higher the quality of the social bond with someone, the more likely one is to ask for and receive social support from that person. For example, if your car broke down on a dark country road in the middle of the night, who could you call for help—and know that the person would do everything possible to get there? Common descriptions of strong social support include the following:[5]

- Being cared for and loved, with shared intimacy
- Being esteemed and valued; having a sense of self-worth
- Sharing companionship, communication, and mutual obligations with others; having a sense of belonging

- Having "informational" support—access to information, advice, community services, and guidance from others

Spiritual Health

It is possible to be mentally, emotionally, and socially healthy and still not achieve optimal psychological well-being. What is missing? For many people, the difficult-to-describe element that gives purpose to life is the spiritual dimension.

According to the National Center for Complementary and Alternative Medicine (NCCAM), *spirituality* is broader in meaning than religion; it goes beyond material values and can be defined as an individual's sense of purpose and meaning in life.[6] Spirituality may be practiced in many ways, including through religion; however, religion does not have to be part of a spiritual life. **Spiritual health** refers to the sense of belonging to something greater than the purely physical or personal dimensions of existence. For some, this unifying force is nature; for others, it is a feeling of connection to other people; for still others, the unifying force is a god or other higher power.

- **What are the dimensions of psychological health?**
- **How do you assess your psychological health in each of the dimensions discussed here?**

Factors That Influence Psychological Health

learning **outcomes**

- **Describe factors that affect your psychological health.**

Psychological health can be influenced by multiple environmental factors, including family, social supports, and community.

The Family

Families have a significant influence on psychological development. Healthy families model and help develop the cognitive and social skills necessary to solve problems, communicate emotions in socially acceptable ways, manage stressors, and develop a sense of self-worth and purpose in life. Consistent love and nurturing from family members develop our capacity to value ourselves and to relate to others with care and respect. Children raised in nurturing homes are more likely to become well-adjusted, productive adults. In adulthood, family support is one of the best predictors of health and happiness.[7] Children brought up in **dysfunctional families**—

in which there is violence; distrust; anger; deprivation; drug abuse; parental discord; or sexual, physical, or emotional abuse—may have a harder time adapting to life and run an increased risk of psychological problems. Yet not everyone raised in dysfunctional families becomes psychologically unhealthy, and not everyone from healthy environments becomes well adjusted.

Social Supports

Initial social support may be provided by family, but as we develop the support of peers becomes more and more important. We rely on friends to help us figure out who we are and what we want to do with our lives. A recent study involving college students demonstrated that the availability of a social network (a sense of belonging) predicted health.[8] Think about questions you may be asking yourself—"What major should I choose?" "Should I take my relationship to the next level?" or "Is partying affecting my grades?" Such challenges require us to consider our goals and values, recognize our emotional responses, think through our options, and make decisions. We often bounce ideas off friends as we do so.

Community

Our communities can affect our psychological health through collective actions. *Collective efficacy* occurs when a group expects that it can achieve a goal through collective action.[9] For example, neighbors may come together to pick up trash, participate in a neighborhood watch, or initiate a community picnic. You are part of a campus community, which may support psychological health by creating a safe environment in which to develop your mental, emotional, social, and spiritual dimensions. Participation in sports, academic support services, a fraternity or sorority, campus religious organizations, student health services, campus counseling services, student government, performing arts groups, or campus cultural centers may be a part of the collective efficacy of your campus community.

How do others influence my psychological well-being?

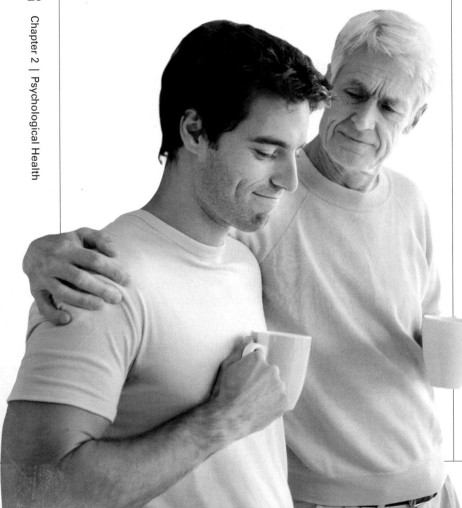

Your outlook on life is determined in part by your social and cultural surroundings, and your general sense of well-being can be strongly affected by the positive or negative nature of your social bonds. In particular, family members shape your psychological health. As you were growing up, they modeled behaviors and skills that helped you develop cognitively and socially. Their love and support can give you a sense of self-worth and encourage you to treat others with compassion and care.

75%

of the general U.S. population is estimated to be extroverted, as measured by the Meyer-Briggs Type Indicator personality test.

Self-Efficacy and Self-Esteem

During our formative years, successes and failures in school, athletics, friendships, relationships, jobs, and every other aspect of life subtly shape our beliefs about our personal worth and abilities. These beliefs in turn become influences on our psychosocial health.

Self-efficacy describes a person's belief about whether he or she can successfully engage in and execute a specific behavior. *Self-esteem* refers to one's sense of self-respect or self-worth. People with high levels of self-efficacy and self-esteem tend to express a positive outlook on life.

Our self-esteem is a result of the relationships we have with our parents and family during our formative years; with our friends as we grow older; with our significant others as we form intimate relationships; and with our teachers, coworkers, and others throughout our lives.

Psychologist Martin Seligman proposed that people who continually experience failure may develop a pattern of responding known as **learned helplessness,** in which they give up and fail to take action to help themselves. Seligman ascribes this response in part to society's tendency toward *victimology*—blaming one's problems on other people and circumstances.[10] Although viewing ourselves as victims may make us feel better temporarily, it does not address the underlying causes of a problem. Ultimately, it can erode self-efficacy.

Many self-help programs use elements of Seligman's principle of **learned optimism**—the idea that by changing our self-talk, examining our reactions, and blocking negative thoughts, we can "unlearn" negative thought processes that have become habitual.

Personality

Your personality is the unique mix of characteristics that distinguishes you from others, as influenced by heredity, environment, culture, and experience. Personality determines how we react to the challenges of life, interpret our feelings, and resolve conflicts.

Most recent psychological theories promote the idea that we have the power to understand and change our behavior, thus molding our own personalities. The following traits are often related to psychological well-being:[11]

- **Extroversion**—the ability to adapt to a social situation and demonstrate assertiveness as well as power or interpersonal involvement
- **Agreeableness**—the ability to conform, be likable, and demonstrate friendly compliance and love
- **Openness to experience**—the willingness to demonstrate curiosity and independence (also referred to as inquiring intellect)
- **Emotional stability**—the ability to maintain emotional control

- **Conscientiousness**—the qualities of being dependable and demonstrating self-control, discipline, and a need to achieve
- **Resiliency**—the ability to adapt to change and stressful events in healthy and flexible ways

Emotional Control and Maturity

Our temperaments change as we grow, as illustrated by the extreme emotions that children and many young teens experience. Most of us learn to control our emotions as we age. The college years mark a transition period for young adults as they move away from families and become independent. This transition is easier for those who have accomplished earlier developmental tasks such as learning how to solve problems, make and evaluate decisions, define and adhere to personal values, and establish both casual and intimate relationships. People who have not fulfilled these earlier tasks may find their lives interrupted by recurrent crises left over from earlier stages. For example, those who did not learn to trust others in childhood may have difficulty establishing intimate relationships as adults.

Skills for Behavior Change

BUILD YOUR SELF-EFFICACY AND SELF-ESTEEM

- Pay attention to your needs and wants. Listen to what your body, mind, and heart tell you.
- List things that make you happy; do something from your list every day.
- Do things you are good at, and enjoy the satisfaction in a job well done.
- Do something you've been putting off, such as cleaning out your closet or paying a bill that you've been ignoring, to give yourself a sense of accomplishment.
- Acknowledge that you're a good person by rewarding yourself regularly.
- Don't engage in self-criticism.
- Write down good things about yourself and practice positive affirmations.
- Spend time with people who make you feel good about yourself. Avoid people who treat you poorly.
- Keep items that inspire you to reflect on your achievements, your friends, or special times.
- Take advantage of opportunities to learn something new.
- Do something for others. There is no greater way to feel better about yourself than to help someone in need.

---

check yourself

- **What are four factors that affect your psychological health?**
- **Give an example of the interrelationship among the various factors that affect psychological health.**

The Mind–Body Connection

- **Describe the interaction between psychological well-being and health.**

Can negative emotions make us physically ill? Can positive emotions help us stay well? Researchers are exploring the interaction between emotions and health, especially in conditions of stress. In fact, more and more large research projects explore the link between mind and body. At the core of the mind–body connection is the study of **psycho-neuroimmunology (PNI)**, or how the brain and behavior affect the body's immune system.

One area that appears to be particularly promising in enhancing physical health is *happiness*—a collective term for positive states in which individuals actively embrace the world around them.[12] In examining the characteristics of happy people, scientists have found that happiness, and related mental states such as hopefulness, optimism, and contentment, can have a profound impact on the body—appearing to reduce the risk or limit the severity of cardiovascular disease, pulmonary disease, diabetes, hypertension, colds, and other infections. Laughter can promote increases in heart and respiration rates and can reduce levels of stress hormones in much the same way as light exercise can. For this reason, it has been promoted as a possible risk reducer for people with hypertension and other forms of cardiovascular disease.[13]

Subjective well-being is that uplifting feeling of inner peace or an overall "feel-good" state, which includes happiness. It is defined by three components: satisfaction with present life, relative presence of positive emotions, and relative absence of negative emotions.[14] You don't have to be happy all the time to achieve subjective well-being. Everyone experiences disappointments, unhappiness, and times when life seems unfair. However, people with a high level of subjective well-being are typically resilient, able to look on the positive side and get back on track fairly quickly, and less likely to fall into despair over setbacks.

Scientists suggest that some people may be biologically predisposed to happiness. Psychologist Richard Davidson has proposed that neurotransmitters, the chemicals that transfer messages between neurons, may function more efficiently in happy people.[15] Other psychologists suggest that we can develop happiness by practicing positive psychological actions.[16]

Skills for **Behavior Change**

USING POSITIVE PSYCHOLOGY TO ENHANCE YOUR HAPPINESS

Try these strategies to enhance happiness and employ a more positive outlook:

- **Develop gratitude.** Gratitude is thankfulness and appreciation for the good things in life as well as for life's lessons. For 1 week, write down three positive things that happened each day, then answer the question, "Why did this good thing happen?"
- **Use capitalization.** Focus on the good things that happen to you, and share them with others. Research indicates that telling others about a positive experience increases the positive emotion associated with it and prolongs good feelings.
- **Know when to say when.** Find a level of achievement that you will be satisfied with, make sure it is realistic, and stick to it.
- **Grow a signature strength.** Traits such as wisdom, courage, humanity, hope, vitality, curiosity, and love are believed among the most important to overall health.

Sources: R. Biswas-Diener, *Practicing Positive Psychology Coaching: Assessment, Activities, and Strategies for Success* (New York: Wiley, 2010); C. Peterson, *Primer of Positive Psychology* (New York: Oxford University Press, 2006).

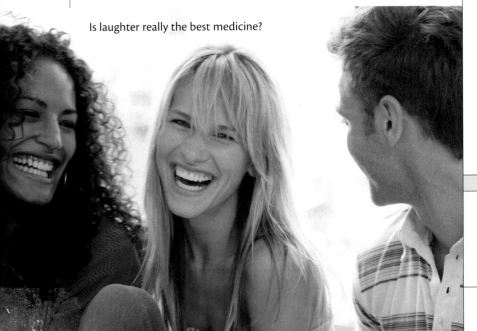

Is laughter really the best medicine?

- **How does a person's psychological state affect his or her health?**
- **Give an example in which your emotional state affected your health.**

Strategies to Enhance Psychological Health

learning outcomes

- **Describe behavior change strategies to improve psychological health.**

As we have seen, psychological health involves four dimensions. Attaining self-fulfillment is a lifelong, conscious process that involves enhancing each of these components. Strategies include building self-efficacy and self-esteem, understanding and controlling emotions, maintaining support networks, and learning to solve problems and make decisions. Try the following strategies to support and improve your own psychological health:

- **Find a support group.** The best way to promote self-esteem is through a support group—peers who share your values. A support group can make you feel good about yourself and force you to take an honest look at your actions and choices. Keeping in contact with old friends and important family members can provide a foundation of unconditional love that will help you through life transitions.
- **Complete required tasks.** A good way to boost your sense of self-efficacy is to learn new skills and develop a history of success. Most college campuses provide study groups and learning centers that can help you manage time, develop study skills, and prepare for tests. Poor grades, or grades that do not meet expectations, are major contributors to emotional distress among college students.
- **Form realistic expectations.** If you expect perfect grades, a steady stream of Saturday-night dates, and the perfect job, you may be setting yourself up for failure. Assess your current resources and the direction in which you are heading. Set small, incremental goals that you can actually meet.
- **Make time for you.** Taking time to enjoy yourself is another way to boost your self-esteem and psychosocial health. View a new activity as something to look forward to and an opportunity to have fun. Anticipate and focus on the fun things that you have to look forward to each day.
- **Maintain physical health.** Regular exercise fosters a sense of well-being. More and more research supports the role of exercise in improved mental health. Nourishing meals can help you stay well and avoid the weight gain and related depression many college students experience.

- **Examine problems and seek help when necessary.** Knowing when to seek help from friends, support groups, family, or professionals is an important factor in boosting self-esteem. Sometimes you can handle life's problems alone; at other times you need assistance. Get help before you feel overwhelmed.
- **Get adequate sleep.** Getting enough sleep on a daily basis is a key factor in physical and psychological health. Not only do our bodies need to rest to conserve energy for our daily activities, but we also need to restore supplies of many of the neurotransmitters that we use up during our waking hours.

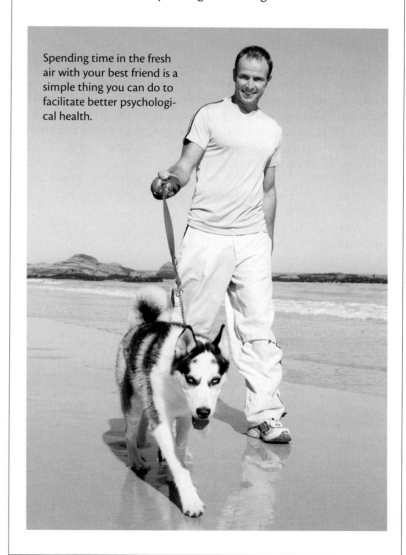

Spending time in the fresh air with your best friend is a simple thing you can do to facilitate better psychological health.

check yourself

- **Give examples of four ways to enhance psychological health. Which of these strategies do you think would be most effective for you?**

What Is Spiritual Health?

- **Define spirituality and describe how religion and values affect spirituality.**
- **Explain how spirituality contributes to physical and psychosocial health.**

Lia's favorite spot on campus is the Japanese garden behind the library. A few minutes in the garden leaves her feeling refreshed and refocused, with greater confidence in her ability to tackle challenges.

Lia's desire to find a sense of purpose, meaning, and harmony in her life is shared by a majority of American college students. According to UCLA's Higher Education Research Institute (HERI), although undergraduates' religious attendance declines during the college years, students show significant growth in a wide spectrum of spiritual and ethical considerations.[17] Data from nearly 15,000 students at more than 136 colleges and universities found that interest in the following goals increased by more than 10 percent during the college years, to levels representing more than half of all students surveyed:
- Attaining inner harmony
- Developing a meaningful philosophy of life
- Seeking beauty in life

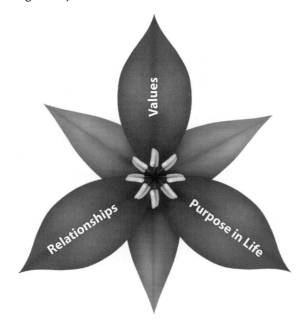

Figure 2.4 Three Facets of Spirituality
Most of us are prompted to explore our spirituality because of questions relating to our relationships, values, and purpose in life. At the same time, these three facets together constitute spiritual well-being.

- Becoming a more loving person

Researchers also found that, compared with first-year students, juniors and seniors were more desirous of reducing pain and suffering in the world, were more thankful for all that had happened to them, and expressed higher levels of ecumenical worldviews—views expressing tolerance and respect for other religions and philosophies.

What Is Spirituality?

Spirituality tends to defy the boundaries that strict definitions impose. The word's root, *spirit*, in many cultures refers to *breath*, or the force that animates life. When you're "inspired," your energy flows. You're not held back by doubts about the meaning of your work and life. Many definitions incorporate this sense of transcendence; the National Center for Complementary and Alternative Medicine (NCCAM) defines **spirituality** as an individual's sense of purpose and meaning in life, beyond material values.[18] Harold G. Koenig, MD, one of the foremost researchers of spirituality and health, defines spirituality as the personal quest for understanding answers to ultimate questions about life, meaning, and relationship with the sacred or transcendent.[19]

Spirituality may include participation in organized **religion**—a system of beliefs, practices, rituals, and symbols designed to facilitate closeness to the sacred or transcendent.[20] Most Americans consider spirituality to be important in their lives, but not necessarily in the form of religion: A recent survey of more than 35,000 Americans revealed that 92 percent believe in some kind of "higher power," but not all of these identified themselves as being affiliated with a particular religion.[21]

Elements of Spirituality

Brian Luke Seaward, a professor at the University of Northern Colorado and author of several books on spirituality and mind–body healing, identifies the core of human spirituality as consisting of three elements: relationships, values, and purpose in life (**Figure 2.4**).[22]

Have you ever wondered if someone you were attracted to were right for you, or if you should break off a relationship? Have you wished you had more friends, or that you were a better friend to yourself? Have you ever tried to make a connection with a "higher self"? Such questions about relationships and yearnings are often triggers for spiritual growth.

Our **values** are our principles—the set of fundamental rules by which we conduct our lives. When we attempt to clarify our values, and to live according to them, we're engaging in spiritual work.

What career do you plan to pursue? Do you hope to marry? Do you plan to have or adopt children? What things make you feel "complete"? Contemplating such questions about purpose in life fosters spiritual growth. People who are spiritually healthy are able

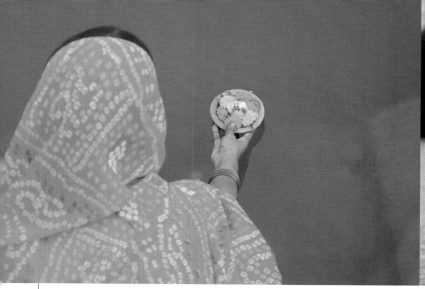
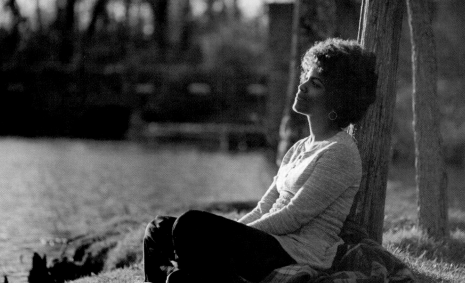

Is spirituality the same as religion?

Spirituality and religion are not the same. Many people find that religious practices, such as attending services or making offerings—such as the flowers this Hindu woman is preparing to place in the sacred Ganges River—help them to focus on their spirituality. However, religion does not have to be part of a spiritual person's life.

to articulate their purpose, and to make choices that manifest that purpose.

Our relationships, values, and sense of purpose together contribute to our overall **spiritual intelligence (SI)**. This term was introduced by physicist and philosopher Danah Zohar, who defined it as "the intelligence that makes us whole, that gives us our integrity . . . the intelligence of the deep self."[23] Zohar includes self-awareness, spontaneity, and compassion in her definition, explaining that SI helps us use adversity in a positive way and live according to our values.

Contributions to Health

The importance of spirituality to wellness and health is based on hundreds of published studies.[24] The NCCAM cites evidence of its influence on general health and longevity, and suggests that the connection may be due to improved immune function, cardiovascular function, and/or other physiological changes.[25] And Americans who attend religious services regularly, particularly those whose religious tenets restrict smoking, alcohol use, and engaging in other risk behaviors, live longer—on average—than those who do not. It isn't attendance per se that is the key;[26] such things as kindness, balance, harmony, selflessness, and respect for others are probably the most important contributors. Some researchers believe that improved health and longer life in spiritually healthy people is a product of self-control—increased capacity to refrain from overeating, smoking, and abusing alcohol and other drugs, and to be disciplined about getting adequate exercise and sleep.[27]

When we do get sick, contends the National Cancer Institute (NCI), spiritual or religious well-being may help restore health and improve quality of life by:[28]

- Decreasing anxiety, depression, anger, discomfort, and feelings of isolation
- Decreasing alcohol and drug abuse

Does spirituality influence health?

Spirituality is widely acknowledged to have a positive impact on health and wellness. The benefits range from reductions in overall morbidity and mortality to improved abilities to cope with illness and stress.

- Decreasing blood pressure and the risk of heart disease
- Increasing ability to cope with the effects of illness and medical treatments
- Increasing feelings of hope and optimism, freedom from regret, satisfaction with life, and inner peace

Several studies show an association between spiritual health and ability to cope with physical illness;[29] a study of people living with chronic pain and fatigue showed a benefit of spiritual health.[30] Another study of people with HIV showed slower disease progression over a period of 4 years in people who become more spiritually focused after their diagnosis.[31]

Research also suggests that spiritual health contributes to psychosocial health, reducing anxiety and depression.[32] Practices such as yoga, deep meditation, and prayer can positively affect brain chemistry much as conventional antianxiety and antidepressant medications do.[33] People who have found a spiritual community also benefit from social support and avoid isolation, reinforcing feelings of security and belonging.

Both the NCCAM and the NCI cite stress reduction as one probable mechanism among spiritually healthy people for improved health and longevity and for better coping with illness,[34] whereas other studies support the contentions that positive religious coping supports stress management[35] and mindfulness meditation reduces stress levels in both sick and healthy people.[36]

check yourself

- **What are some components of spirituality and spiritual intelligence?**
- **List three benefits of spiritual health.**

Strategies for Cultivating Spiritual Health

■ **Describe several strategies for improving spiritual health.**

Cultivating your spiritual side takes just as much work as becoming physically fit. Here, we introduce some ways to develop your spiritual health by training your body, expanding your mind, tuning in and reaching out.

Train Your Body

For thousands of years, throughout the world, seekers have cultivated transcendence through physical means. A foremost example is the practice of **yoga**. Although in the West we think of yoga as involving controlled breathing and physical postures, traditional forms also emphasize meditation, chanting, and other practices believed to cultivate unity with the *Atman*, or Absolute.

If you're interested in yoga, sign up for a class. Some forms, such as *hatha yoga*, focus on developing flexibility, deep breathing, and tranquility; others, such as *ashtanga yoga*, are fast paced and demanding. The instructor will likely lead you through warm-up poses; more challenging poses designed to align, stretch, and invigorate; and relaxation and deep breathing exercises.

Training your body to improve spiritual health doesn't necessarily require a formal practice; any exercise can contribute to spiritual health. Begin by acknowledging gratitude for your body's strength and speed. Throughout the session, try to stay mindful of your breathing.

You can also cultivate spirituality through engaging or restricting your senses. Viewing artwork or listening to music can calm the mind and soothe the spirit. Alternatively, closing your eyes and sitting in silence removes visual and auditory distractions, helping you to focus. Try turning off your phone and taking a solitary walk, or spending a weekend at a retreat center (for options, see www.SpiritSite.com).

Expand Your Mind

For many people, psychological counseling is a step toward spiritual health. Ther-

apy helps you let go of past hurts, accept limitations, manage stress and anger, reduce anxiety and depression, and take control of your life—all steps toward spiritual growth.

You can also study the sacred texts of the world's major religions and spiritual practices, explore on-campus meditation groups, take classes in spirituality or comparative religions, go to different churches in your area, attend public lectures, and check out the websites of spiritual and religious organizations.

Tune in to Yourself and Your Surroundings

Focusing on spiritual health has been likened to tuning in on a radio: Inner wisdom is available, but if we fail to tune our "receiver," we won't hear it for all the "static" of daily life. Four ancient practices used throughout the world can help you tune in—contemplation, mindfulness, meditation, and prayer.

In the domain of spirituality, **contemplation** usually refers to a practice of concentrating the mind on a spiritual or ethical subject, a view of the natural world, or an icon or other image representative of divinity. For instance, a Zen Buddhist might contemplate a riddle called a *koan*. A Sufi might contemplate the 99 names of God. A Catholic might contemplate an image of the Virgin Mary. Others might contemplate nature, a favorite poem, or an ethical question, or keep a gratitude journal. Many traditions advocate contemplating gratitude, forgiveness, and unconditional love.

A practice of focused, nonjudgmental observation, **mindfulness** is the ability to be fully present in the moment rather than focused on past or future[37] (**Figure 2.5**). If you've ever "forgotten yourself" while watching the sunset, listening to music, or performing challenging work, you've experienced mindfulness.

So how do you practice mindfulness? According to guru of mindfulness Jon Kabat-Zinn, living mindfully means "making more of your ordinary moments notable and noteworthy by taking note of them."[38]

For instance, the next time you eat an orange, pay attention. What does it feel like to pierce the skin with your thumbnail? Do you smell the fragrance of the orange as you peel it? How does the juice splatter as you separate the segments? How does the taste change from the first bite to the last?

Almost any endeavor that requires concentration can help you develop mindfulness. Consider arts such as sculpting, painting, writing, dancing, or playing a musical instrument. Even household activities such as cooking and cleaning can foster mindfulness—as long as you pay attention while you do them.

Meditation is a practice of cultivating stillness and quieting the mind's noise. For thousands of years, many cultures have found that daily meditative stillness enhances spiritual health. Brain scans have shown that experienced meditators show significantly increased *empathy*, the ability to understand and share another person's experience.[39]

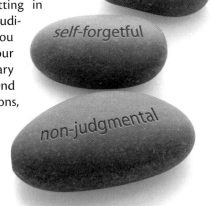

Figure 2.5 Qualities of Mindfulness

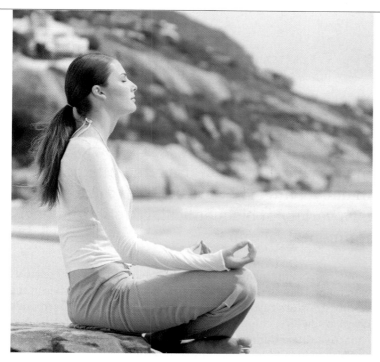

Is meditation boring?

Once you get the hang of it, meditation is anything but boring. As expert Jon Kabat-Zinn notes, "[When] you pay attention to boredom, it gets unbelievably interesting."

Another recent study showed increased capacity for forgiveness.[40] Meditation also improves the brain's ability to process information, reduces stress, improves sleep, and relieves chronic pain.[41]

So how do you meditate? Detailed instructions are beyond the scope of this text, but most teachers advise sitting where you won't be interrupted. You may want to assume a modified lotus position, in which your legs are crossed in front of you. Lying down is not recommended; you may fall asleep. Beginners may find it easier to meditate with eyes closed. Now start emptying your mind; different schools of meditation teach different methods to achieve this:

- **Object meditation.** With your eyes open, focus on an object such as a religious symbol, or a flower or stone. Allow your eyes to soften. Treat distractions as for other forms of meditation.
- **Breath meditation.** Count each breath: Pay attention to each inhalation, the brief pause that follows, and the exhalation; these equal one breath. When you have counted 10 breaths, return to 1. As distractions arise, release them and return to the breath.
- **Color meditation.** When your eyes are closed, you may perceive a field of color, such as a deep blue "pearl" or "flame." Focus on this color. Treat distractions as for other forms of meditation.
- **Mantra meditation.** Focus on a *mantra*, a word such as *Om, Amen, Love*, or *God*. Keep repeating it silently to yourself. When a distracting thought arises, simply set it aside. It may help to imagine the thought as a leaf, and mentally place it on a flowing stream that carries it away. Don't fault yourself for becoming distracted. Simply notice the thought, release it, and return to your mantra.

After several minutes, with practice you may come to experience a sensation, sometimes described as "dropping down," in which you feel yourself release into the meditation. In this state, distracting thoughts are less likely and you may receive surprising insights.

When you're starting out, try meditating for just 10 to 20 minutes, once or twice a day. You may find yourself feeling more rested and less stressed, and you may begin to experience increased empathy.

In **prayer**, rather than emptying the mind, an individual focuses it in communication with a transcendent Presence. For many, prayer offers a sense of comfort; a sense that we are not alone; and an avenue for expressing concern for others, admitting transgressions, seeking forgiveness, and renewing hope and purpose. Focusing on gratitude can provide strength in challenging times.

Reach out to Others

Altruism, the giving of oneself out of genuine concern for others, is a key aspect of a spiritually healthy life. Volunteering to help others, working for a nonprofit organization, donating money or other resources, picking up litter—all are ways to serve others and enhance your own spiritual health.

Altruism can also take the form of **environmental stewardship**, which the Environmental Protection Agency (EPA) defines as the responsibility for environmental quality shared by all those whose actions affect the environment.[42] Simple actions such as reducing and recycling packaging, turning off unused lights, and taking shorter showers are part of environmental stewardship.

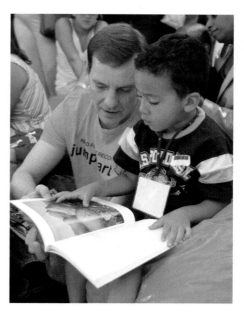

Volunteering can be a fun and fulfilling way to broaden your experience, connect with your community, and focus on your spiritual health.

check yourself

- **How do physical, mental, and contemplative strategies affect spiritual health?**
- **What are some of the benefits of including spiritual health among the dimensions of health?**

When Psychological Health Deteriorates

- **Define mental illness and discuss its prevalence.**

Sometimes circumstances overwhelm us to such a degree that we need help to get back on track. Stress, anxiety, loneliness, financial upheavals, and other traumatic events can derail our coping resources, causing us to turn inward or act in ways outside the norm; chemical imbalances, drug interactions, trauma, neurological disruptions, and other physical problems may also contribute.

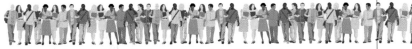

Felt overwhelmed by all they needed to do 83.6%

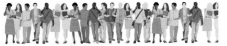

Thought things were hopeless 43.9%

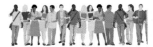

Had difficulty functioning because of depression 28.4%

Seriously considered suicide 6.0%

Intentionally injured themselves 5.1%

 = 2%

Attempted suicide 1.3%

Figure 2.6 Mental Health Concerns of American College Students, Past 12 Months

Source: Data are from American College Health Association, *American College Health Association–National College Health Assessment II (ACHA-NCHA II) Reference Group Data Report Fall 2010* (Baltimore: ACHA, 2011).

Mental illnesses are disorders that disrupt thinking, feeling, moods, and behaviors, causing varying degrees of impaired functioning in daily living. They are believed to be caused by a variety of biochemical, genetic, and environmental factors.[43]

Risk factors for mental illness include having biological relatives with mental illness; malnutrition or exposure to viruses while in the womb; stressful situations such as financial problems, a loved one's death, or divorce; chronic medical conditions; combat; taking psychoactive drugs during adolescence; childhood abuse or neglect; and lack of friendships or healthy relationships.[44]

As with physical disease, mental illnesses can range from mild to severe and can exact a heavy toll on quality of life, both for people with the illnesses and those in contact with them.

The basis for diagnosing mental disorders in the United States is the *Diagnostic and Statistical Manual of Mental Disorders*, Fourth Edition, Text Revision (*DSM-IV-TR*). An estimated 26.2 percent of Americans 18 and older—approximately 57.7 million people—suffer from a diagnosable mental disorder in a given year; nearly half of those have more than one mental illness at once.[45] Of this group, about 1 in 17 suffer from serious mental illness requiring close monitoring, residential care in many instances, and medication. Mental disorders are the leading cause of disability in the United States and Canada for people 15 to 44.[46]

Mental health problems are common among college students.[47] The most recent National College Health Assessment survey found that 28.4 percent of undergraduates reported "feeling so depressed it was difficult to function" at least once in the past year, while 6.0 percent reported "seriously considering attempting suicide" in the past year.[48] Figure 2.6 shows more results from this survey. Students surveyed met the DSM-IV-TR criteria for at least one mental disorder in the previous year.[49] Although such data may appear alarming, increases in help-seeking behavior rather than actual increases in prevalence of disorders may be contributing to these trends. More effective psychotropic medications, combined with young people having more access to effective treatments during adolescence that allow them to function well enough to attend college, may lead to more persons with mental disorders attending college.[50]

- **What is mental illness?**
- **Is mental illness more or less common than you expected?**

Anxiety Disorders

learning outcomes

- **Describe common anxiety disorders, including causes and treatments.**

Anxiety disorders, which are characterized by persistent feelings of threat and worry, are the number-one mental health problem in the United States, affecting more than 40 million people 18 and older each year, or about 18 percent of all adults.[51] Among U.S undergraduates, 9.2 percent report being diagnosed with or treated for anxiety in the past year.[52]

To be diagnosed with **generalized anxiety disorder (GAD)**, one must exhibit at least three of the following symptoms for more days than not during a 6-month period: restlessness or feeling on edge; being easily fatigued; difficulty concentrating or mind going blank; irritability; muscle tension; sleep disturbances.[53] GAD often runs in families and is readily treatable.

Panic disorders are characterized by **panic attacks,** acute anxiety bringing on an intense physical reaction. Approximately 6 million Americans 18 and older experience panic attacks each year.[54] Although highly treatable, panic attacks can become debilitating, particularly if they happen often and lead sufferers to avoid interacting with others. An attack typically starts abruptly, lasts about 30 minutes, and leaves the person tired and drained.[55] Symptoms include increased respiration, chills, hot flashes, shortness of breath, stomach cramps, chest pain, difficulty swallowing, and a sense of doom or impending death. Although researchers aren't sure what causes panic attacks, heredity, stress, and certain biochemical factors may play a role. Some researchers believe that sufferers are experiencing an overreactive fight-or-flight response.

Phobias, or phobic disorders, involve persistent and irrational fear of a specific object, activity, or situation, often out of proportion to circumstances. About 9 percent of American adults suffer from phobias such as fear of spiders, snakes, or public speaking.[56]

Another 7 percent suffer from **social phobia**, or social anxiety disorder,[57] characterized by persistent avoidance of social situations for fear of being humiliated, embarrassed, or even looked at. Some social phobias cause difficulty only in specific situations, such as speaking in front of a group. In extreme cases, sufferers avoid all contact with others.

People compelled to perform rituals over and over again; who are fearful of dirt or contamination; who have an unnatural concern about order and exactness; or who have persistent intrusive thoughts that they can't shake may suffer from **obsessive-compulsive disorder (OCD)**. Approximately 2 million Americans 18 and over have OCD.[58] Sufferers often see their behaviors as irrational and senseless yet feel powerless to stop them. For a person to be diagnosed with OCD, the obsessions must consume more than 1 hour per day and interfere with normal life. The exact cause is unknown; genetics, biological abnormalities, learned behaviors, and environmental factors have been considered. Onset is usually in adolescence or early adulthood; median age of onset is 19.

People who have experienced or witnessed a natural disaster, violent assault, or other traumatic event may develop **post-traumatic stress disorder (PTSD)**. Often PTSD affects soldiers returning from war. In a survey of personnel deployed to Iraq, 1 in 8 reported symptoms of PTSD.[59] Unfortunately, less than half of those sought help, fearing stigma and damage to their careers.

Symptoms of PTSD include the following:

- Dissociation, or perceived detachment of the mind from the emotional state or even the body
- Intrusive recollections of the traumatic event—flashbacks, nightmares, or recurrent thoughts
- Acute anxiety or nervousness, in which the person is hyper-aroused and may cry easily or experience mood swings
- Insomnia and difficulty concentrating
- Intense physiological reactions, such as shaking or nausea, when reminded of the traumatic event

Although these are common initial responses to traumatic events, PTSD may be diagnosed if a person experiences them for at least 1 month following the event. In some cases, symptoms may not appear until months or years later.

Anxiety disorders vary in complexity and degree, and scientists have yet to find clear reasons why one person develops them and another doesn't. The following are cited as possible causes:[60]

- **Biology.** Positron-emission tomography (PET) scans can identify areas of the brain that react during anxiety-producing events. We may inherit tendencies toward anxiety disorders.
- **Environment.** Although genetic tendencies may exist, experiencing a repeated pattern of reaction to certain situations programs the brain to respond in a certain way. For example, if a parent screamed whenever a large spider crept into view, you might be predisposed to react with anxiety to spiders later in life.
- **Social and cultural roles.** Because men and women are taught to assume different roles in society (man as protector, woman as victim), women may find it more acceptable to express extreme anxiety. Men, in contrast, may have learned to repress such anxieties rather than act on them.

check yourself

- **What are the most common anxiety disorders?**
- **What are causes and treatments for anxiety disorders?**

Mood Disorders

- **Describe common mood disorders, including causes and treatments.**

Chronic mood disorders are disorders affecting one's emotional state. In any given year, approximately 10 percent of Americans 18 or older—or 20.9 million people—suffer from a mood disorder.[61]

Major Depression

Major depression, the most common mood disorder, affects approximately 14.8 million American adults, or about 7 percent of the U.S. population[62]—though many are misdiagnosed or underdiagnosed. Characterized by a combination of symptoms that interfere with work, study, sleep, appetite, relationships, and enjoyment of life, major depression is not only having a bad day or feeling down after a negative experience; it can't just be willed away. Symptoms can last for weeks, months, or years[63] and can include the following:

- Sadness and despair
- Loss of motivation or interest in pleasurable activities

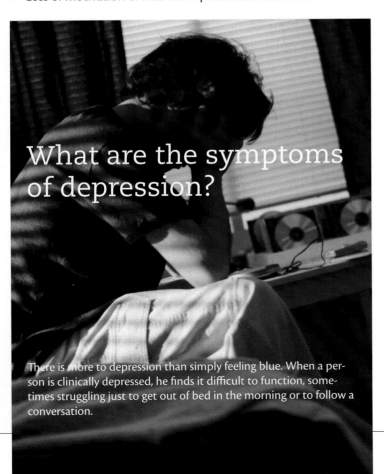

What are the symptoms of depression?

There is more to depression than simply feeling blue. When a person is clinically depressed, he finds it difficult to function, sometimes struggling just to get out of bed in the morning or to follow a conversation.

- Preoccupation with failures and inadequacies
- Difficulty concentrating; indecisiveness; memory lapses
- Loss of sex drive or interest in close interactions with others
- Fatigue and loss of energy; slow reactions
- Sleeping too much or too little; insomnia
- Feeling agitated, worthless, or hopeless
- Withdrawal from friends and family
- Diminished or increased appetite
- Significant weight loss or gain
- Recurring thoughts that life isn't worth living; thoughts of death or suicide

Depression in College Students Depression has gained increasing recognition on campus. Stressors such as anxiety over relationships, pressure over grades and social acceptance, abuse of alcohol and other drugs, poor diet, and lack of sleep can overwhelm even resilient students. In a recent survey, 8.3 percent of students reported having been diagnosed with depression.[64]

Being far from home can exacerbate problems and make coping difficult; international students are particularly vulnerable to depression and other mental health concerns. Most campuses have counseling centers, cultural centers, and other services available, though many students do not use them because of persistent stigma.

Other Mood Disorders

Dysthymic disorder (dysthymia) is chronic, mild depression. Though dysthymic individuals may function acceptably, they may lack energy, be short-tempered and pessimistic, or not feel up to par without any overt symptoms. People with dysthymia may cycle into major depression over time. For a diagnosis, symptoms must persist for at least 2 years in adults (1 year in children). This disorder affects approximately 1.5 percent of the U.S. population 18 and older in a given year, or about 3.3 million American adults.[65]

People with **bipolar disorder**, also called *manic depression*, often have severe mood swings, ranging from extreme highs (mania) to extreme lows (depression). Swings can be dramatic and rapid, or more gradual. When in the manic phase, people may be overactive, talkative, and have tons of energy; in the depressed phase, they may experience symptoms of major depression.

Although the exact cause of bipolar disorder is unknown, biological, genetic, and environmental factors, such as drug abuse and stressful or psychologically traumatic events, seem to be triggers. Once diagnosed, persons with bipolar disorder have several counseling and pharmaceutical options; most can live a healthy, functional life while being treated. Bipolar disorder affects 5.7 million adults in the United States, or approximately 2.6 percent of the population.[66]

Seasonal affective disorder (SAD) strikes during the winter and is associated with reduced exposure to sunlight. People with SAD suffer from irritability, apathy, carbohydrate craving and weight gain, increased sleep, and general sadness. Factors implicated in SAD include disruption in circadian rhythms and changes in levels of the hormone melatonin and the brain chemical serotonin.[67]

The most beneficial treatment for SAD is light therapy, using lamps that simulate sunlight. Eighty percent of patients experience relief within 4 days. Other treatments include diet change, increased exercise, stress management, sleep restriction (limiting hours slept in a 24-hour period), psychotherapy, and prescription medications.

Causes of Mood Disorders

Mood disorders are caused by the interaction of factors including biological differences, hormones, inherited traits, life events, and trauma.[68] The biology of mood disorders is related to levels of brain chemicals called *neurotransmitters*. Several types of depression, including bipolar disorder, appear to have a genetic component. Depression can also be triggered by serious loss, difficult relationships, financial problems, and pressure to succeed. Early trauma, such as loss of a parent, may cause permanent changes in the brain, making one more prone to depression. Research has also shown that changes in physical health can be accompanied by mental changes, particularly depression. Stroke, heart attack, cancer, Parkinson's disease, chronic pain, diabetes, certain medications, alcohol, hormonal disorders, and a range of other afflictions can trigger depression.

Depression across Gender, Age, and Ethnicity

Although depression affects a wide range of people, it does not always manifest itself in the same way across populations. Women are almost twice as likely to experience depression as men are, possibly due to hormonal changes. Women often face stressors related to multiple responsibilities—work, childrearing, single parenthood, household work, and eldercare—at rates higher than those of men. Researchers have observed gender differences in coping strategies (responses to certain events or stimuli) and proposed that some women's strategies make them more vulnerable to depression.[69]

Depression in men is often masked by alcohol or drug abuse, or by the socially acceptable habit of working excessively. Typically, depressed men present as irritable, angry, and discouraged. Men are less likely to admit they are depressed, and doctors are less likely to suspect it. Depression is associated with increased risk of heart disease in both men and women, but with a higher risk of *death* by heart disease in men. Men are also more likely to act on suicidal feelings, and to succeed at suicide; suicide rates among depressed men are four times those among depressed women.[70]

Depression in children is increasingly reported, with 1 in 10 children between ages 6 and 12 experiencing persistent feelings of sadness, the hallmark of depression. Depressed children may pretend to be sick, refuse to go to school or have a sudden drop in school performance, sleep incessantly, engage in self-mutilation, abuse drugs or alcohol, or attempt suicide. Before adolescence, girls and boys experience depression at about the same rate, but by adolescence and young adulthood, the rate among girls is higher. This may be due to biological and hormonal changes; girls' struggles with self-esteem and perceptions of success and approval; and an increase in girls' exposure to traumas such as childhood sexual abuse and poverty.[71]

As adults reach their middle and older years, most are emotionally stable and lead active and satisfying lives. However, when depression does occur, it is often undiagnosed or untreated, particularly in people in lower income groups or without access to resources. Depression is the most common mental disorder of people 65 and older. Older adults may be less likely to discuss feelings of sadness and loss, or may attribute depression to aging.[72]

Rates of depression among Latinos, African Americans, and Asian Americans/Pacific Islanders are difficult to determine; members of these groups may have difficulty accessing mental health services because of economic barriers, social and cultural differences, language barriers, and lack of culturally competent providers. Data from the 2008 U.S. National Health and Wellness Survey indicated that when whites report depression symptoms to a health care provider, they are much more likely to be officially diagnosed with depression. Seventy-six percent of whites reporting symptoms were officially diagnosed, versus 58.7 percent of African Americans, 62.7 percent of Latinos, and 47.4 percent of Asian Americans.[73]

Skills for Behavior Change

DEALING WITH AND DEFEATING DEPRESSION

If you feel you have depression symptoms, make an appointment with a counselor. Depression is often a biological condition that you can't just "get over" on your own. You may need talk therapy, sometimes combined with antidepressant medication, to help you reach a place where you can play a greater role in getting well. Once you've started along a path of therapy and healing, these strategies may help you feel better faster:

- Be realistic and responsible in setting appropriate personal goals.
- Break large tasks into small ones, set priorities, and do what you can as you can.
- Try to be with other people and to confide in someone.
- Mild exercise and religious or social activities may help.
- Try meditation, yoga, tai chi, or another mind–body practice. These disciplines can help you connect with your feelings, release tension, and clear your mind.
- Expect your mood to improve gradually, not immediately.
- Before deciding to make a significant transition, change jobs, or get married or divorced, discuss it with others who know you well.
- Let family and friends help you.
- Continue working with your counselor. If he or she isn't helpful, look for another.

check yourself

- **What are the most common mood disorders?**
- **What are causes and treatments for mood disorders?**

Other Psychological Disorders

- **Describe personality disorders, schizophrenia, and ADHD, including causes and treatments.**

Personality Disorders

A **personality disorder** is an "enduring pattern of inner experience and behavior that deviates markedly from the expectation of the individual's culture and is pervasive and inflexible."[74] About 9 percent of adults in the United States have some form of personality disorder.[75] People dealing with individuals suffering from personality disorders often find interactions with them challenging and destructive.

Paranoid personality disorder involves pervasive, unfounded mistrust of others, irrational jealousy, and secretiveness, often with delusions of being persecuted by everyone from family members to the government. *Narcissistic personality disorders* involve an exaggerated sense of self-importance and self-absorption; sufferers are overly needy and demanding and feel "entitled" to nothing but the best.

Borderline personality disorder (BPD) is characterized by risky behaviors such as gambling sprees, unsafe sex, use of illicit drugs, and daredevil driving.[76] Characteristics include mood swings and the tendency to see everything in black-and-white terms. Seventy to 80 percent of persons diagnosed with BPD engage in **self-injury,** or deliberately causing harm to one's own body—such as by cutting or burning—to cope with emotions.[77]

Researchers estimate that between 2 and 8 million Americans have engaged in self-harm; the prevalence in college students is between 17 and 38 percent. Many people who inflict self-harm have experienced abuse as children or adults. If you or someone you know is engaging in self-injury, seek professional help. Not only must the behavior be stopped, but the sufferer must also learn to recognize and manage the feelings that triggered it.[78]

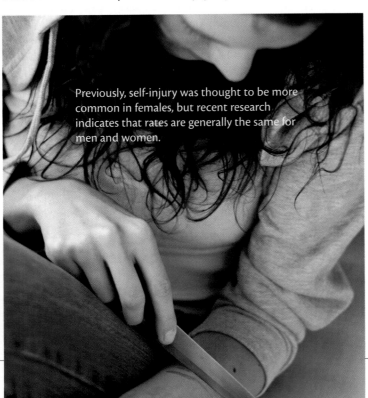

Previously, self-injury was thought to be more common in females, but recent research indicates that rates are generally the same for men and women.

Schizophrenia

Perhaps the most frightening psychological disorder is **schizophrenia,** which affects about 1 percent of the U.S. population.[79] Schizophrenia is characterized by alterations of the senses (including auditory and visual hallucinations); the inability to sort out incoming stimuli and make appropriate responses; an altered sense of self; and radical changes in emotions, movements, and behaviors. Typical symptoms include delusional behavior, hallucinations, incoherent speech, inability to think logically, erratic movement, and difficulty with daily living.[80]

Schizophrenia is a biological disease, perhaps due to brain damage as early as the second trimester of fetal development. Symptoms usually appear in men in their late teens and twenties and in women in their late twenties and early thirties.[81]

At present, schizophrenia is treatable but not curable. With proper medication, public understanding, support of loved ones, and access to therapy, many schizophrenics lead normal lives—though without such assistance, many have great difficulty.

ADHD

Attention-deficit/hyperactivity disorder (ADHD) is a common neurobehavioral disorder that affects 5 to 8 percent of school-aged children. In as many as 60 percent of cases, symptoms persist into adulthood. In any given year, 4.1 percent of adults are identified as having ADHD.

People with ADHD are often hyperactive or distracted. Even when they try to concentrate, they find it hard to pay attention. They have a hard time organizing things, listening to instructions, remembering details, and controlling their behavior. ADHD may look like a willpower problem, but it's essentially a chemical problem in the brain's management systems. People with ADHD are also six times more likely than the general population to have another psychiatric or learning disorder.

Untreated, ADHD can disrupt health, work, finances, and relationships.[82] If you suspect you or someone close to you has ADHD, see www.chadd.org for information and support.

- **What are causes and treatments for personality disorders, schizophrenia, and ADHD?**

Psychological Health Through the Lifespan: Successful Aging

- **Describe psychological conditions associated with aging.**
- **Explain the impact of loss on psychological health.**

Most older adults lead healthy, fulfilling lives. However, some older people do suffer from mental and emotional disturbances. Depression is the most common psychological problem facing older adults—though the rate of major depression is lower among older than younger adults. Regardless of age, people who have a poor perception of their health, have multiple chronic illnesses, take many medications, abuse alcohol and other drugs, lack social support, and do not exercise face more challenges that may require emotional strength.

Memory failure, errors in judgment, disorientation, or erratic behavior can occur at any age and for various reasons. The terms *dementing diseases*, or **dementias**, are used to describe either reversible symptoms or progressive forms of brain malfunctioning.

One of the most common dementias is **Alzheimer's disease (AD)**. Affecting an estimated 5.4 million Americans,[83] the disease "kills twice": through slow loss of personhood (memory loss, disorientation, personality changes, and eventual loss of independent functioning), then through deterioration of body systems.

Patients with AD live for an average of 4 to 6 years after diagnosis, although the disease can last for up to 20 years.[84] Although often associated with the aged, AD has been diagnosed in people in their forties. In AD, areas of the brain that affect memory, speech, and personality develop "tangles" that impair nerve cell communication causing cell death. It progresses in stages marked by increasingly impaired memory and judgment. In later stages, many patients become depressed, combative, and aggressive. In the final stage, the person becomes dependent on others; identity loss and speech problems are common. Eventually, control of bodily functions may be lost.

Researchers are investigating possible causes including genetic predisposition, immune malfunction, a slow-acting virus, chromosomal or genetic defects, chronic inflammation, uncontrolled hypertension, and neurotransmitter imbalance. No treatment can stop AD, but medications can slow or relieve some symptoms.[85]

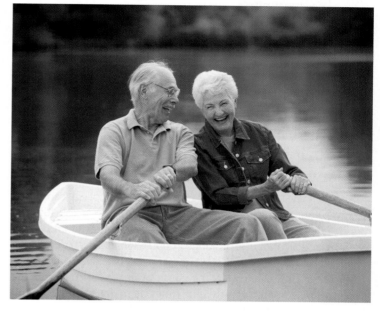

People who have aged successfully usually are resilient and able to cope well with physical, social, and emotional changes. They live independently and are actively engaged in mentally challenging and stimulating activities and in social and productive pursuits.

39

Coping with Loss

Coping with the loss of a loved one is extremely difficult. Understanding feelings and behaviors related to death can help you comprehend the emotional processes associated with it.

Bereavement is the loss or deprivation a survivor experiences when a loved one dies. The death of a parent, spouse, sibling, child, friend, or pet will result in different feelings for different people. Loneliness and despair may envelop survivors. Understanding of these normal reactions, time, patience, and support from loved ones can help the bereaved heal and move on, even though they will not forget.

Grief occurs in reaction to significant loss, including one's own impending death, the death of a loved one, or a loss (such as the end of a relationship or job) involving separation or change in identity. Grief may be a mental, physical, social, or emotional reaction, and often includes changes in eating, sleeping, working, and even thinking. Symptoms vary in severity and duration. However, the bereaved person can benefit from emotional and social support.

- **What are three particular psychological issues associated with aging?**

When Psychological Problems Become Too Much: Suicide

- **Identify warning signs associated with suicide.**
- **Discuss strategies for suicide prevention.**

Each year there are more than 34,000 reported suicides in the United States.[86] Experts estimate there may be closer to 100,000; it is difficult to determine the causes of many deaths.

Suicide is the second leading cause of death on college campuses. However, young adults not attending college are also at risk. Risk factors include family history of suicide, previous suicide attempts, excessive drug and alcohol use, prolonged depression, financial difficulties, serious illness in oneself or a loved one, and loss of a loved one.

Suicide is the seventh leading cause of death for men and the fifteenth for women.[87] Nearly four times as many men die by suicide than women. Firearms, suffocation, and poison are by far the most common methods of suicide. Men are almost twice as likely as women to use firearms, whereas women are almost three times as likely to use poisoning.[88]

Warning Signs

Seventy-five to 80 percent of people who commit suicide indicate their intentions, though warnings aren't always recognized.[89] Anyone expressing a desire to kill himself or herself or who has made an attempt is at risk. Signs that one may be contemplating suicide include the following:[90]

- Recent loss and a seeming inability to let go of grief
- A history of depression
- Change in personality—withdrawal, irritability, anxiety, tiredness, apathy
- Change in behavior—inability to concentrate, loss of interest in classes or work, unexplained demonstration of happiness following a period of depression
- Sexual dysfunction (such as impotence) or diminished sexual interest
- Expressions of self-hatred and excessive risk-taking
- Change in sleep or eating habits or in appearance
- A direct statement such as "I might as well end it all"
- An indirect statement such as "You won't have to worry about me anymore"
- Final preparations such as writing a will or giving away prized possessions
- Preoccupation with death

Preventing Suicide

Most people who attempt suicide want to live but see death as the only way out of an intolerable situation. Crisis counselors and suicide

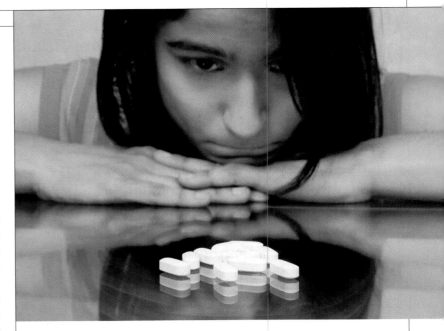

If you notice warning signs of suicide in someone you know, it is imperative that you take action.

hotlines may help temporarily, but the best way to prevent suicide is to get rid of conditions and substances that may precipitate attempts, including alcohol, drugs, isolation, and access to guns.

If someone you know threatens suicide or displays warning signs of doing so:[91]

- **Monitor signals.** Ensure there is someone around the person as often as possible. Don't leave him or her alone.
- **Take threats seriously.** Don't brush them off as "just talk."
- **Let the person know how much you care.** Say you're there to help.
- **Listen.** Try not to discredit or be shocked by what the person says. Empathize, sympathize, and keep the person talking.
- **Ask directly,** "Are you thinking of hurting or killing yourself?"
- **Don't belittle feelings.** Don't tell the person he or she doesn't mean it or couldn't commit suicide. To some, such comments offer the challenge of proving you wrong.
- **Help think about alternatives.** Offer to go for help along with the person. Call a suicide hotline, and use all available community and campus resources.
- **Tell your friend's spouse, partner, parents, siblings, or counselor.** Don't keep your suspicions to yourself.

- **What are five warning signs that someone may be contemplating suicide?**
- **What are five specific actions you can take to prevent suicide?**

Seeking Professional Help

learning outcomes

- **Recognize feelings and behaviors that may warrant seeking help from a mental health professional.**
- **Describe possible treatment options for psychological problems.**

A physical ailment will readily send most people to the nearest health professional, but many resist seeking help for psychological problems. However, nearly 1 in 5 Americans now seeks such help. Consider seeking help if:

- You feel you need help.
- You feel out of control or experience wild mood swings or inappropriate responses to normal stimuli.
- Your fears or feelings of guilt distract you.
- You have hallucinations.
- You feel worthless, or feel life is not worth living.
- Your life seems nothing but a series of crises.
- You're considering suicide.
- You turn to drugs or alcohol to escape.

Deciding to Seek Treatment

Common misconceptions about people with mental illness: they're dangerous, irresponsible, or "need to get over it." The stigma of mental illness often leads to shame and isolation. Many people with mental illness report that the stigma was more disabling at times than the illness itself.[92] The group Active Minds (www.activeminds .org) works to end the stigma of mental illness and encourage those at risk to seek care.

If you're considering treatment for a psychological problem, first see a health professional for an evaluation that should include:

1. A *physical checkup*, to rule out other issues that can result in depression-like symptoms
2. A *psychiatric history*, to trace the apparent disorder, genetic or family factors, and any past treatments
3. A *mental status examination*, including tests for other psychiatric symptoms

Type of Mental Health Professionals

The most common types of mental health professionals are psychiatrists, psychologists, social workers, counselors, psychoanalysts, and licensed marriage and family therapists. Which one you choose depends on your needs and goals. When choosing a therapist, the most important criterion is whether you feel you can work with him or her. Questions to ask the therapist and yourself:

- **Can you interview the therapist before starting treatment?** An initial meeting will help determine whether this person is a good fit for you.
- **Do you like the therapist?** Can you talk to him or her comfortably?
- **Does the therapist demonstrate professionalism?** Be concerned if your therapist frequently breaks appointments, suggests outside social interaction, talks inappropriately about himself or herself, has questionable billing practices, or resists releasing you from therapy.
- **Will the therapist help set goals?** A good professional should help you set small goals to work on between sessions.

Pharmacological Treatment

Drug therapy can be important in treatment of many psychological disorders. Such medications aren't, however, without side effects and contraindications. For example, the FDA recently proposed new warnings about suicidal thinking and behavior in young adults taking antidepressants.[93]

Talk to your health care provider to understand the risks and benefits of any medication prescribed; tell your doctor of any adverse effects. With some therapies, such as antidepressants, you may not feel effects for several weeks. Finally, compliance with your doctor's recommendations for beginning or ending a course of any medication is very important.

What to Expect in Therapy

Before meeting, briefly explain your needs. Ask about the fee. Arrive on time and expect your visit to last about an hour. The therapist will ask about your history and what brought you to therapy. Answer honestly; it's critical that you trust this person enough to be open and honest.

Many types of counseling exist, including individual therapy and group therapy. *Cognitive therapy* focuses on the impact of thoughts on feelings and behavior. It helps a person correct habitually pessimistic or faulty thinking patterns. *Behavioral therapy* focuses on what we do, using the concepts of stimulus, response, and reinforcement to alter behavior patterns. *Psychotherapeutic treatment* often combines cognitive-behavioral therapies with drug therapies.

check yourself

- **Give four examples of feelings and behaviors that may warrant seeking help from a mental health professional.**
- **What are some advantages and disadvantages to the various treatment options described?**

How Psychologically Healthy Are You?

An interactive version of this assessment is available online. Download it from the Live It! section of www.pearsonhighered.com/donatelle.

Being psychologically healthy requires both introspection and the willingness to work on areas that need improvement. Begin by completing the following assessment scale. Use it to determine how well each statement describes you. When you're finished, ask someone who is very close to you to take the same test and respond with his or her own perceptions of you. Carefully assess areas in which your responses differ from those of your friend or family member. Which areas need some work? Which are in good shape?

	Never	Rarely	Fairly Frequently	Most of the Time	All of the Time
1. My actions and interactions indicate that I am confident in my abilities.	1	2	3	4	5
2. I am quick to blame others for things that go wrong in my life.	1	2	3	4	5
3. I am spontaneous and like to have fun with others.	1	2	3	4	5
4. I am able to give love and affection to others and show my feelings.	1	2	3	4	5
5. I am able to receive love and signs of affection from others without feeling uneasy.	1	2	3	4	5
6. I am generally positive and upbeat about things in my life.	1	2	3	4	5
7. I am cynical and tend to be critical of others.	1	2	3	4	5
8. I have a large group of people whom I consider to be good friends.	1	2	3	4	5
9. I make time for others in my life.	1	2	3	4	5
10. I take time each day for myself for quiet introspection, having fun, or just doing nothing.	1	2	3	4	5
11. I am compulsive and competitive in my actions.	1	2	3	4	5
12. I handle stress well and am seldom upset or stressed out	1	2	3	4	5
13. I try to look for the good in everyone and every situation before finding fault.	1	2	3	4	5
14. I am comfortable meeting new people and interact well in social settings.	1	2	3	4	5

	Never	Rarely	Fairly Frequently	Most of the Time	All of the Time
15. I would rather stay in and watch TV or read than go out with friends or interact with others.	1	2	3	4	5
16. I am flexible and can adapt to most situations, even if I don't like them.	1	2	3	4	5
17. Nature, the environment, and other living things are important aspects of my life.	1	2	3	4	5
18. I think before responding to my emotions.	1	2	3	4	5
19. I tend to think of my own needs before those of others.	1	2	3	4	5
20. I am consciously trying to be a better person.	1	2	3	4	5
21. I like to plan ahead and set realistic goals for myself.	1	2	3	4	5
22. I accept others for who they are.	1	2	3	4	5
23. I value diversity and respect others' rights, regardless of culture, race, sexual orientation, religion, or other differences.	1	2	3	4	5
24. I try to live each day as if it might be my last.	1	2	3	4	5
25. I have a great deal of energy and appreciate the little things in life.	1	2	3	4	5
26. I cope with stress in appropriate ways.	1	2	3	4	5
27. I get enough sleep each day and seldom feel tired.	1	2	3	4	5
28. I have healthy relationships with my family.	1	2	3	4	5

29. I am confident that I can do most things if I put my mind to them.

	Never	Rarely	Fairly Frequently	Most of the Time	All of the Time
	1	2	3	4	5

30. I respect others' opinions and believe that others should be free to express their opinions, even when they differ from my own.

	Never	Rarely	Fairly Frequently	Most of the Time	All of the Time
	1	2	3	4	5

Interpreting Your Scores

Look at items 2, 7, 11, 15, and 19. Add up your score for these five items and divide by 5. Is your average for these items above or below 3? Did you score a 5 on any of these items? Do you need to work on any of these areas? Now look at your scores for the remaining items (there should be 25 items). Total these scores and divide by 25. Is your average above or below 3? On which items

did you score a 5? Obviously you're doing well in these areas. Now remove these items from this grouping of 25 (scores of 5), and add up your scores for the remaining items. Then divide your total by the number of items included. Now what is your average?

Do the same for the scores completed by your friend or family member. Which scores, if any, are different, and how do they differ? Which areas do you need to work on? What actions can you take now to improve your ratings in these areas?

Your Plan for Change

The Assess Yourself activity gave you the chance to look at various aspects of your psychological health and compare your self-assessment with a friend's perceptions. Now that you have considered these results, you can take steps to change behaviors that may be detrimental to your psychological health.

Today, You Can:

◯ Evaluate your behavior and identify patterns and specific things you are doing that negatively affect your psychological health. What can you change now? What can you change in the near future?

◯ Start a journal and note changes in your mood. Look for trends and think about ways you can change your behavior to address them.

◯ Make a list of the things that bring you joy—friends, family, activities, entertainment, nature. Commit yourself to making more room for these joy-givers in your life.

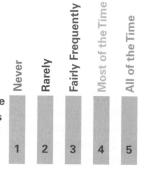

Within the Next 2 Weeks, You Can:

◯ Visit your campus health center and find out about the counseling services they offer. If you are feeling overwhelmed, depressed, or anxious, make an appointment with a counselor.

◯ Pay attention to the negative thoughts that pop up throughout the day. Note times when you find yourself devaluing or undermining your abilities, and notice when you project negative attitudes on others. Bringing your awareness to these thoughts gives you an opportunity to stop and reevaluate them.

By the End of the Semester, You Can:

◯ Make a commitment to an ongoing therapeutic practice aimed at improving your psychological health. Depending on your current situation, this could mean anything from seeing a counselor or joining a support group to practicing meditation or attending religious services.

◯ Volunteer regularly with a local organization you care about. Focus your energy and gain satisfaction by helping to improve others' lives or the environment.

Summary

- Psychological health is a complex phenomenon involving mental, emotional, social, and spiritual dimensions.
- Many factors influence psychological health, including life experiences, family, the environment, other people, self-esteem, self-efficacy, and personality.
- The mind–body connection is an important link in overall health and well-being. Positive psychology emphasizes happiness as a key factor in determining overall reaction to life's challenges.
- Developing self-esteem and self-efficacy, making healthy connections, having a positive outlook, and maintaining physical health enhance psychological health.
- College is a high-risk time for developing depression or anxiety disorders because of high stress levels, pressures for grades, and financial problems, among others.
- Mood disorders include major depression, dysthymic disorder, bipolar disorder, and seasonal affective disorder. Anxiety disorders include generalized anxiety disorder, panic disorders, phobic disorders, obsessive-compulsive disorder, and post-traumatic stress disorder. Personality disorders include paranoid, narcissistic, and borderline personality disorders.
- Suicide is a result of negative psychosocial reactions to life. People intending to commit suicide often give signs of their intentions. Such people can often be helped.
- Mental health professionals include psychiatrists, psychoanalysts, psychologists, social workers, and counselors. Many therapy methods exist, including group, individual, cognitive, and behavioral therapies.

Pop Quiz

1. A person with high self-esteem
   a. possesses feelings of self-respect and self-worth.
   b. believes he or she can successfully engage in a specific behavior.
   c. believes external influences shape psychosocial health.
   d. has a high altruistic capacity.

2. All the following traits have been identified as related to psychological well-being *except*
   a. conscientiousness.
   b. introversion.
   c. openness to experience.
   d. agreeableness.

3. Subjective well-being includes all the following components *except*
   a. spirituality.
   b. satisfaction with present life.
   c. relative presence of positive emotions.
   d. relative absence of negative emotions.

4. People who have experienced repeated failures at the same task may eventually quit trying altogether. This pattern of behavior is termed
   a. post-traumatic stress disorder.
   b. learned helplessness.
   c. self-efficacy.
   d. introversion.

5. The term that most accurately refers to the feeling or subjective side of psychological health is
   a. social health.
   b. mental health.
   c. emotional health.
   d. spiritual health.

6. Which of the following statements is *false*?
   a. One in four adults in the United States suffers from a diagnosable mental disorder in a given year.
   b. Mental disorders are the leading cause of disability in the United States.
   c. Dysthymia is an example of an anxiety disorder.
   d. Bipolar disorder can also be referred to as manic depression.

7. This disorder is characterized by a need to perform rituals over and over.
   a. Personality disorder
   b. Obsessive-compulsive disorder
   c. Phobic disorder
   d. Post-traumatic stress disorder

8. What is the number one mental health problem in the United States?
   a. Depression
   b. Anxiety disorders
   c. Alcohol dependence
   d. Schizophrenia

9. Every winter, Stan suffers from irritability, apathy, weight gain, and sadness. He most likely has
   a. panic disorder.
   b. generalized anxiety disorder.
   c. seasonal affective disorder.
   d. chronic mood disorder.

10. Which of these is *not* an element of spirituality?
   a. relationships
   b. focus on the past
   c. values
   d. meaningful purpose in life

Answers to these questions can be found on page A-1.

Web Links

1. **American Foundation for Suicide Prevention.** Resources for suicide prevention; support for family and friends of those who have committed suicide. www.afsp.org
2. **American Psychological Association Help Center.** Information on psychology at work, the mind–body connection, psychological responses to war, and other topics. http://apahelpcenter.org
3. **National Alliance on Mental Illness.** Support and advocacy for families and friends of people with severe mental illnesses. www.nami.org
4. **National Institute of Mental Health (NIMH).** An overview of mental health information and research. www.nimh.nih.gov
5. **Helpguide.** Resources for improving mental and emotional health, plus information on topics such as self-injury, sleep, depressive disorders, and anxiety disorders. www.helpguide.org

Stress

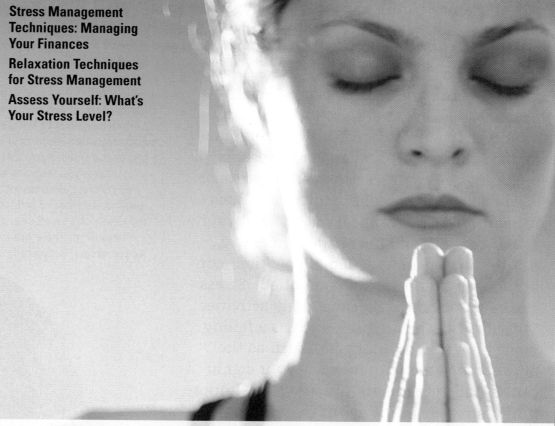

Rising tuition, difficult roommates, dating anxiety, grades, money, worries about what to do with your life—they all add up to STRESS. In today's 24/7 world, stress can lead us to feel overwhelmed. But it can also cause us to push ourselves to improve, bring excitement into an otherwise humdrum life, and leave us exhilarated. While we work, play, socialize, and sleep, stress affects us in myriad ways, many of which we may not even notice.

According to a recent American Psychological Association poll, a majority of American adults reported experiencing moderate to high levels of stress in the past month.[1] Although the exact toll stress exerts on us during a lifetime of overload is unknown, we do know that stress is a significant health hazard. It can rob the body of needed nutrients, damage the cardiovascular system, raise blood pressure, increase the risk of cancer and diabetes, and dampen immune defenses. It can also drain our emotional reserves; contribute to depression, anxiety, fatigue, and irritability; and punctuate our social interactions with hostility and anger.

Is too much stress inevitable? Fortunately, the answer is no. To tame stress, we can learn to anticipate and recognize personal stressors—and develop skills to reduce or manage those we cannot avoid or control. First, we must understand what stress is and what effects it has on the body.

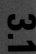

What Is Stress?

learning outcomes

■ **Define stress-related key terms.**

Most current definitions state that **stress** is the mental and physical response and adaptation by our bodies to the real or perceived changes and challenges in our lives. A **stressor** is any real or perceived physical, social, or psychological event or stimulus that causes our bodies to react or respond.[2] Several factors influence one's response to stressors, including the *characteristics of the stressor* (Can you control it? Is it predictable? Does it occur often?); *biological factors* (e.g., your age or gender); and *past experiences* (e.g., things that have happened to you, their consequences, and how you responded). Stress can be associated with most daily activities. Stressors may be tangible, such as a failing grade on a test, or intangible, such as the angst associated with meeting your significant other's parents for the first time. Importantly, stress is in the eye of the beholder: Each person's unique combination of heredity, life experiences, personality, and ability to cope influences how the person perceives an event and what meaning he or she attaches to it. What "stresses out" one person may not even bother the next person.

And stress isn't necessarily bad for you. Although events that cause prolonged negative stress, such as a natural disaster, can undermine your health, positive, yet stressful, events can have positive effects on your growth and well-being. Generally, positive stress is called **eustress**. Eustress presents the opportunity for personal growth and satisfaction and can actually improve health. It can energize you, motivate you, and raise you up when you are down. Events such as getting married, having a child, getting a promotion at work, or winning a major competition can give rise to the pleasurable rush associated with eustress. In general, people perform at their best and live their lives to the fullest when they experience a moderate level of stress—just enough to keep them challenged and motivated—and deal with that stress in a productive manner. Just as too much stress can be detrimental to your health, too little stress leaves you stagnant and unfulfilled.

In contrast, **distress**, or negative stress, is caused by events that result in debilitative tension and strain, such as financial problems, the death of a loved one, academic difficulties, and the breakup of a relationship. There are two kinds of distress: acute and chronic. **Acute stress** is typically intense, flares quickly, and disappears

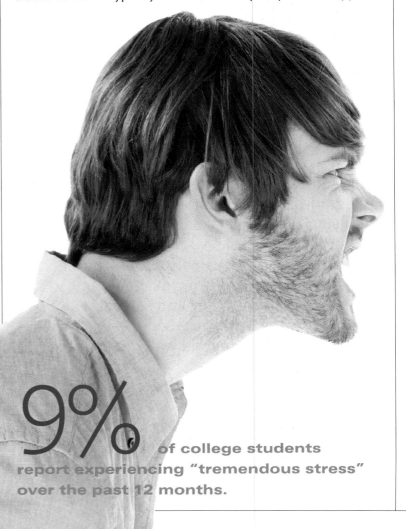

9% of college students report experiencing "tremendous stress" over the past 12 months.

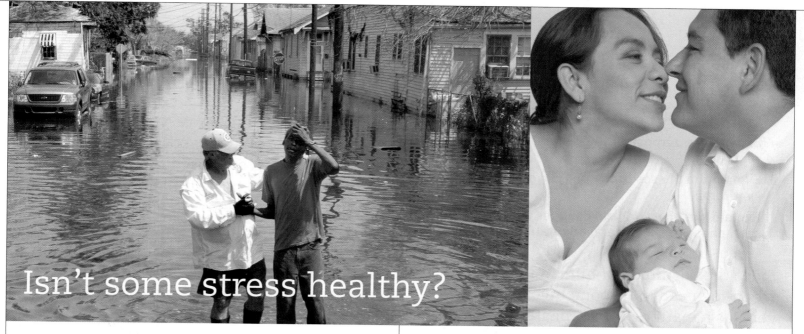

Isn't some stress healthy?

A moderate level of stress—especially eustress arising from new experiences—can actually help you live life to the fullest. Too much stress can affect your health for the worst, such as what is experienced by survivors of a natural disaster, but so can too little stress; we need change and challenge to keep us fulfilled and growing.

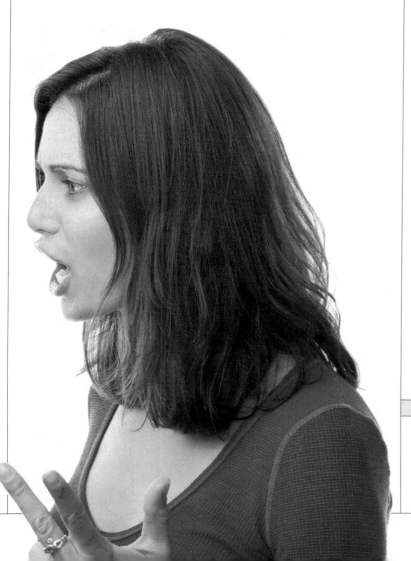

quickly. If you view a TV program in which a knife-wielding murderer lurks in a bedroom closet and watches a sleeping victim, your stress response might zoom into overdrive for a short time, only to be relieved when the CSI team swoops in and intervenes. Although **chronic stress** may not feel as intense, it can linger indefinitely and wreak silent havoc on your body's systems. Losing your mother after her long battle with breast cancer can cause prolonged stress responses in your body. For months after her death, you may struggle to balance the need to process emotions such as anger, grief, loneliness, and guilt, while focusing to stay caught up in classes and with your life.[3]

On any given day, we all experience both eustress and distress, each triggered by a wide range of both obvious and not-so-obvious sources. Several studies in recent years have examined sources of stress among various populations in the United States and globally. One of the most comprehensive is conducted annually by the American Psychological Association; the 2010 survey found that concerns over money, work, family, and health were major sources of stress among American adults.[4] College students, in particular, face stressors that come from internal sources, as well as external pressures to succeed in a competitive environment that is often geographically far removed from the support of family and lifelong friends.

Awareness of the sources of the stress in your life can do much to help you develop a plan to avoid, prevent, and control the things that cause you stress.

check yourself

- **How do distress and eustress differ?**
- **Do you have more trouble managing acute stress or chronic stress? Why?**

Your Body's Response to Stress

- **Explain the purpose of the general adaptation syndrome.**
- **Explain the phases of the general adaptation syndrome.**
- **Explain the physiological changes that occur during each phase of the general adaptation syndrome.**

Since the beginning of human life on Earth, when the need to respond quickly to danger was a matter of life or death, the body's physiological responses have evolved to protect humans from harm. Back then, a person who didn't respond by fighting or fleeing was all too likely to be eaten by a saber-toothed tiger or killed by a marauding enemy clan. Today, although such life-or-death encounters are thankfully far more rare, at least for those of us in industrialized countries, each of us nonetheless faces metaphorical tigers every day. Whether it's the city bus that sent a mud puddle flying across your new outfit, an e-mail from an angry boss, or an insidious insult from a supposed friend, ordinary "attacks" provoke these same, very real, physiological responses—which our bodies must then process, contain, or repress. Continually having to "stuff" our reactions rather than letting our physiological responses run their course can harm our health over time.

The General Adaptation Syndrome

When stress levels are low, the body is often in a state of **homeostasis**: All body systems are operating smoothly to maintain equilibrium. Stressors trigger a "crisis-mode" physiological response, after which the body attempts to return to homeostasis by means of an **adaptive response**. First characterized by Hans Selye in 1936, the internal fight to restore homeostasis in the face of a stressor is known as the **general adaptation syndrome**, or **GAS** (Figure 3.1). The GAS has three distinct phases: alarm, resistance, and exhaustion.[5] It's important to note that regardless of whether positive or negative events cause your eustress or distress, similar physiological changes will occur in your body.

Alarm Phase Suppose you are walking to your residence hall after a night class on a dimly lit campus. As you pass a particularly dark area, you hear someone cough behind you, and you sense someone approaching rapidly. You walk faster, only to hear the quickened footsteps of the other person. Your senses become increasingly alert, your breathing quickens, your heart races, and you begin to perspire. In desperation you stop, rip off your backpack, and prepare to fling it at your attacker to defend yourself. You turn around quickly and let out a blood-curdling yell. To your surprise, the only person you see is a classmate: She has been trying to stay close to you out of her own anxiety about walking alone in the dark. She screams and backs off the sidewalk into the bushes, and you both stare at each other in startled embarrassment. You have just experienced the alarm phase of the GAS. Also known as the **fight-or-flight response**, this physiological reaction is one of our most basic, innate survival instincts.[6]

How does this work, exactly? When the mind perceives a real or imaginary stressor, the cerebral cortex, the region of the brain that interprets the nature of an event, triggers an **autonomic nervous system (ANS)** response that prepares the body for action. The ANS is the portion of the central nervous system that regulates body functions that we do not normally consciously control, such as heart and glandular functions and breathing.

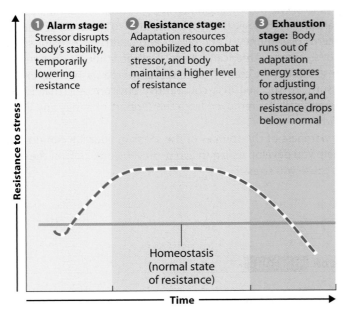

① Alarm stage: Stressor disrupts body's stability, temporarily lowering resistance

② Resistance stage: Adaptation resources are mobilized to combat stressor, and body maintains a higher level of resistance

③ Exhaustion stage: Body runs out of adaptation energy stores for adjusting to stressor, and resistance drops below normal

Resistance to stress

Homeostasis (normal state of resistance)

Time

Figure 3.1 The General Adaptation Syndrome (GAS)
The GAS describes the body's method of coping with prolonged stress.

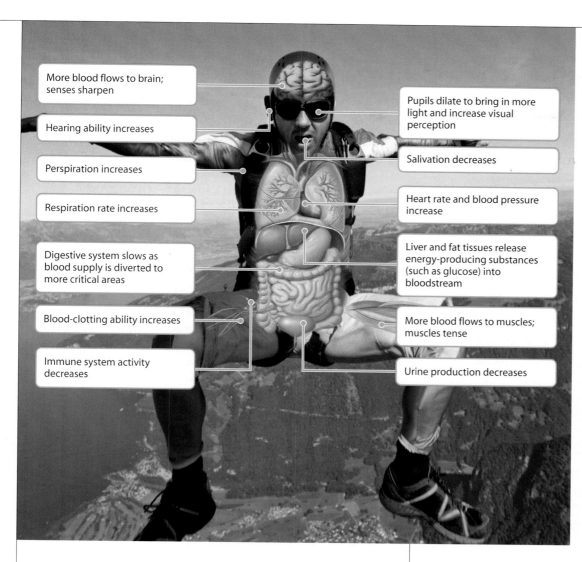

More blood flows to brain; senses sharpen

Hearing ability increases

Perspiration increases

Respiration rate increases

Digestive system slows as blood supply is diverted to more critical areas

Blood-clotting ability increases

Immune system activity decreases

Pupils dilate to bring in more light and increase visual perception

Salivation decreases

Heart rate and blood pressure increase

Liver and fat tissues release energy-producing substances (such as glucose) into bloodstream

More blood flows to muscles; muscles tense

Urine production decreases

Figure 3.2 The Body's Acute Stress Response
Exposure to stress of any kind causes a complex series of involuntary physiological responses.

release a powerful hormone, *adrenocorticotropic hormone (ACTH)*. ACTH signals the adrenal glands to release **cortisol**, a hormone that makes stored nutrients more readily available to meet energy demands. Finally, other parts of the brain and body release endorphins, which relieve pain that a stressor may cause.

Resistance Phase In the resistance phase of the GAS, the body tries to return to homeostasis by resisting the alarm responses. However, because some perceived stressor still exists, the body does not achieve complete calm or rest. Instead, the body stays activated or aroused at a level that causes a higher metabolic rate in some organ tissues. For example, if a loved one develops an aggressive form of cancer, you may be wild with grief or anxiety after hearing the diagnosis, and all of your systems may respond in the alarm phase. As you get used to the diagnosis, you calm down somewhat, but your body does not return completely to rest. The organs and systems of resistance are working overtime.

Exhaustion Phase A prolonged effort to adapt to the stress response leads to **allostatic load**, or exhaustive wear and tear on the body.[7] In the exhaustion phase of the GAS, the physical and emotional energy used to fight a stressor have been depleted. As the body adjusts to chronic unresolved stress, the adrenal glands continue to release cortisol, which remains in the bloodstream for longer periods of time as a result of slower metabolic responsiveness. Over time, cortisol can reduce **immunocompetence**, or the ability of the immune system to respond to attack. Blood pressure can remain dangerously elevated, you may catch colds more easily, or your body's ability to control blood glucose levels can be affected.

The ANS has two branches: sympathetic and parasympathetic. The **sympathetic nervous system** energizes the body for fight or flight by signaling the release of several stress hormones. The **parasympathetic nervous system** slows all the systems stimulated by the stress response; in effect, it counteracts the actions of the sympathetic branch.

The responses of the sympathetic nervous system to stress involve a series of biochemical exchanges between different parts of the body. The **hypothalamus**, a structure in the brain, functions as the control center of the sympathetic nervous system and determines the overall reaction to stressors. When the hypothalamus perceives that extra energy is needed to fight a stressor, it stimulates the adrenal glands, which are located near the top of the kidneys, to release the hormone **epinephrine**, also called *adrenaline*. Epinephrine causes more blood to be pumped with each beat of the heart, dilates the airways in the lungs to increase oxygen intake, increases the breathing rate, stimulates the liver to release more glucose (which fuels muscular exertion), and dilates the pupils to improve visual sensitivity (see Figure 3.2). The body is then poised to act immediately.

In addition to the fight-or-flight response, the alarm phase can also trigger a longer-term reaction to stress. The hypothalamus uses chemical messages to trigger the pituitary gland within the brain to

check yourself

- **How does the general adaptation syndrome help us understand our reaction to stressors?**
- **What are the phases of the general adaptation syndrome?**
- **How does the body react during each phase of the general adaptation syndrome?**

Effects of Stress on Your Life

learning outcomes

- **Specify negative health outcomes associated with chronic stress.**
- **Describe the impact of stress on intellectual and psychological functioning.**

Stress is often described as a "disease of prolonged arousal" that leads to a cascade of negative health effects whose likelihood increases with ongoing stress. Nearly all body systems become potential targets, and the long-term effects may be devastating. Some warning symptoms of prolonged stress are shown in Figure 3.3.

Physical Effects of Stress

Studies show that 40 percent of deaths and 70 percent of diseases in the United States are related, in whole or in part, to stress.[8] Ailments related to chronic stress include heart disease, diabetes, cancer, headaches, ulcers, low back pain, depression, and the common cold. Increases in rates of suicide, homicide, and domestic violence across the United States are additional symptoms of a nation under stress.

Stress and Cardiovascular Disease Perhaps the most documented health consequence of unresolved stress is cardiovascular disease (CVD).

Research has demonstrated the impact of chronic stress on heart rate, blood pressure, heart attack, and stroke.[9] The INTERHEART Study, which followed almost 30,000 participants in 52 countries, identified stress as one of the key modifiable risk factors for heart attack.[10]

Historically, the increased risk of CVD from chronic stress has been linked to arterial plaque buildup due to elevated cholesterol, hardening of the arteries, alterations in heart rhythm, increased and fluctuating blood pressures, and difficulties in cardiovascular responsiveness.[11] Research has also shown direct links between CVD and external stressors.[12]

Stress and Weight Gain You're not imagining it—you *are* more likely to gain weight when stressed. Higher stress levels may increase cortisol levels in the bloodstream, contributing to hunger and activating fat-storing enzymes; studies also support the theory that cortisol plays a role in increased belly fat and eating behaviors.[13]

Stress and Hair Loss The most common stress-induced hair loss is *telogen effluvium*. Often seen in individuals who have suffered a death in the family, had a difficult pregnancy, or experienced severe weight loss, this condition pushes colonies of hair into a resting phase in which much more hair falls out than grows. A similar condition, *alopecia areata*, occurs when stress triggers white blood cells to attack and destroy hair follicles.[14]

Stress and Diabetes Controlling stress is critical for preventing development of type 2 diabetes, as well as for successful diabetes management.[15] People under severe stress often don't get enough sleep, don't eat well, and may drink or take other drugs. These behaviors can alter blood sugar levels and promote development of diabetes.

Stress and Digestive Problems The causes of digestive disorders are often unknown; most likely, an underlying illness, pathogen, injury, or inflammation is exacerbated by stress, triggering nausea, vomiting, stomach cramps, or diarrhea.[16]

Why do I always get sick during finals week?

Prolonged stress can compromise your immune system, leaving you vulnerable to infection. If you spend exam week in a state of high stress—sleeping too little, studying too hard, and worrying a lot—chances are you'll reduce your body's ability to fight off any cold or flu bugs you may encounter.

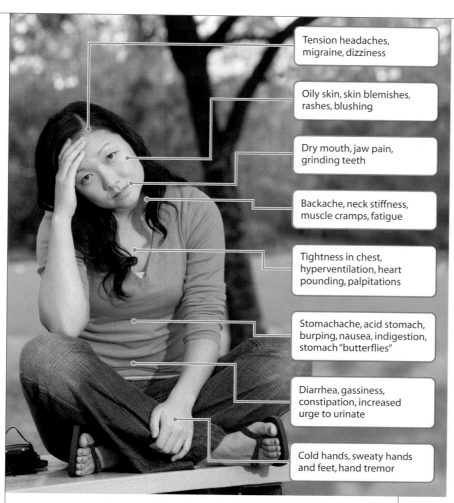

Tension headaches, migraine, dizziness

Oily skin, skin blemishes, rashes, blushing

Dry mouth, jaw pain, grinding teeth

Backache, neck stiffness, muscle cramps, fatigue

Tightness in chest, hyperventilation, heart pounding, palpitations

Stomachache, acid stomach, burping, nausea, indigestion, stomach "butterflies"

Diarrhea, gassiness, constipation, increased urge to urinate

Cold hands, sweaty hands and feet, hand tremor

Figure 3.3 Common Physical Symptoms of Stress
You may not even notice how stressed you are until your body starts sending you signals. Do you frequently experience any of these physical symptoms of stress?

Stress and Impaired Immunity A growing area of investigation known as *psychoneuroimmunology (PNI)* analyzes the relationship between stress and immune function. Research suggests that increased stress over time can affect cellular immune response.[17] Acute stressors can impair immunity for as much as 6 months;[18] prolonged stressors such as loss of a spouse, caregiving, and unemployment also have been shown to impair immune response over time.[19]

Stress and Libido Stress can throw a wrench into your sex life at any age. In both men and women, sexual drive, or libido, can be influenced by psychological and physiological factors, including time pressures, concerns over appearance, anxiety over performance, exhaustion from work, lack of sleep, and the multiple demands of classes and social life. In men, high stress can lead to declines in testosterone production, affecting their ability to get or maintain an erection. In women, stress can disrupt reproductive hormones, affecting mood, anxiety, sleep, and libido. And in both men and women, virtually any extreme or prolonged stressor, from illness to intense grief, can trigger a decline in desire.[20]

28% of college students reported that stress negatively affected their individual academic performance.

Intellectual and Psychological Effects of Stress

In a recent national survey of college students, 50 percent of respondents had felt overwhelmed by all they had to do within the past 2 weeks. Thirty-nine percent felt they had been under more than average stress in the past 12 months, with 8.7 percent reporting tremendous stress during that period. Not surprisingly, these same students rated stress as their number one impediment to academic performance, followed by lack of sleep.[21] Stress can play a huge role in whether a student stays in school, gets good grades, and succeeds on a career path. It can also wreak havoc on a person's ability to concentrate, remember, and understand and retain complex information.

Stress, Memory, and Concentration Animal studies provide compelling indicators of how *glucocorticoids*—stress hormones released from the adrenal cortex—affect memory. In humans, acute stress has been shown to impair short-term memory, particularly verbal memory.[22] Prolonged exposure to *cortisol* (a key stress hormone) has been linked to shrinking of the hippocampus, the brain's major memory center. In chronically stressed rats, decision-making regions of the brain shriveled, while brain sectors responsible for habitual behaviors not reliant on memory increased.[23]

Stress is an enormous contributor to mental disability and emotional dysfunction in industrialized nations. Studies have linked rates of mental disorders, particularly depression and anxiety, to environmental stressors, including divorce, marital conflict, and economic hardship.[24] Stressful life events and inadequate social support contribute to mental disorders among people aged 15 to 24 more than among other age groups. Researchers suggest that individuals moving from adolescence into adulthood face increased stressors of all kinds.[25] The high incidence of suicide among college students is assumed to indicate high personal and societal stress in the lives of young people, as is the increasing rate of anxiety disorders.[26]

check yourself

- **What are four possible effects of stress on your physical and psychological health?**

- **Give an example of an instance in which psychological stress had a physical effect on you.**

Stress and Headaches

learning outcomes

- **Describe common types of headaches.**
- **Explain possible connections between stress and headaches.**

Millions of people see their doctors for headaches each year; millions more put up with the pain or take pain relievers to blunt the symptoms. The good news: most headaches are not a sign of serious diseases or underlying conditions. The vast majority are either tension-type headaches or migraines.

Nearly 80 percent of adults (slightly more women than men) have this type of headache at some time in their lives.[27] Symptoms may include dull pain; a sensation of tightness; tender scalp, neck, and shoulder muscles; and occasionally loss of appetite.[28]

Typically, chemical and neuronal imbalances in the brain and/or muscular tension result in pain in the head or neck. Frequency and severity of symptoms varies, with occurrences categorized as epi-

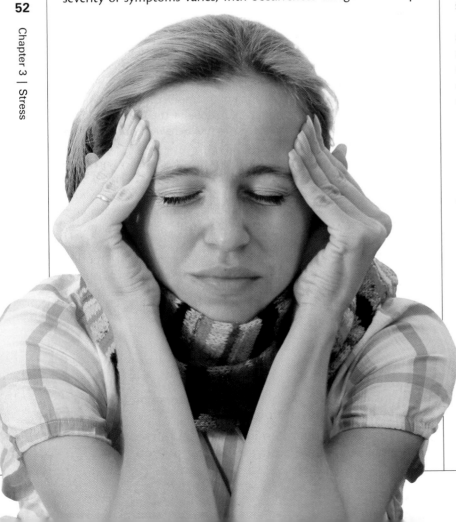

sodic (less than once a month; triggered by stress, anxiety, fatigue, or anger), frequent (1 to 15 days per month), and chronic (more than 15 days per month; often associated with depression or other emotional problems). Possible triggers include red wine, lack of sleep, fasting, menstruation, and food preservatives.

Such headaches are most often helped by reducing triggers. If stress is a trigger, try a range of relaxation techniques, such as those described later in the module "Relaxation Techniques for Stress Management." Exercise can relieve some tension headaches, as can over-the-counter pain relievers. Frequent headaches that are unresponsive to over-the-counter medications are probably *chronic tension headaches*; these warrant a doctor visit to assess underlying causes.

Nearly 30 million Americans suffer from **migraines**, headaches whose severe, debilitating symptoms include moderate to severe pain on one or both sides of the head, throbbing pain, pain that worsens with or interferes with activity, nausea, and sensitivity to light and sound.[29] Usually migraine incidence peaks between ages 20 and 45.[30]

Migraines appear to run in families: If both your parents have migraines, you have a 75 percent chance of experiencing them; one parent, a 50 percent chance.[31] Three times as many women as men suffer from migraines.[32]

Whereas all headaches can be painful, migraines can be disabling. Symptoms vary greatly by change to migraines individual, and attacks can last anywhere from 4 to 72 hours. In about 25 percent of cases, migraines are preceded by a warning sign called an *aura*—most often flickering vision, blind spots, tingling in the arms or legs, or a sensation of odor or taste.[33]

Prescription drugs such as pain relievers or sumatriptans often help migraine sufferers. See your doctor or the National Headache Foundation (www.headaches.org) for more information.

What triggers a migraine headache?

Patients report that migraines can be triggered by emotional stress, too much or not enough sleep, fasting, caffeine, alcohol, hormonal changes, altitude, weather, chocolate or other foods, and a litany of other causes. There is tremendous variability, and what triggers a migraine in one person may relieve it in another.

check yourself

- **What are three common types of headaches?**
- **How could effective stress management contribute to headache reduction?**

Stress and Sleep Problems

learning outcomes

- **Describe the importance of sleep to good health.**
- **List strategies for ensuring restful sleep.**

In a recent survey, 10.4 percent of students reported that in the past week they did not get enough sleep to feel rested on even a single day.[34]

Sleep is much more important than most people realize. Sleep conserves body energy and restores you physically and mentally. Colds, flu, and many other ailments are more common when your immune system is depressed by lack of sleep. High blood pressure is more common in people who get fewer than 7 hours of sleep a night, and poor or reduced sleep increases the risk of heart disease and stroke.[35] Sleep also contributes to healthy metabolism, which helps you maintain a healthy body weight.

Restricting sleep can cause attention lapses, slow or poor memory, reduced cognitive ability, and a tendency for thinking to get "stuck in a rut."[36] Your ability not only to remember facts but also to integrate those facts, make meaningful generalizations about them, and consolidate what you've learned requires adequate sleep.[37]

Sleep also has a restorative effect on motor function, affecting one's ability to perform tasks such as driving a car.[38] Researchers contend that a night without sleep impairs motor skills and reaction time as much as driving drunk.[39]

Certain brain regions, including the cerebral cortex (your "master mind"), achieve some form of essential rest only during sleep.

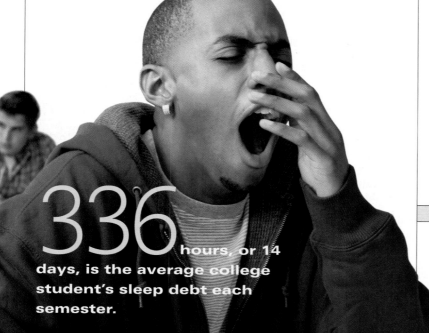

336 hours, or 14 days, is the average college student's sleep debt each semester.

You're also more likely to feel stressed out, worried, or sad when you're sleep deprived. Stress and sleep problems can reinforce or exacerbate each other.[40]

Seven to 8 hours is considered "average" sleep time, and the vast majority of people need this much.[41] Individual variations do occur according to age (kids need more), gender (women need more), and other factors. In addition, when trying to figure out your sleep needs, you have to consider your body's physiological need plus your **sleep debt**—the total hours of missed sleep you're carrying. The good news is that you can catch up, if you do it sensibly over time. Ways to ensure a good night's sleep include:

- **Let there be light.** Stay in sync with your circadian rhythm by spending time in the daylight.
- **Stay active.** Get plenty of regular activity. But note that strenuous exercise within several hours of bedtime makes it harder to fall asleep.
- **Sleep tight.** Comfortable pillows, bedding, and mattress can help you sleep more soundly.
- **Create a sleep "cave."** As bedtime approaches, keep your bedroom quiet, cool, and dark. Turn off electronic devices and block light with shades or curtains.
- **Condition yourself into better sleep.** Go to bed and get up at the same time each day.
- **Allow at least 3 hours between dinner and bedtime.** If you're hungry before bed, have a light snack.
- **Don't toss and turn.** If you're not asleep after 20 minutes, read or listen to gentle music. Once you feel sleepy, go back to bed.
- **Don't nap in the late afternoon or evening,** and don't nap for longer than 30 minutes.
- **Don't read, study, watch TV, use your laptop, talk on the phone, eat, or smoke in bed.** In fact, don't smoke at all; it disturbs sleep. Emotionally intense phone conversations can also make it hard to calm yourself enough to sleep.
- **Don't use caffeine or alcohol before bedtime.** It takes your body about 6 hours to clear just *half* of a caffeinated drink from your system.[42] Alcohol interferes with your natural sleep stages and can cause you to awaken in the middle of the night.
- **Don't drink large amounts of liquid before bed,** to prevent having to get up in the night to use the bathroom.
- **Don't take sleeping pills,** unless prescribed by your health care provider. Over-the-counter sleep aids can interfere with progression through the stages of sleep.

53

check yourself

- **Why is it important for your health to sleep well?**
- **What are three common reasons for poor sleep, and how can you overcome them?**

Psychosocial Causes of Stress

learning outcomes

■ **Discuss and classify psychosocial sources of stress.**

Psychosocial stressors refer to the factors in our daily routines and in our social and physical environments that cause us to experience stress. Which of these are most common in your life?

Adjustment to Change Any time change occurs in your normal routine, whether good or bad, you experience some level of stress. The more changes you experience and the more adjustments you must make, the greater the chances are that stress will have an impact on your health. The enormous changes associated with starting college, while exciting, can also be among the most stressful you will face in your life. Moving away from home, trying to fit in and make new friends from diverse backgrounds, adjusting to a new schedule, learning to live with strangers in housing that is often lacking in the comforts of home: All of these things can cause sleeplessness and anxiety and keep your body in a continual fight-or-flight mode.

Hassles Some psychologists have proposed that little stressors, frustrations, and petty annoyances, known collectively as *hassles*, can be just as stressful as major life changes.[43] Listening to classmates who talk too much during lecture, having to hear someone airing dirty laundry on a loud cell phone call, not finding parking on campus, and a host of other small but bothersome situations can trigger frustration, anger, and fight-or-flight responses.[44]

Technostress Technostress is stress created by a dependence on technology and the constant state of connection, which can include a perceived obligation to always respond or be ever present. Much good comes from technology. For some folks, however, technomania can become obsessive. Although technology can allow us to work on the go and communicate in new ways, there are some clear downsides to all of that "virtual" interaction—the dangers of distracted driving, repetitive stress injuries, and even what authors Michell Weil and Larry Rosen call *technosis*, a syndrome in which people become so immersed in technology that they risk losing their own identities.[45]

To reduce technostress, set limits on your technology use, and make sure that you devote sufficient time to face-to-face interactions with people you care about, cultivating and nurturing

your relationships. You don't always need to answer your phone or respond to a text or e-mail immediately. Leave your devices at home or turn them off when you are out with others or on vacation. Tune in to your surroundings, your loved ones and friends, your job, and your classes.

The Toll of Relationships Relationships can trigger enormous fight-or-flight reactions—whether we're talking about the exhilaration of new love or the pain of a breakup, the result is often lack of focus, lack of sleep, and an inability to focus on anything but the love interest. And although we may think first of love relationships, even relationships with friends, family members, and coworkers can be the sources of overwhelming struggles, just as they can be sources of strength and support. These relationships can make us strive to be the best that we can be and give us hope for the future, or they can diminish our self-esteem and leave us reeling from a destructive interaction.

Academic and Financial Pressure Putting a group of top high school graduates into a college or university and encouraging them

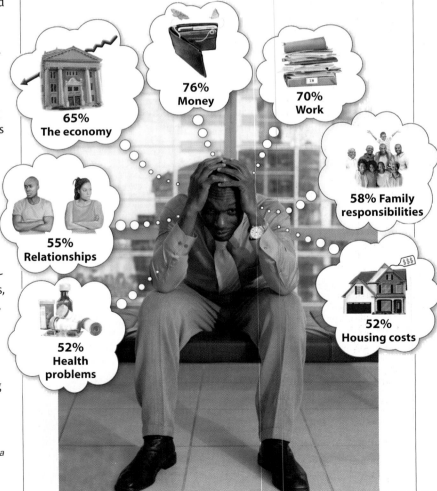

Figure 3.4 What Stresses Us?
Respondents indicated the events and issues that cause stress for them.
Source: Data are from the American Psychological Association, *Stress in America 2010, Key Findings,* 2010, Available at www.apa.org/news/press/releases/stress/key-findings.pdf.

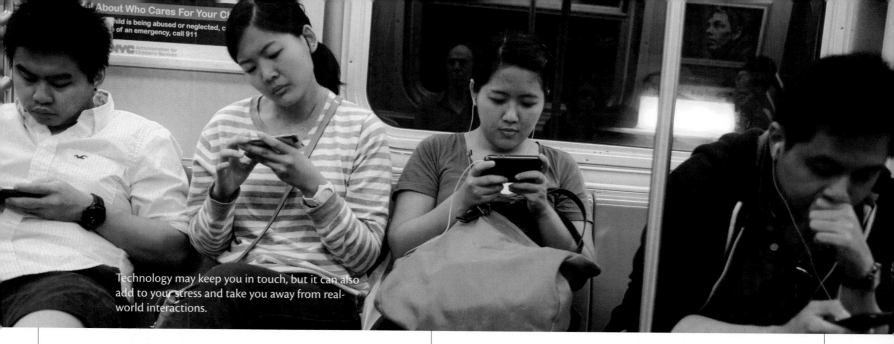
Technology may keep you in touch, but it can also add to your stress and take you away from real-world interactions.

to compete for grades, athletic positions, and job offers can lead to immense pressure.

Financial pressures are also increasing, on nearly everyone. Over the past few years, the annual Stress in America survey has indicated that American adults are increasingly experiencing money, work, and housing concerns as major sources of stress in their lives (Figure 3.4).[46] Students aren't immune, either. Challenging classes can be tough enough, but many students also work at least part time to pay the bills. Even in times of economic prosperity, students often have a hard time meeting all of their costs and obligations on limited budgets; a tough economic downturn like today's can increase those daily stresses.

Frustrations and Conflicts Disparity between our goals (what we hope to obtain in life) and our behaviors (actions that may or may not lead to these goals) can trigger frustration. Conflicts occur when we are forced to decide among competing motives, impulses, desires, and behaviors, or to face demands incompatible with our own values and sense of importance. College students away from their families and familiar communities for the first time may face conflicts among parental values, their own beliefs, and the beliefs of those different from themselves.

Overload We've all experienced times when the combined demands of work, responsibilities, and relationships seem to be pulling us under—and our physical, mental, and emotional reserves are insufficient to deal with it all. Students suffering from **overload** may experience depression, sleeplessness, mood swings, frustration, and anxiety.[47] Unrelenting overload can lead to a state of physical and mental exhaustion known as *burnout*.

Stressful Environments For many students, the environment around them can cause significant stress. Unscrupulous landlords have been known to exploit struggling students by leasing them substandard, even unhealthy, apartments. Conflict with difficult roommates can also cause major environmental stress. Although rare, natural disasters such as flooding, earthquakes, hurricanes, blizzards, and tornadoes can disrupt students' ability to conduct their daily lives. Often equally damaging are environmental **back-ground distressors**—including noise, air, and water pollution; allergy-aggravating pollen and dust; and second-hand smoke—that trigger a constant resistance phase.

Bias and Discrimination Diversity of students, faculty members, and staff enriches everyone's educational experience. It also challenges us to examine our attitudes and biases. Those perceived as dissimilar due to race, ethnicity, religious affiliation, age, sexual orientation—or differences in viewpoint, appearance, behavior, or background—may become victims of subtle and not-so-subtle bigotry, insensitivity, harassment, or hostility, or may simply be ignored.[48]

Evidence of the health effects of excessive stress in minority groups abounds. For example, African Americans suffer higher rates of hypertension, CVD, and most cancers than do whites.[49] Although poverty and socioeconomic status have been blamed for much of the spike in hypertension rates for African Americans and other marginalized groups, this chronic, physically debilitating stress may reflect real and perceived effects of harassment in society even more than it reflects actual poverty.[50]

International students experience unique adjustment issues related to language barriers, cultural barriers, and a lack of social support, among other challenges. Academic stress may pose a particular problem for the more than 690,000 international students who have left family and friends in their native countries to study in the United States. Yet many international students refrain from seeking emotional support from others because of cultural norms, feelings of shame, or the belief that seeking support is a sign of weakness. This, coupled with language barriers, cultural conflicts, and other stressors, can lead international students to suffer significantly more stress-related illnesses than their American counterparts.[51]

check yourself

- **What are five sources of psychosocial stress?**
- **Which psychosocial sources of stress do you encounter most frequently?**

Internal Causes of Stress

learning **outcomes**

■ **Discuss and classify internal causes of stress.**

Although stress can come from the environment and other external sources, it can result from internal factors as well. Internal stressors such as negative appraisal, low self-esteem, and low self-efficacy can cause unsettling thoughts or feelings, and can ultimately affect your health.[52] It is important to address and manage these internal stressors.

Appraisal and Stress Throughout life, we encounter many different demands and potential stressors—some biological, some psychological, and others sociological. In any case, it is our **appraisal** of these demands, rather than the demands themselves, that results in our experiencing stress. Appraisal is defined as the interpretation and evaluation of information provided to the brain by the senses. Appraisal is not a conscious activity, but rather a natural process that the brain constantly performs. As new information becomes available, appraisal helps us recognize stressors, evaluate them on the basis of past experiences and emotions, and decide how to cope with them. When you perceive that your coping resources are sufficient to meet life's demands, you experience little or no stress. By contrast, when you perceive that life's demands exceed your coping resources, you are likely to feel strain and distress.

Self-Esteem and Self-Efficacy *Self-esteem* refers to how you feel about yourself. Self-esteem varies; it can and does continually change.[53] When you feel good about yourself, you are less likely to respond to or interpret an event as stressful. Conversely, if you place little or no value on yourself and believe you have inadequate coping skills, you become susceptible to stress and strain.[54] Of particular concern, research with high school and college students has found that low self-esteem and stressful life events significantly predict **suicidal ideation**, a desire to die and thoughts about suicide. On a more positive note, research has also indicated that it is possible to increase an individual's ability to cope with stress by increasing self-esteem.[55]

Self-efficacy is another important factor in the ability to cope with life's challenges. Self-efficacy refers to belief or confidence in one's skills and performance abilities.[56] Self-efficacy is considered one of the most important personality traits that influences psychological and physiological stress responses and has been found to predict a number of health behaviors in college students.[57]

Developing self-efficacy is also vital to coping with and overcoming academic pressures and worries. For example, by learning to handle anxiety around testing situations, you improve your chances of performing well; the more you feel yourself capable of handling testing situations, the greater will be your sense of academic self-efficacy.

Type A and Type B Personalities It should come as no surprise to you that personality can have an impact on whether you are happy and socially well adjusted or sad and socially isolated. However, your personality may affect more than just your social interactions: It may be a critical factor in your stress level, as well as in your risk for CVD, cancer, and other chronic and infectious diseases.

In 1974, physicians Meyer Friedman and Ray Rosenman published a book indicating that Type A individuals had a greatly increased risk of heart disease.[58] *Type A* personalities are defined as hard-driving, competitive, time-driven perfectionists. In contrast, *Type B* personalities are described as being relaxed, noncompetitive, and more tolerant of others.

Today, most researchers recognize that none of us will be wholly Type A or Type B all of the time. We might exhibit either type as we respond to the various challenges of our daily lives. In addition, recent research indicates that not all Type A people experience negative health consequences; in fact, some hard-driving

People with Type A personalities—hard-driving, competitive perfectionists—often have high levels of stress.

individuals seem to thrive on their supercharged lifestyles. Only those Type A individuals who exhibit a "toxic core"—who have disproportionate amounts of anger; are distrustful of others; and have a cynical, glass-half-empty approach to life, in total, a set of characteristics referred to as **hostility**—are at increased risk for heart disease.[59]

Type C and Type D Personalities In addition to CVD risks, personality types have been linked to increased risk for a variety of illnesses ranging from asthma to cancer. *Type C* personality is one such type. Typically, Type C people are stoic and tend to deny feelings. They have a tendency to conform to the wishes of others (or to be "pleasers"), a lack of assertiveness, and an inclination toward feelings of helplessness or hopelessness. Possibly as a result of these characteristics, research indicates they are more susceptible to illnesses such as asthma, multiple sclerosis, autoimmune disorders, and cancer.[60] These are the "nice" guys and gals who really do finish last when it comes to their health.

A more recently identified personality type is *Type D* (distressed), characterized by a tendency toward excessive negative worry, irritability, gloom, and social inhibition. Several recent studies have shown that Type D people may be up to eight times more likely to die of a heart attack or sudden cardiac death.[61]

Psychological Hardiness According to psychologist Susanne Kobasa, **psychological hardiness** may negate self-imposed stress associated with Type A behavior. Psychologically hardy people are characterized by control, commitment, and willingness to embrace challenge.[62] People with a sense of control are able to accept responsibility for their behaviors and change those that they discover to be debilitating. People with a sense of commitment have good self-esteem and understand their purpose in life. Those who embrace challenge see change as a stimulating opportunity for personal growth. The concept of hardiness has been studied extensively, and many researchers believe it is the foundation of an individual's ability to cope with stress and remain healthy.[63]

Patterns of Thinking People fall into patterns and ways of thinking that can cause stress and increase their levels of anxiety. The fact is, your thought patterns can be your own worst enemy. If you can become aware of the internal messages you are giving yourself, you can recognize them and work to change them. Some strategies for doing this include:

- **Reframe a distressing event from a positive perspective.** Reframing is a stress-management technique that helps you change your perspective on a situation to a more positive vantage point. For example, if you feel perpetually frustrated that you can't be the best in every class, reframe the issue to highlight your strengths.
- **Break the worry habit.** If you are preoccupied with "what if's" and worst case scenarios, doubts and fears can sap your strength and send your stress levels soaring. The following suggestions can help slow the worry drain:
  - If you must worry, create a "worry period"—a 20 minute time period each day when you can journal or talk about it. After that, move on.

- Try to focus on the many things that are going right, rather than the one thing that might go wrong.
- Learn to accept what you cannot change. Chronic worriers want to be in control, but each of us must learn to live with some uncertainty.
- **Look at life as being fluid.** If you accept that change is a natural part of living and growing, the jolt of changes will become less stressful.
- **Moderate your expectations.** Aim high, but be realistic about your circumstances and motivation.
- **Weed out trivia.** Cardiologist Robert Eliot offers two rules for coping with life's challenges: "Don't sweat the small stuff," and remember, "It's all small stuff."
- **Tolerate mistakes by yourself and others.** Rather than getting angry or frustrated by mishaps, evaluate what happened and learn from it.

Skills for Behavior Change

OVERCOMING TEST-TAKING ANXIETY

Here's an example of how to increase self-efficacy in a familiar situation—an academic exam. Try these helpful hints when approaching your next exam, and you might just reduce your stress levels as well as improve your grade.

Before the Exam
- **Manage your study time. Start studying a week before your test to reduce anxiety. Do a limited review the night before, get a good night's sleep, and arrive for the exam early.**
- **Build your test-taking self-esteem. On an index card, write down three reasons you will pass the exam. Keep the card with you and review it whenever you study. When you get the test, write your three reasons on the test or on a piece of scrap paper.**
- **Eat a balanced meal before the exam. Avoid sugar and rich or heavy foods, as well as foods that might upset your stomach. You want to feel your best.**
- **If you feel that you are a slow reader and need more time, discuss this in advance with your teacher or test administrator.**

During the Test
- **Manage your time during the test. Decide how much time you need to take the test, review your answers, and go back over questions you might be stuck on. Hold to this schedule.**
- **Slow down and pay attention. When you open your test book, always write "RTFQ" (Read the Full Question) at the top. Make sure you understand the question before answering.**
- **Stay on track. If you begin to get anxious, reread your three reasons for success.**

check yourself

- **What are five causes of internal stress?**
- **Which internal causes of stress do you experience most frequently?**

Stress Management Techniques: Mental and Physical Approaches

- **Examine mental and physical approaches to stress management.**

Being on your own in college may pose challenges, but it also lets you take control of and responsibility for your life and take steps to reduce negative stressors. **Coping** is the act of managing events or conditions to lessen the physical or psychological effects of excess stress.[64] One of the most effective ways to combat stressors is to build coping strategies and skills, known collectively as *stress-management techniques*.

Practicing Mental Work to Reduce Stress

Your perceptions often contribute to your stress, so assessing your "self-talk," beliefs, and actions are good first steps. Here's how:

- Make a list of things you're worried about.
- Examine the causes of your problems and worries. Perceptions are often part of the problem; try assessing your "self-talk," beliefs, and actions.
- Consider the size of each problem. What are the consequences of doing nothing? Of taking action?

- List your options, including ones you may not like much.
- Outline a plan, then act. Even little things can make a big difference.
- Evaluate. How did you do? Do you need to change your actions to achieve a better outcome next time? How?

One way to anticipate and prepare for specific stressors is a technique known as **stress inoculation**. Suppose speaking in front of a class scares you. To prevent freezing up during a presentation, practice in front of friends or a video camera. Dealing with such specific fears helps you develop resistance; larger fears then seem less overwhelming.

Negative self-talk can take the form of *pessimism*, or focusing on the negative; *perfectionism*, or expecting superhuman standards; *should-ing*, or reprimanding yourself for things you should have done; *blaming* yourself or others for circumstances and events; and *dichotomous thinking*, in which everything is seen as either entirely good or bad.[65] To combat negative self-talk, become aware of an irrational or overreactive thought, interrupt it by saying "stop" (under your breath or out loud), then replace it with positive thoughts—a process called **cognitive restructuring**.

Taking Physical Action

Physical activities can complement your mental and emotional strategies of stress management:

- **Exercise regularly.** The human stress response is intended to end in physical activity; exercise "burns off" stress hormones by directing them toward their intended metabolic function[66] and can combat stress by raising levels of endorphins—mood-elevating, painkilling hormones—in the bloodstream.
- **Get enough sleep.** Adequate sleep allows you to cope with multiple stressors more effectively, and be more productive.
- **Learn to relax.** You can use simple relaxation techniques at any time. As your body relaxes, your heart rate slows and your blood pressure and metabolic rate decrease.
- **Eat healthfully.** A balanced, healthy diet will help provide the stamina you need to get through problems while stress-proofing you in ways not yet fully understood. Undereating, overeating, and eating the wrong foods can create distress in the body. In particular, avoid **sympathomimetics**, foods that produce (or mimic) stresslike responses, such as caffeine.

Are college students more stressed out than other groups?

The combination of a new environment, peer and parental pressure, and the demands of course work, campus activities, and social life contribute to above average stress levels in college students.

- **What are four effective mental or physical approaches to managing stress?**

Stress Management Techniques: Managing Emotional Responses

learning outcomes

■ **Explain how management of emotional responses contributes to stress management.**

We often get upset not by realities, but by our faulty perceptions. Stress management requires examining your emotional responses to interactions with others—and remembering that you are responsible for the emotion and the resulting behaviors. Learning to identify emotions based on irrational beliefs, or expressed and interpreted in an over-the-top manner, can help you stop such emotions or express them in healthy and appropriate ways.

Learn to Laugh, Be Joyful, and Cry Smiling, laughing, and even crying can elevate mood, relieve stress, and improve relationships. In the moment, laughter and joy raise endorphin levels, increase blood oxygen, decrease stress, relieve pain, and enhance productivity; additional evidence for long-term effects on immune function and protection against disease is only starting to be understood.[67]

Fight the Anger Urge Anger usually results when we feel we have lost control of a situation or are frustrated by events we can do little

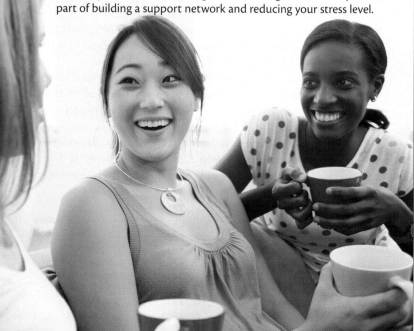

Spending time communicating and socializing can be an important part of building a support network and reducing your stress level.

about. Major sources of anger include (1) perceived *threats* to self or others we care about; (2) *reactions to injustice*; (3) *fear*; (4) *faulty emotional reasoning* or misinterpretation of normal events; (5) *low frustration tolerance*, often fueled by stress, drugs, or lack of sleep; (6) *unreasonable expectations* for ourselves and others; and (7) *people rating*, or applying derogatory ratings to others.

To deal with anger, you can express, suppress, or calm it. Surprisingly, expressing anger is probably the healthiest option, if you do so assertively rather than aggressively. Several strategies can help redirect aggression into assertion:[68]

■ **Recognize anger patterns and learn to de-escalate them.** Note what angers you. What thoughts or feelings led up to your boiling point? Try changing your self-talk, or interrupting anger patterns by counting to 10 or taking deep breaths.

■ **Verbally de-escalate.** When couples fight, using words that suggest thoughtfulness—*think, because, reason, why*—can reduce conflict, demonstrating consideration for one's partner and the issues at hand.[69]

■ **Plan ahead.** Explore ways to minimize your exposure to anger triggers such as traffic jams.

■ **Develop a support system.** Find a few close friends you can confide in or vent your frustration to. Allow them to listen and provide perspective. Don't wear down supporters with continual rants.

■ **Develop realistic expectations.** Anger is often the result of unmet expectations, frustrations, resentments, and impatience. Are your expectations of yourself and others realistic?

■ **Turn complaints into requests.** Try reworking a problem into a request. Instead of screaming because your neighbors' music woke you up at 2 AM, talk with them. Try to reach an agreement.

■ **Leave past anger in the past.** Learn to resolve issues that have caused pain, frustration, or stress. If necessary, seek professional counsel.

Invest in Loved Ones Too often, we don't make time for the people most important to us: friends and family. Cultivate and nurture relationships built on trust, mutual acceptance and understanding, honesty, and caring. Treating others empathically provides them with a measure of emotional security and reduces *their* anxiety.

Cultivate Your Spiritual Side Spiritual health and spiritual practice can link you to a community and offer perspective on the things that truly matter.

check yourself

■ **How can emotions affect your stress levels?**

Stress Management Techniques: Managing Your Time

- **Describe strategies for effective time management.**

Ever put off writing a paper until the night before it was due? If you're like up to 95 percent of all college students, you **procrastinate**, or voluntarily delay doing some task despite expecting to be worse off for it.[70] Procrastination can result in academic difficulties, financial problems, relationship problems, and stress-related ailments.[71] For some, procrastination may stem from fear of failure or a wish to avoid being put on the spot; distraction sends others in pursuit of fun. Afterwards, stress levels increase, sleep goes by the wayside, caffeine intake increases, and emotions flare.

According to psychologist Shane Owens and his colleagues at Hofstra University, one key to beating procrastination is setting clear "implementation intentions."[72] You could specify that you will work on your paper from 6 to 7 PM each night for a week. A plan of action, with interim deadlines and associated rewards, can motivate you along the way.

Try logging your activities for a week—everything from going to class to doing laundry to texting friends—and note the time you spend doing each. Once you've kept track for several days, you can then assess your results and make changes accordingly. Use these time-management tips to help you:

- **Do one thing at a time.** Don't try to watch television, wash clothes, and write your term paper all at once.
  - **Clear your desk.** Toss unnecessary papers; file those you'll need later. Read your mail, recycle what you don't need, and file the rest for later action.
    - **Prioritize tasks.** Make a daily "to do" list and stick to it. List things you must do today, things you must do but not immediately, and "nice to dos" that you can take on if you finish the others or if they include fun.

- **Find a clean, comfortable place to work, and avoid interruptions.** For a project that requires concentration, schedule uninterrupted time. Close your door and turn off your phone—or go to a quiet room in the library or student union.
- **Reward yourself.** Did you finish a task? Do something nice for yourself. Breaks give you time to recharge.
- **Work when you're at your best.** If you're a morning person, study in the morning. Take breaks when you start to slow down.
- **Break overwhelming tasks into small pieces, and allocate time to each.** If you're floundering on a task, move on and come back to it when you're refreshed.
- **Remember that time is precious.** Try to value each day in the moment.

Skills for **Behavior Change**

LEARN TO SAY NO AND MEAN IT!

Is your calendar so full you barely have time to breathe? Do you have difficulty saying no? A bulging calendar can be a misplaced badge of honor. Ditch the idea that you're indispensable or superhuman, and avoid overcommitment.

- **Be sympathetic but firm.** Explain that you can't take on one more project right now. If they pressure you, say it was nice talking, but you have to run.
- **Don't say you want to think about it.** This only leads to more forceful requests later. Say "not this time," and reiterate that you can't take on any more obligations now.
- **Don't give in to guilt.** Stick to your guns. You don't owe anyone your time.
- **Avoid spontaneous "yes" responses to new projects.** Make a rule that you will take at least a day to think about committing your time. Then, if you still think it's a good idea, choose something to take off your plate in exchange.
- **Schedule time for yourself first.** Stop and prioritize. Keep two or three "must dos" on your list each day. Cross off "I don't have to, but I said yes" events; admit you overcommitted and bow out. Add one or two "I really want to" items.
- **Remember that there are 24 hours in every day and you need at least 8 for sleep.** Consider how each list item will help you grow personally or professionally, or will contribute to society. Choose wisely.

- **What are some time management strategies that could help reduce your stress levels?**

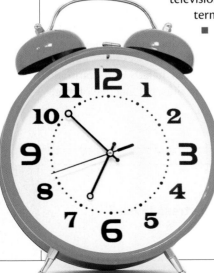

Stress Management Techniques: Managing Your Finances

■ **Describe strategies for effective time management.**

Higher education can impose a huge financial burden on parents, students, and communities. In recent studies, nearly two-thirds of students indicated that the "current economic situation significantly affected my college choice." Fifty-three percent of incoming students used loans to help pay for college, and 73 percent used grants and scholarships—both significant increases over past years, with more students than ever using multiple strategies to make ends meet.[73] The economic downturn of the past few years is likely pushing already financially stressed students closer to the breaking point.

Several factors are converging to increase today's students' financial woes. First, a recession has caused many parents to lose their jobs. Faced with dwindling resources at home, many students are being forced to look for part-time or even full-time work. These students may encounter increasing competition for even the lowest-paying jobs as displaced workers take these jobs to stay afloat financially. Already known to carry a disproportionate level of credit card debt, students are resorting to using plastic to pay for essentials, leading to more debt and higher stress.

Consider Downshifting

Today's lifestyles are hectic and pressure packed, and stress often comes from trying to keep up. Many people, questioning whether "having it all" is worth it, are taking a step back and

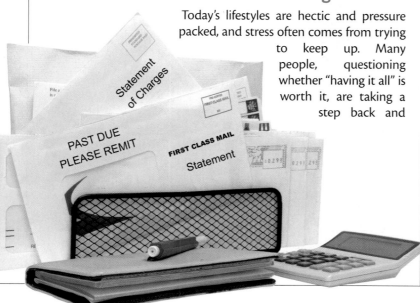

35%

of college students report that their finances have been very difficult to handle during the past 12 months.

simplifying their lives. This trend has been labeled *downshifting,* or *voluntary simplicity.* Moving from a large urban area to a smaller town or leaving a high-stress job for one that makes you happy are examples of downshifting.

Downshifting involves a fundamental alteration in values and honest introspection about what is important in life. It means cutting down on shopping habits, buying only what you need to get by, and living within modest means. When you contemplate any form of downshift or perhaps even start your career this way, it's important to move slowly and consider the following:

■ **Plan for health care costs.** Make sure that you budget for health insurance and basic preventive health services if you're not covered under your parents' plan. Understand your coverage, and keep on top of shifting health care policy and skyrocketing rates. This should be a top priority.

■ **Determine your ultimate goal.** What is most important to you, and what will you need to reach that goal? What can you do without?

■ **Make both short- and long-term plans for simplifying your life.** Set up your plans in doable steps, and work slowly toward each step.

■ **Complete a financial inventory.** How much money will you need to do the things you want to do? Will you live alone or share costs with roommates? Do you need a car, or can you rely on public transportation? Pay off your debt, and get used to paying with cash. If you don't have the cash, don't buy.

■ **Select the right career.** Look for work that you enjoy and that isn't necessarily driven by salary. Can you be happy taking a lower-paying job if it is less stressful or gives you satisfaction?

■ **Consider options for saving money.** Downshifting doesn't mean renouncing money; it means choosing not to let money dictate your life. Saving is still important. If you're just getting started, you need to prepare for emergencies and for future plans.

■ **Resist credit card offers.** Racking up debt in school can affect your finances for years to come.

■ **Which of these strategies can be used to improve your current financial situation?**

Relaxation Techniques for Stress Management

learning outcomes

- **Discuss relaxation techniques that can reduce stress.**

Relaxation techniques to reduce stress have been practiced for centuries, and there is a wide array of practices from which to choose. Common techniques include yoga, qigong, tai chi, deep breathing, meditation, visualization, progressive muscle relaxation, massage therapy, biofeedback, and hypnosis.

Yoga Yoga is an ancient practice that combines meditation, stretching, and breathing exercises designed to relax, refresh, and rejuvenate. It began about 5,000 years ago in India and has been evolving ever since. In the United States today, some 20 million adults practice many versions of yoga.

Classical yoga is the ancestor of nearly all modern forms of yoga. Breathing, poses, and verbal mantras are often part of classical yoga. Of the many branches of classical yoga, *Hatha yoga* is the most well known because it is the most body focused. This style of yoga involves the practice of breath control and *asanas*—held postures and choreographed movements that enhance strength and flexibility.

Qigong *Qigong* (pronounced "chee-kong") is one of the fastest-growing and most widely accepted forms of mind-body health exercises. Some of the country's largest health care organizations, such as Kaiser Permanente, include this relaxation technique in their systems, particularly for people suffering from chronic pain or stress. Qigong is an ancient Chinese practice that involves becoming aware of and learning to control *qi* (or *chi*, pronounced "chee"), or vital energy in your body. According to Chinese medicine, a complex system of internal pathways called *meridians* carry *qi* throughout your body. If your *qi* becomes stagnant or blocked, you'll feel sluggish or powerless. Qigong incorporates a series of flowing movements, breath techniques, mental visualization exercises, and vocalizations of healing sounds designed to restore balance and integrate and refresh the mind and body.

Tai Chi *Tai chi* (pronounced "ty-chee") is sometimes described as "meditation in motion." Originally developed in China as a form of self-defense, this graceful form of exercise has existed for about 2,000

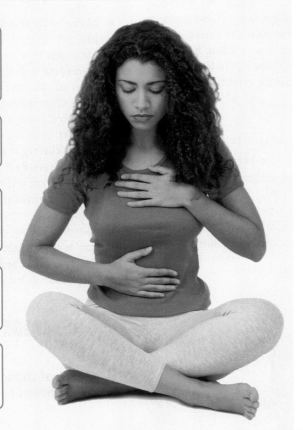

Figure 3.5 Diaphragmatic Breathing
This exercise will help you learn to breathe deeply as a way to relieve stress. Practice this for 5 to 10 minutes several times a day, and soon diaphragmatic breathing will become natural for you.

1 Assume a natural, comfortable position either sitting up straight with your head, neck, and shoulders relaxed, or lying on your back with your knees bent and your head supported. Close your eyes and loosen binding clothes.

2 In order to feel your abdomen moving as you breathe, place one hand on your upper chest and the other just below your rib cage.

3 Breathe in slowly and deeply through your nose. Feel your stomach expanding into your hand. The hand on your chest should move as little as possible.

4 Exhale slowly through your mouth. Feel the fall of your stomach away from your hand. Again, the hand on your chest should move as little as possible.

5 Concentrate on the act of breathing. Shut out external noise. Focus on inhaling and exhaling, the route the air is following, and the rise and fall of your stomach.

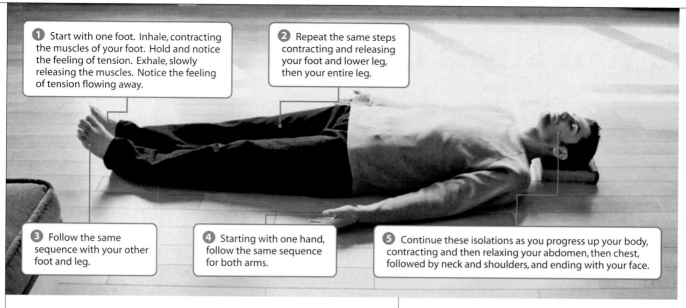

① Start with one foot. Inhale, contracting the muscles of your foot. Hold and notice the feeling of tension. Exhale, slowly releasing the muscles. Notice the feeling of tension flowing away.

② Repeat the same steps contracting and releasing your foot and lower leg, then your entire leg.

③ Follow the same sequence with your other foot and leg.

④ Starting with one hand, follow the same sequence for both arms.

⑤ Continue these isolations as you progress up your body, contracting and then relaxing your abdomen, then chest, followed by neck and shoulders, and ending with your face.

Figure 3.6
Progressive Muscle Relaxation
Sit or lie down in a comfortable position and follow the steps described to increase your awareness of tension in your body.

years. Tai chi is noncompetitive and self-paced. To do tai chi, you perform a defined series of postures or movements in a slow, graceful manner. Each movement or posture flows into the next without pause. Tai chi has been widely practiced in China for centuries and is becoming increasingly popular around the world, both as a basic exercise program and as a complement to other health care methods. Health benefits include stress reduction, improved balance, and increased flexibility.

Diaphragmatic or Deep Breathing Typically, we breathe using only the upper chest and thoracic region rather than involving the abdominal region. Simply stated, diaphragmatic breathing is deep breathing that maximally fills the lungs by involving the movement of the diaphragm and lower abdomen. This technique is commonly used in yoga exercises and in other meditative practices. Try the diaphragmatic breathing exercise in Figure 3.5 right now and see if you feel more relaxed!

Meditation There are many different forms of **meditation**. Most involve sitting quietly for 15 minutes or longer, focusing on a particular word or symbol or observing one's thoughts, and controlling breathing. Practiced by Eastern religions for centuries, meditation is seen as an important form of introspection and personal renewal. In stress management, it can calm the body and quiet the mind, creating a sense of peace.

Visualization Often it is our own thoughts and imagination that provoke distress by conjuring up worst-case scenarios. Our imagination, however, can also be tapped to reduce stress. In **visualization**, you create mental scenes using your imagination. The choice of mental images is unlimited, but natural settings such as ocean beaches and mountain lakes are often used, because they call to mind places people often go to escape the stresses of home, school, or work. Recalling specific physical senses of sight, sound, smell, taste, and touch can replace stressful stimuli with peaceful or pleasurable thoughts.

Progressive Muscle Relaxation Progressive muscle relaxation involves systematically contracting and relaxing different muscle groups in your body. The standard pattern is to begin with the feet and work your way up your body, contracting and releasing as you go (Figure 3.6). The process is designed to teach awareness of the different feelings of muscle tension and muscle release. With practice, you can quickly identify tension in your body when you are facing stressful situations, then consciously release that tension to calm yourself.

Massage Therapy If you have ever had someone massage your stiff neck or aching feet, you know that massage is an excellent way to relax. Techniques vary from deep-tissue massage to gentler acupressure.

Biofeedback **Biofeedback** involves monitoring your physical responses to stress via a machine. A typical biofeedback machine records perspiration, heart rate, respiration rate, blood pressure, surface body temperature, muscle tension, and other stress responses. You use various relaxation techniques while hooked up to the machine, and then, through trial and error and feedback signals from the machine, you learn to lower your stress responses. Eventually, you develop the ability to recognize and lower stress responses without the help of the machine.

Hypnosis **Hypnosis** requires a person to focus on one thought, object, or voice, thereby freeing the right hemisphere of the brain to become more active. The person then becomes unusually responsive to suggestion. Whether self-induced or induced by someone else, hypnosis can reduce certain types of stress.

check yourself

- **What are three potential benefits to learning a variety of relaxation techniques?**
- **Which relaxation technique is the most effective for you? Why?**

Assessyourself

What's Your Stress Level?

An interactive version of this assessment is available online. Download it from the Live It! section of www.pearsonhighered.com/donatelle.

1 The Student Stress Scale

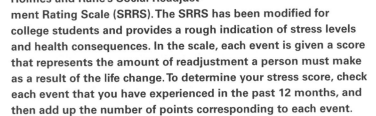

The **Student Stress Scale** represents an adaptation of Holmes and Rahe's Social Readjustment Rating Scale (SRRS). The SRRS has been modified for college students and provides a rough indication of stress levels and health consequences. In the scale, each event is given a score that represents the amount of readjustment a person must make as a result of the life change. To determine your stress score, check each event that you have experienced in the past 12 months, and then add up the number of points corresponding to each event.

1. Death of a close family member	____	100
2. Death of a close friend	____	73
3. Divorce between parents	____	65
4. Jail term	____	63
5. Major personal injury or illness	____	63
6. Marriage	____	58
7. Firing from a job	____	50
8. Failure of an important course	____	47
9. Change in health of a family member	____	45
10. Pregnancy	____	45
11. Sex problems	____	44
12. Serious argument with close friend	____	40
13. Change in financial status	____	39
14. Change of major	____	39
15. Trouble with parents	____	39
16. New girlfriend or boyfriend	____	37
17. Increase in workload at school	____	37
18. Outstanding personal achievement	____	36
19. First quarter/semester in school	____	36
20. Change in living conditions	____	31
21. Serious argument with an instructor	____	30
22. Lower grades than expected	____	29
23. Change in sleeping habits	____	29
24. Change in social activities	____	29
25. Change in eating habits	____	28
26. Chronic car trouble	____	26
27. Change in number of family gatherings	____	26
28. Too many missed classes	____	25
29. Change of college	____	24
30. Dropping of more than one class	____	23
31. Minor traffic violations	____	20
Total:		

SCORING PART 1:

If your score is 300 or higher, you may be at high risk for developing a stress-related illness. If your score is between 150 and 300, you have approximately a 50-50 chance of experiencing a serious health problem within the next 2 years. If your score is below 150, you have a 1 in 3 chance of experiencing a serious health change in the next few years.

Source: Adapted from T. Holmes and R. H. Rahe, "The Social Readjustment Rating Scale," *Journal of Psychosomatic Research* 11, no. 2 (1967): 213–18. Copyright © 1967 Elsevier, Inc. Reprinted with permission from Elsevier.

2 How Do You Respond to Stress?

Read the following scenarios and choose the response that you would most likely have to these stressful events.

1. You've been waiting 20 minutes for a table in a crowded restaurant, and the hostess seats a group that arrived after you.
   a. You yell, "Hey! I was here first!" in an irritated voice.
   b. You say "Excuse me" in a polite voice and inform the other group or the hostess that you were there first.
   c. You walk out of the restaurant in disgust. Obviously the hostess was willfully ignoring you.
2. You come home to find the kitchen looking like a disaster area and your spouse/roommate lounging in front of the TV.
   a. You pick a fight about how your spouse/roommate never does anything and always expects you to clean up after him or her.
   b. You sit down next to your spouse/roommate and ask if he or she would take a 5-minute break from the TV show to help you clean.
   c. You don't say anything but instead tense up and angrily start cleaning the kitchen, making as much noise as possible.

3. You have to present a paper in front of your class, and you are anxious about doing a good job.
   a. You get flustered during the presentation and snap at your fellow classmates when they ask questions about your topic.
   b. You ask a friend to help you practice the presentation ahead of time so you can feel confident going in to class.
   c. You lose sleep worrying about the presentation, and afterward you spend the rest of the day reliving all the mistakes you made.

4. Your partner is seen out with another person and appears to be acting quite close to the person.
   a. You immediately assume your partner is cheating on you. Infuriated, you launch into a stream of accusations the next time you are together.
   b. The next time you see your partner, you calmly mention your concerns and describe your feelings, giving him or her a chance to explain the situation.
   c. You decide your partner no longer cares about you and spend the evening reproaching yourself for being so unlovable.

5. You aren't able to study as much as you'd like for an exam and, when you get it back, you find that you did horribly.
   a. You angrily bad-mouth your professor to your friends and anyone else who will listen.
   b. You make an appointment to talk with the professor and determine what you can do to improve on the next exam.

c. You decide you're just crummy at the subject and don't even bother studying at all the next time.

ANALYZING PART 2

If you chose mostly "a" responses, you are probably a hot reactor who responds to mildly stressful situations with a fight-or-flight adrenaline rush. Before you honk or make obscene gestures at the guy who cuts you off in traffic, remember that the only thing you'll hasten by reacting is a decline in health. Look at ways to change your perceptions and cope more effectively.

If you chose mostly "b" responses, you are probably a cool reactor who tends to roll with the punches when a situation becomes stressful. This usually indicates a good level of coping; overall, you will suffer fewer health consequences when stressed. The key here is that you really are not stressed, and you really are calm and unworried about the situation—not just behaving as though you were.

If you chose mostly "c" responses, you have intense reactions to stress that you are prone to directing inward. This can negatively affect your health just as much as being explosive. To change your approach to stress, work on ways of building your senses of self-efficacy and self-esteem. Changing the way you think about yourself and others can help you approach stress in a more balanced and productive way.

Your Plan for Change

The Assess Yourself activity gave you the chance to look at your stress responses and identify particular situations in your life that cause stress. Now that you are aware of these patterns, you can change behaviors that lead to increased stress.

Today, you can:

◯ Practice one new stress-management technique. For example, you could spend 10 minutes doing a deep-breathing exercise or find a good spot on campus to meditate.

◯ Buy a journal and write down stressful events or symptoms of stress that you experience. Try to focus on intense emotional experiences and explore how they affect you.

Within the next 2 weeks, you can:

◯ Attend a class or workshop in yoga, tai chi, qigong, meditation, or some other stress-relieving activity. Look for beginner classes offered on campus or in your community.

◯ Make a list of the papers, projects, and tests that you have over the coming semester and create a schedule for them. Break projects and term papers into small, manageable tasks, and try to be realistic about how much time you'll need to get these tasks done.

By the end of the semester, you can:

◯ Keep track of the money you spend and where it goes. Establish a budget and follow it for at least a month.

◯ Find some form of exercise you can do regularly. You may consider joining a gym or just arranging regular "walk dates" or pickup basketball games with your friends. Try to exercise at least 30 minutes every day.

Summary

- Stress is an inevitable part of our lives. *Eustress* refers to stress associated with positive events; *distress* refers to negative events.
- The alarm, resistance, and exhaustion phases of the general adaptation syndrome (GAS) involve physiological responses to both real and imagined stressors. Prolonged arousal may be detrimental to health.
- Undue stress for extended periods of time can compromise the immune system. Stress has been linked to cardiovascular disease (CVD), weight gain, hair loss, diabetes, digestive problems, increased susceptibility to infectious diseases, and diminished libido. Psychoneuroimmunology is the science that analyzes the relationship between the mind's reaction to stress and immune function.
- Stress can affect intellectual and psychological health and contribute to depression and anxiety.
- Psychosocial factors contributing to stress include change, hassles, relationships, pressure, conflict, overload, and environmental stressors. Persons subjected to discrimination or bias may face unusually high levels of stress. Some sources of stress are internal and related to appraisal, self-esteem, self-efficacy, personality, and psychological hardiness.
- College can be stressful. Recognizing the signs of stress is the first step toward better health. To manage stress, find coping skills that work for you—probably some combination of managing emotional responses, taking mental or physical action, downshifting, time management, managing finances, and relaxation techniques.

Pop Quiz

1. Even though Andre experienced stress when he graduated from college and moved to a new city, he viewed these changes as an opportunity for growth. What is Andre's stress called?
   a. Strain
   b. Distress
   c. Eustress
   d. Adaptive response

2. The branch of the autonomic nervous system that is responsible for energizing the body for either fight or flight and for triggering many other stress responses is the
   a. central nervous system.
   b. parasympathetic nervous system.
   c. sympathetic nervous system.
   d. endocrine system.

3. During what phase of the general adaptation syndrome has the physical and psychological energy used to fight the stressor been depleted?
   a. Alarm phase
   b. Resistance phase
   c. Endurance phase
   d. Exhaustion phase

4. A state of physical and mental exhaustion caused by excessive stress is called
   a. conflict
   b. overload
   c. hassles
   d. burnout

5. Losing your keys is an example of what psychosocial source of stress?
   a. Pressure
   b. Inconsistent behaviors
   c. Hassles
   d. Conflict

6. After 5 years of 70-hour workweeks, Tom decided to leave his high-paying, high-stress law firm and lead a simpler lifestyle. What is this trend called?
   a. Adaptation
   b. Conflict resolution
   c. Burnout reduction
   d. Downshifting

7. Which of the following test-taking techniques is not recommended to reduce test-taking stress?
   a. Plan ahead and study over a period of time for the test.
   b. Eat a balanced meal before the exam.
   c. Do all your studying the night before the exam so it is fresh in your mind.
   d. Remind yourself of three reasons you will pass the exam.

8. Which of the following is not an example of a time-management technique?
   a. Doing one thing at a time
   b. Rewarding yourself for finishing a task
   c. Practicing procrastination in completing homework assignments
   d. Breaking tasks into smaller pieces

9. Which of the following is an example of a chronic stressor?
   a. Giving a talk in public
   b. Meeting a deadline for a big project
   c. Dealing with a permanent disability
   d. Preparing for a job interview

10. In which stage of the general adaptation syndrome does the fight-or-flight response occur?
    a. Exhaustion stage
    b. Alarm stage
    c. Resistance stage
    d. Response stage

Answers to these questions can be found on page A-1.

Web Links

1. **American College Health Association.** This site provides information and data from the National College Health Assessment survey. www.acha.org

2. **American Psychological Association.** Here you can find current information and research on stress and stress-related conditions. www.apa.org/topics/stress

3. **Higher Education Research Institute.** This organization provides annual surveys of first-year and senior college students that cover academic, financial, and health-related issues. www.heri.ucla.edu

4. **National Institute of Mental Health.** This site from the National Institutes of Health is a resource for information on all aspects of mental health, including the effects of stress. www.nimh.nih.gov

Relationships and Sexuality

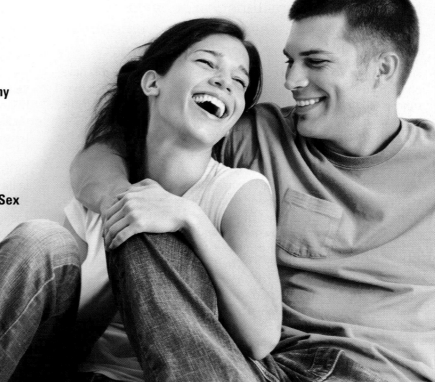

Humans are social animals—we have a basic need to belong and to feel loved. We can't live without interacting with others in some way. We build "social capital," or networks of friends, family, and significant others, who help us meet life's challenges. Numerous studies have shown that supportive interpersonal relationships are beneficial to health.[1]

All relationships involve a degree of risk. However, only by taking these risks can we grow and experience all life has to offer. This chapter examines healthy relationships and the communication skills necessary to create and maintain them. Expressing ourselves well and knowing how to listen and understand what others are saying are essential for healthy relationships.

Sexuality is a component of some of our most important relationships—and of our understanding of ourselves. How you experience yourself as a sexual person affects everything from your self-image to your identity, happiness, fertility, and health. Sexuality begins with our biological sex, gender, anatomy and physiology, and sexual functions, but it also encompasses values, beliefs, and attitudes about how we see ourselves as sexual beings and how we relate to others.

Characteristics and Types of Intimate Relationships

- **List characteristics of intimate relationships.**
- **Compare and contrast different theories of love.**

Intimate relationships can be defined in terms of four characteristics: *behavioral interdependence, need fulfillment, emotional attachment,* and *emotional availability.*

Behavioral interdependence refers to the impact that people have on each other as their lives intertwine. It may become stronger over time, to the point that each person would feel a great void if the other were gone.

Intimate relationships also provide *need fulfillment.* Through relationships with others, we fulfill our needs for *intimacy* (someone with whom we can share our feelings freely), *social integration* (someone with whom we can share worries and concerns), *nurturance* (someone we can take care of and who will take care of us), *assistance* (someone to help us in times of need), and *affirmation* (someone who will reassure us of our own worth and tell us that we matter).

Intimate relationships also involve strong bonds of *emotional attachment,* or feelings of love. When we hear the word *intimacy,* we often think of a sexual relationship. Although sex can play an important role in emotional attachment, a relationship can be very intimate and yet not sexual. Two people can be emotionally or spiritually intimate, or they can be intimate friends.

Emotional availability is the ability to give to and receive from others emotionally without fear of being hurt or rejected. At times, we may limit our emotional availability—for example, after a painful breakup, holding back can offer time for healing. However, some people who have experienced intense trauma find it difficult to be available emotionally.

Family Relationships

A family is a group whose central focus is to care for and love one another. The family is a dynamic institution that changes as society changes, and the definition of *family* changes over time. Historically, most families have been made up of people related by blood, marriage or long-term committed relationships, or adoption. Yet today, many other groups are recognized and functioning as family units. It is from our **family of origin**, those in our household during our first years, that we initially learn about feelings, problem solving, love, intimacy, and gender roles. We learn to negotiate relationships and have opportunities to communicate, develop attitudes and values, and explore spiritual beliefs. When we establish relationships outside the family, we often rely on experiences and skills modeled by our family of origin.

Relating to Yourself

You have probably heard that you must love yourself before you can honestly love someone else. Most of us begin to develop a healthy sense of self growing up with our families—a sense of being loved, being able to reach out to others, being able to accomplish our goals. That positive sense of self grows as we are accepted by others; forming loving relationships is a natural part of that growth and development for many.

Two qualities important to any good relationship are *accountability* and *self-nurturance.* **Accountability** entails recognizing that you are responsible for your own decisions, choices, and actions. **Self-nurturance** means developing individual potential through a balanced and realistic appreciation of self-worth and ability. Individuals on a path of accountability and self-nurturance have a much better chance of maintaining satisfying relationships with others.

Self-Esteem and Self-Acceptance Factors that affect your ability to nurture yourself and maintain healthy relationships include how you define yourself (*self-concept*) and evaluate yourself (*self-esteem*).

Your perception of yourself influences your relationship choices. If you feel unattractive or inferior to others, you may choose not to interact with them. Or you may unconsciously seek out

Does an intimate relationship have to be sexual?

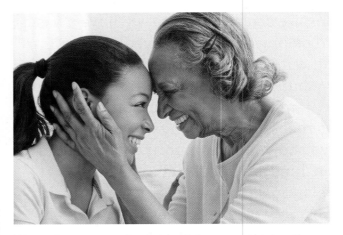

We may be accustomed to hearing *intimacy* used to describe romantic or sexual relationships, but intimate relationships can take many forms. The emotional bonds that characterize intimate relationships often span generations and give insight into each other's worlds.

individuals who confirm your view of yourself by treating you poorly. Conversely, a positive self-concept makes it easier to form relationships with people who nurture you and to interact with others in a healthy, balanced way.

Friendships

Friendships are often the first relationships we form outside our immediate families, and they can be some of our most stable and enduring. Being able to establish and maintain strong friendships may be a good predictor of success in establishing love relationships, because each requires shared interests and values, mutual acceptance, trust, and respect.

Getting to know someone well requires time, effort, and commitment. A good friend can be an honest and trustworthy companion, someone who honors and respects your strengths and weaknesses, who can share your joys and sorrows, and whom you can count on for support.

Romantic Relationships

Most people choose at some point to enter into an intimate romantic and sexual relationship with another person. Romantic relationships typically include all the characteristics of friendship as well as the following:

- **Fascination.** Lovers are often preoccupied by the other and want to think about, talk to, or be with the other.
- **Exclusiveness.** Lovers have a relationship that usually precludes having the same relationship with a third party. The love relationship often takes priority over all others.
- **Sexual desire.** Lovers desire physical intimacy and want to touch, hold, and engage in sexual activities with the other.
- **Giving the utmost.** Lovers care enough to give the utmost when the other is in need.
- **Being an advocate.** Lovers actively champion each other's interests and attempt to ensure that the other succeeds.

Theories of Love Love may mean different things to different people, depending on cultural values, age, gender, and situation. Many social scientists maintain that love may be of two kinds: *companionate* and *passionate*. Companionate love is a secure, affectionate, and trusting attachment, similar to what we may feel for family or close friends. *Passionate love* is an intense state of wanting to bond with another. It has three components. In the cognitive component, one has a preoccupation with, idealizes, and has an intense desire to know a person. The emotional component includes strong feelings, physiological arousal and attraction, and a desire for sexual intimacy. The behavioral component encompasses actions to know the other person's feelings, maintain physical closeness, and be helpful to the other.[2]

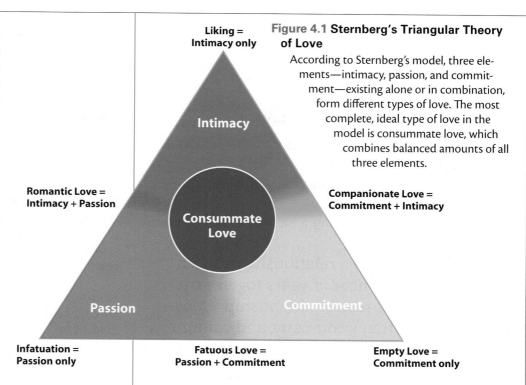

Figure 4.1 Sternberg's Triangular Theory of Love According to Sternberg's model, three elements—intimacy, passion, and commitment—existing alone or in combination, form different types of love. The most complete, ideal type of love in the model is consummate love, which combines balanced amounts of all three elements.

Liking = Intimacy only

Intimacy

Romantic Love = Intimacy + Passion

Companionate Love = Commitment + Intimacy

Consummate Love

Passion

Commitment

Infatuation = Passion only

Fatuous Love = Passion + Commitment

Empty Love = Commitment only

In his Triangular Theory of Love, psychologist Robert Sternberg proposes three key components to loving relationships (**Figure 4.1**):[3]

- **Intimacy.** The emotional component, which involves closeness, sharing, and mutual support.
- **Passion.** The motivational component, which includes lust, attraction, sexual arousal, and sharing.
- **Commitment.** The cognitive component, which includes the decision to be open to love in the short term and commitment to the relationship in the long term.

Sternberg uses the term *consummate love* to describe a combination of intimacy, passion, and commitment.

In an alternate theory, anthropologist Helen Fisher, among others, has hypothesized that attraction and love follow a fairly predictable pattern based on (1) *imprinting,* in which our evolutionary patterns, genetic predispositions, and past experiences trigger a romantic reaction; (2) *attraction,* in which neurochemicals produce feelings of euphoria and elation; (3) *attachment,* in which endorphins—natural opiates—cause lovers to feel peaceful, secure, and calm; and (4) production of a *cuddle chemical,* in which the brain secretes the hormone oxytocin, stimulating sensations during lovemaking and eliciting feelings of satisfaction and attachment.[4]

check yourself

- **What are the common characteristics of intimate relationships?**
- **What are the strengths and weaknesses of the proposed theories of love?**

Strategies for Success in Relationships

- **Compare characteristics of healthy and unhealthy relationships.**
- **Discuss factors affecting the choice of a romantic partner.**
- **Identify factors in achieving a healthy relationship.**

Although success in a relationship is often defined by the number of years together, it is factors such as respect, friendship, enjoyment of each other's company, and communication that are true measures of success.

What Makes A Healthy Relationship?

Satisfying and stable relationships share traits such as good communication, intimacy, and friendship (**Figure 4.2**). A key ingredient is trust, the degree of confidence each person feels in a relationship. Trust includes three fundamental elements:

1. **Predictability.** You can predict your partner's behavior, based on the knowledge that he or she acts in consistently positive ways.
2. **Dependability.** You can rely on your partner for support, particularly in situations where you feel threatened with hurt or rejection.
3. **Faith.** You feel certain about your partner's intentions and behavior.

How do you know whether you're in a healthy relationship?

- Do you love and care for yourself to the same extent you did before the relationship? Do you feel you can be yourself in the relationship?
- Do you share interests, values, and opinions? Is there mutual respect for, and civil discussion of, differences?
- Is there mutual encouragement and emotional support? Do you trust each other?
- Are you honest with each other? Can you comfortably express feelings, needs, and desires?
- Is there genuine caring and goodwill? Are you there for each other?
- Is there room for growth as you evolve and mature?

Choosing a Romantic Partner

The choice of partner is influenced by more than just chemical and psychological processes. One important factor is *proximity*—the more often you see someone, the more likely interaction will occur. We often choose partners based on similarities (in attitudes, values, intellect, interests, education, and socioeconomic status); the adage that "opposites attract" usually isn't true.

Also playing a significant role is *physical attraction*. Attraction is complex and influenced by social, biological, and cultural factors.[5]

Meeting People Online The Internet has revolutionized how we communicate and how we meet. Here are some online dating guidelines:

- As you get to know someone, ask about things such as hobbies, politics, religion, education, age, family background, and marital history and status. Note the answers you receive and beware of contradictions.
- Be suspicious of anyone who seems too good to be true. Trying too hard to please may mark a manipulative and potentially dangerous personality.
- Be honest about yourself; state your interests and characteristics fairly, including things you think might be less attractive.
- If you exchange pictures, be sure to see photos of the person in a variety of situations and with others to ensure they aren't sending you pictures of someone else. Consider a first meeting over a video link such as Skype.
- If you meet, plan something brief during the day. Set up a group date if possible. Meet in a public place such as a coffee shop. Do not meet with anyone who wants to keep the location and time a secret.
- Tell a friend where and when you're going to meet, and provide information about the person you're meeting.

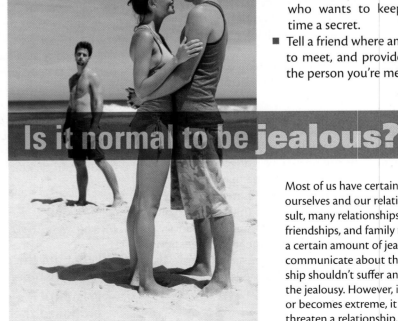

Is it normal to be jealous?

Most of us have certain insecurities about ourselves and our relationships and, as a result, many relationships—including romances, friendships, and family relationships—include a certain amount of jealousy. As long as you communicate about the issue, your relationship shouldn't suffer and you can move past the jealousy. However, if jealousy is ignored or becomes extreme, it can undermine and threaten a relationship.

In an unhealthy relationship...	In a healthy relationship...
You care for and focus on another person only and neglect yourself or you focus only on yourself and neglect the other person.	You both love and take care of yourselves before and while in a relationship.
One of you feels pressure to change to meet the other person's standards and is afraid to disagree or voice ideas.	You respect each other's individuality, embrace your differences, and allow each other to "be yourselves."
One of you has to justify what you do, where you go, and whom you see.	You both do things with friends and family and have activities independent of each other.
One of you makes all the decisions and controls everything without listening to the other's input.	You discuss things with each other, allow for differences of opinion, and compromise equally.
One of you feels unheard and is unable to communicate what you want.	You express and listen to each other's feelings, needs, and desires.
You don't have any personal space and have to share everything with the other person.	You respect each other's need for privacy.
Your partner keeps his or her sexual history a secret or hides a sexually transmitted infection from you, or you do not disclose your history to your partner.	You share sexual histories and information about sexual health with each other.
You feel stifled, trapped, and stagnant. You are unable to escape the pressures of the relationship.	You both have room for positive growth, and you both learn more about each other as you develop and mature.

Figure 4.2 Healthy versus Unhealthy Relationships

Source: Adapted from Advocates for Youth, Washington, DC, 20036, www.advocatesforyouth.org. Copyright © 2000. Reprinted with permission.

Confronting Couple Issues

Couples in long-term relationships must confront issues that can either enhance or diminish their chances of success:

Jealousy **Jealousy** has been described as an aversive reaction evoked by a real or imagined relationship involving one's partner and a third person. Jealousy often indicates underlying problems such as insecurity or possessiveness. Often, jealousy is rooted in past deception and loss. Other common causes:

- **Overdependence.** People with few social ties who rely exclusively on their significant others tend to be fearful of losing them.
- **High value on sexual exclusivity.** People who believe that sexual exclusivity is a crucial indicator of love are more likely to become jealous.
- **Low self-esteem.** People who think poorly of themselves are more likely to fear someone will snatch their partner away.
- **Fear of losing control.** Feeling one may lose attachment to or control over a partner can cause jealousy.

Although a certain amount of jealousy can be expected in any relationship, it doesn't have to threaten a relationship as long as partners communicate openly about it.[6]

Changing Gender Roles Throughout history, women and men have taken on various roles in relationships. Our society has very few gender-specific roles; many couples find it makes more sense to divide tasks based on convenience and preference. However, it rarely works out that the division is equal. Even when women work full time, they tend to bear heavy family and household responsibilities—and to become stressed and frustrated. Men may have expected a more traditional role for their partners. Over time, if couples can't communicate about this, the relationship may suffer.

Sharing Power **Power** can be defined as the ability to make and implement decisions. In traditional relationships, men were the wage earners and consequently had decision-making power. As women have become earners, the dynamics have shifted considerably. In general, successful couples share responsibilities, power, and control. If one partner always has the final say regarding social plans, for example, the unequal distribution of power may affect the relationship.

Unmet Expectations We all have expectations of ourselves and our partners—how we'll spend our time or money, express love, and grow as a couple. If we can't communicate our expectations, we set ourselves up for disappointment. Partners in healthy relationships can communicate wants and needs and have honest discussions when things aren't going as expected.

check yourself

- **What are three characteristics of a healthy relationship? Which do you consider most important?**
- **What factors are involved in the choice of a romantic partner?**
- **What are common obstacles to achieving a successful relationship?**

Skills for Better Communication: Appropriate Self-Disclosure

- **Discuss the role of appropriate self-disclosure in good communication.**

From the moment of birth, we struggle to be understood. By the time we enter adulthood, each of us has developed a unique way of communicating with gestures, words, expressions, and body language. No two people communicate in the exact same way or have the same need for connecting with others. Some of us are outgoing and quick to express our emotions and thoughts. Others are quiet and reluctant to talk about feelings.

Different cultures have different ways of expressing feelings and using body language. Men and women also tend to have different styles of communication, largely dictated by culture and socialization.

Although people differ in how they communicate, no one sex, culture, or group is better at it than another. We must be willing to accept differences and work to keep communication open and fluid. Remaining interested, engaged, and willing to exchange ideas and thoughts are skills typically learned with practice.

When two people begin a relationship, they bring their communication styles with them. How often have you heard someone say, "We just can't communicate" or "You're sending mixed messages"? Communication is a process; our every action, word, expression, gesture, and posture becomes part of our shared experience and part of the evolving impression we make on others. If we are angry in our responses, others will be reluctant to interact with us. If we bring "baggage"

There's more to good communication than just the ability to gab.

from past bad interactions to new relationships, we may be cynical, distrustful, and guarded. If we are positive, happy, and share openly, others will be more likely to communicate openly with us. This ability to communicate assertively is an important skill in relationships. Assertive communicators are in touch with their feelings and values and can communicate their needs directly and honestly.

Sharing personal information with others is called **self-disclosure**. If you want to learn more about someone, you have to be willing to share parts of yourself with that person. Self-disclosure is not storytelling or sharing secrets; rather, it is revealing how you are reacting to the present situation and giving any information about the past that is relevant to the other person's understanding of your current reactions.

If you sense that sharing feelings and thoughts will result in a closer relationship, you will likely take such a risk. But if you believe that the disclosure may result in rejection or alienation, you may not open up so easily. If the confidentiality of shared information has been violated, you may hesitate to disclose yourself in the future.

However, the risk in not disclosing yourself to others is that you will lack intimacy in relationships. Psychologist Carl Rogers believed that weak relationships were characterized by inhibited self-disclosure.[7]

If self-disclosure is such a key to creating healthy communication, but fear is a barrier to that process, what can we do? The following suggestions can help:

- **Get to know yourself.** The more you know about your feelings, beliefs, thoughts, and concerns, the more likely you'll be able to communicate with others about yourself.
- **Become more accepting of yourself.** No one is perfect, or has to be.
- **Be willing to discuss your sexual history.** In a culture that puts taboos on discussions of sex, it's no wonder we find it hard to disclose our sexual feelings. However, with the soaring rate of sexually transmitted infections and the ever-looming threat of AIDS, there has never been a more important time to disclose sexual feelings and history before you become intimate.
- **Choose a safe context for self-disclosure.** When and where you make such disclosures and to whom may greatly influence the response. Choose a setting in which you feel safe to let yourself be known.

- **How can appropriate self-disclosure contribute to healthy communication?**

Skills for Better Communication: Understanding Gender Differences

learning outcomes

- **Describe differences and similarities in communication patterns between men and women.**

Men and women may communicate in ways somewhat distinctive to their genders—though these lines have begun to blur. According to Dr. Cynthia Burggraf Torppa at Ohio State University, differences in communication by gender are quite minor; what is

with their mates, perhaps because society expects women to be responsible for regulating intimacy. Men are more sensitive to subtle messages about status; societal expectations dictate that they negotiate hierarchy.[9]

Within our society, some gender-specific communication patterns are obvious to the casual observer. Recognizing these differences and how they make us unique is a good step in avoiding unnecessary frustrations and irritations.

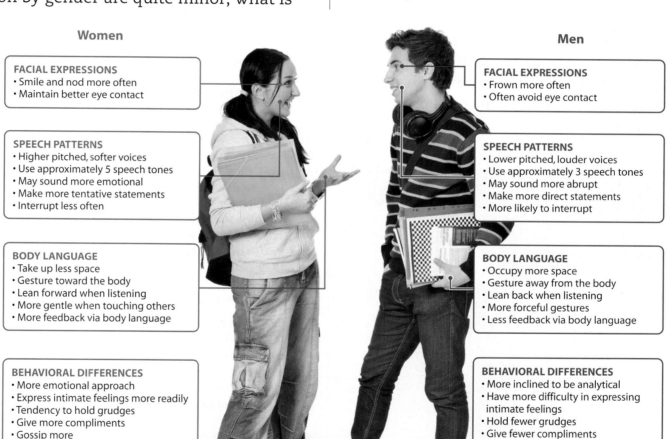

Women

FACIAL EXPRESSIONS
- Smile and nod more often
- Maintain better eye contact

SPEECH PATTERNS
- Higher pitched, softer voices
- Use approximately 5 speech tones
- May sound more emotional
- Make more tentative statements
- Interrupt less often

BODY LANGUAGE
- Take up less space
- Gesture toward the body
- Lean forward when listening
- More gentle when touching others
- More feedback via body language

BEHAVIORAL DIFFERENCES
- More emotional approach
- Express intimate feelings more readily
- Tendency to hold grudges
- Give more compliments
- Gossip more
- More likely to ask for help
- Tend to take rejection more personally
- Apologize more frequently
- Talk is primarily a means of rapport, establishing connections, and negotiating relationships

Men

FACIAL EXPRESSIONS
- Frown more often
- Often avoid eye contact

SPEECH PATTERNS
- Lower pitched, louder voices
- Use approximately 3 speech tones
- May sound more abrupt
- Make more direct statements
- More likely to interrupt

BODY LANGUAGE
- Occupy more space
- Gesture away from the body
- Lean back when listening
- More forceful gestures
- Less feedback via body language

BEHAVIORAL DIFFERENCES
- More inclined to be analytical
- Have more difficulty in expressing intimate feelings
- Hold fewer grudges
- Give fewer compliments
- Gossip less
- Less likely to ask for help
- Tend to take rejection less personally
- Apologize less often
- Talk is primarily a means of preserving independence and negotiating and maintaining status

important is how men and women interpret the same message.[8] Studies support the idea that women are more sensitive to the interpersonal meanings of messages exchanged

check yourself

- **How would you describe communication patterns among men and women?**

Skills for Better Communication: Listening and Nonverbal Skills

- **Explain the importance of listening for good communication.**
- **List and describe forms of nonverbal communication.**

Listening allows us to share feelings, express concerns, communicate wants and needs, and make our thoughts and opinions known. Improving our speaking and listening skills can enhance our relationships. We listen best when (1) we believe that the message is important and relevant to us; (2) the speaker holds our attention through humor, dramatic effect, etc.; and (3) we are free of distractions and worries.

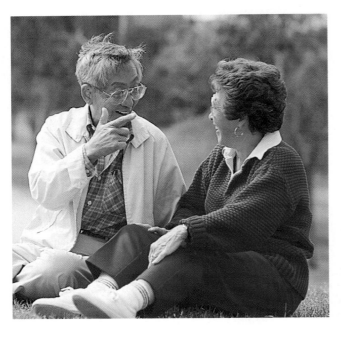

How can I communicate better?

One way to communicate better is to pay attention to your body language. Researchers have found that 93 percent of communication effectiveness is determined by nonverbal cues. Laughing, smiling, and gesturing all help convey meaning and assure your partner you are actively engaged in communicating.

Becoming a Better Listener

To become a better listener, practice these skills on a daily basis:

- Be present in the moment. Good listeners acknowledge what the other person is saying through nonverbal cues such as nodding, smiling, saying "yes" or "uh-huh," and asking questions at appropriate times.
- Show empathy and sympathy.
- Ask for clarification if you aren't sure what the speaker means, or paraphrase what you think you heard.
- Control the desire to interrupt. Try taking a deep breath, then holding it for another second and really listening to what is being said as you exhale.
- Avoid snap judgments based on what other people look like or say.
- Resist the temptation to "set the other person straight."
- Focus on the speaker. Hold back the temptation to launch into a story about your own experience in a similar situation.

Using Nonverbal Communication

Smiling, eye contact or its lack, movements and gestures—these nonverbal clues influence how conversational partners interpret messages. **Nonverbal communication** includes all unwritten and unspoken messages, intentional and unintentional. Ideally, nonverbal communication matches and supports verbal communication. Research shows that when verbal and nonverbal communications don't match, we are more likely to believe the nonverbal cues.[10] It's important to be aware of the nonverbal cues we use and understand how others might interpret them.

Nonverbal communication can include the following:[11]

- **Touch.** This can be a handshake, a hug, a hand on the shoulder, or a kiss on the cheek.
- **Gestures.** These can include mannerisms such as a thumbs-up or a wave, or movements that augment verbal communication, such as fanning your face when you are hot.
- **Interpersonal space.** This is the amount of physical space separating two people. Getting too close can be offensive.
- **Facial expressions.** Expressions such as frowns, smiles, and grimaces signal moods and emotions.
- **Body language.** This includes actions such as folding your arms, crossing your legs, leaning forward, and shaking your head no.
- **Tone of voice.** This refers to elements of speaking such as pitch, volume, and speed.

- **Why is listening an important part of communication?**
- **How do nonverbal cues affect interactions?**

Skills for Better Communication: Managing Conflict

- **Identify strategies for managing and resolving conflict.**

A **conflict** is an emotional state that arises when the behavior of one person interferes with that of another. Some conflict is inevitable, and not all conflict is bad; airing feelings and resolving differences can strengthen relationships. **Conflict resolution** and conflict management form a systematic approach to resolving differences fairly and constructively.

Prolonged conflict can destroy relationships unless the parties agree to resolve points of contention. As two people learn to negotiate and compromise, the number and intensity of conflicts should diminish.

During a heated conflict, try to pause before responding, consider the possible impact of your comments or actions, and state your point constructively. You can also say, "I can see we aren't going to resolve this right now. Let's talk when we've both cooled off."

E-mail messages are easily misunderstood because we can't see or hear the person talking. In general, when you're tempted to send a nasty response to an e-mail, stop. Observe the 24-hour rule—don't hit Send until the next day. Usually, you'll find it's better to hit Delete and move on, or to talk in person.

Rudeness or inconsiderate behavior usually develops when one person fails to recognize the feelings or rights of another. Try to see the other person's point of view, listen actively, avoid interrupting, and avoid gestures such as head-shaking or finger-pointing. Key elements of conflict management include validating others' opinions and treating others as you would like to be treated.

Here are some strategies for conflict resolution:

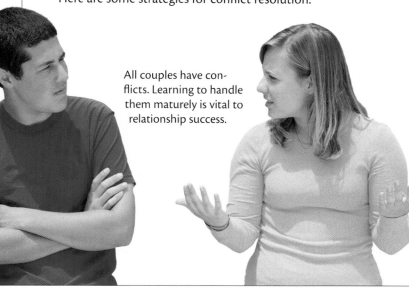

All couples have conflicts. Learning to handle them maturely is vital to relationship success.

1. **Identify the problem.** Talk together to clarify the conflict or problem. Say what you want and listen to what the other person wants. Use "I" messages; avoid blaming "you" messages. Be an active listener—repeat what the other person has said and ask questions for clarification or information.
2. **Generate possible solutions.** Brainstorm ways to address the problem. Base your search on goals and interests identified in the first step. Come up with several alternatives, but avoid evaluating them for now.
3. **Evaluate solutions.** Review the possible solutions. Narrow your list to one or two that work for both parties. Focus on finding a solution you both feel is satisfactory.
4. **Decide on the best solution.** Choose an alternative acceptable to both parties. You must both commit to the decision for it to be effective.
5. **Implement the solution.** Discuss how the decision will be carried out. Establish who is responsible to do what and when.
6. **Follow up.** Check in and evaluate whether a solution is working. If it's not working as planned, or if circumstances have changed, revise your plan. Remember that both parties must agree to any changes, as to the original idea.

Skills for **Behavior Change**

COMMUNICATING WHEN EMOTIONS RUN HIGH

These guidelines can help you express your feelings more effectively in an emotionally charged situation:

- Try to be specific rather than general about how you feel.
- When expressing anger or irritation, describe the specific behavior you don't like, then your feelings.
- If you have mixed feelings, say so; express and explain each feeling.
- Use "I" messages, rather than "you" statements that can cast blame or imply fault. With "I" messages, the speaker takes responsibility for communicating his or her feelings, thoughts, and beliefs.
- Avoid judgmental statements.
- Avoid lecturing or projecting superiority.
- Don't ask for feedback unless you want an honest answer.

- **Which strategy for conflict resolution do you find most effective? Why?**

Committed Relationships

learning **outcomes**

■ **List different forms of committed relationships.**

Commitment in a relationship means an intent to act over time in a way that perpetuates the well-being of the other person, oneself, and the relationship. Such commitment can take several forms, including marriage, cohabitation, and gay or lesbian partnerships.

Marriage

In many societies, traditional committed relationships take the form of marriage. In the United States, marriage means entering into a legal agreement that includes shared finances and responsibility for raising children. Many Americans also view marriage as a religious commitment.

Nearly 90 percent of Americans marry at least once; at any given time, close to 60 percent of U.S. adults are married (**Figure 4.3**). However, since 1960, annual marriages have steadily declined,[12] possibly due to factors including delay of first marriage, an increase in cohabitation, and fewer remarriages. In 1960, the median age for first marriage was 23 for men and 20 for women; by 2009, it had risen to 28.1 for men and 25.9 for women.[13]

Many Americans believe that marriage involves **monogamy**, or exclusive sexual involvement with one partner. In fact, the lifetime pattern for many Americans appears to be **serial monogamy**, where a person has a monogamous sexual relationship with one partner before moving on to another. Some people prefer **open relationships**, in which partners agree that each may be sexually involved with others outside their relationship.

Considerable research indicates that married people live longer, feel happier, remain mentally alert longer, and suffer fewer physical and mental health problems.[14] Healthy marriage contributes to less stress via financial stability, expanded support networks, and improved personal behaviors. Married adults are about half as likely to smoke as other adults,[15] and less likely to be heavy drinkers or to engage in risky sexual behavior. The one negative health indicator for married people is body weight. Married adults, particularly men, weigh more than do single adults.

Choosing Whether to Have Children Choosing to raise children changes a marriage or other relationship. It can bring joy and meaning to your lives. However, it is also highly stressful: time, energy, and money are split many ways, and you will no longer be able to give each other undivided attention. Having a child does not save a bad relationship—in fact, it seems only to compound problems that already exist.

Changing patterns in family life affect the way children are raised. Today, either partner may choose to provide primary childcare. Nearly half a million children each year become part of blended families when their parents remarry.[16] In addition, many individuals have children in a family structure other than heterosexual marriage. Single women or lesbian couples can choose adoption or alternative insemination; single men or gay couples can choose to adopt, or obtain the services of a surrogate mother. According to the U.S. Census Bureau, in 2009 over 26 percent of all children under age 18 lived in families headed by an adult raising a child alone.[17]

Regardless of structure, certain factors remain important to a family's well-being: consistency, communication, affection, and respect. Good parenting does not necessarily come naturally. Many people parent as they were parented, using strategies that may or may not follow sound child-rearing principles. A positive, respectful parenting style sets the stage for healthy family growth and development.

Finally, potential parents must consider the financial implications of having a child. It is estimated that a family with a child born in 2009 will spend $200,000 to $475,000 on the child over the next 17 years, not including the cost of college.[18] Prospective parents should think about how they will handle child rearing both financially and practically—who will work less or not at all, or how will they pay for childcare?

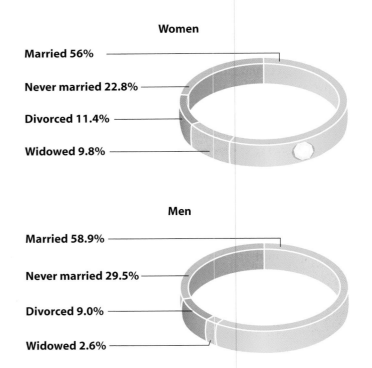

Figure 4.3 Marital Status of the U.S. Population by Sex

Source: U.S. Census Bureau, *The 2011 Statistical Abstract*, table 57, "Marital Status of the Population by Sex and Age: 2009," 2011, Available at www.census.gov/compendia/statab.

46%

of couples living together in a given year are doing so as a precursor to marriage. Within 5 to 7 years, 52% of those couples will have actually married and 31% will have split up.

Cohabitation

Cohabitation is a relationship in which two unmarried people with an intimate connection live together. In some states, cohabitation lasting a designated number of years (usually 7) legally constitutes a **common-law marriage** for purposes of sharing many financial obligations.

Cohabitation can offer many of the same emotional benefits as marriage. Some people may also cohabit for financial reasons. The past 20 years has seen a large increase in the number of persons who have ever cohabited; cohabitation is increasingly the first coresidential partnership formed by young adults.[19]

Cohabitation isn't a clear predictor of marriage success or failure; in one large study, 71 percent of men who were engaged when they moved in with their fiancées were still married after 10 years.[20] For men who didn't cohabit first, the rate was 69 percent. Sixty-five percent of cohabiting engaged women made it to 10 years, versus 66 percent of women who waited until marriage.

Cohabitation can be a prelude to marriage, but for some it is an alternative. It is more common among those of lower socioeconomic status, those who are less religious, those who have been divorced, and those who have experienced parental divorce or high parental conflict during childhood. Many cohabitants are young, but some older adults choose cohabitation because they would lose income, such as Social Security, if they were to marry. Cohabitation has both advantages and drawbacks. Perhaps the greatest disadvantage is the lack of societal validation for the relationship, especially if the couple subsequently has children. Many cohabitants also deal with difficulties obtaining insurance and tax benefits and legal issues over property.

Gay and Lesbian Partnerships

Lesbians and gay men seek the same things in committed relationships that heterosexuals do: love, friendship, communication, validation, and stability. A 2008 survey identified an estimated 564,743 same-sex couples in the United States.[21]

Challenges to successful lesbian and gay relationships often stem from discrimination and difficulties dealing with social, legal, and religious doctrines. For lesbian and gay couples, obtaining benefits such as tax deductions, power-of-attorney rights, partner health insurance, and child custody rights is a challenge—one that continues to be fought over in the courts and in public opinion.

At the time of this writing in 2011, New York, Massachusetts, Connecticut, Iowa, New Hampshire, Vermont, and the District of Columbia grant same-sex couples full marriage equality. Five other states have laws that extend to same-sex couples all, or nearly all, the state rights and responsibilities of married heterosexuals, whether "civil unions" or "domestic partnerships," and an additional five provide more limited rights and protections.[22] Worldwide, the number of countries that have legalized same-sex marriages or approved same-sex civil unions or domestic partnerships continues to grow.

Staying Single

Increasing numbers of adults of all ages are electing to marry later or remain single altogether. According to data from 2009, 52.1 percent of women and 62 percent of men aged 20 to 34 have never married.[23] Many singles live rewarding lives and maintain a network of close friends and families.

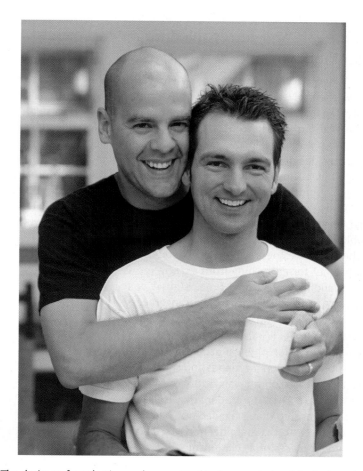

The desire to form lasting and committed intimate relationships is shared by most adults, regardless of sexual orientation.

check yourself

- **What forms can committed relationships take?**

When Relationships Falter

- **Discuss common reasons that relationships end.**
- **Provide examples of how to cope with a failed relationship.**

Breakdowns in relationships usually begin with a change in communication, however subtle. Either partner may stop listening and cease to be emotionally present for the other. In turn, the other feels ignored, unappreciated, or unwanted. Unresolved conflicts increase, and unresolved anger can cause problems in sexual relations.

When a couple who previously enjoyed spending time together find themselves continually in the company of others, spending time apart, or preferring to stay home alone, it may be a sign that the relationship is in trouble. Of course, the need for individual privacy is not a cause for worry—it's essential to health. If, however, a partner decides to change the amount and quality of time spent together without the input or understanding of the other, it may be a sign of hidden problems.

College students, particularly those who are socially isolated or far from family and hometown friends, may be particularly vulnerable to staying in unhealthy relationships. They may become emotionally dependent on a partner for everything from sharing meals to spending recreational time. Mutual obligations, such as shared rental arrangements, transportation, and child care, can make it tough to leave. It's also easy to mistake sexual advances for physical attraction or love. Without a network of friends and supporters to talk with, to obtain validation for feelings, or to share concerns, a student may feel stuck in a relationship that is headed nowhere.

Honesty and verbal affection are usually positive aspects of a relationship. In a troubled relationship, however, they can be used to cover up irresponsible or hurtful behavior.

"At least I was honest" is not an acceptable substitute for acting in a trustworthy way. "But I really do love you" is not a license for being inconsiderate or rude. Relationships that are lacking in mutual respect and consideration can become physically or emotionally abusive.

Recognizing a Potential Abuser

Is that new "item" in your life really what he or she appears to be? Your new love interest may seem like the perfect catch in the beginning. He or she appears sensitive, gentle, caring, respectful, and considerate—all the things you've been looking for. It can be hard to tell what someone is really like early on, as that person tries to make a good impression on you. To avoid getting into a long-term relationship with an abuser, watch carefully and trust your instincts. Ask others about the person and find out about his or her history with partners, friends, and family. All are important indicators of an emotionally and socially healthy person.

When you are beginning a relationship, be immediately wary if your partner demonstrates any of the following red flags:

- Gets extremely angry and swears at you or others.
- Hurts you by making fun of you or putting you down.
- Takes too much control. In a healthy relationship, partners share decision making.

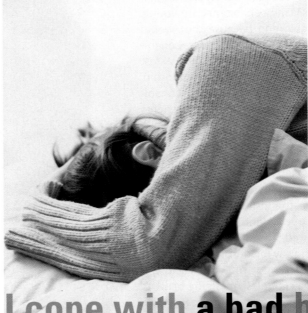

It may feel as if there is no end to the sorrow, anger, and guilt that often attend a difficult breakup, but time is a miraculous healer. Acknowledging your feelings, finding healthful ways to express them, spending time with friends, and allowing yourself to take as much time as you need to recover are all helpful strategies for dealing with the end of a romantic relationship.

How do I cope with **a bad breakup?**

- Displays excessive jealousy. Someone who is constantly jealous may lack the self-esteem to have a healthy relationship.
- Tries to shut out people you want to see, and wants to spend more and more time alone with you.
- Expresses continual negativity. Sulks, angers easily, throws tantrums when things don't go his or her way.
- Pushes you verbally or physically to have unwanted sex or intimacy.
- Damages your property in fits of anger.
- Threatens you.
- Verbally or physically hurts children or animals.
- Is always in trouble or fighting with someone.

The list above is not exhaustive, and there are degrees of seriousness for each. However, if someone you have known only for a short time displays any sign of physical anger or pushes, shoves, slaps, restrains, or threatens you early on, it's time to walk.

When and Why Relationships End

In the last decade, overall divorce rates have declined in the United States to between 41 to 50 percent (depending on how rates are calculated). Perhaps more important than these overall percentages is the fact that there are huge disparities in divorce rates by education and socioeconomic status.[24] College-educated individuals who delay marriage until after they have obtained their degrees tend to be less likely to divorce, less likely to experience infidelity, and less likely to have babies out of wedlock. In striking contrast, Americans who do not hold college degrees tend to have higher divorce rates, higher rates of infidelity, and much higher rates of childbirth outside of marriage.[25] Although it is widely reported that the chances of divorce increase with subsequent marriages, the actual sources of these statistics remain elusive.

The divorce rate, however, represents only a portion of the actual number of failed relationships. Many people whose marriages fail never go through a legal divorce process; as a result, they are not counted in these statistics. Cohabitants and unmarried partners who raise children, own homes together, and exhibit all the outward appearances of marriage without the license are also not included.

Why do relationships end? There are many reasons, and many factors, including illness, financial concerns, and career problems. Other breakups arise from unmet expectations. Many people enter a relationship with certain expectations about how they and their partner will behave. Failure to communicate these beliefs can lead to resentment and disappointment. Differences in sexual needs may also contribute to the demise of a relationship. Under stress, communication and cooperation between partners can break down. Conflict, negative interactions, and a general lack of respect between partners can erode even the most loving relationship.

Coping with Failed Relationships

No relationship comes with a guarantee, no matter how many promises partners make to be together forever. Losing a love is as much a part of life as falling in love. That being said, the uncoupling process can be very painful. Whenever we risk getting close to another, we also risk being hurt if things don't work out. Remember that knowing, understanding, and feeling good about oneself before entering a relationship is very important. Consider these tips for coping with a failed relationship:

- **Recognize and acknowledge your feelings.** These may include grief, loneliness, rejection, anger, guilt, relief, and sadness. Seek professional help and support, as needed.
- **Find healthful ways to express your emotions, rather than turning them inward.** Go for a walk, talk to friends, listen to music, work out at the gym, volunteer with a community organization, or write in a journal.
- **Spend time with current friends, or reconnect with old friends.** Get reacquainted with yourself, what you enjoy doing, and the people whose company you enjoy.
- **Don't rush into a "rebound" relationship.** You need time to resolve your past experience rather than escape from it. You can't be trusting and intimate in a new relationship if you are still working on getting over a past relationship.

Skills for Behavior Change

HOW DO YOU END IT?

Relationship endings are just as important as their beginnings. Healthy closure affords both parties the opportunity to move on without wondering or worrying about what went wrong and whose fault it was. If you need to end a relationship, do so in a manner that preserves and respects the dignity of both partners. If you are the person "breaking up," you have probably had time to think about the process and may be at a different stage from your partner.

Here are some tips for ending a relationship in a respectful and caring way:

- Arrange a time and quiet place where you can talk without interruption.
- Say in advance that there is something important you want to discuss.
- Accept that your partner may express strong feelings and be prepared to listen quietly.
- Consider in advance if you might also become upset and what support you might need.
- Communicate honestly using "I" messages and without personal attacks. Explain your reasons as much as you can without being cruel or insensitive.
- Don't let things escalate into a fight, even if you have very strong feelings.
- Provide another opportunity to talk about the end of the relationship when you both have had time to reflect.

check yourself

- **What are some common reasons that relationships end?**
- **What are three ways to cope with a failed relationship?**

Your Sexual Identity: More than Biology

- **Define sexual identity.**
- **Discuss the major components of sexual identity.**

Sexual identity, the recognition and acknowledgment of oneself as a sexual being, is determined by the interaction of genetic, physiological, environmental, and social factors.

The beginning of sexual identity occurs at conception with the combining of chromosomes. All eggs (ova) carry an X chromosome; sperm may carry either an X or a Y chromosome, and thus determine sex. If a sperm carrying an X fertilizes an egg, the resulting combination of chromosomes (XX) produces a female. If a sperm carrying a Y fertilizes an egg, the XY combination produces a male.

The genetic instructions included in the sex chromosomes lead to the differential development of male and female **gonads** (reproductive organs). Once the male gonads (testes) and the female gonads (ovaries) develop, they play a key role in all future sexual development, being responsible for production of sex hormones. The primary female sex hormones are estrogen and progesterone; the primary male sex hormone is testosterone. The release of testosterone in a maturing fetus signals the development of a penis and other male genitals. If no testosterone is produced, female genitals form.

At the time of **puberty**, hormones released by the pituitary gland, the gonadotropins, stimulate the testes and ovaries to make appropriate sex hormones. The increase of estrogen production in females and testosterone production in males leads to the development of secondary sex characteristics, features that distinguish the sexes but that have no direct reproductive function. For males, these include deepening of the voice, development of facial and body hair, and growth of the skeleton and musculature. For females, they include growth of breasts, widening of hips, and development of pubic and underarm hair.

Another important component of sexual identity is **gender**, which refers to characteristics and actions typically associated with men or women (masculine or feminine) as defined by culture. Our sense of masculine and feminine traits is largely a result of **socialization** during childhood. **Gender roles** are the behaviors and activities we use to express maleness or femaleness in ways that conform to society's expectations. For example, you may learn to play with dolls or trucks, based on how your parents influence your actions. For some, gender roles can be confining when they lead to stereotyping. Boundaries established by **gender-role stereotypes** can make it difficult to express one's identity. Men are traditionally expected to be independent, aggressive, logical, and in control of emotions. Women are traditionally expected to be passive, nurtur-

ing, intuitive, and emotional. **Androgyny** refers to the combination of traditional masculine and feminine traits in a single person; each of us is in small or large ways androgynous. Highly androgynous people do not always follow traditional sex roles.

Whereas gender roles are an expression of cultural expectations for behavior, **gender identity** refers to a sense or awareness of being male or a female. A person's gender identity does not always match his or her biological sex; this is called being **transgendered**. There is a broad spectrum of expression among transgendered persons that reflects degree of dissatisfaction with sexual anatomy. Some transgendered persons are comfortable with their bodies and content simply to dress and live as the other gender. At the other end of the spectrum are **transsexuals**, who feel extremely trapped in their bodies and may opt for interventions such as sex reassignment surgery.

Sexual Orientation

Sexual orientation refers to a person's enduring emotional, romantic, sexual, or affectionate attraction to others. You may be primarily attracted to members of the opposite sex **(heterosexual)**, the same sex **(homosexual)**, or both sexes **(bisexual)**. Many homosexuals prefer the terms **gay,** queer, or **lesbian** to describe their sexual orientation. *Gay* and *queer* can apply to both men and women, but *lesbian* refers specifically to women.

Researchers today agree that sexual orientation is best understood using a model that incorporates biological, psychological, and socioenvironmental factors. Biological explanations focus on

The presence of gay and lesbian celebrities in the media contributes to the increasing acceptance of gay relationships in everyday life. Talk show host Ellen DeGeneres and actress Portia de Rossi married in 2008.

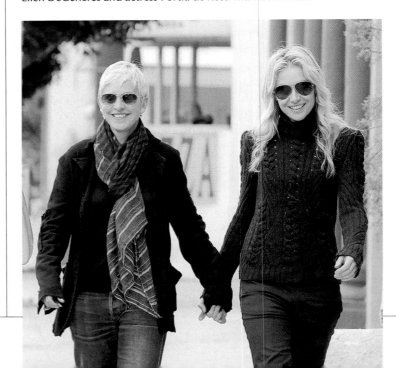

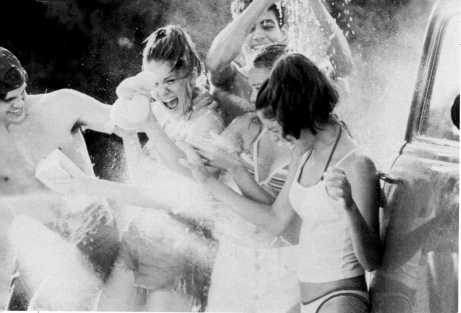

What influences sexual identity besides biology?

How you perceive yourself as a sexual being is influenced by socialization and personal experience. Your understanding of gender roles, your contact with people of various gender identities or sexual orientations, and your own degree of emotional maturity can all affect your sense of sexual identity.

research into genetics, hormones, and differences in brain anatomy, whereas psychological and socioenvironmental explanations examine parent–child interactions, sex roles, and early sexual and interpersonal interactions. Collectively, this growing body of research suggests that the origins of homosexuality, like heterosexuality, are complex. To diminish the complexity of sexual orientation to "a choice" is a clear misrepresentation of current research. Homosexuals do not "choose" their sexual orientation any more than heterosexuals do.

Gay, lesbian, and bisexual persons are often the targets of **sexual prejudice** (or *sexual bias*). Prejudice refers to negative attitudes and hostile actions directed at a social group. Hate crimes, discrimination, and hostility toward sexual minorities are evidence of ongoing sexual prejudice. Bias regarding sexual orientation is the motivation for approximately 18.5 percent of all hate crimes reported.[26]

Sexual orientation is often viewed as based entirely on whom one has sex with, but this is inaccurate and overly simplistic. Researcher Fritz Klein developed a questionnaire that looks at not only whom one is sexually attracted to, fantasizes about, and has sex with, but also factors such as whom one feels close to emotionally and socializes with, and in which "community" one feels comfortable. From this viewpoint, there are not just three (homosexual, heterosexual, bisexual) orientations, but a range of complex, interacting, and fluid factors influencing sexuality over time.

Disorders of Sexual Development

Sometimes chromosomes are added, lost, or rearranged at conception, and the sex of the offspring is unclear, a condition known as **intersex.** *Disorders of sexual development* (*DSDs*) is a less confusing term that has been recommended to refer to intersex conditions, which may occur as often as 1 in 1,500 live births.[27]

People with DSDs are born with various levels of male and female biological characteristics, ranging from different chromosomal arrangements to altered hormone production to variation in primary and secondary sex characteristics. Whereas most people are born with either XX or XY chromosomes, some are born with XXY or XO chromosomes (where O signifies a missing or damaged chromosome). In some people, gonads do not develop fully into ovaries or

testicles, although there may be no external signs to indicate this; in others, external genitalia may be ambiguous.

Many, but not all, DSDs require some degree of hormonal or surgical intervention to ensure physical health. It is also necessary to "assign" a gender to children as early as possible to ensure psychological health. If this assignment is later found to be inconsistent with the child's own sense of gender, he or she may adopt a different gender identity. Most people born with DSDs today are allowed to grow up, establish their own gender identity, and choose as adults whether to have additional surgeries to alter any sexual tissues they feel that are incongruent with their gender.[28]

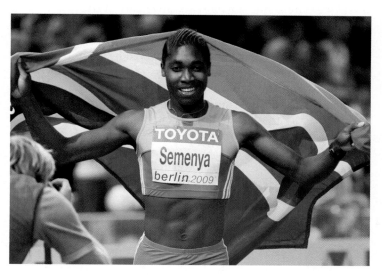

After South African middle-distance runner Caster Semenya won the gold medal in the 800-meter race at the 2009 World Championships, she was required to undergo gender testing and was subsequently barred from competition. Officials wanted to determine whether Semenya has a DSD resulting in testosterone levels that give her an unfair athletic advantage over other women competitors. After 11 months, a panel of medical experts announced that Semenya was again eligible to compete against other women. Her case highlights the challenges facing athletes and other people with both male and female characteristics.

check yourself

- **What is sexual identity?**
- **What are the major components of sexual identity?**

Female Sexual Anatomy and Physiology

- **Identify the major features and functions of female sexual anatomy and physiology.**

The female reproductive system includes two major groups of structures, the external genitals and the internal organs (Figure 4.4).

The external female genitals are collectively known as the **vulva**. The **mons pubis** is a pad of fatty tissue covering and protecting the pubic bone; after the onset of puberty, it becomes covered with coarse hair. The **labia majora** are folds of skin and erectile tissue that enclose the urethral and vaginal openings; the **labia minora**, or inner lips, are folds of mucous membrane found just inside the labia majora.

The **clitoris** is located at the upper end of the labia minora and beneath the mons pubis; its only known function is to provide sexual pleasure and is the most sensitive part of the genital area. Directly below the clitoris is the **urethral opening**, through which urine is expelled from the body; below it is the vaginal opening. In some women, the vaginal opening is covered by a thin membrane called the **hymen.** The hymen can be stretched or torn by physical activity, and is not present in all women to begin with. The **perineum** is the area of smooth tissue between the vulva and the anus. The tissue in this area has many nerve endings and is sensitive to touch; it can play a part in sexual excitement.

The internal female genitals include the vagina, uterus, fallopian tubes, and ovaries. The **vagina** is a tubular organ that serves as a passageway from the uterus to the outside of the body. It allows menstrual flow to exit from the uterus during a woman's monthly cycle, receives the penis during intercourse, and serves as the birth canal during childbirth. The **uterus (womb)** is a hollow, muscular, pear-shaped organ. Hormones acting on the inner lining of the uterus (the **endometrium**) either prepare the uterus for implantation and development of a fertilized egg or signal that no fertilization has taken place, in which case the endometrium deteriorates and becomes menstrual flow.

The lower end of the uterus, the **cervix**, extends down into the vagina. Its actual opening is the *cervical os*. The **ovaries**, almond-sized organs on either side of the uterus, produce the hormones estrogen and progesterone and are the reservoir for immature eggs. (All the eggs a woman will ever have are present in her ovaries at birth.) Extending from the upper end of the uterus are two thin, flexible tubes called the **fallopian tubes** (or **oviducts**). The fallopian tubes capture eggs as they are released from the ovaries during ovulation and are the site where sperm and egg meet and fertilization takes place. They then serve as the passageway to the uterus, where the fertilized egg becomes implanted.

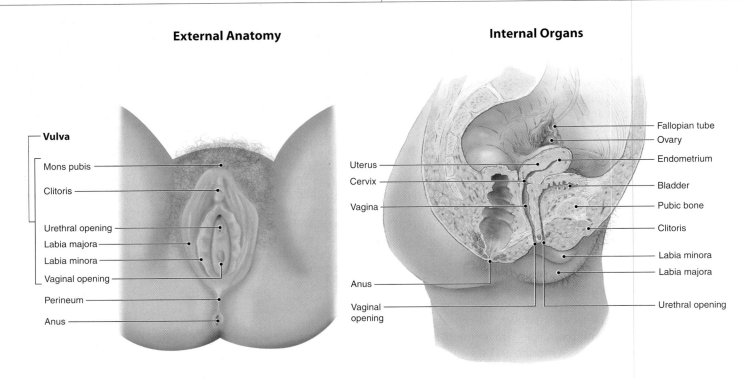

External Anatomy

Vulva
- Mons pubis
- Clitoris
- Urethral opening
- Labia majora
- Labia minora
- Vaginal opening

Perineum

Anus

Internal Organs

Fallopian tube
Ovary
Endometrium
Uterus
Cervix
Bladder
Vagina
Pubic bone
Clitoris
Anus
Labia minora
Labia majora
Vaginal opening
Urethral opening

Figure 4.4 Female Reproductive System

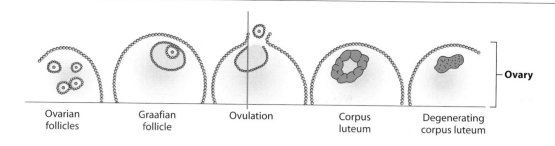

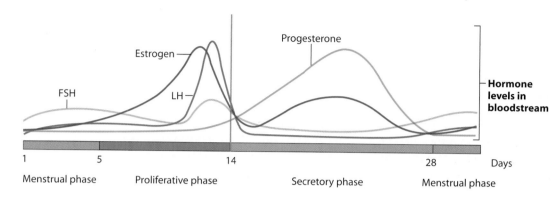

Figure 4.5 **Hormonal Control and Phases of the Menstrual Cycle**

Ovary

Ovarian follicles   Graafian follicle   Ovulation   Corpus luteum   Degenerating corpus luteum

Progesterone

Estrogen

FSH   LH

Hormone levels in bloodstream

1   5   14   28   Days

Menstrual phase   Proliferative phase   Secretory phase   Menstrual phase

The Onset of Puberty and the Menstrual Cycle

With the onset of puberty, the female reproductive system matures, and **secondary sex characteristics,** including breasts, widened hips, and underarm and pubic hair, develop. The first sign of puberty is the beginning of breast development, around age 11. The **pituitary gland, hypothalamus,** and ovaries all secrete hormones that act as chemical messengers among them.

Around the same time, the hypothalamus receives a message to begin secreting *gonadotropin-releasing hormone (GnRH)*. This, in turn, signals the pituitary gland to release hormones called *gonadotropins.* Two specific gonadotropins, *follicle-stimulating hormone (FSH)* and *luteinizing hormone (LH)*, signal the ovaries to start producing **estrogens** and **progesterone.** The age range for the onset of the first menstrual period, or **menarche,** is 9 to 17 years, with the average 11 to 13 years. Body fat heavily influences the onset of puberty, and increasing rates of obesity in children may account for the fact that girls seem to be reaching puberty much earlier than they used to.[29]

The average menstrual cycle lasts 28 days and consists of the proliferative, secretory, and menstrual phases (**Figure 4.5**). The *proliferative phase* begins with the end of menstruation. During this time, the endometrium develops, or proliferates. The hypothalamus, sensing low levels of estrogen and progesterone in the blood, increases its secretions of GnRH, which, in turn, triggers the pituitary gland to release FSH. When FSH reaches the ovaries, it signals several **ovarian follicles** to begin maturing. Normally, only one of the follicles, the **graafian follicle,** reaches full maturity in the days preceding ovulation. While the follicles mature, they begin producing estrogen, which, in turn, signals the endometrial lining of the uterus to proliferate. High estrogen levels signal the pituitary to slow down FSH production and increase release of LH. Under the influence of LH, the graafian follicle rup-

tures and releases a mature **ovum** (plural: *ova*), a single egg cell, near a fallopian tube. This event, which usually occurs around day 14 of the cycle, is referred to as **ovulation.** The other ripening follicles degenerate and are reabsorbed by the body. Occasionally, two ova mature and are released during ovulation. If both are fertilized, fraternal (nonidentical) twins develop. Identical twins develop when one fertilized ovum (called a *zygote*) divides into two separate zygotes.

The phase following ovulation is called the *secretory phase.* The ruptured graafian follicle, which has remained in the ovary, is transformed into the **corpus luteum** and begins secreting large amounts of estrogen and progesterone. These secretions peak around the twentieth day of the cycle and cause the endometrium to thicken. If fertilization and implantation take place, cells surrounding the developing embryo release *human chorionic gonadotropin (HCG)*, increasing estrogen and progesterone secretions that maintain the endometrium and signal the pituitary not to start a new menstrual cycle. If no implantation occurs, the hypothalamus signals the pituitary to stop producing FSH and LH, peaking the levels of progesterone in the blood. The corpus luteum begins to decompose, leading to rapid declines in estrogen and progesterone, the hormones needed to sustain the uterine lining. Without them, the endometrium is sloughed off in the menstrual flow, beginning the *menstrual phase.* Low estrogen levels signal the hypothalamus to release GnRH, which acts on the pituitary to secrete FSH—and the cycle begins again.

check yourself

- **What are the major features and functions of female sexual anatomy and physiology?**
- **Describe a 28-day menstrual cycle, starting with the proliferative phase.**

Menstrual Problems and Menopause

■ **Discuss possible menstrual problems.**

Premenstrual Syndrome

Premenstrual syndrome (PMS) is a term used for a collection of physical, emotional, and behavioral symptoms that many women experience 7 to 14 days prior to their menstrual period. The most common symptoms are tender breasts, food cravings, fatigue, irritability, and depression. It is estimated that 75 percent of menstruating women experience some signs and symptoms of PMS each month. For the majority of women, these disappear as their period begins, but for a small subset of women (3–5%), symptoms are severe enough to affect daily routines and activities to the point of being disabling. This severe form of PMS has its own designation, **premenstrual dysphoric disorder (PMDD)**, with symptoms that include severe depression, hopelessness, anger, anxiety, low self-esteem, difficulty concentrating, irritability, and tension.

Several natural approaches to managing PMS can also help PMDD. These include eating more carbohydrates (grains, fruits, and vegetables), reducing caffeine and salt intake, exercising regularly, and taking measures to reduce stress. Recent investigation into methods of controlling severe emotional swings has led to the use of antidepressants for treating PMDD, primarily selective serotonin reuptake inhibitors (e.g., Prozac, Paxil, and Zoloft).

Dysmenorrhea

Dysmenorrhea is a medical term for menstrual cramps, the pain or discomfort in the lower abdomen that many women experience just before or after menstruation. Along with cramps, some women can experience nausea and vomiting, loose stools, sweating, and

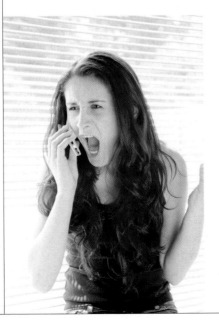

Do all women get PMS?

About 75 percent of menstruating women experience some PMS symptoms every month, but for most women these symptoms are mild and short-lived. Stress reduction, regular exercise, and a healthy diet are all good strategies for coping with PMS symptoms, which can include irritability and moodiness, fatigue, breast tenderness, and food cravings.

dizziness. Primary dysmenorrhea doesn't involve any physical abnormality and usually begins 6 months to a year after a woman's first period, whereas secondary dysmenorrhea has an underlying physical cause such as endometriosis or uterine fibroids.[30] If you experience primary dysmenorrhea, you can reduce discomfort by using over-the-counter nonsteroidal anti-inflammatory drugs (NSAIDs) such as aspirin, ibuprofen (Advil or Motrin), or naproxen (Aleve). Soaking in a hot bath or using a heating pad on your abdomen may also ease cramps. For severe cramping, your health care provider may recommend a low-dose oral contraceptive to prevent ovulation, which, in turn, may reduce the production of prostaglandins and therefore the severity of cramps. Managing secondary dysmenorrhea involves treating the underlying cause.

Toxic shock syndrome (TSS), although rare today, is still something women should be aware of. It is caused by a bacterial infection facilitated by tampon or diaphragm use. Symptoms, which occur during one's period or a few days afterward, can be hard to recognize because they mimic the flu and include sudden high fever, vomiting, diarrhea, dizziness, fainting, or a rash that looks like sunburn. Proper treatment usually assures recovery in 2 to 3 weeks.

Changes in the Menstrual Cycle: Menopause

Just as menarche signals the beginning of a woman's potential reproductive years, **menopause**—the permanent cessation of menstruation—signals the end. Generally occurring between the ages of 40 and 60, menopause results in decreased estrogen levels, which may produce symptoms such as decreased vaginal lubrication, hot flashes, headaches, dizziness, and a decline in **libido,** or sex drive.

Hormones, such as estrogen and progesterone, have long been prescribed as **hormone replacement therapy** to relieve menopausal symptoms and reduce the risk of heart disease and osteoporosis. (The National Institutes of Health prefers the term **menopausal hormone therapy**, because hormone therapy is not a replacement and does not restore the physiology of youth.) However, recent studies suggest that hormone therapy may actually do more harm than good.[31] All women need to discuss the risks and benefits of menopausal hormone therapy with their health care provider to make an informed decision. A healthy lifestyle including regular exercise, a balanced diet, and adequate calcium intake can also help protect postmenopausal women from heart disease and osteoporosis.

■ **What are some common problems associated with menstruation?**

Male Sexual Anatomy and Physiology

- **Identify major features and functions of male sexual anatomy and physiology.**

The structures of the male reproductive system are divided into external and internal genitals (Figure 4.6).

The external genitals are the penis and the scrotum. The **penis** is the organ that deposits sperm in the vagina during intercourse. The urethra, which passes through the center of the penis, acts as the passageway for both semen and urine to exit the body. During sexual arousal, the spongy tissue in the penis becomes filled with blood, making the organ stiff (erect). Further sexual excitement leads to **ejaculation**, a series of rapid, spasmodic contractions that propels semen out of the penis.

Situated behind the penis and also outside the body is a sac called the **scrotum**. The scrotum encases the testes, protecting them and helping control their internal temperature, which is vital to proper sperm production. The **testes** (singular: *testis*) manufacture sperm and **testosterone**, the hormone responsible for development of male secondary sex characteristics, including deepening of the voice and growth of facial, body, and pubic hair.

The development of sperm is referred to as **spermatogenesis**. Like the maturation of eggs in the female, this process is governed by the pituitary gland. Follicle-stimulating hormone (FSH) is secreted into the bloodstream to stimulate the testes to manufacture sperm. Immature sperm are released into a comma-shaped structure on the back of each testis called the **epididymis** (plural: *epididymides*), where they ripen and reach full maturity.

Each epididymis contains coiled tubules that gradually "unwind" to become the **vas deferens**. The two vasa deferentia make up the tubes whose sole function is to store and move sperm. Along the way, the **seminal vesicles** provide sperm with nutrients and other fluids that compose **semen**.

The vasa deferentia eventually connect each epididymis to the **ejaculatory ducts**, which pass through the prostate gland and empty into the urethra. The **prostate gland** contributes more fluids to the semen, including chemicals that help the sperm fertilize an ovum and neutralize the acidic environment of the vagina to make it more conducive to sperm motility and potency. Just below the prostate gland are two pea-shaped nodules called the **Cowper's glands**. The Cowper's glands secrete a fluid that lubricates the urethra and neutralizes any acid that may remain in the urethra after urination. During ejaculation of semen, a small valve closes off the tube to the urinary bladder.

Debate continues over the practice of *circumcision*, the surgical removal of a fold of skin covering the end of the penis known as the *foreskin*. Approximately 56 percent (1.1 million) of all newborn boys are circumcised in the United States each year. Circumcision can be a controversial issue for parents, who must balance personal, cultural, and health issues in deciding whether to circumcise a son.[32]

Arguments for circumcision include religious or cultural reasons (Jewish and Muslim cultures have historically circumcised), the belief that a son's penis should look the same as his father's, and easier genital hygiene. There is also a lower risk of penile cancer (though it is rare to begin with), urinary tract infections during infancy, and foreskin infections.

Arguments against circumcision include the possibility of pain during the surgery and potential complications such as infection or improper healing. Families may feel the foreskin is needed for reasons of identity, culture, or sexual pleasure.

Men do not experience a rapid hormone decline in middle age as women do during menopause. Instead, men typically experience a gradual decline in testosterone levels throughout adulthood, averaging 1 percent a year after age 30.[33] Many doctors use the term *andropause* to describe age-related hormone changes in some men, with symptoms including reduced sexual desire, infertility, changes in sleep patterns or insomnia, increased body fat, reduced muscle bulk, decreased bone density, and hair loss. Men may also experience emotional changes such as decreased motivation, depression, or memory problems.[34] For some men, testosterone therapy relieves bothersome symptoms. For others, especially older men, the benefits aren't clear.

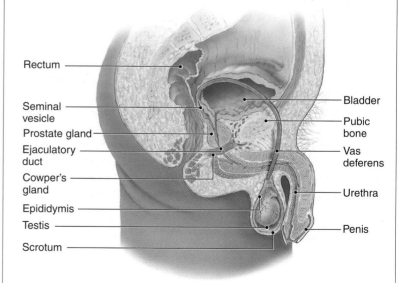

Figure 4.6 Male Reproductive System

- **Identify major features and functions of male sexual anatomy and physiology.**

Human Sexual Response and Expression

learning outcomes

- **Describe the human sexual response.**
- **Discuss examples of human sexual expression.**

For both men and women, sexual response is a physiological process of four stages: excitement/arousal, plateau, orgasm, and resolution; of course, individuals can vary in their experiences of this pattern.

During *excitement/arousal*, **vasocongestion** (increased blood flow causing swelling in the genitals) stimulates genital responses. The vagina begins to lubricate, and the penis becomes partially erect.

During the *plateau phase,* initial responses intensify. Voluntary and involuntary muscle tensions increase. The woman's nipples and the man's penis become erect. The penis secretes a few drops of pre-ejaculatory fluid, which may contain sperm.

During the *orgasmic phase,* vasocongestion and muscle tension reach their peak, and rhythmic contractions occur through the genital regions. In women, these contractions are centered in the uterus, outer vagina, and anal sphincter. In men, the contractions occur in two stages. First, contractions within the prostate gland begin propelling semen through the urethra. In the second stage, the muscles of the pelvic floor, urethra, and anal sphincter contract. Semen usually, but not always, is ejaculated from the penis.

Muscle tension and congested blood subside in the *resolution phase* as the genital organs return to prearousal states. Both sexes usually experience feelings of well-being and profound relaxation. Many women can become rearoused and experience additional orgasms; most men experience a refractory period of a few minutes to a few hours, during which they are incapable of subsequent arousal.

Although men and women experience the same stages in the sexual response cycle, time spent in any one stage varies; one partner may be in the plateau phase while the other is in the excitement/arousal or orgasmic phase. Such variations are entirely normal.

Sexual Responses among Older Adults

Older adults are commonly stereotyped as incapable of or uninterested in sex. In truth, although we do experience physical changes as we age, they generally do not cause us to stop enjoying sex.

In women, the most significant physical changes follow menopause. Skin becomes less elastic; vaginal lubrication may decrease. (Use of artificial lubricants usually resolves this problem.) Men's bodies also change; they require more direct and prolonged stimulation to achieve erection and are slower to reach orgasm, with less intense ejaculation.

Sexual Behavior: What Is "Normal"?

Which sexual behaviors are considered normal? Whose criteria should we use? Every society sets standards and attempts to regulate sexual behavior. Some common sociocultural standards for sexual behavior in Western culture today include the following:[35]

- **The coital standard.** Penile–vaginal intercourse (coitus) is viewed as the ultimate sex act.
- **The orgasmic standard.** Sexual interaction should lead to orgasm.
- **The two-person standard.** Sex is an activity to be experienced by two people.
- **The romantic standard.** Sex should be related to love.
- **The safer-sex standard.** If we choose to be sexually active, we should act to prevent unintended pregnancy or disease transmission.

These are not rules, but social scripts. Sexual standards often shift over time, and many people choose not to follow them. Rather than making blanket judgments, we might ask: Is a sexual behavior healthy and fulfilling for a particular person? Is it safe? Does it involve exploitation of others? Does it take place between responsible, consenting adults?[36]

In this way, we can view behavior along a continuum that takes into account many individual factors.

Options for Sexual Expression

The range of human sexual expression is virtually infinite. What you find enjoyable may not be an option for someone else. How you meet your sexual needs may change over time. Accepting yourself as a sexual person with individual desires and preferences is the first step in achieving sexual satisfaction.

Celibacy is avoidance of or abstention from sexual activities with others. Some people choose celibacy for religious or moral reasons. Others may be celibate for a period of time due to illness, the breakup of a long-term relationship, or lack of an acceptable partner. For some, celibacy is lonely, but others find it an opportunity for introspection and personal growth.

Autoerotic behaviors involve sexual self-stimulation. **Sexual fantasies** are sexually arousing thoughts and dreams. Fantasies may reflect real-life experiences, forbidden desires, or the opportunity to practice new or anticipated sexual experiences. The fact that you fantasize about a particular experience does not mean that you want to, or have to, act it out. **Masturbation,** or self-stimulation of the genitals, is one of the most common ways humans seek sexual pleasure. In one survey of college students, 48 percent of women and 92 percent of men reported masturbating.[37]

Kissing and erotic touching are two common forms of nonverbal sexual communication. Both men and women have **erogenous zones,** areas of the body that lead to sexual arousal when touched. These may include genital as well as areas such as the earlobes,

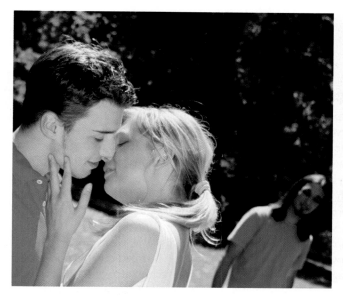

You may think everyone else on campus is having more sex with more partners than you are, but generally speaking, the actual numbers don't measure up to college students' perceptions.

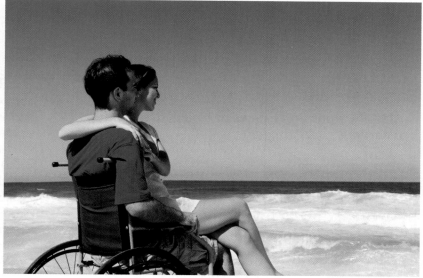

Whether able-bodied or disabled, we are all sexual beings deserving of intimacy and fulfilling sexual relationships.

mouth, breasts, and inner thighs. Spending time with your partner to explore and learn about his or her erogenous areas is a pleasurable and safe means of sexual expression.

Manual Stimulation Both men and women can be sexually aroused and achieve orgasm through manual stimulation of the genitals. For many women, orgasm is more likely through manual stimulation than through intercourse. *Sex toys* (such as vibrators and dildos) can be used alone or with a partner. Toys must be cleaned after each use.

Oral–Genital Stimulation **Cunnilingus** refers to oral stimulation of a woman's genitals and **fellatio** to oral stimulation of a man's genitals. Many partners find oral stimulation intensely pleasurable. Forty-two percent of college students reported having oral sex in the past month.[38] Note that HIV and other sexually transmitted infections (STIs) can be transmitted via unprotected oral–genital sex just as through intercourse. Use of an appropriate barrier device is strongly recommended if either partner's health status is in question.

Vaginal Intercourse The term *intercourse* generally refers to **vaginal intercourse** (*coitus*, or insertion of the penis into the vagina), the most frequently practiced form of sexual expression. More than 45 percent of college students reported having vaginal intercourse in the past month.[39] Whatever your circumstances, you should practice safer sex to avoid disease and unintended pregnancy.

Anal Intercourse The anal area is highly sensitive to touch, and some couples find pleasure in stimulation there. **Anal intercourse** is insertion of the penis into the anus. Over 20 percent of college-aged men and women have had anal sex.[40] Stimulation of the anus by the mouth, fingers, or sex toys is also practiced. If you enjoy this form of sexual expression, use condoms and/or dental dams

to avoid transmitting disease. Also, anything inserted into the anus should not then be directly inserted into the vagina, as bacteria commonly found in the anus can cause vaginal infections.

Variant Sexual Behavior

Although attitudes toward sexuality have changed substantially over time, some people still believe that any sexual behavior other than heterosexual intercourse is abnormal. People who study sexuality prefer to use the neutral term **variant sexual behavior** to describe sexual behaviors that most people do not engage in. Examples include group sex (sexual activity involving more than two people), transvestism (wearing the clothing of the opposite sex), and fetishism (sexual arousal achieved by looking at or touching inanimate objects, such as underclothing or shoes).

Some variant sexual behaviors can be harmful to the individual, to others, or to both Examples include: exhibitionism (exposing one's genitals to strangers in public places), voyeurism (observing other people for sexual gratification), sadomasochism [getting gratification from inflicting pain (verbal or physical) on a partner, or by being the object of such infliction], and pedophilia (sexual activity or attraction between an adult and a child). Autoerotic asphyxiation is the practice of reducing oxygen to the brain, usually by tying a cord around one's neck while masturbating to orgasm. Tragically, some individuals accidentally strangle themselves.

check yourself

- **What are the steps of the typical human sexual response?**
- **What are three examples of sexual expression?**

Sexual Dysfunction

- **Classify types and causes of sexual dysfunction disorders.**

Sexual dysfunction, problems that can hinder sexual functioning, is common. You can have breakdowns involving sexual function just as in any other body system. Sexual dysfunction can be divided into disorders of sexual desire, sexual arousal, orgasm, sexual performance, and sexual pain. All can be treated successfully.

The most frequent reason people seek out a sex therapist is **inhibited sexual desire**,[41] a lack of interest and pleasure in sexual activity. A low sex drive (decreased libido) may be caused by a drop in estrogen in women or testosterone in men and women or by fatigue, stress, depression, or anxiety. Antidepressant medications (e.g., Prozac, Zoloft, Paxil) can often reduce sexual desire.[42] **Sexual aversion disorder** is characterized by sexual phobias (unreasonable fears) and anxiety about sexual contact. Causes may include the psychological stress of a punitive upbringing, a rigid religious background, or a history of physical or sexual abuse.

The most common sexual arousal disorder is **erectile dysfunction (ED)**—difficulty achieving or maintaining a penile erection sufficient for intercourse. At some time, every man experiences ED. Risk factors include many medical conditions, medications, and treatments; being overweight; injuries; psychological conditions, drug, alcohol, or tobacco use; and prolonged bicycling.[43] Some 30 million men in the United States, half under age 65, suffer from ED. The condition generally becomes more common with age, affecting 1 in 4 men over 65.[44] Drugs treat ED by relaxing the smooth muscle cells in the penis, allowing increased blood flow to erectile tissues.

Premature ejaculation—ejaculation that occurs before or very soon after insertion of the penis into the vagina—affects up to 50 percent of men at some time. Treatment first involves physical examination to rule out organic causes. If the cause is not physiological, therapy can help a man learn how to control timing of his ejaculation. Fatigue, stress, performance pressure, and alcohol use can all contribute to this problem.

In a woman, the inability to achieve orgasm is called **female orgasmic disorder**. A woman with this disorder often blames herself and learns to fake orgasm to avoid embarrassment or preserve her partner's ego. The first step is a physical exam to rule out organic causes. However, the problem is often solved by self-exploration to learn more about self-stimulation. Once a woman has become orgasmic through masturbation, she learns to communicate her needs to her partner.

Both men and women can experience **sexual performance anxiety**. A man may become anxious and unable to maintain an erection or experience premature ejaculation. A woman may be unable to achieve orgasm or to allow penetration because of involuntary contraction of vaginal muscles. Both can overcome performance anxiety by learning to focus on immediate sensations rather than orgasm.

Dyspareunia is pain experienced by a woman during intercourse, which may be caused by endometriosis, uterine tumors, chlamydia, gonorrhea, or urinary tract infections. Damage to tissues during childbirth and insufficient lubrication during intercourse may also cause discomfort. Dyspareunia can also be psychological in origin. As with other sexual problems, dyspareunia can be treated, with good results.

Vaginismus is the involuntary contraction of vaginal muscles, making penile insertion painful or impossible. Most cases are related to fear of intercourse or to unresolved sexual conflicts. Treatment involves teaching a woman to achieve orgasm through nonvaginal stimulation.

Sexual dysfunctions are most common in the early adult years. The incidence of dysfunction increases again during perimenopause and postmenopause years in women and in older age for both men and women.[45] Don't be afraid to talk to a counselor or medical professional; most colleges and universities have services available. The American Association of Sex Educators, Counselors, and Therapists (AASECT) also lists highly trained and certified counselors, sex therapists, and clinics that treat sexual dysfunctions at www.aasect.org.

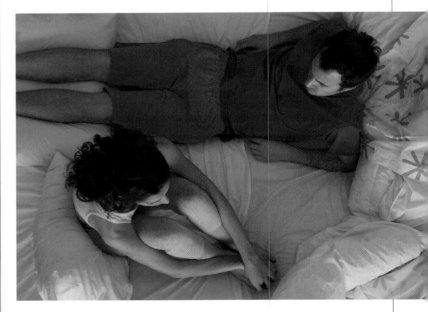

Sexual disorders can have both physical and psychological roots. Interpersonal problems can contribute to dysfunction as well.

check yourself

- **What are some types and causes of sexual dysfunction?**

- **Would you consider physical or psychological causes of sexual dysfunction easer to treat? Why?**

Alcohol, Drugs, and Sex

- **Examine the negative outcomes associated with combining sex with drugs or alcohol.**

Because psychoactive drugs and alcohol affect the body's entire physiological functioning, it is only logical that they affect sexual behavior. Promises of increased pleasure make drugs very tempting to people seeking greater sexual satisfaction. Too often, however, drugs and alcohol become central to sexual activities and damage the relationship.

Drug and alcohol use can also lead to undesired sexual activity, as well as a tendency to blame the drug for negative behavior or unsafe sexual activities. "I can't help what I did last night because I was drunk" is a statement that demonstrates sexual immaturity. A sexually mature person carefully examines risks and benefits and makes decisions accordingly. If drugs are necessary to increase erotic feelings, it is likely that the partners are being dishonest about their feelings for each other. Good sex should not depend on chemical substances.

Alcohol is notorious for reducing inhibitions and promoting feelings of well-being and desirability. At the same time, alcohol inhibits sexual response—the mind may be willing, but not the body.

In addition to alcohol use, an increasing number of young men have begun experimenting with recreational use of drugs intended to treat erectile dysfunction, including Viagra, Cialis, and Levitra. Young men who take this type of medication are hoping to increase their sexual stamina or counteract sexual performance anxiety or the effects of alcohol or other drugs. However, these drugs probably have only a placebo effect in men with normal erections, and combining them with other drugs, such as cocaine, MDMA (Ecstasy), amyl nitrate ("poppers"), or methamphetamine, can lead to potentially fatal drug interactions. In particular, when combined with amyl nitrate these drugs can lead to a sudden drop in blood pressure and possible cardiac arrest.[46]

12%

of college men and 10% of college women who drank alcohol in the past year reported having **unprotected sex as a consequence of their drinking.**

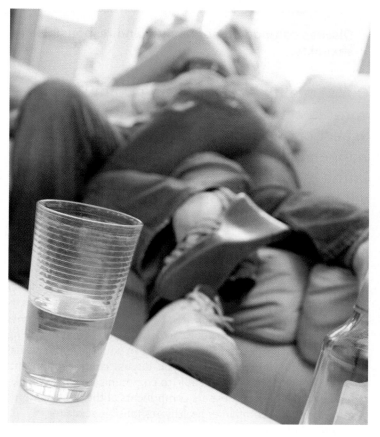

Drugs and alcohol can lead to decisions that you later regret.

"Date rape" drugs have been a growing concern in recent decades. They have become prevalent on college campuses, where they are often used in combination with alcohol. Rohypnol ("roofies," "rope," "forget pill"), GHB (gamma hydroxybutyrate, or "liquid X," "Grievous Bodily Harm," "easy lay," "Mickey Finn"), and ketamine ("K," "Special K," "cat valium") have all been used to facilitate rape. Rohypnol and GHB are difficult-to-detect drugs that depress the central nervous system. Ketamine can cause dreamlike states, hallucinations, delirium, amnesia, and impaired motor function. These drugs are often introduced to unsuspecting women through alcoholic drinks to render them unconscious and vulnerable to rape. This problem is so serious that the U.S. Congress passed the Drug-Induced Rape Prevention and Punishment Act of 1996 to increase federal penalties for using drugs to facilitate sexual assault.

- **Give three potential negative outcomes from combining sex with drugs or alcohol.**

Responsible and Satisfying Sexual Behavior

■ **Discuss components of healthy and responsible sexuality.**

Our sexuality is a fascinating, complex, contradictory, and sometimes frustrating aspect of our lives. Healthy sexuality doesn't happen by chance. It is a product of assimilating information and skills, of exploring values and beliefs, and of making responsible and informed choices. Healthy and responsible sexuality includes the following:

■ **Good communication as the foundation.** Open and honest communication with your partner is the basis for establishing respect, trust, and intimacy. Do you communicate with your partner in caring and respectful ways? Can you share your thoughts and emotions freely with your partner? Do you talk about being sexually active and what that means? Can you share your sexual history with your partner? Do you discuss contraception and disease prevention? Are you able to communicate what you like and don't like? All of these are components of the open communication that accompanies healthy, responsible sexuality.

■ **Acknowledging that you are a sexual person.** People who can see and accept themselves as sexual beings are more likely to make informed decisions and take responsible actions. If you see yourself as a potentially sexual person, you will plan ahead for contraception and disease prevention. If you are comfortable being a sexually active person, you will not need or want your sexual experiences clouded by alcohol or other drug use. If you choose not to be sexually active, you do so consciously, as a personal decision based on your convictions. Even if you are not sexually active, it is important to acknowledge that sex is a natural aspect of everyone's life and to recognize that you are in charge of your own decisions about your sexuality.

■ **Understanding sexual structures and their functions.** If you understand how your body works, sexual pleasure and response will not be mysterious events. You will be able to pleasure yourself as well as communicate to your partner how best to please you. You will understand how pregnancy and STIs can be prevented. You will be able to recognize sexual dysfunction and take responsible actions to address the problem.

■ **Accepting and embracing your gender identity and your sexual orientation.** "Being comfortable in your own skin" is an old saying that is particularly relevant when it comes to sexuality. It is difficult to feel sexually satisfied if you are conflicted about your gender identity or sexual orientation. You should explore and address questions and feelings you may have about your gender identity and/or your sexual orientation. Having good communication skills, acknowledging that you are a sexual person, and understanding your sexual structures and their functions will allow you to do so.

Skills for **Behavior Change**

TAKING STEPS TOWARD HEALTHY SEXUALITY

Healthy and responsible sexuality means having information and skills, exploring values and beliefs, and making responsible and informed choices. The following tips can help you:

■ Give some thought to your own sexuality. Do you choose to be sexually active now, or are you more comfortable waiting? If you are sexually active, which sexual practices are you comfortable with, and with whom?

■ Get to know sexual structures and their functions in order to make communicating easier and sex better. If you understand the workings of your body and your partner's, it can improve your sexual satisfaction and your relationship as a whole.

■ If you have a partner now, sit down and talk about your sexual relationship. Are you both comfortable and satisfied with all aspects of the relationship? Discuss what you like and don't like, and what you might like to change.

■ Explore and address any questions and feelings you may have about your gender identity and/or your sexual orientation.

■ **What are three components of healthy and responsible sexuality?**

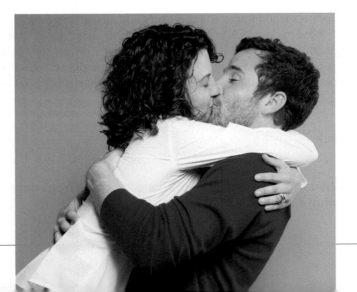

How Well Do You Communicate?

An interactive version of this assessment is available online. Download it from the Live It! section of www.pearsonhighered.com/donatelle.

Imagine that you are in each of the situations below and indicate how confident and satisfied you are that you could communicate competently using the following scale:

1. Very dissatisfied with my ability to communicate
2. Somewhat dissatisfied with my ability to communicate
3. Not sure how effectively I could communicate
4. Somewhat satisfied that I could communicate competently
5. Very satisfied that I could communicate competently

_____ 1. Someone asks you personal questions that you feel uncomfortable answering. You'd like to tell the person that you don't want to answer.

_____ 2. You think a friend is drinking more alcohol than is healthy, and you want to bring the topic up with her.

_____ 3. Your colleague asks you to write him a letter of recommendation. You don't think he is well suited for the position to which he's applying.

_____ 4. During a heated discussion about social issues, the person with whom you are talking says, "You're not listening to anything I'm saying!"

_____ 5. A friend shares his creative writing with you. You don't think the writing is very good, but you need to respond to his request for an opinion.

_____ 6. Your roommate's bad habits are really getting on your nerves. You want to tell her you're bothered and that you'd like her to stop.

_____ 7. You arrive at a party and discover that you don't know anyone there.

_____ 8. A classmate asks you for notes for the classes he missed, but you realize he has missed half the classes and expects you to bail him out.

_____ 9. The person you have been dating declares, "I love you." You care about her, but you don't love her, at least not yet.

_____ 10. A friend comes to you with his problems, and you give him attention and advice. However, when you want to discuss your problems, he doesn't seem to have the time. You value the friendship, but you don't like feeling it's one way.

_____ Total

Interpreting Your Score

If your score indicates that you are moderately satisfied (25–39) or dissatisfied (10–24) with your communication skills, notice whether your answers are extremes (1s and 5s). Focus on improving your skills in the situations that make you uneasy.

Source: Based on Julia Wood and Stephanie Coopman's Instructor's Resource Manual for Wood's text, *Interpersonal Communication: Everyday Encounters*, 5th ed. Copyright © 2006, Cengage Learning.

Your Plan for Change

The Assess Yourself activity gave you the chance to look at how you communicate. Now that you have considered your responses, you can take steps toward becoming a better communicator and improving your relationships.

Today, you can:

◯ Call a friend you haven't talked to in a while or arrange a coffee date with a new acquaintance you'd like to get to know better.

◯ Start a journal in which you keep track of communication and relationship issues that arise. Look for trends and think about ways you can change your behavior to address them.

Within the next 2 weeks, you can:

◯ Spend some time letting the people you care about know how important their relationship is to you.

◯ If there is someone with whom you have a conflict, arrange a time to sit down with that person in a neutral setting away from distractions to talk about the issues.

By the end of the semester, you can:

◯ Practice being an active listener and notice when your mind wanders while you are listening to someone.

◯ Take note of your nonverbal messages. Work on maintaining good eye contact and using open body language and inviting facial expressions.

Summary

- Characteristics of intimate relationships include behavioral interdependence, need fulfillment, emotional attachment, and emotional availability.
- Characteristics of satisfying and successful relationships include good communication, intimacy, friendship, and trust. Issues that can cause problems in relationships include jealousy, differences over gender roles, power struggles, and unmet expectations.
- To improve our ability to communicate, we need to learn how to use self-disclosure, listen effectively, convey and interpret nonverbal communication, establish a proper climate for communicating, and manage and resolve conflicts.
- For most people, commitment is an important ingredient in successful relationships. Committed relationships include marriage, cohabitation, and gay and lesbian partnerships.
- Life decisions such as whether to marry or have children require serious consideration. Remaining single is more common than ever before.
- By recognizing signs of relationship problems and taking action to change behaviors, partners may save and enhance their relationships.
- The major structures of the female sexual anatomy include the mons pubis, labia minora and majora, clitoris, vagina, uterus, cervix, fallopian tubes, and ovaries. The major structures of the male sexual anatomy are the penis, scrotum, testes, epididymides, vasa deferentia, ejaculatory ducts, urethra, and the accessory glands (seminal vesicles, prostate gland, and Cowper's glands).
- Physiologically, both males and females experience four stages of sexual response: excitement/arousal, plateau, orgasm, and resolution.
- Biological sex, gender identity, gender roles, and sexual orientation are all blended into our *sexual identity*. *Sexual orientation* refers to a person's enduring emotional, romantic, sexual, or affectionate attraction to other persons.
- People can express themselves sexually in a variety of ways.
- Responsible and satisfying sexuality involves good communication, recognition of yourself as a sexual being, understanding sexual structures and functions, and acceptance of your gender identity and sexual orientation.

Pop Quiz

1. Intimate relationships fulfill our psychological need for someone to listen to our worries and concerns. This is known as our need for
   a. dependence.
   b. social integration.
   c. enjoyment.
   d. spontaneity.

2. Lovers tend to pay attention to the other person even when they should be involved in other activities. This is called
   a. inclusion.
   b. exclusivity.
   c. fascination.
   d. authentic intimacy.

3. Terms such as *behavioral interdependence, need fulfillment,* and *emotional availability* describe which type of relationship?
   a. Dysfunctional
   b. Sexual
   c. Intimate
   d. Behavioral

4. All of the following are typical causes of jealousy EXCEPT
   a. overdependence on the relationship.
   b. low self-esteem.
   c. a past relationship that involved deception.
   d. belief that relationships can easily be replaced.

5. Jamie has just broken up with her boyfriend. Which is a recommended way to cope with the break up?
   a. Initiate a new relationship as soon as possible to recover.
   b. Cut off contact with friends, who will be painful reminders of the relationship.
   c. Avoid dwelling on sad feelings.
   d. Find ways to express emotions through exercise or listening to music.

6. Your personal inner sense of maleness or femaleness is known as your
   a. sexual identity.
   b. sexual orientation.
   c. gender identity.
   d. gender.

7. The most sensitive or erotic spot in the female genital region is the
   a. mons pubis.
   b. vagina.
   c. clitoris.
   d. labia.

8. When a woman is ovulating,
   a. she has released an egg cell.
   b. she has menstrual bleeding.
   c. an egg has been fertilized.
   d. the lining of her uterus thins.

9. A condition in which a woman experiences pain when menstruating is known as
   a. premenstrual syndrome.
   b. dysmenorrhea.
   c. premenstrual dysphoric disorder.
   d. amenorrhea.

10. What is the role of testosterone in the male reproductive system?
    a. It is used to produce sperm for reproduction.
    b. It is the hormone that stimulates development of secondary male sex characteristics.
    c. It allows the penis to harden during sexual arousal.
    d. It secretes the seminal fluid preceding ejaculation.

Answers to these questions can be found on page A-1.

Web Links

1. **Relationship Growth Online.** Information on how to build better relationships. www.relationshipweb.com
2. **The Conflict Resolution Information Source.** Resources for resolving conflicts. www.crinfo.org
3. **SmarterSex.org.** Student-friendly information on sexual health targeted at 18- to 24-year-olds. www.smartersex.org

Reproductive Choices

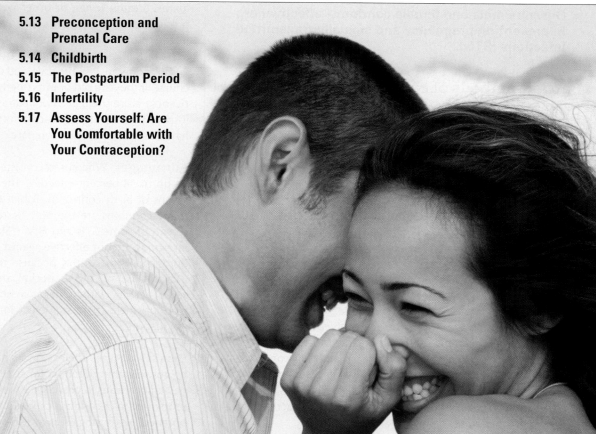

Today, we understand the intimate details of reproduction and possess technologies to control **fertility**. Along with information comes choice and responsibility, and one measure of maturity is the ability to discuss birth control with one's sexual partner. Too often, no one brings up the topic, and unprotected sex is the result. In fact, only 50 percent of college students (52% of women and 47% of men) report having used contraception the last time they had sexual intercourse.[1] The sad outcome is too many unwanted pregnancies and **sexually transmitted infections (STIs)**. If you're thinking about becoming sexually active, or you are but haven't used birth control, visit your health clinic to discuss contraceptives.

Birth control (or **contraception**) refers to methods of preventing **conception**, which occurs when a sperm fertilizes an egg. To evaluate a contraceptive method's effectiveness, look at its **perfect-use failure rate**, or percentage of pregnancies likely in the first year of use if the method is used entirely without error. Even more important, and more useful, is its **typical-use failure rate**, the percentage of pregnancies likely in the first year with *typical* use—that is, with the normal number of errors, memory lapses, and so on.

Barrier Methods: Male and Female Condoms

- **List the advantages and disadvantages of the male and female condoms.**
- **Describe male and female condoms' effectiveness in preventing pregnancy and sexually transmitted infections (STIs).**

Barrier methods of contraception work on the principle of preventing sperm from reaching the egg by use of a physical or chemical barrier during intercourse. Some barrier methods prevent semen from having contact with the woman's body, whereas others prevent sperm from going past the cervix. In addition, many barrier methods contain, or are used in combination with, a substance that kills sperm.

The Male Condom

The **male condom** is a thin sheath designed to cover the erect penis and catch semen before it enters the vagina. Most male condoms are made of latex, though polyurethane or lambskin condoms are also available. Condoms in a wide variety of styles may be purchased in pharmacies, supermarkets, public bathrooms, and many health clinics. A new condom must be used for each act of vaginal, oral, or anal intercourse.

A condom must be rolled onto the penis before the penis touches the vagina and must be held in place when removing the penis from the vagina after ejaculation (see **Figure 5.1**). Condoms come with or without **spermicide** and with or without lubrication.

Spermicide can cause irritation for some users, and there is no evidence that using it with condoms reduces the risk of pregnancy. If desired, users can lubricate their own condoms with contraceptive foams, creams, jellies, or other water-based lubricants. Never use products such as baby oil, cold cream, petroleum jelly, vaginal yeast infection medications, or body lotion with a condom. These products contain mineral oil and will cause the latex to disintegrate.

Condoms are less effective, and more likely to break during intercourse, if they are old or improperly stored. To maintain their effectiveness, store them in a cool place (not in a wallet or pocket), and inspect them for small tears before use. Discard all condoms that have passed their expiration date.

Advantages When used consistently and correctly, condoms can be up to 98 percent effective. The condom is the only temporary means of birth control available for men, and latex and polyurethane condoms are the only barriers that effectively prevent the spread of some STIs and HIV. ("Skin" condoms, made from lamb intestines, are not effective against STIs.) Many people choose condoms for birth control because they are inexpensive and readily available without a prescription, and their use is limited to times of sexual activity, with no negative health effects. Some men find that condoms help them stay erect longer or help prevent premature ejaculation.

Disadvantages The easy availability of condoms is accompanied by considerable potential for user error; the typical use effectiveness of condoms in preventing pregnancy is around 85 percent. Improper use of a condom can lead to breakage, leakage, or slipping, potentially exposing users to STIs or an unintended pregnancy. Even when used perfectly, a condom doesn't protect against STIs that may have external areas of infection (e.g., herpes). Some people feel that condoms ruin the spontaneity of sex because stopping to put one on may break the mood. Others report that condoms decrease

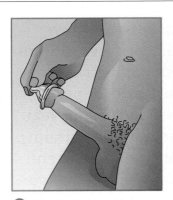

❶ Pinch the air out of the top half-inch of the condom to allow room for semen.

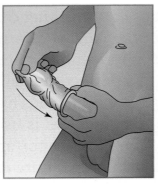

❷ Holding the tip of the condom with one hand, use the other hand to unroll it onto the penis.

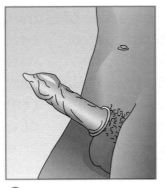

❸ Unroll the condom all the way to the base of the penis, smoothing out any air bubbles.

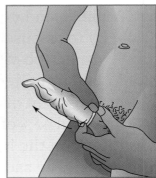

❹ After ejaculation, hold the condom around the base until the penis is totally withdrawn to avoid spilling any semen.

Figure 5.1 How to Use a Male Condom

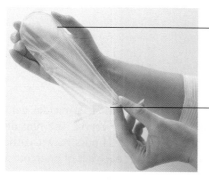

Inner ring is used for insertion and to help hold the sheath in place during intercourse.

Outer ring covers the area around the opening of the vagina.

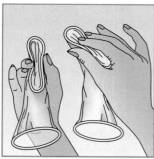

1 Grasp the flexible inner ring at the closed end of the condom, and squeeze it between your thumb and second or middle finger so it becomes long and narrow.

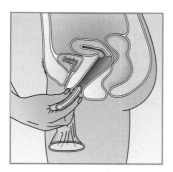

2 Choose a comfortable position for insertion: squatting, with one leg raised, or sitting or lying down. While squeezing the ring, insert the closed end of the condom into your vagina.

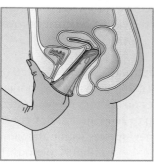

3 Placing your index finger inside of the condom, gently push the inner ring up as far as it will go. Be sure the sheath is not twisted. The outer ring should remain outside of the vagina.

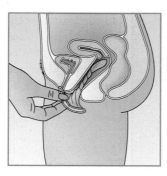

4 During intercourse, be sure that the penis is not entering on the side, between the sheath and the vaginal wall. When removing the condom, twist the outer ring so that no semen leaks out.

Figure 5.2 How to Use a Female Condom

sensation. These inconveniences and perceptions contribute to improper use or avoidance of condoms altogether. Partners who apply a condom as part of foreplay are generally more successful with this form of birth control. As a new condom is required for each act of intercourse, some users find it difficult to be sure to have a condom available when needed.

The Female Condom

The **female condom** is a single-use, soft, loose-fitting polyurethane sheath for internal vaginal use. It is designed as one unit with two flexible rings. One ring lies inside the sheath and serves as an insertion mechanism and internal anchor. The other remains outside the vagina once the device is inserted and protects the labia and the base of the penis from infection. **Figure 5.2** shows proper use of the female condom.

Advantages Used consistently and correctly, female condoms can be up to 95 percent effective. They also can prevent the spread of HIV and other STIs, including those that can be transmitted by external genital contact. The female condom can be inserted up to 8 hours in advance, so its use doesn't have to interrupt lovemaking. Some women choose the female condom because it gives them more personal control over prevention of pregnancy and STIs or because they cannot rely on their partners to use the male condom. Because the polyurethane is thin and pliable, there is less loss of sensation with the female condom than with the latex male condom. The female condom is relatively inexpensive, readily available without a prescription, and causes no negative health effects.

Disadvantages As with the male condom, there is potential for user error with the female condom, including possible breaking, slipping, or leaking, all of which could lead to STI transmission or an unintended pregnancy. Because of the potential problems, the typical use effectiveness of the female condom is 79 percent. Some people dislike using the female condom because they find it disruptive, noisy, odd looking, or difficult to use. Some women have reported external or vaginal irritation from using the female condom. A new condom is required for each act of intercourse, so users may not always have one available when needed. The female condom can be used effectively for anal sex, but it is difficult to use in this manner and can be painful. There is also the risk of rectal bleeding, which increases the risk of contracting HIV. Therefore, it's better to use the male condom with plenty of lubricant for anal sex.

check yourself

- **What are the advantages and disadvantages of the male and female condoms?**
- **How effective are the male and female condoms in preventing pregnancy and STIs?**
- **What are some reasons you might give to persuade a partner to use a condom?**

Other Barrier Methods

- **List the advantages and disadvantages of different types of barrier methods.**
- **Describe the effectiveness of barrier methods in preventing pregnancy and STIs.**

There are options beyond the male and female condoms for those who wish to use other barrier methods, including spermicides, the sponge, the diaphragm, and the cervical cap.

Spermicides

Some barrier methods—jellies, creams, foams, suppositories, and film—require no prescription. These are spermicides, substances designed to kill sperm. The active ingredient in most is nonoxynol-9 (N-9).

Jellies and creams come in tubes and foams in aerosol cans with applicators for vaginal insertion. They must be inserted far enough to cover the cervix, providing both a chemical barrier that kills sperm and a physical barrier that stops sperm from continuing toward an egg.

Suppositories are capsules inserted into the vagina, where they melt. They must be inserted 10 to 20 minutes before intercourse, but no more than 1 hour before or they lose their effectiveness. Additional contraceptive chemicals must be applied for each subsequent act of intercourse.

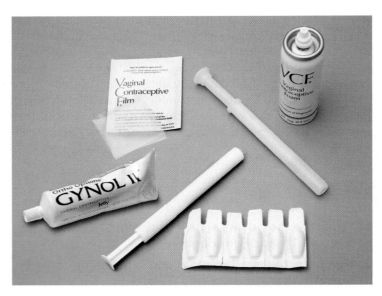

Spermicides come in many forms, including jellies, creams, films, foam, and suppositories.

With vaginal film, a thin film infused with spermicidal gel is inserted into the vagina so that it covers the cervix. The film dissolves into a spermicidal gel effective for up to 3 hours. As with other spermicides, a new film must be inserted for each act of intercourse.

Advantages Spermicides are most effective when used with another barrier method (condom, diaphragm, etc.). When used alone, they offer only 71 percent (typical use) to 82 percent (perfect use) effectiveness at preventing pregnancy. Spermicides are inexpensive, require no prescription or pelvic examination, and are available over the counter. They are simple to use and use is limited to the time of sexual activity.

Disadvantages Spermicides can be messy and must be reapplied for each act of intercourse. Some people experience irritation or allergic reactions to spermicides, and studies indicate that spermicides containing N-9 are ineffective in preventing transmission of STIs such as gonorrhea, chlamydia, and HIV. In fact, frequent use of N-9 spermicides can cause irritation and breaks in the mucous layer or skin of the genital tract, creating a point of entry for viruses and bacteria.[2] Spermicides containing N-9 have also been associated with increased risk of urinary tract infection.

The Sponge

The **Today sponge** is made of polyurethane foam and contains nonoxynol-9. Before insertion, it is moistened with water to activate the spermicide. It is then inserted into the vagina, where it fits over the cervix and creates a barrier against sperm.

Advantages The sponge is fairly effective (91% perfect use; 84% typical use) when used consistently and correctly. A main advantage of the sponge is convenience; it requires no doctor's fitting. Protection begins on insertion and lasts for up to 24 hours. It is not necessary to reapply spermicide or insert a new sponge within the same

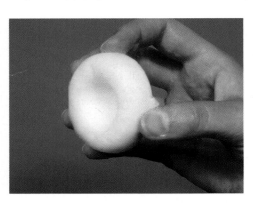

The Today sponge is a combination barrier method and spermicide that is most effective when used in conjunction with male condoms.

24-hour period; it must be left in place for at least 6 hours after last intercourse. Like the diaphragm and cervical cap, the sponge offers limited protection from some STIs.

Disadvantages The sponge is less effective for women who have given birth (80% perfect use; 68% typical use). Allergic

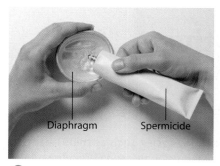

① Place spermicidal jelly or cream inside the diaphragm and all around the rim.

Diaphragm   Spermicide

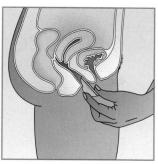

② Fold the diaphragm in half and insert dome-side down (spermicide-side up) into the vagina, pushing it along the back wall as far as it will go.

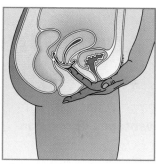

③ Position the diaphragm with the cervix completely covered and the front rim tucked up against your pubic bone; you should be able to feel your cervix through the rubber dome.

Figure 5.3 The Proper Use and Placement of a Diaphragm

reactions, such as vaginal irritation, are more common than with other barrier methods. Should the vaginal lining become irritated, the risk of yeast infections and other STIs may increase. Some cases of toxic shock syndrome have been reported in women using the sponge; precautions should be taken as with the diaphragm and cervical cap. Some women find the sponge difficult or messy to remove.

The Diaphragm

Invented in the mid-nineteenth century, the **diaphragm** was the first widely used birth control method for women. The device is a soft, shallow cup made of thin latex rubber. Its flexible, rubber-coated ring is designed to fit behind the pubic bone in front of the cervix and over the back of the cervix on the other side. Diaphragms must be used with spermicidal cream or jelly that is applied to the inside of the diaphragm before inserting. A diaphragm may be inserted up to 6 hours before intercourse. The diaphragm holds the spermicide in place, creating a physical and chemical barrier against sperm (**Figure 5.3**). Diaphragms come in different sizes and must be fitted by a trained practitioner, who should ensure that the user knows how to insert her diaphragm correctly before leaving the practitioner's office.

Advantages If used consistently and correctly, diaphragms can be 94 percent effective in preventing pregnancy. When used with spermicidal jelly or cream, the diaphragm also offers protection against gonorrhea and possibly chlamydia and human papillomavirus (HPV). After the initial fitting, the only ongoing expense is spermicide. Because the diaphragm can be inserted up to 6 hours in advance and used for multiple acts of intercourse, some users find it less disruptive than other barrier methods.

Disadvantages Although the diaphragm can be left in place for multiple acts of intercourse, additional spermicide must be applied each time, and the diaphragm must then stay in place for 6 to 8 hours afterward to allow the chemical to kill any sperm remaining in the vagina. Some women find insertion awkward. When inserted incorrectly, diaphragms are much less effective. A diaphragm may

also slip out of place, be difficult to remove, or require refitting (e.g., following pregnancy or significant weight gain or loss).

The Cervical Cap

One of the oldest methods used to prevent pregnancy, early **cervical caps** were made from beeswax, silver, or copper. The currently available FemCap is a clear silicone cup that fits over the cervix. It comes in three sizes and must be fitted by a practitioner. The FemCap is designed for use with spermicidal jelly or cream. It is held in place by suction created during application and works by blocking sperm from the uterus.

Advantages Cervical caps can be reasonably effective (86%) with typical use. They may also offer some protection against transmission of gonorrhea, HPV, and possibly chlamydia. They are relatively inexpensive—the only ongoing cost is for spermicide.

The FemCap can be inserted up to 6 hours before intercourse, making it potentially less disruptive than other barrier methods. The device must be left in place for 6 to 8 hours afterward; after that, if removed and cleaned, it can be reinserted immediately. Because the FemCap is made of silicon rubber, it is a suitable alternative for people allergic to latex.

Disadvantages The FemCap is somewhat more difficult to insert than a diaphragm because of its size. Like a diaphragm, it requires a fitting and may require subsequent refitting if a woman's cervix size changes, as after giving birth. Because the FemCap can become dislodged during intercourse, placement must be checked frequently. It cannot be used during the menstrual period or for longer than 48 hours because of the risk of *toxic shock syndrome (TSS)*. Some women report unpleasant vaginal odors after use.

check yourself

- **What are the advantages and disadvantages of different types of barrier methods?**
- **How effective are barrier methods in preventing pregnancy and STIs?**

learning **outcomes**

- **List the advantages and disadvantages of oral contraceptives.**
- **Describe the effectiveness of oral contraceptives in preventing pregnancy and STIs.**

The term *hormonal contraception* refers to birth control containing synthetic estrogen and/or progestin. These ingredients are similar to the hormones estrogen and progesterone, which a woman's ovaries produce naturally for the process of ovulation and the menstrual cycle. In recent years, hormonal contraception has become available in a variety of forms (transdermal, injection, and oral). All forms require a prescription from a health care provider.

Hormonal contraception alters a woman's biochemistry, preventing ovulation (release of the egg) from taking place and producing changes that make it more difficult for the sperm to reach the egg if ovulation does occur. Many hormonal contraceptives contain estrogen and progestin (synthetic progesterone); several contain just progestin. Synthetic estrogen works to prevent the ovaries from releasing an egg. If no egg is released, there is nothing to be fertilized by sperm and pregnancy cannot occur. Progestin, too, can prevent ovulation. It also thickens cervical mucus, which hinders sperm movement, inhibits the egg's ability to travel through the fallopian tubes, and suppresses sperm's ability to unite with the egg. Progestin also thins the uterine lining, rendering the egg unlikely to implant in the uterine wall.

Oral Contraceptives

Oral contraceptive pills were first marketed in the United States in 1960. Their convenience quickly made them the most widely used reversible method of fertility control. Most modern pills are up to 99 percent effective at preventing pregnancy with perfect use. Today, oral contraceptives are the most commonly used birth control method among college women (**Table 5.1**).[3]

Most oral contraceptives work through the combined effects of synthetic estrogen and progesterone (*combination pills*). Combination pills are taken in a cycle. At the end of each 3-week cycle, the user discontinues the drug or takes placebo pills for 1 week. The resultant drop in hormones causes the uterine lining to disintegrate; the user then has a menstrual period, usually within 1 to 3 days. Menstrual flow is generally lighter than for women who don't use the pill, because the hormones in the pill prevent thick endometrial buildup.

Several new pills have extended cycles, such as the 91-day Seasonale and Seasonique. A woman using this type of regimen takes active pills for 12 weeks, followed by 1 week of placebos. Under this cycle, women can expect to have a menstrual period every 3 months. Women often have increased occurrence of spotting or bleeding in the first few cycles.[4] Lybrel, another extended-cycle pill, is taken continuously for 1 year, eliminating menstruation completely.

Advantages Combination pills are highly effective at preventing pregnancy: 99.7 percent with perfect use and 92 percent with typical use. It is easier to achieve perfect use with pills than with barrier contraceptives, because there is less room for user error. Aside from its effectiveness, much of the pill's popularity is due to convenience and discreetness. Users like the fact that it does not interfere with lovemaking.

In addition to preventing pregnancy, the pill may lessen menstrual difficulties such as cramps and premenstrual syndrome (PMS). Oral contraceptives also lower the risk of conditions including

TABLE 5.1	Top Reported Means of Contraception Sexually Active Students or Their Partner Used the Last Time They Had Intercourse		
Method	**Male**	**Female**	**Total**
Any form of hormonal contraceptive (pills, injection, patch, ring, implant) excluding IUD	*71.9%*	*68.1%*	*69.6%*
Male condom	68.3%	61.3%	63.6%
Birth control pills (monthly or extended cycle)	60.1%	59.1%	59.4%
Male condom plus another method	*49.7%*	*45.0%*	*46.5%*
Withdrawal	27.1%	29.7%	28.8%
Any two or more methods (excluding male condoms)	*26.9%*	*27.1%*	*27.1%*
Fertility awareness (calendar, mucus, basal body temperature)	5.2%	5.5%	5.4%
Spermicide (foam, jelly, cream)	7.8%	3.8%	5.1%
Intrauterine device	3.9%	4.5%	4.3%
Vaginal ring	4.4%	4.2%	4.3%

Note: Survey respondents could select more than one method. Italicized rows are aggregates of the data.
Source: American College Health Association, *American College Health Association—National College Health Assessment II: Reference Group Report Fall 2010* (Baltimore: American College Health Association, 2011).

endometrial and ovarian cancers, noncancerous breast disease, osteoporosis, ovarian cysts, pelvic inflammatory disease (PID), and iron-deficiency anemia.[5] Many different brands of combination pills are on the market, some of which contain progestins that offer benefits such as reducing acne or minimizing fluid retention. Less-expensive generic versions are also available for many brands. With the extended-cycle pills, the major additional benefit is reduction in or absence of menstruation and associated cramps or PMS symptoms. Users of these pills also like that they don't need to remember when to stop or start a cycle of pills, or when to use placebos.

Disadvantages The estrogen in combination pills is associated with the risk of several serious health problems, including blood clots (which can lead to strokes or heart attacks) and an increased risk of high blood pressure. The risk is low for most healthy women under the age of 35 who don't smoke; it increases with age and especially with cigarette smoking. Early warning signs of serious medical complications are severe abdominal pain; chest pain with breathing difficulty; severe headache, weakness, or numbness; vision or speech problems; or severe calf or thigh pain.[6] If you use the pill and experience any of these symptoms, contact your health care provider immediately. Women over the age of 35 should especially be aware of these warning signs and should take them seriously.

Different brands of pills can cause varying minor side effects. Some of the most common are spotting between periods (particularly with extended-cycle regimens), breast tenderness, and nausea. With most pills, these clear up within a few months. Other potential side effects include change in sexual desire, acne, weight gain, and hair loss or growth. Because so many brands are available, most women who wish to use the pill are able to find one that works for them with few side effects.

The pill's other major disadvantage is that it must be taken every day. If a woman misses one pill, she should use an alternative form of contraception for the remainder of that cycle. A backup method of birth control is also necessary during the first week of use. After a woman discontinues the pill, return of fertility may be delayed, though the pill is not known to cause infertility. Another drawback is that the pill does not protect against STIs. Cost may also be a problem for some women. Some teenagers report that the requirement to have a complete gynecological examination in order to get a prescription for the pill is an obstacle.

Progestin-Only Pills

Progestin-only pills (or minipills) contain small doses of synthetic progesterone and no estrogen. These pills are taken continuously (no placebo pills are included in each pack).

Advantages Progestin-only pills are a good choice for women who are at high risk for estrogen-related side effects or who cannot take estrogen-containing pills because of diabetes, high blood pressure, or other cardiovascular conditions. They can also be used safely by women over 35 and breastfeeding mothers. Their effectiveness rate is 96 percent with perfect use, slightly lower than that of estrogen-containing pills. Progestin-only pills share some health benefits associated with combination pills and carry no estrogen-related

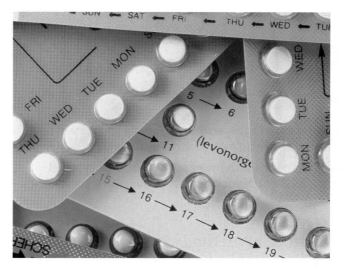

Does the birth control pill cause any side effects?

There are many different brands and regimens of oral contraceptives available to women today, some of which are associated with various health benefits such as acne reduction or lessening of PMS symptoms. Some women experience minor side effects from pill use—the most common being headaches, breast tenderness, nausea, and breakthrough bleeding—but these usually clear up within 2 to 3 months. If you experience any side effects from pill use, talk to your health care provider about them, as she may be able to recommend another brand of pill or method of birth control that will work better for you.

99

cardiovascular risks. Also, some typical side effects of combination pills, including nausea and breast tenderness, seldom occur with progestin-only pills. With progestin-only pills, menstrual periods generally become lighter or stop altogether.

Disadvantages Because of the lower dose of hormones in progestin-only pills, it is especially important that they be taken at the same time each day. If a woman takes a pill 3 or more hours later than usual, she will need to use a backup method of contraception for the next 48 hours. The most common side effect of progestin-only pills is irregular menstrual bleeding or spotting. Less common side effects include mood changes, changes in sex drive, and headaches. As with all oral contraceptives, progestin-only pills do not protect against STI transmission.

check yourself

- **What are the advantages and disadvantages of oral contraceptives?**

- **How effective are oral contraceptives in preventing pregnancy and STIs?**

Hormonal Methods: The Patch, Ring, Injections, and Implants

- **List the advantages and disadvantages of various hormonal methods of contraception.**
- **Describe the effectiveness of various hormonal methods of contraception in preventing pregnancy and STIs.**

Some hormonal methods, such as oral contraceptives, require the user to remember to take the pill every day. Others, such as the skin patch, ring, injections, and implants, do not require daily action.

Contraceptive Skin Patch

Ortho Evra is a square transdermal (through the skin) adhesive patch. It is as thin as a plastic strip bandage, is worn for 1 week, and is replaced on the same day of the week for 3 consecutive weeks; the fourth week is patch-free. Ortho Evra works by delivering continuous levels of estrogen and progestin through the skin and into the bloodstream. The patch can be worn on one of four areas of the body: buttocks, abdomen, upper torso (front and back, excluding the breasts), or upper outer arm.

Advantages Ortho Evra is 99.7 percent effective with perfect use. As with other hormonal methods, there is less room for user error than with barrier methods. Women who choose to use the patch often do so because they find it easier to remember than taking a daily pill, and they like the fact that they need to change the patch only once a week. Ortho Evra probably offers similar potential health benefits as combination pills (reduction in risk of certain cancers and diseases, lessening of PMS symptoms, etc.). Like other hormonal methods, the patch regulates a woman's menstrual cycle.

Disadvantages Using the patch requires an initial exam and prescription, weekly patch changes, and the ongoing monthly expense of patch purchase. A generic version is not currently available. A backup method is required during the first week of use. Similar to other hormonal methods of birth control, the patch offers no protection against HIV or other STIs. Some women experience minor side effects, such as those associated with combination pills. The estrogen in the patch is associated with cardiovascular risks, particularly in women who smoke and women over the age of 35. In 2005, amidst evidence that the patch may increase a woman's risk for life-threatening blood clots, the U.S. Food and Drug Administration (FDA) mandated an additional warning label explaining that patch use exposes women to about 60 percent more total estrogen than if they were taking a typical combination pill. Recently, the FDA released another warning for users, indicating more conclusive evidence of an increased risk of blood clots among regular users.[7]

Vaginal Contraceptive Ring

NuvaRing is a soft, flexible plastic hormonal contraceptive ring about 2 inches in diameter. The user inserts the ring into her vagina, leaves it in place for 3 weeks, and removes it for 1 week for her menstrual period. Once the ring is inserted, it releases a steady flow of estrogen and progestin.

Advantages When used properly, the ring is 99.7 percent effective. Advantages of NuvaRing include less likelihood of user error, protection against pregnancy for 1 month, no pill to take daily or patch to change weekly, no need to be fitted by a clinician, no requirement to use spermicide, and rapid return of fertility when use is stopped. It also exposes the user to a lower dosage of estrogen than do the patch and some combination pills, so it may have fewer estrogen-related side effects. It probably offers some of the same potential health benefits as combination pills and, like other hormonal contraceptives, it regulates a woman's menstrual cycle.

Disadvantages NuvaRing requires an initial exam and prescription, monthly ring changes, and the ongoing monthly expense of purchasing the ring (a generic version is not currently available). A backup method must be used during the first week, and the ring provides no protection against STI transmission. Like combination pills, the ring poses possible minor side effects and potentially more serious health risks for some women. Possible side effects unique to the ring include increased vaginal discharge and vaginal irritation or infection. Oil-based vaginal medicines to treat yeast infections cannot be used when the ring is in place, and a diaphragm or cervical cap cannot be used as a backup method for contraception.

Ortho Evra is an adhesive patch that delivers estrogen and progestin through the skin for 3 weeks.

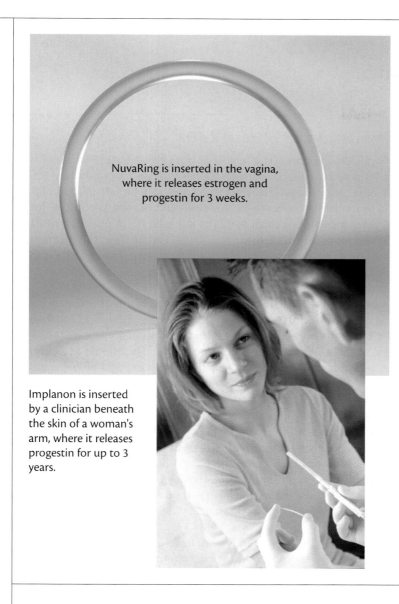

NuvaRing is inserted in the vagina, where it releases estrogen and progestin for 3 weeks.

Implanon is inserted by a clinician beneath the skin of a woman's arm, where it releases progestin for up to 3 years.

Contraceptive Injections

Depo-Provera is a long-acting synthetic progesterone that is injected intramuscularly every 3 months by a health care provider. It prevents ovulation, thickens cervical mucus, and thins the uterine lining—all of which prevent pregnancy from occurring.

Advantages Depo-Provera takes effect within 24 hours of the first shot, so there is usually no need to use a backup method. There is little room for user error with the shot (because it is administered by a clinician every 3 months): with perfect use the shot is 99.7 percent effective, and with typical use it is 97 percent effective. Some women feel Depo-Provera encourages sexual spontaneity, because they do not have to remember to take a pill or insert a device. With continued use of this method, a woman's menstrual periods become lighter and may eventually stop altogether. No estrogen-related health risks are associated with Depo-Provera, and it offers the same potential health benefits as progestin-only pills. Unlike estrogen-containing hormonal methods, Depo-Provera can be used by women who are breast-feeding.

Disadvantages Using Depo-Provera requires an initial exam and prescription, as well as follow-up visits every 3 months to have the shot administered. It offers no protection against transmission of STIs. The main disadvantage of Depo-Provera use is irregular bleeding, which can be troublesome at first, but within a year most women are amenorrheic (have no menstrual periods). Weight gain (an average of 5 pounds in the first year) is common. Depo-Provera comes with a warning that prolonged use is linked with loss of bone density. Other possible side effects include dizziness, nervousness, and headache. Unlike other methods of contraception, this method cannot be stopped immediately if problems arise, and the drug and its side effects may linger for up to 6 months after the last shot. Also, after the final injection, it may take women who wish to get pregnant up to a year to conceive.

Contraceptive Implants

A single-rod implantable contraceptive, **Implanon** is a small (about the size of a matchstick), soft plastic capsule that is inserted just beneath the skin on the inner side of a woman's upper underarm by a health care provider. Implanon continually releases a low, steady dose of progestin for up to 3 years, suppressing ovulation during that time.

Advantages After insertion, Implanon is generally not visible, making it a discreet method of birth control. The main advantages of Implanon are that it is highly effective (99.95%), it is not subject to user error, and it needs to be replaced only every 3 years. It has similar benefits to those of other progestin-only forms of contraception, including the lightening or cessation of menstrual periods, the lack of estrogen-related side effects, and safety for use by breast-feeding women. Fertility usually returns quickly after removal of the implant.

Disadvantages Insertion and removal of Implanon must be performed by a clinician. The initial cost is higher for this method, and it may not be covered by all health plans. Potential minor side effects include irritation, allergic reaction, swelling, or scarring around the area of insertion; there is also a possibility of infection or complications with removal. As with other progestin-only contraceptives, users can experience irregular bleeding. Implanon offers no protection against transmission of STIs, and it may require a backup method during the first week of use.

check yourself

- **What are the advantages and disadvantages of the various hormonal methods of contraception?**
- **How effective are various hormonal methods of contraception in preventing pregnancy and STIs?**
- **The methods of contraception discussed in this module remain in place for days or weeks. What are the benefits and drawbacks of this characteristic?**

Intrauterine Contraceptives

learning outcomes

- **List the advantages and disadvantages of intrauterine contraceptives.**
- **Describe the effectiveness of intrauterine contraceptives in preventing pregnancy and STIs.**

The **intrauterine device (IUD)** is a small, plastic, flexible device with a nylon string attached that is placed in the uterus through the cervix and left there for 5 to 10 years at a time. The exact mechanism by which it works is not clearly understood, but researchers believe IUDs affect the way sperm and egg move, thereby preventing fertilization and/or affecting the lining of the uterus to prevent a fertilized ovum from implanting.

The IUD was once extremely popular in the United States; however, most brands were removed from the market because of serious complications, such as pelvic inflammatory disease and infertility. Worldwide, newer IUDs are again very popular, though they have not experienced the same resurgence of popularity among U.S. women.

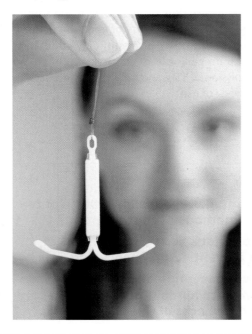

Mirena IUD is a flexible plastic device inserted by a clinician into a woman's uterus, where it releases progestin for up to 5 years.

ParaGard and Mirena IUDs

Two IUDs are currently available in the United States. *ParaGard* is a T-shaped plastic device with copper wrapped around the shaft. It does not contain any hormones and can be left in place for 10 years before replacement. A newer IUD, *Mirena*, is effective for 5 years and releases small amounts of progestin. A physician must fit and insert an IUD. One or two strings extend from the IUD into the vagina so the user can check to make sure that her IUD is in place. The device is removed by a practitioner when desired.

Advantages The IUD is a safe, discreet, and highly effective method of birth control (99.4%). It is effective immediately and needs to be replaced only every 10 years (ParaGard) or every 5 years (Mirena). ParaGard has the benefit of containing no hormones at all, and so has none of the potential negative health impacts of hormonal contraceptives. Mirena probably offers some of the same potential health benefits as other progestin-only methods. Both IUDs can be used by breastfeeding women. With Mirena, periods become lighter or stop altogether. The IUDs are fully reversible; after removal, there is usually no delay in return of fertility. Both of these methods offer sexual spontaneity, because there is no need to keep supplies on hand or to interrupt lovemaking. The devices begin working immediately, and there is a low incidence of side effects. The IUD can be removed at any time by a clinician.

Disadvantages Disadvantages of IUDs include possible discomfort, cost of insertion, and potential complications. Also, the IUD does not protect against STIs. In some women, the device can cause heavy menstrual flow and severe cramps for the first few months. With Mirena, menstrual periods tend to become shorter and lighter over time. Other side effects include acne, headaches, nausea, breast tenderness, mood changes, uterine cramps, and backache, which seems to occur most often in women who have never been pregnant. Women using IUDs have a higher risk of benign ovarian cysts. The devices are not usually recommended for use by women who have never had children because of an increased incidence of side effects and risk of infection with possible resultant infertility.

check yourself

- **What are the advantages and disadvantages of intrauterine contraceptives?**
- **How effective are intrauterine contraceptives in preventing pregnancy and STIs?**

Emergency Contraception

learning outcomes

- **Describe how emergency contraception prevents pregnancy.**

The most common **emergency contraceptive pills (ECPs)** are combination estrogen–progestin pills and progestin-only pills. ECPs are used to prevent pregnancy after unprotected intercourse, sexual assault, or failure of another birth control method.

ECPs are sometimes referred to as "morning-after pills." They are not the same as the "abortion pill," although the two are often confused. ECPs are used after unprotected intercourse, but before a woman misses her period. A woman takes ECPs to prevent pregnancy; the method will not work if she is already pregnant, nor will it harm an existing pregnancy. In contrast, Mifeprex or mifepristone (formerly known as RU-486), the *early abortion pill*, is used to terminate a pregnancy that is already established—after a woman is sure she is pregnant. It and other methods of abortion are discussed later in the chapter.

ECPs prevent pregnancy by delaying or inhibiting ovulation, inhibiting fertilization, or blocking implantation of a fertilized egg, depending on the phase of the menstrual cycle. Although ECPs use the same hormones as birth control pills, not all brands of pills can be used for emergency contraception. When taken within 24 hours, ECPs reduce the risk of pregnancy by up to 95 percent; when taken 2 to 5 days later, ECPs reduce the risk of pregnancy by 75 to 89 percent.[8]

Three brands of ECPs are available in the United States. Plan B One-Step and its generic equivalent, Next Choice, are available over the counter for those 17 and older. For anyone under 17, a prescription is required. Nine states have laws permitting a pharmacist to provide emergency contraception to customers under 17 without a prescription under certain conditions. Seven states have laws allowing pharmacists to distribute it to minors if they are working in collaboration with a physician under state-approved protocols.[9] These progestin-only pills should be taken as soon as possible (but not later than 72 hours, or 3 days) after unprotected intercourse.

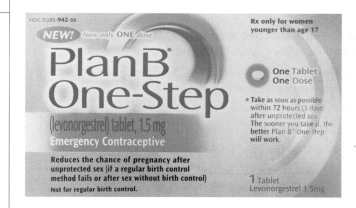

What is emergency contraception?

Emergency contraception is the use of a contraceptive—either hormone-containing pills or an IUD—after an act of unprotected intercourse. Plan B One-Step and Next Choice are the two brands of emergency contraceptive currently available without a prescription to American consumers aged 17 or older. A third choice, ella, is available only by prescription.

In August 2010, the FDA approved ella, a new ECP available only by prescription. A progesterone receptor modulator, ella works by inhibiting or preventing ovulation. It can prevent pregnancy when taken up to 120 hours (5 days) following unprotected intercourse.

Although ECPs are no substitute for proper precautions before sex, their potential for reducing unintended pregnancy, and ultimately abortion, is strong. According to recent surveys, 67 percent of all college health centers provide emergency contraception and 15.8 percent of sexually active college students reported using (or their partner using) it within the past year.[10]

ECPs are hormone-based, and so they can have the same physical side effects as other hormonal contraceptives. Among some women, they can cause an upset stomach and vomiting. Other women may experience breast tenderness, irregular bleeding, dizziness, and headaches. If ECPs are used frequently, their hormonal effects can lead to irregular menstrual periods.

A copper-wrapped IUD may also be used as emergency contraception if inserted by a doctor or a trained clinician within 5 days after intercourse.

check yourself

- **How does emergency contraception prevent pregnancy?**
- **What, if any, do you think the restrictions should be on providing emergency contraception?**

103

- **List the advantages and disadvantages of behavioral and fertility awareness methods.**

- **Describe the effectiveness of behavioral and fertility awareness methods in preventing pregnancy and STIs.**

Some methods of contraception rely on one or both partners altering their sexual behavior. In general, these methods require more self-control, diligence, and commitment, making them more prone to user error than other methods.

Withdrawal, or *coitus interruptus*, involves removing the penis from the vagina just prior to ejaculation. In a recent survey, approximately 29 percent of respondents reported using withdrawal the last time they had intercourse.[11] This statistic is startlingly high, considering the very high risk of pregnancy or contracting an STI associated with this method. Withdrawal is highly unreliable, even with "perfect" use—there can be up to half a million sperm in the drop of fluid at the tip of the penis *before* ejaculation. Timing withdrawal is also difficult. Withdrawal offers no protection against transmission of STIs.

Strictly defined, **abstinence** means "deliberately avoiding intercourse," which would allow one to engage in such forms of intimacy as massage, kissing, and solitary masturbation. However, many people today have broadened the definition to include all forms of sexual contact. Couples engaging in activities such as oral–genital sex and mutual masturbation are sometimes said to be engaging in "outercourse."

Abstinence is the only method of avoiding pregnancy that is 100 percent effective. It is also the only one 100 percent effective against transmitting disease. Outercourse can be 100 percent effective for birth control as long as the male does not ejaculate near the vaginal opening, though it is not 100 percent effective against STIs. Oral–genital contact can transmit disease, although the practice can be made safer by using a condom on the penis or a dental dam on the vaginal opening. Both abstinence and outercourse may be difficult to sustain over long periods of time.

Fertility awareness methods (FAMs) of birth control rely on altering sexual behavior during certain times of the month (**Figure 5.4**) based on the facts that an ovum can survive for up to 48 hours after ovulation and sperm can live for up to 5 days in the vagina. Strategies include the *cervical mucus method*, which requires tracking changes in vaginal secretions; the *body temperature method*, which requires tracking subtle changes in a woman's basal body temperature; and the *calendar method*, which involves recording the menstrual cycle for 12 months and assuming that ovulation occurs during the midpoint

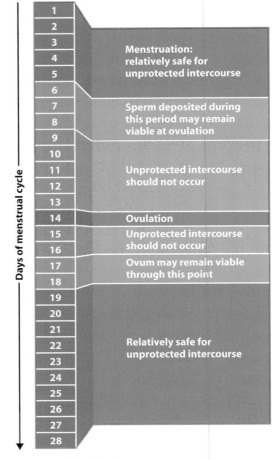

Figure 5.4 The Fertility Cycle

It is important to remember that most women do not have a consistent 28-day cycle.

of the cycle. All these methods require abstaining from penis–vagina contact during fertile times.

Fertility awareness methods are the only birth control complying with certain religious teachings, including those of the Roman Catholic Church. They require no medical visit or prescription and have no negative health effects. Their effectiveness depends on diligence and self-discipline; they are only 75 percent effective with typical use. They offer no STI protection and may not work for women with irregular menstrual cycles.

- **What are the advantages and disadvantages of behavioral and fertility awareness methods?**

- **How effective are these methods in preventing pregnancy and STIs?**

Surgical Methods

learning outcomes

- **List the advantages, disadvantages, and effectiveness of surgical methods in preventing pregnancy and STIs.**

In the United States, **sterilization** has become the second leading method of contraception for women of all ages and the leading method among married women and women over 35.[12] Because sterilization is permanent, anyone considering it should think through possibilities such as divorce and remarriage or improvement in financial status that might make a pregnancy desirable.

Female Sterilization

In **tubal ligation**, the woman's fallopian tubes are sealed to block sperm's access to released eggs (**Figure 5.5**). The operation is usually done laparoscopically on an outpatient basis and takes less than an hour. Tubal ligation does not affect ovarian and uterine function. The menstrual cycle continues; released eggs disintegrate and are absorbed by the lymphatic system. As soon as her incision heals, the woman may resume intercourse with no fear of pregnancy.

A newer procedure, Essure, involves placement of microcoils into the fallopian tubes via the vagina. The microcoils expand, promoting growth of scar tissue that blocks the tubes. Essure is recommended for women who cannot have a tubal ligation because of health conditions such as obesity or heart disease. With Adiana, another new method, a small flexible instrument is used to place a tiny insert into each fallopian tube. The body's tissue grows around the insert and eventually blocks the tubes.

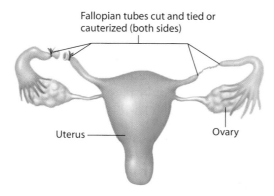

Fallopian tubes cut and tied or cauterized (both sides)

Uterus — — Ovary

Figure 5.5 Female Sterilization: Tubal Ligation

A **hysterectomy**, or removal of the uterus, is a method of sterilization requiring major surgery. It is usually done only when a woman's uterus is diseased or damaged.

The main advantage to female sterilization is that it is highly effective and permanent. Afterward, no other cost or action is required. Sterilization has no negative effect on sex drive. The Essure and Adiana methods require no incision. As with any surgery, there are risks involved. Sterilization offers no protection against STIs and is initially expensive.

Male Sterilization

Sterilization in men is less complicated. A **vasectomy** is frequently done on an outpatient basis, using a local anesthetic (see **Figure 5.6**). It involves making a small incision in each side of the scrotum to expose the vasa deferentia, cutting and either tying or cauterizing the ends. Because sperm constitute only a small percentage of semen, the amount of ejaculate is not changed significantly. The testes continue to produce sperm, which disintegrate and are absorbed into the lymphatic system.

A vasectomy is highly effective and permanent: After 1 year, the pregnancy rate in women whose partners have had vasectomies is 0.15 percent.[13] The procedure requires minimal recovery time, and afterward no cost or action is required. Vasectomy has no effect on sex drive or sexual performance.

Male sterilization offers no protection against STI transmission. Also, a vasectomy is not immediately effective; because sperm are stored in other areas besides the vasa deferentia, couples must use alternative birth control for at least 1 month afterward. A physician's semen analysis determines when unprotected intercourse can take place. As with any surgery, there are some risks. Very infrequently the vas deferens may create a new path, negating the procedure.

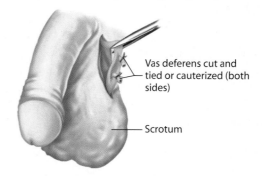

Vas deferens cut and tied or cauterized (both sides)

Scrotum

Figure 5.6 Male Sterilization: Vasectomy

check yourself

- **What are the advantages, disadvantages, and effectiveness of surgical methods in preventing pregnancy and STIs?**

Choosing a Method of Contraception

- **Explore questions to consider when choosing a method of contraception.**
- **Determine strategies for discussing contraception with a partner.**

With all the options available, how does a person or a couple decide what method of contraception is best? Take some time to research the various methods, ask questions of your health care provider, and be honest with yourself and your partner about your own preferences. Questions to ask yourself include the following:

- **How comfortable would I be using a particular method?** If you aren't at ease with a method, you may not use it consistently, and it probably will not be a reliable choice for you. Think about whether the method may cause discomfort for you or your partner, and consider your own comfort level with touching your body. For women, methods such as the diaphragm, sponge, and NuvaRing require inserting an apparatus into the vagina and taking it out. For men, using a condom requires rolling it onto the penis.
- **Will this method be convenient for me and my partner?** Some methods require more effort than do others. Be honest with yourself about how likely you are to use the method consistently. Are you willing to interrupt lovemaking, to abstain from sex during certain times of the month, or to take a pill every day? You may feel condoms are easy and convenient to use, or you

may prefer something that requires little ongoing thought, such as Depo-Provera or an IUD.

- **Am I at risk for the transmission of STIs?** If you have multiple sex partners or are uncertain about the sexual history or disease status of your current sex partner, then you are at risk for transmission of STIs and HIV (the virus that causes AIDS). Condoms (both male and female) are the *only* birth control methods that protect against STIs and HIV (although some other barrier methods offer limited protection). Condoms reduce your risk of STIs as well as HIV. Condoms alone are not a highly effective birth control method; to avoid both STI infection and pregnancy, combine a condom with a more effective birth control method.
- **Do I want to have a biological child in the future?** If you are unsure about your plans for future childbearing, you should use a temporary birth control method rather than a permanent one such as sterilization. Keep in mind that you may regret choosing a permanent method if you are young, if you have few or no children, if you are choosing this method because your partner wants you to, or if you believe this option will fix relationship problems. If you know you want to have children in the future, consider how soon that will be, because some methods, such as Depo-Provera, cause a delay in return to fertility.
- **How would an unplanned pregnancy affect my life?** If an unplanned pregnancy would be a potentially devastating event for you or would have a serious impact on your plans for the future, then you should choose a highly effective birth control method, for example, the pill, patch, ring, implant, or IUD. If, however, you are in a stable relationship, have a reliable source of income, are planning to have children in the future, and would embrace a pregnancy should it occur now, then you may be comfortable with a less reliable method such as the diaphragm, cervical cap, or spermicides.
- **What are my religious and moral values in relation to contraception?** Fertility awareness methods are a good option if you are morally or spiritually opposed to using certain other birth control methods. When both partners are motivated to use these methods, they can be successful at preventing unintended pregnancy. If you are considering this option, sign up for a class to get specific training on using the method effectively.
- **How much will the birth control method cost?** Some contraceptive methods involve an initial outlay of money and few continuing costs (e.g., sterilization, IUD), whereas others are fairly inexpensive but must be purchased repeatedly (e.g., condoms, spermicides, monthly pill prescriptions). You should consider whether a method will be cost-effective for you in the long run. Remember that any prescription methods require routine checkups, which may involve some cost to you.
- **Do I have any health factors that could limit my choice?** Hormonal birth control methods can pose potential health risks to women with certain preexisting conditions, such as high

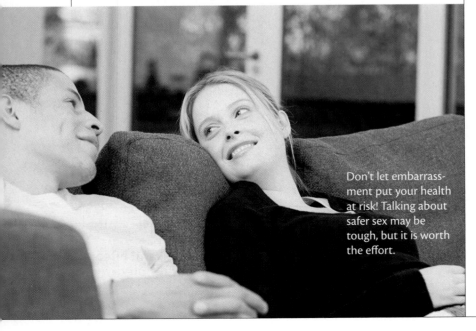

Don't let embarrassment put your health at risk! Talking about safer sex may be tough, but it is worth the effort.

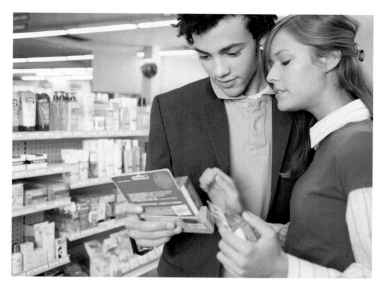

How do I choose a method of birth control?

Many different methods of birth control are on the market: barrier methods, hormonal methods, surgical methods, and other options. When you choose a method, you'll need to consider several factors, including cost, comfort level, convenience, and health risks. All of these factors together will influence your ability to consistently and correctly use the contraceptive and prevent unwanted pregnancy.

blood pressure, a history of stroke or blood clots, liver disease, migraines, or diabetes. You should discuss this issue with your health care provider when considering birth control methods. In addition, women who smoke or are over the age of 35 are at risk from complications of combination hormonal contraceptives. Breastfeeding women can use progestin-only methods, but should avoid methods containing estrogen. Men and women with latex allergies may need to use polyurethane, silicon, or plastic barrier methods.

■ **Are there any additional benefits I'd like to get from my contraceptive?** Hormonal birth control methods can have desirable secondary effects, such as the reduction of acne or the lessening of premenstrual symptoms. Certain pills are marketed as having specific effects, so it is possible to choose one that is known to clear skin or reduce mood changes caused by menstruation. Hormonal birth control methods are also associated with reduced risks of certain cancers. Extended-cycle pills and some progestin-only methods cause menstrual periods to be less frequent or to stop altogether, which some women find desirable. Condoms carry the added health benefit of protecting against STIs.

Communicating about Contraception

Communication is key to a healthy relationship, and it is especially so between those who are sexually intimate. It is a sign of care and respect for your own body and your partner's and it empowers both of you to be assertive about your individual needs, likes, limits, and desires in the sexual relationship. Open communication also creates a safe environment to ask about your partner's sexual history, sexually transmitted infection (STI) testing, and sexual expectations.

You may feel awkward or uncomfortable discussing sex, and you may believe that talking beforehand ruins the naturalness or spontaneity of sex. Some people are concerned that their partner will misinterpret the conversation and feel accused of infidelity, distrust, promiscuity, or lack of love in the relationship. Try to address these concerns in an honest and open manner. And remember: Sexual communication is about protecting both of your bodies and ensuring that you are clear about your needs and concerns.

If you are afraid that talking about sex beforehand is going to make your partner think you don't trust him or her, take some time to examine the strength of your relationship. Trust is about being open and honest. If you're afraid to talk with your partner, the chances are you actually don't trust your partner and you might be better off with a partner you do trust.

Before you talk with your partner, it's a good idea to talk with your health care provider about your options for practicing safer sex. Remember, you need to think about getting pregnant and avoiding STIs.

With your partner, try to find a time and place where you are both comfortable, free of distractions, and you have time to have a full conversation. It's generally better to have this conversation outside of the bedroom, so that you're not pressured by the heat of the moment to do things you don't want to do.

Some tips to boost your confidence in negotiating safer sex include the following:

■ It can be helpful to have condoms and/or dental dams around, so when things start to really heat up you will be ready.
■ Talk to your partner about using protection before getting intimate. This will help both of you be more comfortable and prepared to use a condom or dental dam when the time comes.
■ Practice makes perfect. The best way to learn how to use condoms correctly and guarantee their effectiveness is to practice putting them on yourself or your partner. A staggering 98 percent of all "condom malfunctions" (breaks, leaks, tears, slips) are due to user error. The two most essential keys to using a condom are consistently and correctly.
■ If you are concerned about the interruption of using either condoms or dental dams, try to incorporate them into your foreplay. By helping your partner put on protection together, you both will stay aroused and in the moment.

check yourself

■ **What are some questions to consider when choosing a method of contraception?**
■ **What are some potential obstacles to communicating about contraception, and how can you overcome them?**

Abortion

- **Summarize historic legal decisions surrounding abortion.**
- **Summarize the various types of abortion procedures.**

The vast majority of abortions occur because of unintended pregnancies.[14] Even the best birth control methods can fail; other pregnancies are terminated because they are a consequence of rape or incest. Other commonly cited reasons are not being ready financially or emotionally to care for a child at the time.[15]

In 1973, the landmark U.S. Supreme Court decision in *Roe v. Wade* stated that the "right to privacy . . . founded on the Fourteenth Amendment's concept of personal liberty . . . is broad enough to encompass a woman's decision whether or not to terminate her pregnancy."[16] The decision maintained that during the first trimester of pregnancy a woman and her practitioner have the right to terminate the pregnancy through **abortion** without legal restrictions. It allowed individual states to set conditions for second-trimester abortions. Third-trimester abortions were ruled illegal unless the mother's life or health was in danger. Prior to this, women wishing to terminate a pregnancy had to travel to a country where the procedure was legal, consult an illegal abortionist, or perform their own abortions. These procedures sometimes led to death from hemorrhage or infection or infertility from internal scarring.

The Debate over Abortion

Abortion is a highly charged issue in America. Pro-choice individuals feel it is a woman's right to make decisions about her own body and health, including the decision to continue or terminate a pregnancy. On the other side of the issue, pro-life, or anti-abortion, individuals believe that the embryo or fetus is a human being with rights that must be protected. Pro-life groups lobby for laws prohibiting the use of public funds for abortion and abortion counseling at the same time that pro-choice groups lobby for laws that make abortions more widely available. At times, violence has arisen as a result of this controversy in the form of attacks on clinics or on individual physicians who perform abortions.

In recent years, new legislation has given states the right to impose certain restrictions on abortions. The procedure cannot be performed in publicly funded clinics in some states; others have laws requiring parental notification before a teenager can obtain an abortion.

Even without specific parental involvement laws, 6 in 10 minors who have had an abortion report that at least one parent knew about it.[17]

On the federal level, the U.S. Congress has banned access to abortion funding for virtually all women receiving health care through the federal government. Since the Federal Abortion Ban was signed in 2003, it has been challenged across the country on the grounds that it is unconstitutional, based on claims that the broad language could ban abortion as early as the twelfth week of pregnancy and that it does not include exceptions to protect women's health.[18] The U.S. Supreme Court struck down an identical law as unconstitutional in 2000, and the ban was found unconstitutional by six federal courts before the Supreme Court ruled in April 2007 that it was constitutional and could be enforced.[19] This decision represented a monumental departure from prior cases, as the Court effectively eliminated one of *Roe v. Wade*'s core protections: that a woman's health must always be paramount.

Emotional Aspects of Abortion

The best scientific evidence published indicates that among adult women who have an unplanned pregnancy the risk of mental health problems is no greater if they have an abortion than if they deliver a baby. Although feelings such as regret, guilt, sadness, relief, and happiness are normal, no evidence has shown that an abortion causes long-term negative mental health outcomes.[20] Researchers found that the best predictor of a woman's emotional well-being following an abortion was her emotional well-being prior to the procedure.[21] Factors that place a woman at higher risk for negative psychological responses following an abortion include perception of stigma, need for secrecy, low levels of social support for the abortion decision, prior mental health issues, low self-esteem, and avoidance and denial coping strategies.[22] Certainly a support network is helpful to any woman struggling with the emotional aspects of her abortion decision.

Methods of Abortion

The choice of abortion procedure is determined by how many weeks the woman has been pregnant. Length of pregnancy is calculated from the first day of her last menstrual period.

Surgical Abortions The majority of abortions performed in the United States today are surgical. If performed during the first trimester of pregnancy, abortion presents a relatively low health risk to the mother. About 88 percent of abortions occur during the first 12 weeks of pregnancy (see **Figure 5.7**).[23] The most commonly used method of first-trimester abortion is **suction curettage** (**Figure 5.8**). Approximately 87 percent of abortions in the United States are done using this procedure, usually under local anesthetic. The cervix is dilated with instruments or by placing laminaria, a sterile seaweed product, into the cervical canal. A tube is inserted into the uterus through the cervix, and gentle suction removes fetal tissue from the uterine walls.

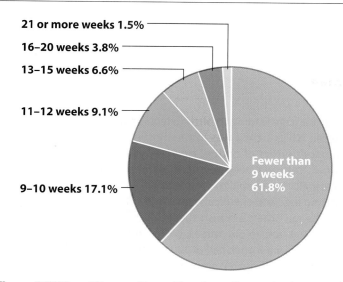

21 or more weeks 1.5%
16–20 weeks 3.8%
13–15 weeks 6.6%
11–12 weeks 9.1%
9–10 weeks 17.1%
Fewer than 9 weeks 61.8%

Figure 5.7 When Women Have Abortions (in weeks from the last menstrual period)

Source: Data are from Guttmacher Institute, *Facts on Induced Abortions in the United States*, May 2010, Available at www.guttmacher.org/pubs/fb_induced_abortion.html

Pregnancies in the second trimester (after week 12) can be terminated through **dilation and evacuation (D&E)**. For this procedure, the cervix is dilated for 1 to 2 days and a combination of instruments and vacuum aspiration is used to empty the uterus. Second-trimester abortions may be done under general anesthetic. A D&E can be performed on an outpatient basis, with or without pain medication; it may cause uterine cramping and blood loss.

Two less common methods used in second-trimester abortions are prostaglandin and saline **induction abortions**. Prostaglandin hormones or saline solution is injected into the uterus, which kills the fetus and initiates labor contractions. After 24 to 48 hours, the fetus and placenta are expelled from the uterus. A **hysterotomy**, or surgical removal of the fetus from the uterus, may be used during emergencies, when the mother's life is in danger, or when other types of abortions are deemed too dangerous.

One surgical method that abortion opponents target is **intact dilation and extraction (D&X)**, sometimes referred to by the nonmedical term *partial-birth abortion*. This procedure, used after 21 weeks of gestation, is rarely performed but is considered when other abortion methods could injure the mother and when there are severe fetal abnormalities. Two days before the procedure, laminaria is inserted vaginally to dilate the cervix. The water should break on the third day, and the woman should return to the clinic. The fetus is rotated to a breech (feet first) position, and forceps are used to pull the legs, shoulders, and arms through the birth canal. The head is collapsed to allow it to pass through the cervix. Then the fetus is completely removed.

The risks associated with surgical abortion include infection, incomplete abortion (when parts of the placenta remain in the uterus), missed abortion, excessive bleeding, and cervical and uterine trauma. Follow-up and attention to danger signs decrease the chances of long-term problems.

The mortality rate for women undergoing first-trimester abortions in the United States averages 1 death per every 1,000,000 procedures at 8 or fewer weeks. At 16 to 20 weeks, the mortality rate

is 1 per 29,000; at 21 weeks or more, it increases to 1 per 11,000.[24] This higher rate later in the pregnancy is due to the increased risk of uterine perforation, bleeding, infection, and incomplete abortion; these can happen because the uterine wall becomes thinner as the pregnancy progresses.

Medical Abortions Unlike surgical abortions, **medical abortions** are performed without entering the uterus. Mifepristone, formerly called RU-486 and currently sold in the United States under the name Mifeprex, is a steroid hormone that induces abortion by blocking the action of progesterone, which maintains the lining of the uterus. As a result, the uterine lining and embryo are expelled from the uterus, terminating the pregnancy.

This treatment actually involves more steps than a suction curettage abortion, which takes approximately 15 minutes followed by physical recovery of about 1 day. With mifepristone, a first visit involves a physical exam and a dose of three tablets, which may cause minor side effects, such as nausea, headaches, weakness, and fatigue. The patient returns 2 days later for a dose of prostaglandins (misoprostol; brand name Cytotec), which causes uterine contractions that expel the fertilized egg. The patient is required to stay under observation for 4 hours and to make a follow-up visit 12 days later.[25]

Ninety-two percent of women who use this method during the first 9 weeks of pregnancy will experience a complete abortion.[26] Approximately 1 in 1,000 women requires a blood transfusion because of severe bleeding.

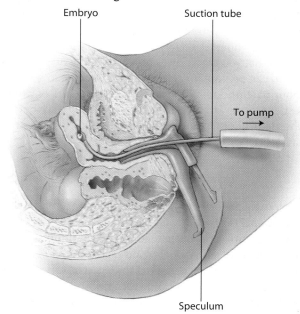

Embryo   Suction tube
To pump
Speculum

Figure 5.8 Suction Curettage Abortion
This procedure, in which a long tube with gentle suction is used to remove fetal tissue from the uterine walls, can be performed up to the twelfth week of pregnancy.

check yourself

- **What is the current legal status of abortion?**
- **What are the various types of abortion procedures?**

109

Planning a Pregnancy

- **Discuss key issues to consider when planning a pregnancy.**

The many methods available to control fertility give you choices that did not exist when your parents—and even you—were born. If you are in the process of deciding whether, or when, to have children, take the time to evaluate your emotions, finances, and physical health.

Emotional Health

First and foremost, consider why you want to have a child. To fulfill an inner need to carry on the family? Because it's expected? Other reasons? Then, consider the responsibilities involved with becoming a parent. Are you ready to make all the sacrifices necessary to bear and raise a child? Can you care for this new human being in a loving and nurturing manner?

If you feel that you are ready to be a parent, the next step is preparation. You can prepare for this change in your life in several ways: Read about parenthood, take classes, talk to parents of children of all ages, spend time with friends' children, and join a support group. If you choose to adopt, you will find many support groups available to you as well.

Maternal Health

Before becoming pregnant, a woman should have a thorough medical examination. **Preconception care** should include an assessment of potential complications that could occur during pregnancy. Medical problems such as diabetes and high blood pressure should be discussed, as well as any genetic disorders that run in the family. Additional suggestions for preparing for a healthy pregnancy can be found in the Skills for Behavior Change feature.

Paternal Health

It is common wisdom that mothers-to-be should steer clear of toxic chemicals that can cause birth defects, should eat a healthy diet, and should stop smoking and drinking alcohol. Now, similar precautions are recommended for fathers-to-be. New research suggests that a man's exposure to chemicals influences not only his ability to father a child, but also the future health of that child.

Fathers-to-be have been overlooked in past preconception and prenatal studies for several reasons. Researchers assumed that the genetic damage leading to birth defects and other health problems occurred while a child was in the mother's womb or were caused by random errors of nature. However, it now appears that some disorders can be traced to sperm damaged by chemicals. Sperm are naturally vulnerable to toxic assault and genetic damage. Many drugs and ingested chemicals can readily invade the testes from the bloodstream; others ambush sperm after they leave the testes and pass through the epididymides, where they mature and are stored. By one route or another, half of 100 chemicals studied so far (including byproducts of cigarette smoke) apparently harm sperm.[27]

Financial Evaluation

Finances are another important consideration. Are you prepared to go out to dinner less often, forgo a new pair of shoes, or drive an older car? What about health insurance, disability insurance, life insurance, child care, and preschool? Clothes and shoes that are outgrown every 3 to 12 months? Maybe even orthodontia, glasses, summer camp, college savings accounts? These are important questions to ask yourself when considering the financial aspects of being a parent. Can you afford to give your child the life you would like him or her to enjoy?

First, check your medical insurance: Does it provide pregnancy and delivery benefits? If not, you can expect to pay, on average, $14,000 for a normal delivery and up to $35,000 for even a nonemergency cesarean section birth. These costs don't include prenatal medical care, and complications can increase the cost substantially. Both partners should investigate their employers' policies concerning parental leave, including length of leave available and conditions for returning to work.

The U.S. Department of Agriculture estimates that it can cost between $11,610 and $13,480 annually for a middle-class married couple to raise a child (housing costs and food are the two largest expen-

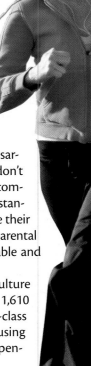

Being in good physical shape will help prepare you for the demands of pregnancy.

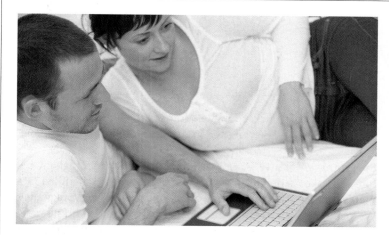

How can I prepare to be a parent?

Following a doctor-approved exercise program during pregnancy is just one aspect of healthy preparation for parenthood. Even before they conceive, prospective mothers and fathers should evaluate their emotional, physical, social, and financial well-being and implement healthy change where needed to better ready themselves for bringing a child into the world.

ditures).[28] These costs tend to increase with the age of the child. It is also more expensive to raise a child in the urban Northeast than in the South and rural areas. These figures do not include college, which can now run over $40,000 per year at a private institution, with room and board. Also consider the cost and availability of quality child care. How much family assistance can you realistically expect with a new baby, and is nonfamily child care available? How much does part-time or full-time child care cost? Prices vary by region and type of care. According to the National Association of Child Care Resource and Referral Agencies (NACCRRA), day care costs for an infant in the United States range from $4,560 to $15,895 a year.[29]

Choosing a Prenatal Care Practitioner

A woman should carefully choose a practitioner who will attend her pregnancy and delivery. If possible, she should do this before she becomes pregnant. Recommendations from friends and from one's family physician are a good starting point. She should consider a practitioner's philosophy about pain management during labor, experience handling complications, and willingness to accommodate her personal beliefs on these issues.

Several different types of practitioners are qualified to care for a woman through pregnancy, birth, and the postpartum period, including obstetrician-gynecologists, family practitioners, and midwives. Obstetrician-gynecologists are MDs. They are specialists trained to handle all types of pregnancy- and delivery-related emergencies. They generally can perform deliveries only in a hospital setting and cannot serve as the baby's physician after birth. Family practitioners provide care for people of all ages, so they can serve as the baby's physician after birth. However, they may pro-

vide pregnancy care only to low-risk pregnancies and rarely perform home births. Midwives may be lay or certified. Certified midwives can oversee deliveries in nonhospital settings and have access to traditional medical facilities. They cannot provide any medication and may need to refer high-risk pregnancies to a clinician. Lay midwives are educated through informal routes such as apprenticeship and may not have training to handle an emergency.

Ideally, a woman should begin medical checkups as soon as possible after becoming pregnant (within the first 3 months). This early care reduces infant mortality and low birth weight. On the first visit, the practitioner should obtain a complete medical history of the mother and her family and note any hereditary conditions that could put a woman or her fetus at risk. Regular checkups to measure weight gain and blood pressure and to monitor the fetus's size and position should continue throughout the pregnancy. The American College of Obstetricians and Gynecologists recommends seven or eight prenatal visits for women with low-risk pregnancies.

Skills for Behavior Change

PREPARING FOR PREGNANCY

Before becoming pregnant, parents-to-be should take stock of, and possibly improve, their own health to help ensure the health of their child. Among the most important factors to consider are the following:

For Women:

- If you smoke, drink alcohol, or use drugs, stop.
- Reduce or eliminate your caffeine intake.
- Maintain a healthy weight; lose or gain weight, if necessary.
- Avoid X rays and environmental chemicals, such as lawn and garden herbicides and pesticides.
- Take multivitamins or prenatal vitamins, which are especially important in providing adequate folic acid.

For Men:

- If you smoke, quit.
- Drink alcohol only in moderation, and avoid drug use.
- Get checked for sexually transmitted infections and seek treatment if you have one.
- Avoid exposure to toxic chemicals in your work or home environment.
- Maintain a healthy weight; lose or gain weight, if necessary.

check yourself

- **What are key issues to consider when planning a pregnancy?**
- **Of the issues discussed, which do you think are the most important?**
- **When considering the lifestyle changes needed for a successful pregnancy, which do you think would be the most challenging to implement?**

The Process of Pregnancy

learning outcomes

- **Describe the process of pregnancy, from ovulation to implantation.**
- **Discuss physical changes experienced by a mother during the three trimesters of pregnancy.**

Pregnancy is an important event in a woman's life. Actions taken before, as well as behaviors engaged in during, pregnancy can significantly affect the health of both infant and mother.

The process of pregnancy begins the moment a sperm fertilizes an ovum in the fallopian tubes (**Figure 5.9**). From there, the single fertilized cell, now called a zygote, multiplies and becomes a sphere-shaped cluster of cells called a blastocyst that travels toward the uterus, a journey that may take 3 to 4 days. Upon arrival, the embryo burrows into the thick, spongy endometrium—in a process called implantation—and is nourished from this carefully prepared lining.

Pregnancy Testing A woman may suspect she is pregnant before she takes a pregnancy test. A pregnancy test scheduled in a medical office or birth control clinic will confirm the pregnancy. Women who wish to know immediately can purchase home pregnancy test kits, sold over the counter in drugstores. A positive test is based on the secretion of **human chorionic gonadotropin (HCG)**, which is found in the woman's urine.

Home pregnancy tests can be used as early as 2 weeks after conception and are about 85 to 95 percent reliable. Instructions must be followed carefully. If the test is done too early in the pregnancy, it may show a false negative. Other causes of false negatives are unclean test tubes, ingestion of certain drugs, and vaginal or urinary tract infections. Accuracy also depends on the quality of the test itself and the user's ability to perform it and interpret the results. Blood tests administered and analyzed by a medical laboratory are more accurate.

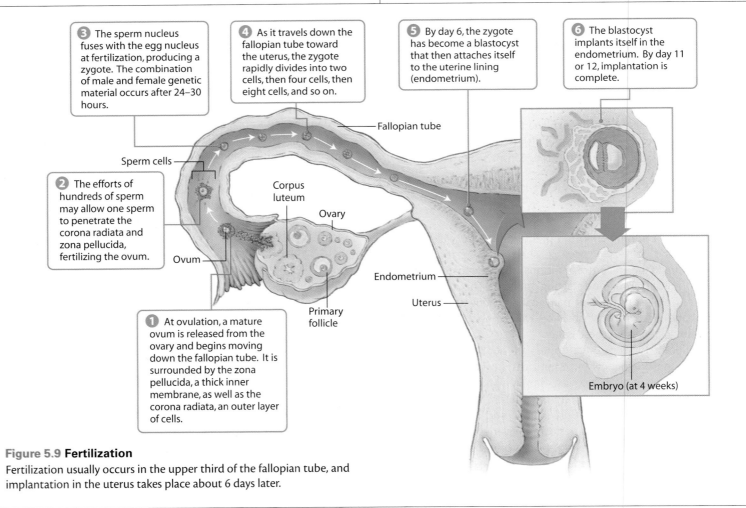

3 The sperm nucleus fuses with the egg nucleus at fertilization, producing a zygote. The combination of male and female genetic material occurs after 24–30 hours.

4 As it travels down the fallopian tube toward the uterus, the zygote rapidly divides into two cells, then four cells, then eight cells, and so on.

5 By day 6, the zygote has become a blastocyst that then attaches itself to the uterine lining (endometrium).

6 The blastocyst implants itself in the endometrium. By day 11 or 12, implantation is complete.

2 The efforts of hundreds of sperm may allow one sperm to penetrate the corona radiata and zona pellucida, fertilizing the ovum.

1 At ovulation, a mature ovum is released from the ovary and begins moving down the fallopian tube. It is surrounded by the zona pellucida, a thick inner membrane, as well as the corona radiata, an outer layer of cells.

Fallopian tube

Sperm cells

Corpus luteum

Ovary

Ovum

Primary follicle

Endometrium

Uterus

Embryo (at 4 weeks)

Figure 5.9 Fertilization
Fertilization usually occurs in the upper third of the fallopian tube, and implantation in the uterus takes place about 6 days later.

Early Signs of Pregnancy A woman's body undergoes substantial changes during the course of a pregnancy (Figure 5.10). The first sign of pregnancy is usually a missed menstrual period (although some women "spot" in early pregnancy, which may be mistaken for a period). Other signs include breast tenderness, emotional upset, extreme fatigue, sleeplessness, as well as nausea and vomiting, especially in the morning.

Pregnancy typically lasts 40 weeks and is divided into three phases, or **trimesters**, of approximately 3 months each. The due date is calculated from the expectant mother's last menstrual period.

The First Trimester During the first trimester, few visually noticeable changes occur in the mother's body. She may urinate more frequently and experience morning sickness, swollen breasts, or undue fatigue. These symptoms may or may not be frequent or severe, so she may not even realize she is pregnant unless she takes a pregnancy test.

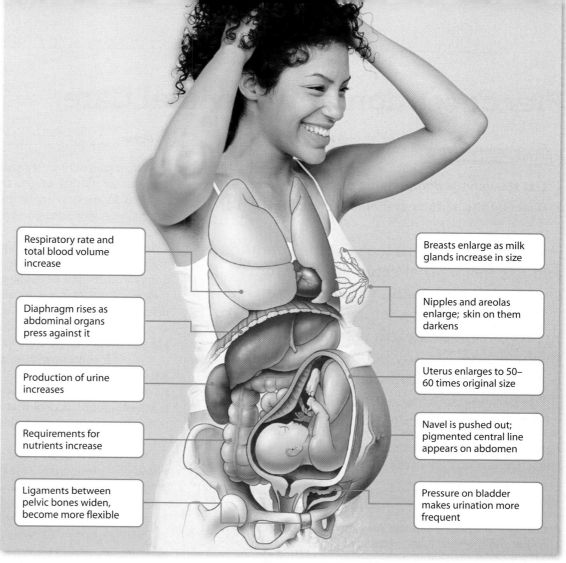

Respiratory rate and total blood volume increase

Diaphragm rises as abdominal organs press against it

Production of urine increases

Requirements for nutrients increase

Ligaments between pelvic bones widen, become more flexible

Breasts enlarge as milk glands increase in size

Nipples and areolas enlarge; skin on them darkens

Uterus enlarges to 50–60 times original size

Navel is pushed out; pigmented central line appears on abdomen

Pressure on bladder makes urination more frequent

Figure 5.10 Changes in a Woman's Body during Pregnancy

During the first 2 months after conception, the **embryo** differentiates and develops its various organ systems, beginning with the nervous and circulatory systems. At the start of the third month, the embryo is called a **fetus**, a term indicating that all organ systems are in place. For the rest of the pregnancy, growth and refinement occur in each major body system so that each can function independently, yet in coordination with all the others, at birth.

The Second Trimester At the beginning of the second trimester, physical changes in the mother become more visible. Her breasts swell and her waistline thickens. During this time, the fetus makes greater demands on the mother's body. In particular, the **placenta**, the network of blood vessels that carries nutrients and oxygen to the fetus and fetal waste products to the mother, becomes well established.

The Third Trimester From the end of the sixth month through the ninth month is the third trimester. This is the period of greatest fetal growth, when the fetus gains most of its weight. During this time, the fetus must get large amounts of calcium, iron, and nitrogen from food the mother eats. Approximately 85 percent of the calcium and iron the mother digests goes into the fetal bloodstream.

Although the fetus may live if it is born during the seventh month, it needs the layer of fat it acquires during the eighth month and time for the organs (especially respiratory and digestive organs) to develop fully. Infants born prematurely usually require intensive medical care.

Emotional Changes Of course, the process of pregnancy involves much more than the changes in a woman's body and the developing fetus. Many important emotional changes occur from the time a woman learns she is pregnant through the "fourth trimester" (the first 6 weeks of an infant's life outside the uterus). Throughout pregnancy, women may experience fear of complications, anxiety about becoming a parent, and wonder and excitement over the developing baby.

check yourself

- **What is the process of pregnancy, from ovulation to implantation?**
- **What are some physical changes experienced by a mother during the three trimesters of pregnancy?**

Preconception and Prenatal Care

learning outcomes

- **List the various components of prenatal care.**
- **Describe the various available prenatal tests.**

Preconception health looks at the conditions and risk factors that could affect a woman if she becomes pregnant, with a focus on factors that can affect a fetus or infant. The key to preconception health is to combine good medical care, healthy behaviors, strong support, and safe environments.[30]

Preconception care is important because the fetus is most susceptible to certain problems in the 4 to 10 weeks after conception. Many women, unaware they are pregnant until after this critical time, cannot reduce risks to their own and their baby's health unless intervention begins before conception.[31]

Prenatal Care

A successful pregnancy depends on a mother who takes good care of herself and her fetus. Good nutrition and exercise; avoiding drugs, alcohol, and other harmful substances; and regular medical checkups from the beginning of pregnancy are essential. Early detection of fetal abnormalities, identification of high-risk mothers and infants, and a complication-free pregnancy are the major goals of prenatal care.

A woman should choose a practitioner to attend her pregnancy and delivery. Recommendations from friends and from one's family physician are a good starting point; she should also consider philosophy about pain management during labor, experience handling complications, and willingness to accommodate her personal beliefs on these and other issues. Practitioners qualified to care for a woman through pregnancy, birth, and the postpartum period include obstetrician-gynecologists, family practitioners, and midwives.

Ideally, a woman should begin medical checkups as soon as possible after becoming pregnant. Regular checkups to measure weight gain and blood pressure and to monitor the fetus's size and position should continue throughout the pregnancy.

Nutrition Pregnant women need additional protein, calories, vitamins, and minerals. Special attention should be paid to getting enough folic acid (found in dark leafy greens), iron (dried fruits, meats, legumes, liver, egg yolks), calcium (nonfat or low-fat dairy products and some canned fish), and fluids. Babies born to poorly nourished mothers run high risks of substandard mental and physical development. Folic acid, when consumed before and during early pregnancy, reduces the risk of spina bifida, a congenital birth defect resulting from failure of the spinal column to close.

Weight gain during pregnancy helps nourish a growing baby. For a woman of normal weight, the recommended gain during pregnancy is 25 to 35 pounds; these numbers vary slightly for overweight or underweight women or for those carrying twins.

Drugs and Alcohol A woman should avoid all types of drugs during pregnancy. Even some common over-the-counter medications can damage a developing fetus. During the first 3 months of pregnancy, the fetus is especially subject to the **teratogenic** (birth-defect-causing) effects of drugs, environmental chemicals, X rays, and diseases. The fetus can also develop an addiction to or tolerance for drugs that the mother uses.

Maternal consumption of alcohol is detrimental to a growing fetus. Symptoms of **fetal alcohol syndrome (FAS)** include mental retardation, slowed nerve reflexes, and small head size. The exact amount of alcohol that causes FAS is not known; therefore, researchers recommend abstinence during pregnancy.

Smoking Tobacco use, and smoking in particular, harms every phase of reproduction. Smokers have more difficulty becoming pregnant and a higher risk of infertility. Women who smoke during pregnancy have a greater chance of complications, premature births, low-birth-weight infants, stillbirth, and infant mortality.[32]

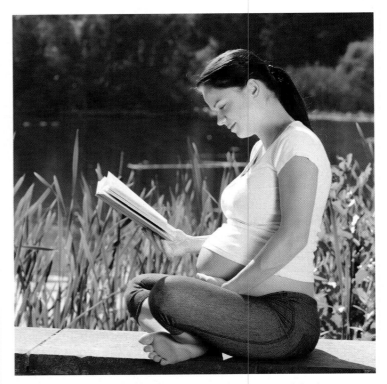

A pregnant woman who exercises, eats well, avoids harmful substances, and has regular medical checkups is more likely to have a successful pregnancy.

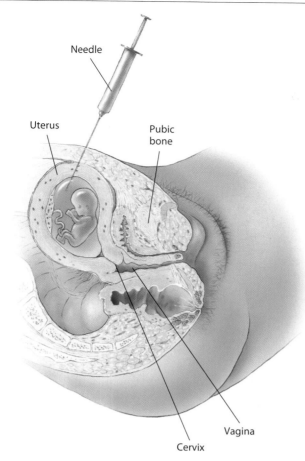

Figure 5.11 Amniocentesis
The process of amniocentesis, in which a long needle is used to withdraw a small amount of amniotic fluid for genetic analysis, can detect certain congenital problems as well as the fetus's sex.

Smoking restricts blood supply to the developing fetus, limiting oxygen and nutrition delivery and waste removal. Tobacco use appears to be a significant factor in the development of cleft lip and palate.

Studies also show that secondhand smoke is detrimental to both mother and unborn child. An exposed fetus is more likely to experience low birth weight, increased susceptibility to childhood diseases, and sudden infant death syndrome.[33]

Other Teratogens A pregnant woman should avoid exposure to X rays, toxic chemicals, heavy metals, pesticides, gases, and other hazardous compounds. She shouldn't clean cat litter boxes; cat feces can contain organisms that cause **toxoplasmosis**—a disease that can cause a baby to be stillborn or suffer mental retardation or other birth defects.

If she has never had rubella (German measles), a woman should be immunized for it before becoming pregnant. A mother's rubella infection can kill a fetus or cause blindness or hearing disorders in the infant. Sexually transmitted infections such as genital herpes or HIV are also risk factors. A woman should inform her physician of any infectious condition so proper precautions and treatment can be taken. Contact with an active herpes infection during birth can be fatal to a baby.

Miscarriage Unfortunately, not every pregnancy ends in delivery. In the United States, 15 to 20 percent of pregnancies end in **miscarriage** (also referred to as *spontaneous abortion*).[34] Most miscarriages occur during the first trimester.

Reasons for miscarriage vary. In some cases, the fertilized egg has failed to divide correctly. In others, genetic abnormalities, maternal illness, or infections are responsible. In most cases, the cause is not known.

Stillbirth One of the most traumatic events a couple can face is a **stillbirth**, the death of a fetus *after* the twentieth week of pregnancy but before delivery. Each year in the United States, there is about 1 stillbirth in every 160 births.[35] Birth defects, placental problems, poor fetal growth, infections, and umbilical cord accidents all may contribute to stillbirth.

Maternal Age The average age at which a woman has her first child has been rising. Although births to women in their twenties are declining, the rate of first births to women between the ages of 30 and 39 is the highest in four decades, and births to women over 39 have increased slightly.[36] Many doctors note that older mothers tend to be more conscientious about self-care during pregnancy and are more psychologically mature and ready to include an infant in their family than are some younger women.

Prenatal Testing and Screening Modern technology enables detection of fetal health defects as early as the fourteenth weeks of pregnancy. One common test is **ultrasonography**, or **ultrasound**, which uses high-frequency sound waves to create a *sonogram* of the fetus in the uterus—a visual image used to determine the fetus's size and position; sonograms can also detect birth defects in the central nervous and digestive systems.

Chorionic villus sampling (CVS) involves snipping tissue from the developing fetal sac. It can be used at 10 to 12 weeks of pregnancy and is an attractive option for couples at high risk for having a baby with Down syndrome or a debilitating hereditary disease.

The **triple marker screen (TMS)** is a maternal blood test done at 16 to 18 weeks. TMS can detect susceptibility to a birth defect or genetic abnormality, but is not meant to diagnose any condition.

Amniocentesis, a common test recommended for women over 35, involves inserting a needle through the abdominal and uterine walls into the **amniotic sac** surrounding the fetus (**Figure 5.11**). The needle draws out 3 to 4 teaspoons of fluid, which is analyzed for genetic information. Amniocentesis can be performed between weeks 14 and 18.

If a test reveals a serious birth defect, parents are advised to undergo genetic counseling. In the case of a chromosomal abnormality such as Down syndrome, the parents are usually offered the option of a therapeutic abortion. Some parents choose this option; others research the disability and decide to go ahead with the pregnancy.

check yourself

- **What are the key components of prenatal care?**
- **Which, if any, prenatal tests would you choose if you or your partner were pregnant? Why?**

learning outcomes

- **Describe the three stages of labor.**

During the few weeks preceding delivery, the baby normally shifts to a head-down position, and the cervix begins to dilate (widen). The pubic bones loosen to permit expansion during birth. Strong uterine contractions signal the beginning of labor. Another common signal is the breaking of the amniotic sac (commonly referred to as "water breaking"). The birth process (Figure 5.12) can last from several hours to more than a day.

If the baby is in physiological distress, a **cesarean section (C-section)**—a surgical procedure that involves making an incision across the mother's abdomen and through the uterus to remove the baby—may be used. A C-section may also be performed if labor is extremely difficult, maternal blood pressure falls rapidly, the placenta separates from the uterus too soon, or other problems occur. A C-section can be traumatic if the mother is not prepared for it. Risks are the same as for any major abdominal surgery, and recovery takes considerably longer afterward.

The rate of C-section delivery in the United States increased from 5 percent in the mid-1960s to 32 percent in 2007.[37] Although C-sections are sometimes necessary, some feel they are performed too frequently. Natural birth advocates suggest that hospitals driven by profits and worried about malpractice are too quick to intervene in the birth process. Some doctors attribute the increase to demand from mothers.

Complications of Pregnancy and Childbirth

Pregnancy carries the risk of complications that can interfere with fetal development or threaten the health of mother and child. **Preeclampsia** is characterized by high blood pressure, protein in the urine, edema, and swelling in the hands and face. Symptoms may include sudden weight gain, headache, nausea or vomiting, changes in vision, racing pulse, mental confusion, and stomach or right shoulder pain. If untreated, preeclampsia can cause *eclampsia*, with outcomes including seizures, liver and kidney damage, internal bleeding, stroke, poor fetal growth, and fetal and maternal death. Preeclampsia tends to occur in the late second or third trimester. The cause is unknown. The incidence is higher in first-time mothers; women over 40 or under 18; women carrying multiple fetuses; and women with a history of chronic hypertension, diabetes, kidney disorder, or previous preeclampsia.

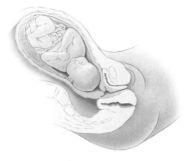

1 Stage I: Dilation of the cervix Contractions in the abdomen and lower back push the baby downward, putting pressure on the cervix and dilating it. The first stage of labor may last from a couple of hours to more than a day for a first birth, but it is usually much shorter during subsequent births.

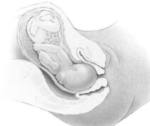

2 End of Stage I: Transition The cervix becomes fully dilated, and the baby's head begins to move into the vagina (birth canal). Contractions usually come quickly during transition, which generally lasts 30 minutes or less.

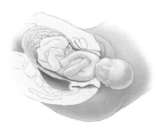

3 Stage II: Expulsion Once the cervix has become fully dilated, contractions become rhythmic, strong, and more intense as the uterus pushes the baby headfirst through the birth canal. The expulsion stage lasts 1 to 4 hours and concludes when the infant is finally pushed out of the mother's body.

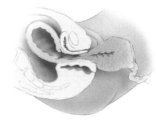

4 Stage III: Delivery of the placenta In the third stage, the placenta detaches from the uterus and is expelled through the birth canal. This stage is usually completed within 30 minutes after delivery.

Figure 5.12 The Birth Process
The entire process of labor and delivery usually takes from 2 to 36 hours. Labor is generally longer for a woman's first delivery and shorter for subsequent births.

Implantation of a fertilized egg in the fallopian tube or pelvic cavity is called an **ectopic pregnancy**. If an ectopic pregnancy goes undiagnosed and untreated, the fallopian tube can rupture, putting the woman at risk of hemorrhage, peritonitis (abdominal infection), and even death.

check yourself

- **What are the stages of labor, from Stage I to Stage III?**

The Postpartum Period

learning outcomes

■ **Describe the postpartum period.**

The postpartum period typically lasts 4 to 6 weeks. During this period, many women experience fluctuating emotions and physical challenges.

For many new mothers, the physical stress of labor, dehydration and blood loss, and other stresses challenge their stamina. Many experience the "baby blues," characterized by sadness, anxiety, headache, sleep disturbances, and irritability. For most women, these symptoms disappear after a short while. About 10 percent of new mothers experience **postpartum depression**, a more disabling syndrome, characterized by mood swings, lack of energy, crying, guilt, and depression, that can happen any time within the first year after childbirth. Mothers who experience postpartum depression should seek professional treatment.[38]

Breast-feeding Although the new mother's milk will not begin to flow for 2 or more days after delivery, her breasts secrete a yellow fluid called *colostrum*. Because colostrum contains vital antibodies to help fight infection, the newborn should be allowed to suckle.

The American Academy of Pediatrics strongly recommends that infants be breast-fed for at least 6 months, ideally for 12 months or more. Breastfed babies have fewer illnesses and a much lower hospi-

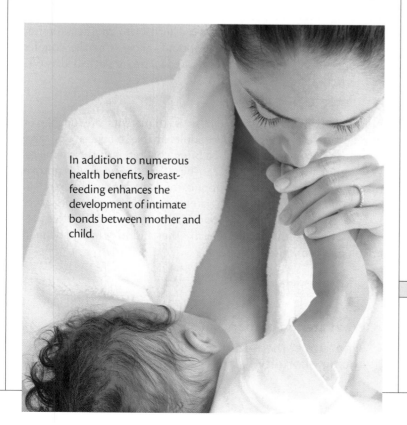

In addition to numerous health benefits, breast-feeding enhances the development of intimate bonds between mother and child.

talization rate; breast milk contains maternal antibodies and immunological cells that stimulate the infant's immune system. When breastfed babies do get sick, they recover more quickly. They are less likely to be obese than babies fed on formula and have fewer allergies. Researchers also theorize that breast milk contains substances that enhance brain development.[39] There is also a potential environmental advantage to breast-feeding. Compounds found in baby bottles and formula cans, including bisphenol-A, are under intense scrutiny following research suggesting they can lead to health problems.[40]

Some women are unable or unwilling to breast-feed; women with certain medical conditions or receiving certain medications are advised not to breast-feed. Prepared formulas can provide nourishment that allows a baby to grow and thrive. When deciding whether to breast- or bottle-feed, mothers must consider their own desires and preferences, too. Both feeding methods can supply the physical and emotional closeness so essential to the parent–child relationship.

Infant Mortality After birth, infant death can be caused by birth defects, low birth weight, injuries, or unknown causes. In the United States, the unexpected death of a child under 1 year of age, for no apparent reason, is called **sudden infant death syndrome (SIDS)**. This is the leading cause of death for children 1 month to 1 year; most common in babies under 6 months, SIDS is responsible for about 2,500 deaths a year.[41] SIDS is not a specific disease; rather, it is ruled a cause of death after all other possibilities are ruled out. A SIDS death is sudden and silent; death occurs quickly, often during sleep, with no signs of suffering.

The exact cause of SIDS is unknown, but researchers have discovered trends that may help them understand it. For instance, babies placed to sleep on their backs are less likely to die from SIDS than those placed on their stomachs. In addition, babies are more likely to die from SIDS when they are placed on or covered by soft bedding. Troublingly, African American babies are two times more likely, and American Indian babies three times more likely, to die from SIDS than white babies.[42]

The American Academy of Pediatrics' Back to Sleep campaign gives parents the following advice when putting a baby down to sleep: Lay infants down on their backs; place them on a firm sleep surface; keep soft objects, toys, and bedding out of the sleep area; don't allow smoking around the baby; and, if the baby uses one, offer a clean, dry pacifier.

check yourself

■ **What are the advantages and drawbacks of breast-feeding?**

■ **What steps can be taken to reduce the risk of SIDS?**

Infertility

- **Discuss the primary causes of and treatments for infertility.**

An estimated 1 in 6 American couples experiences **infertility**, the inability to conceive after trying for a year or more. Both partners should be evaluated; in about 20 percent of cases, infertility is due to a cause involving only the male partner, and in about 30 to 40 percent of cases, both partners.[43]

Reasons for high levels of infertility in the United States include the trend toward delaying childbirth (older women are less likely to conceive), endometriosis, pelvic inflammatory disease, and low sperm count. Environmental contaminants known as *endocrine disrupters*, such as some pesticides and emissions from burning plastics, appear to affect fertility in both men and women. Stress, anxiety, obesity, and diabetes also have reproductive implications.

Most infertility in women results from problems with ovulation. The most common is polycystic ovary syndrome (PCOS). When an egg is mature, its follicle breaks open, releasing it to travel to the uterus for fertilization. In women with PCOS, follicles bunch together to form cysts. Eggs mature, but their follicles don't open to release them. Approximately 5 to 10 percent of women of childbearing age have PCOS.[44]

In *premature ovarian failure*, the ovaries stop functioning before natural menopause. In **endometriosis**, parts of the endometrial lining of the uterus block the fallopian tubes. In **pelvic inflammatory disease (PID)**, chlamydia, or gonorrhea, bacteria invade the fallopian tubes, forming scar tissue that blocks the movement of eggs into the uterus. About 1 in 10 women with PID becomes infertile.[45]

Among men, the largest fertility problem is **low sperm count**.[46] Although only one viable sperm is needed, other sperm in the ejaculate aid in fertilization. There are normally 60 to 80 million sperm per milliliter of semen; below 20 million, fertility declines. Low sperm count may be attributable to environmental factors (such as exposure of the scrotum to intense heat or cold, radiation, or altitude) or even to wearing excessively tight pants. Other factors, such as the mumps virus, can also damage the cells that make sperm.

Infertility Treatments

Medical treatment can identify the cause of infertility in about 90 percent of cases. The chances of becoming pregnant after a cause is determined range from 30 to 70 percent, depending on the cause.[47] The expense, countless tests, and invasion of privacy that characterize some couples' efforts to conceive can put stress on an otherwise healthy relationship.

Fertility drugs stimulate ovulation in women who are not ovulating. Following administration of fertility drugs, 60 to 80 percent of women begin to ovulate; of those, about half conceive.[48] The drugs sometimes trigger the release of more than one egg, with a 1 in 10 chance of multiple births.

Other treatment options include **alternative insemination** (or *artificial insemination*) of a woman with her partner's sperm or that of a donor. In **in vitro fertilization (IVF)**, the most common type of *assisted reproductive technology (ART)*, eggs and sperm are combined in a laboratory dish to fertilize; fertilized eggs (zygotes) are then transferred to the uterus. Other ART techniques may combine an egg and sperm at different points, inside or outside the body.

In *nonsurgical embryo transfer*, a donor egg is fertilized by the man's sperm and implanted in the woman's uterus. In *embryo transfer*, an egg donor is artificially inseminated by the man's sperm, and the resulting embryo is transplanted into birth mother's uterus. Another alternative—embryo adoption—allows infertile couples to adopt excess fertilized eggs generated by treatments such as IVF.

Adoption

Adoption benefits children whose birth parents are unable or unwilling to raise them, and gives adults unable to conceive or carry a pregnancy to term a means to bring children into their families. Waiting for a child to adopt can be a lengthy process. Approximately 2 percent of the adult population has adopted children.[49] In *confidential adoption*, the birth parents and adoptive parents never know each other. In *open adoption*, birth parents and adoptive parents know some things about each other and may have a defined ongoing relationship.

- **What are the primary causes of infertility?**
- **What are some options available for people experiencing infertility?**

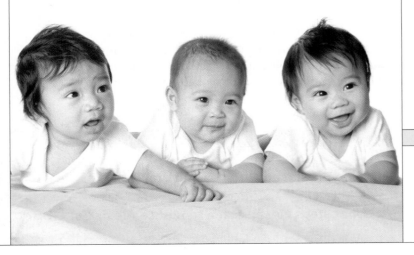

Assessyourself

Are You Comfortable with Your Contraception?

An interactive version of this assessment is available online. Download it from the Live It! section of www.pearsonhighered.com/donatelle

These questions will help you assess whether your current method of contraception or one you may consider using in the future will be effective for you. Answering yes to any of these questions predicts potential problems. If you have more than a few yes responses, consider talking to a health care provider, counselor, partner, or friend to decide whether to use a given method or to learn how to use it so that it will really be effective.

Method of contraception you use now or are considering:

_____

1. Have I or my partner ever become pregnant while using this method? Ⓨ Ⓝ

2. Am I afraid of using this method? Ⓨ Ⓝ

3. Would I really rather not use this method? Ⓨ Ⓝ

4. Will I have trouble remembering to use this method? Ⓨ Ⓝ

5. Will I have trouble using this method correctly? Ⓨ Ⓝ

6. Does this method make menstrual periods longer or more painful for me or my partner? Ⓨ Ⓝ

7. Does this method cost more than I can afford? Ⓨ Ⓝ

8. Could this method cause serious complications? Ⓨ Ⓝ

9. Am I, or is my partner, opposed to this method because of any religious or moral beliefs? Ⓨ Ⓝ

10. Will using this method embarrass me or my partner? Ⓨ Ⓝ

11. Will I enjoy intercourse less because of this method? Ⓨ Ⓝ

12. Am I at risk of being exposed to HIV or other sexually transmitted infections if I use this method? Ⓨ Ⓝ

Total number of yes answers: _____

Source: Adapted from R. A. Hatcher et al., *Contraceptive Technology,* 19th Revised ed. Copyright © 2007 by R. A. Hatcher. Reprinted with permission of Ardent Media, Inc.

Your Plan for Change

The Assess Yourself activity gave you the chance to assess your comfort and confidence with a contraceptive method you are using now or may use in the future. Depending on the results of the assessment, you may consider changing your birth control method.

Today, You Can:

◯ Visit your local drugstore and study the forms of contraception that are available without a prescription. Think about which of them you would consider using and why.

◯ If you are not currently using any contraception or are not in a sexual relationship but might become sexually active, purchase a package of condoms (or pick up a few free samples from your campus health center) to keep on hand just in case.

Within the Next 2 Weeks, You Can:

◯ Make an appointment for a checkup with your health care provider. Be sure to ask him or her any questions you have about contraception.

◯ Sit down with your partner and discuss contraception. Decide who will be responsible and which form will work best for you.

By the End of the Semester, You Can:

◯ Periodically reevaluate whether your new or continued contraception is still effective for you. Review your experiences, and take note of any consistent problems you may have encountered.

◯ Always keep a backup form of contraception on hand. Check this supply periodically and throw out and replace any supplies that have expired.

Summary

- Latex or polyurethane male condoms and female condoms, when used correctly for oral sex or intercourse, provide the most effective protection against sexually transmitted infections (STIs). Other contraceptive methods include spermicides, the diaphragm, cervical cap, Today sponge, oral contraceptives, Ortho Evra, NuvaRing, Depo-Provera, Implanon, and intrauterine devices. Emergency contraception may be used within 72 hours of unprotected intercourse or failure of another contraceptive method. Fertility awareness methods rely on altering sexual practices to avoid pregnancy, as do abstinence, outercourse, and withdrawal. All these methods of contraception are reversible; sterilization is permanent.
- Abortion is legal in the United States through the second trimester. Abortion methods include suction curettage, dilation and evacuation (D&E), intact dilation and extraction (D&X), hysterotomy, induction abortion, and medical abortions.
- Parenting is a demanding job. Prospective parents must consider emotional and physical health and financial plans.
- Full-term pregnancy covers three trimesters. Prenatal care includes a complete physical exam within the first trimester, follow up checkups throughout the pregnancy, nutrition and exercise, and avoidance of substances that could have teratogenic effects on the fetus. Prenatal tests can be used to detect birth defects during pregnancy.
- Childbirth occurs in three stages. Partners should choose a labor method early in the pregnancy to be better prepared when labor occurs. Possible complications include preeclampsia/eclampsia and ectopic pregnancy.
- Infertility in women may be caused by pelvic inflammatory disease (PID) or endometriosis. In men, it may be caused by low sperm count. Treatments may include fertility drugs, alternative insemination, in vitro fertilization (IVF), and assisted reproductive technology (ART).

Pop Quiz

1. What lubricant could you safely use with a latex condom?
   a. Mineral oil
   b. Water-based lubricant
   c. Body lotion
   d. Petroleum jelly

2. Which of the following is a barrier contraceptive?
   a. Seasonale
   b. FemCap
   c. Ortho Evra
   d. Contraceptive patch

3. What is the most commonly used method of first-trimester abortion?
   a. Suction curettage
   b. Dilation and evacuation (D&E)
   c. Medical abortion
   d. Induction abortion

4. What is meant by the *failure rate* of contraceptive use?
   a. The number of times a woman fails to get pregnant when she wants to
   b. The number of times a woman gets pregnant when she doesn't want to
   c. The number of pregnancies that occur for women using a particular method of birth control
   d. The reliability of alternative methods of birth control that do not use condoms

5. Toxic chemicals, pesticides, X rays, and other hazardous compounds causing birth defects are called
   a. carcinogens.
   b. teratogens.
   c. mutants.
   d. environmental assaults.

6. In an ectopic pregnancy, the fertilized egg implants itself in the
   a. fallopian tube.
   b. uterus.
   c. vagina.
   d. ovaries.

7. Twenty-year-old Lani is in a monogamous relationship with her boyfriend. She has a hard time remembering to take the pill or to carry her diaphragm with her. Which form of contraception would you recommend that she try?
   a. Female condom
   b. Tubal ligation
   c. Implanon
   d. The FemCap

8. What prenatal test involves snipping tissue from the developing fetal sac?
   a. Fetoscopy
   b. Ultrasound
   c. Amniocentesis
   d. Chorionic villus sampling

9. Why is it recommended not to use lambskin condoms?
   a. They are less elastic than latex condoms.
   b. They cannot be stored for as long as latex condoms.
   c. They don't protect against transmission of STIs.
   d. They're likely to cause allergic reactions.

10. The number of American couples who experience infertility is
    a. 1 in 6.
    b. 1 in 24.
    c. 1 in 60.
    d. 1 in 100.

Answers to these questions can be found on page A-1.

Web Links

1. **Guttmacher Institute.** This nonprofit organization is focused on sexual and reproductive health research, policy analysis, and public education. www.guttmacher.org
2. **Association of Reproductive Health Professionals.** This independent organization, originally the educational arm of Planned Parenthood, provides education for health care professionals and the general public. It includes an interactive tool to help you choose a birth control method that will work for you. www.arhp.org
3. **The American Pregnancy Association.** A wealth of resources to promote reproductive and pregnancy wellness. www.americanpregnancy.org
4. **Planned Parenthood.** A range of up-to-date information on issues such as birth control, the decision of when and whether to have a child, STIs, and safer sex. www.plannedparenthood.org

Addiction and Drug Abuse

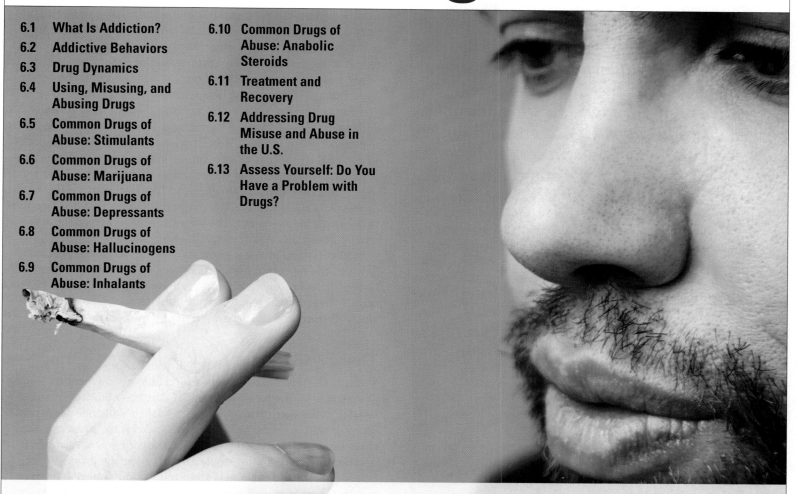

Drug misuse and abuse are enormous problems in our society, and drug addiction wreaks havoc on individuals, families, businesses, and society. Use and abuse of drugs occurs among all income levels, ethnic groups, and ages. According to the most recent statistics, an estimated 21.8 million Americans aged 12 or older—8 percent of the population—were current users of illicit (illegal) drugs.[1] Fourteen percent of people aged 12 or older report having used illicit drugs in the past year, and over 20 percent of high school students have taken prescription drugs without a doctor's permission.[2] Drug misuse and abuse can cause problems ranging from deterioration of relationships to loss of employment to death. It's impossible to put a dollar amount on the pain, suffering, and dysfunction that drugs cause in our everyday lives.

Why do people use drugs? Human beings appear to have a need to alter their consciousness, or mental state, and they do so in many ways: Children spin until they become dizzy; adults enjoy the thrill of extreme sports. Some listen to music, skydive, meditate, pray, or have sex. Others turn to drugs.

What Is Addiction?

- **List the characteristics of addiction.**
- **Distinguish between a habit and an addiction.**

Addiction is a persistent, compulsive dependence on a behavior or substance, despite ongoing negative consequences. Some researchers speak of two types of addictions: *substance addictions* (e.g., alcoholism, drug abuse, and smoking) and *process addictions* (e.g., gambling, shopping, eating, and sex).

Addictive behaviors initially provide a sense of pleasure or stability that is beyond the addict's power to achieve in other ways. With increasing dependence on the addictive behavior comes corresponding deterioration in relationships and in performance at work or school. Eventually, addicts do not find the addictive behavior pleasurable but find it preferable to the unhappy realities they seek to escape. Eventually, the addicted person needs the behavior to feel normal.

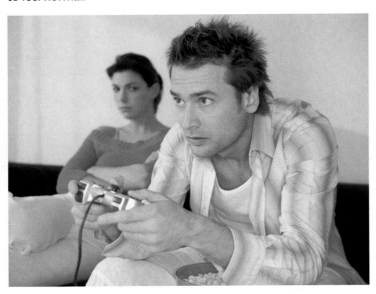

How can I recognize addiction?

Addiction can be difficult to recognize or acknowledge. Symptoms to look for are an obsession or compulsion with a behavior or activity, a loss of control, and negative consequences as a result of the behavior. Another symptom, denial of a problem, may be easy to see in another person but difficult to recognize in yourself.

Physiological dependence, the adaptive state that occurs with regular addictive behavior and results in withdrawal syndrome, is only one indicator of addiction. Chemicals are responsible for the most profound addictions because they cause cellular changes to which the body adapts so well that it eventually requires the chemical to function normally. Psychological dynamics, though, also play an important role. Psychological and physiological dependence are intertwined and nearly impossible to separate; all forms of addiction probably reflect dysfunction of certain biochemical systems in the brain.[3]

Four symptoms are present in both chemical and behavioral addictions: (1) **compulsion** characterized by **obsession**, or excessive preoccupation, with the behavior and an overwhelming need to perform it; (2) **loss of control**, or inability to reliably predict whether any occurrence of the behavior will be healthy or damaging; (3) **negative consequences**, such as physical damage, financial problems, academic failure, and family dissolution, that don't occur with healthy involvement in the behavior; and (4) **denial**, the inability to perceive the behavior as self-destructive.

Addiction also involves elements of **habit**, a repeated behavior in which the repetition may be unconscious. A habit, however, can be broken by becoming aware of its presence and choosing not to do it. With addiction, repetition occurs by compulsion, with considerable discomfort if the behavior is not performed.

The Physiology of Addiction

Virtually all intellectual, emotional, and behavioral functions occur as a result of biochemical interactions in the body. Biochemical messengers called **neurotransmitters** exert their influence at specific receptor sites on nerve cells. Drug use and chronic stress can alter these receptor sites, leading to either production or breakdown of neurotransmitters. Some people's bodies naturally produce insufficient quantities of these neurotransmitters, predisposing them to seek out chemicals, such as alcohol, as substitutes and making them more susceptible to addiction.

Mood-altering substances and experiences produce **tolerance**—when progressively larger doses or more intense involvement are needed to obtain the desired effects. Addicts tend to seek more intense mood-altering experiences and eventually increase the amount and intensity to the point of negative effects.

In **withdrawal**, a drug or activity replaces an effect the body should provide on its own. If the experience is repeated often enough, the body adjusts by *requiring* the drug or experience to obtain the effect. Stopping causes a withdrawal syndrome. Mood-altering chemicals, for example, fill receptor sites for endorphins (the body's "feel-good" neurotransmitters), leading to temporary shutdown of endorphin production. When drug use stops, those receptor sites sit empty, resulting in uncomfortable feelings that remain until the body resumes normal neurotransmitter production or the person consumes more of the drug.

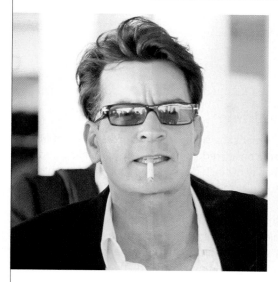
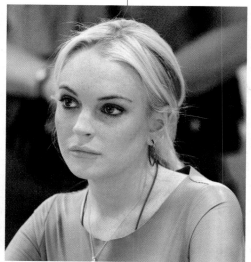

Celebrities Charlie Sheen and Lindsay Lohan have had very public struggles with drug abuse.

Withdrawal symptoms of chemical dependencies are generally the opposite of the effects of the drugs. An addict who feels a high from cocaine will experience a "crash" (depression and lethargy) when he stops taking it. Withdrawal symptoms for addictive behaviors usually involve psychological discomfort and preoccupation with or craving for the behavior.

The Biopsychosocial Model of Addiction

The most effective treatment today is based on the **biopsychosocial model of addiction**, which proposes that addiction is caused not by a single influence but by multiple biological, psychological, social, and environmental factors operating in complex interaction.

Psychological Factors People with low self-esteem, tendencies for risk-taking behavior, or poor coping skills are more likely to develop addictive behavior. Individuals with an external locus of control (those consistently looking outside themselves for solutions and explanations for life events) are more likely to experience addiction.

Biological or Disease Influences Brain processes controlling memory, motivation, and emotional state are subjects for genetic research into risk for addiction, particularly to mood-altering substances. Studies show that drug addicts metabolize these substances differently than do others; for example, genes affecting activity of the neurotransmitters serotonin and GABA (gamma-aminobutyric acid) are likely involved in risk for alcoholism.[4]

Studies also support a genetic influence on addiction. Identical twins, who share the same genes, are about twice as likely as fraternal twins, who share an average of 50 percent of genes, to resemble each other in terms of the presence of alcoholism. Approximately 50 to 60 percent of the risk for alcoholism is genetically determined.[5]

Environmental Influences Cultural expectations and mores help determine whether people engage in certain behaviors. Low rates of alcoholism typically exist in countries, like Italy, where children are gradually introduced to alcohol in diluted amounts, on special occasions, and within a strong family group; intoxication is not viewed as socially acceptable, stylish, or funny.[6] Such traditions and values are less widespread in the United States, where the incidence of alcohol addiction is very high.

Societal attitudes and messages also influence addictive behavior. Media emphasis on appearance and the ideal body plays a significant role in exercise addiction. Societal changes, in turn, influence individual norms. People living in cities characterized by rapid social change or social disorganization often feel disenfranchised and disconnected, leading to increased addiction rates.[7]

Social learning theory proposes that people learn behaviors by watching role models—parents, caregivers, and significant others. Many studies show that modeling by parents and by idolized celebrities exerts a profound influence on young people.[8]

On an individual level, major life events such as marriage, divorce, change in work status, or death of a loved one may trigger addictive behaviors. One thing that makes addictive behaviors so attractive is that they reliably alleviate personal pain, at least for a while—though in the long term they cause more pain than they relieve.

Family members whose needs for love, security, and affirmation are not consistently met; who are refused permission to express feelings or needs; and who frequently submerge their personalities to "keep the peace" are prone to addiction. Children whose parents are not consistently available (physically or emotionally); who are subjected to abuse; or who receive inconsistent or disparaging messages about their self-worth may experience addiction in adulthood.

Effect on Family and Friends

Family and friends of an addicted person often struggle with **codependence**. Codependents find it hard to set healthy boundaries and often live in the chaotic, crisis-oriented mode occurring around addicts. They assume responsibility for meeting others' needs to the point that they subordinate or even cease being aware of their own. Family and friends can also become **enablers**, knowingly or unknowingly protecting addicts from the consequences of their behavior. Both addicts and those around them must learn to see how addicts' behavior affects others and work to establish healthier relationships and boundaries.

check yourself

- **What are the characteristics of addiction?**
- **What is the difference between a habit and an addiction?**
- **How does addiction affect the family and friends of the addict?**

Addictive Behaviors

learning outcomes

- **Give examples of process addictions.**

Process addictions are behaviors known to be addictive because they are mood altering. Traditionally, the word *addiction* was used mainly with regards to psychoactive substances. However, new knowledge suggests that, as far as the brain is concerned, a reward is a reward, whether brought on by a chemical or a behavior.[9]

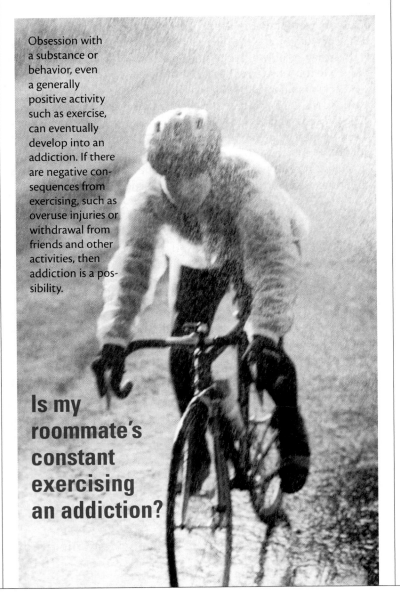

Obsession with a substance or behavior, even a generally positive activity such as exercise, can eventually develop into an addiction. If there are negative consequences from exercising, such as overuse injuries or withdrawal from friends and other activities, then addiction is a possibility.

Is my roommate's constant exercising an addiction?

Disordered Gambling

More than 2 million Americans suffer from **disordered gambling**, and 6 million more are considered to be at risk for gambling addiction.[10] Characteristic behaviors include preoccupation with gambling, unsuccessful efforts to quit, and lying to conceal the extent of one's involvement.

Recent research supports the theory that compulsive gamblers experience neurobiological changes that promote addiction;[11] in fact, the evidence is so compelling that the American Psychiatric Association is likely to list gambling as an addictive disorder in its next diagnostic manual.[12] Most compulsive gamblers seek excitement even more than money. Their cravings can be as intense as those of drug abusers; they show tolerance in their need to increase the amount of bets; and they experience intense highs. Up to half show withdrawal symptoms, including sleep disturbance, sweating, irritability, and craving.

Men, lower-income individuals, those who are divorced, African Americans, Native Americans, older adults, and individuals residing within 50 miles of a casino are more likely to have gambling problems.[13]

Compulsive Buying Disorder

Compulsive buying is estimated to affect up to 16 percent of the U.S. population.[14] **Compulsive shoppers** are preoccupied with shopping and spending and exercise little control over impulses to buy. Signs that a person has crossed the line into compulsive buying include buying more than one of the same item, keeping items with tags still attached, repeatedly buying much more than one needs or can afford, hiding purchases from loved ones, and experiencing euphoria when shopping.[15]

Compulsive buying disorders most often begin in the late teens and early twenties, coinciding with establishment of credit and independence from parents. It can be seasonal (shopping during the winter to alleviate seasonal anxiety and depression) and can occur when people feel depressed, lonely, or angry. Both compulsive gambling and compulsive buying frequently lead to repeated borrowing to help support the addiction.

Technology Addictions

Do you have friends who seem more concerned with texting or Web surfing than with eating, going out, or studying? These attitudes and behaviors are not unusual. An estimated 13 to 18.4 percent of college Internet users experience **Internet addiction**, when smart phone use is taken into account.[16] Approximately 12 percent of college students report that Internet use and computer games have interfered with their academic performance.[17]

What you do online may be as important as how long you spend; some activities, such as gaming and cybersex, seem to be more potentially addictive than others. Signs of Internet addiction include sleep deprivation, depression, neglecting family and friends, lack of physical activity, euphoria when online, uncomfortable feelings when not online, and poor grades or job performance. Addicts may be compensating for loneliness, marital or work problems, a poor social life, or financial problems.

Work Addiction

To understand work addiction, we must understand the concept of healthy work. Healthy work provides a sense of identity; helps develop our strengths; and is a means of satisfaction and mastery. Although work may occasionally keep them from family, friends, and personal interests, healthy workers generally maintain balance in their lives.

Conversely, **work addiction** is the compulsive use of work and the work persona to fulfill needs of intimacy, power, and success. Work addicts usually fail to set boundaries regarding work and feel driven to work even when away from work.[18]

Work addiction, found among all age, racial, and socioeconomic groups, typically develops in people in their forties and fifties. Males outnumber females, but this is changing as women gain more equality in the workforce. Most work addicts come from alcoholic, rigid, violent, or otherwise dysfunctional homes. Work addiction can bring societal admiration, as addicts often excel in their professions. However, it is a major source of marital discord and family breakup in addition to causing problems with friends.[19]

Exercise Addiction

Exercise addicts use exercise compulsively to try to meet needs—for nurturance, intimacy, self-esteem, and self-competency—that an object or activity cannot truly meet. Consequently, addictive or compulsive exercise results in negative consequences similar to those of other addictions: alienation of family and friends, injuries from overdoing it, and craving for more.

Traditionally, women have been perceived as more at risk for

$23,000

is the average amount of debt that a compulsive shopper owes.

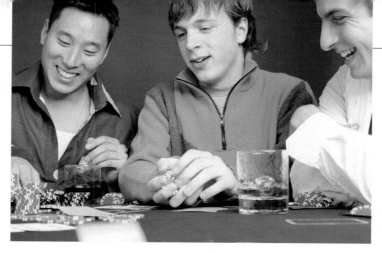

Call, fold, or raise? For increasing numbers of college students, gambling and the debts it can incur are becoming serious problems.

exercise addiction. However, evidence is growing that more men are developing unhealthy exercise patterns. *Muscle dysmorphia* is a pathological preoccupation with being larger and more muscular.[20] Consequences include excessive weightlifting and exercising as well as steroid or supplement abuse.

Sexual Addiction

In **sexual addiction**, people confuse physical arousal with intimacy.[21] They feel nurtured not by the person with whom they have sex, but by the activity itself. Likewise, they are incapable of nurturing another person because sex, not the person, is the object of their affection. In fact, people with sexual addictions may be satisfied by masturbation, whether alone or during phone sex or while reading or watching erotica. They may participate in affairs, sex with strangers, prostitution, voyeurism, exhibitionism, rape, incest, and pedophilia. People addicted to sex frequently experience depression and anxiety fueled by fear of discovery. The toll that sexual addiction exacts is seen in loss of intimacy with loved ones, which frequently leads to family disintegration.

Sexual addictions affect men and women of all ages, married and single people, and people of any sexual preference. Most had dysfunctional childhood families, often characterized by addiction. Many were physically, emotionally, and/or sexually abused.

Multiple Addictions

Although addicts tend to have a "favorite" drug or behavior, the majority of people in treatment have more than one addiction. For example, alcohol addiction and eating disorders are commonly paired in women, whereas individuals trying to break a chemical dependency frequently resort to compulsive eating. Multiple addictions complicate recovery, but don't make it impossible.

check yourself

- **What is an example of a process addiction?**
- **How can a positive behavior such as exercise become addictive?**

Drug Dynamics

learning outcomes

- **Identify the six major categories of drugs.**
- **Discuss interactions that can result from polydrug use.**

Most bodily processes result from chemical reactions or changes in electrical charge. Drugs possess an electrical charge and chemical structure similar to those of chemicals occurring naturally in the body and thus can affect physical functions in many ways.

How Drugs Affect the Brain

Pleasure, which scientists call *reward,* is a powerful biological force for survival. If you do something that you experience as pleasurable, the brain is wired so you tend to do it again. Life-sustaining activities, such as eating, activate a circuit of specialized nerve cells devoted to producing and regulating pleasure. One important set of these cells, which uses a chemical neurotransmitter called *dopamine,* sits at the top of the brain stem in the *ventral tegmental area* (VTA). Here, dopamine-containing neurons relay messages about pleasure to nerve cells in the limbic system—brain structures that regulate emotions. Still other fibers connect to a related part of the frontal region of the cerebral cortex, the area of the brain that plays a key role in memory, perception, thought, and consciousness. So this "pleasure circuit," the *mesolimbic dopamine* system, spans the survival-oriented brain stem, the emotional limbic system, and the thinking frontal cerebral cortex.

All drugs that are addicting can activate the brain's pleasure circuit. Drug addiction is a biological, pathological process that alters how the pleasure center and other parts of the brain function. Almost all **psychoactive drugs** (those that change the way the brain works) do so by affecting chemical neurotransmission—enhancing, suppressing, or interfering with it. Some drugs, such as heroin and lysergic acid diethylamide (LSD), mimic the effects of natural neurotransmitters. Others, such as phencyclidine (PCP), block receptors, preventing neuronal messages from getting through. Still others, such as cocaine, block neurons' reuptake of neurotransmitters, increasing neurotransmitter concentration in the synaptic gap between individual neurons. Finally, some drugs, such as methamphetamine, act by causing neurotransmitters to be released in greater than normal amounts.

Categories of Drugs

Scientists divide drugs into six categories. Each includes some drugs that stimulate the body, some that depress body functions, and others that produce hallucinations (sensory perceptions that are not real). Each category also includes psychoactive drugs:

- *Prescription drugs* can be obtained only with a prescription from a licensed health care practitioner. More than 10,000 prescription drugs are sold in the United States.
- *Over-the-counter drugs* can be purchased without a prescription. More than 300,000 OTC products are available, and an estimated 3 out of 4 people routinely self-medicate with them.[22] Whereas prescription drugs are available at approximately 58,000 pharmacies nationwide, OTC medicines are available at over 750,000 retailers. Americans make more use of widely available OTC medicines each year.[23]
- *Recreational drugs* belong to a category whose boundaries depend upon how the term *recreation* is defined. Generally, recreational drugs contain chemicals used to help people relax or socialize. Most, like alcohol, tobacco, and caffeine, are legal even though they are psychoactive.
- *Herbal preparations* encompass approximately 750 substances, including herbal teas and other products of botanical (plant) origin believed to have medicinal properties.
- *Illicit (illegal) drugs* are the most notorious type of drug. Although laws governing their use, possession, cultivation, manufacture, and sale differ from state to state, illicit drugs are generally recognized as harmful. All are psychoactive.
- *Commercial preparations* are the most universally used, yet least commonly recognized, chemical substances. More than 1,000 exist, including seemingly benign items such as perfumes, cosmetics, household cleansers, paints, glues, inks, dyes, and pesticides.

Routes of Drug Administration

Route of administration refers to how a drug is taken into the body. The route of administration largely determines the rapidity of a drug's effect (**Figure 6.1**). The most common is **oral ingestion**—swallowing a tablet, capsule, or liquid. A drug taken orally may not reach the bloodstream for 30 minutes.

Drugs can also enter the body through the respiratory tract via sniffing, smoking, or **inhalation**. Drugs inhaled and absorbed by the lungs travel the most rapidly of all routes of drug administration. Another rapid form of drug administration is **injection** directly into the bloodstream (intravenously), muscles (intramuscularly), or just under the skin (subcutaneously). Intravenous injection, which involves inserting a hypodermic needle directly into a vein, is the most common method of injection for drug users, due to the speed of effect (within seconds in most cases). It is also the most dangerous, due to the risk of damaging blood vessels and contracting HIV

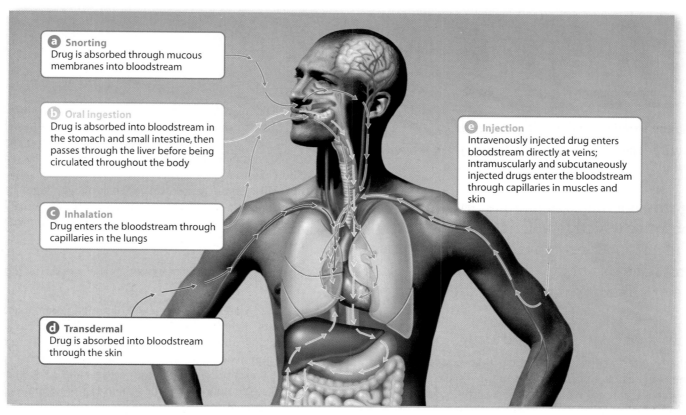

Figure 6.1 Routes of Drug Administration
Drugs are most commonly swallowed, inhaled, or injected. They can also be absorbed through the skin or mucous membranes (as in snorting and suppository use, not shown here).

(human immunodeficiency virus) and hepatitis (a severe liver disease). Drugs can also be absorbed through the skin or tissue lining (**transdermal**)—the nicotine patch is a common example of a drug administered in this manner—or through the mucous membranes, such as those in the nose (snorting) or the vagina or anus (**suppositories**, typically mixed with a waxy medium that melts at body temperature, releasing the drug into the bloodstream).

However a drug enters the system, it eventually finds its way to the bloodstream and is circulated throughout the body to **receptor sites** where chemicals, enzymes, and other substances interact. Psychoactive drugs can cross the blood–brain barrier to reach receptor sites in the brain, where they can affect cognition, emotion, and physiological functioning. Once a drug reaches receptor sites in the brain and other organs, it may remain active for several hours before it dissipates and is carried by the blood to the liver where it is metabolized (broken down by enzymes). The products of enzymatic breakdown, called *metabolites*, are then excreted, primarily through the kidneys (in urine) or bowels (in feces), but also through the skin (in sweat) or lungs (in expired air).

Drug Interactions

Polydrug use—taking several drugs simultaneously—can lead to dangerous health problems. Alcohol in particular frequently has dangerous interactions with other drugs.

Synergism, also called *potentiation*, is an interaction of two or more drugs in which the effects of the individual drugs are multiplied beyond what would normally be expected if they were taken alone. You might think of synergism as 2 + 2 = 10. A synergistic reaction can be very dangerous and even deadly.

Antagonism, though usually less serious than synergism, can also produce unwanted and unpleasant effects. In an antagonistic reaction, drugs work at the same receptor site; one blocks the action of the other. The blocking drug occupies the receptor site and prevents the other drug from attaching, altering its absorption and action.

With **inhibition**, the effects of one drug are eliminated or reduced by the presence of another drug at the receptor site. **Intolerance** occurs when drugs combine in the body to produce extremely uncomfortable reactions. The drug Antabuse (disulfiram), used to help alcoholics give up alcohol, works by producing this type of interaction. A final type of interaction, **cross-tolerance**, occurs when a person develops a physiological tolerance to one drug and shows a similar tolerance to certain other drugs as a result.

check yourself

- **What are the six major categories of drugs?**
- **What is polydrug use, and what are its risks?**

learning **outcomes**

- **Discuss trends in the misuse of drugs**
- **Identify factors associated with drug use by college students**

Drug misuse involves using a drug for a purpose for which it was not intended. This is not too far removed from **drug abuse**, or excessive use of any drug. Misuse or abuse of any drug may lead to addiction.

Abuse of Over-the-Counter Drugs

Over-the-counter medications are drugs that require no prescription; they can be bought in drugstores or supermarkets. OTC medications can be abused, with resultant health complications and potential addiction. Most vulnerable to abusing these drugs are teenagers, young adults, and people over 65.

OTC drugs are abused when the drug is taken in more than the recommended dosage, combined with other drugs, or taken over a longer time than recommended. Tolerance from continued use can create unintended dependence. Teenagers and young adults sometimes abuse OTC medications in search of a cheap high—by drinking large amounts of cough medicine, for instance. Several types of OTC drugs are subject to misuse and abuse:

- **Sleep aids.** In excess, these drugs can cause sleep problems, weaken areas of the body, or induce narcolepsy (excessive, intrusive sleepiness). Continued use can lead to tolerance and dependence.
- **Cold medicines (cough syrups and tablets).** Dextromethorphan (DXM) is present in about 125 OTC medications; as many as 6 percent of high school seniors report taking drugs containing DXM to get high.[24] Large doses can cause hallucinations, loss of motor control, and "out-of-body" sensations. Other effects include impaired judgment, blurred vision, dizziness, paranoia, excessive sweating, slurred speech, irregular heartbeat, and numbness of fingers and toes. Abuse can lead to seizures, brain damage, and death. Some states have passed laws limiting the amount of products containing DXM a person can purchase or prohibiting sale to individuals under 18.[25]

  Pseudoephedrine is another cold and allergy medication ingredient that is frequently abused, most commonly in illegal methamphetamine manu-

facture. U.S. law limits the amount of products containing this drug that an individual may purchase and requires that the product be sold "behind the counter" (without a prescription, but only through a pharmacist). Pharmacists must keep a record of purchasers.[26]

- **Diet pills.** Some teens use diet pills to get high. Diet pills often contain a stimulant such as caffeine, or an herbal ingredient claimed to promote weight loss such as *Hoodia gordonii*.

Nonmedical Use or Abuse of Prescription Drugs

In the United States today, the abuse of prescription medications is at an all-time high; only marijuana is more widely abused.[27]

Over 48 million Americans 12 and older have used prescription drugs for nonmedical reasons.[28] Of these, 7 percent report abusing controlled prescription drugs in the past year.[29] In 2009, 6 percent of people 18 to 25 reported nonmedical use of prescription drugs in the previous month.[30]

Prescription drugs are often easier to obtain than illegal ones. In some cases, unscrupulous pharmacists or other medical professionals steal the drugs or sell fraudulent prescriptions. Abusers visit several doctors to obtain multiple prescriptions, fake or exaggerate symptoms to get prescriptions, or call pharmacies with fraudulent prescriptions.

College Students and Prescription Drug Abuse College students' prescription drug abuse has increased dramatically over the past decade. Many students see prescription drugs as safer than illicit drugs. However, when these drugs are misused they can be even more unsafe than illegal drugs.

From 1993 to 2005, the rate of student abuse of prescription painkillers rose 343 percent,[31] of prescription stimulants, 93 percent; of prescription tranquilizers, 450 percent; and of sedatives 225 percent.[32]

Of particular concern on campuses is increased abuse of stimulants, such as Adderall and Ritalin, intended to treat attention-deficit/hyperactivity disorder (ADHD). Students primarily report using ADHD drugs for academic gain. A recent study on two campuses revealed that 9 percent of students had used ADHD drugs without a prescription at some point in college.[33] Between 16 and 29 percent of students with prescribed stimulant medications for ADHD reported having sold, traded, or been asked for their medications.[34]

Over-the-counter cough syrup is frequently abused by young people seeking a high from the ingredient DXM.

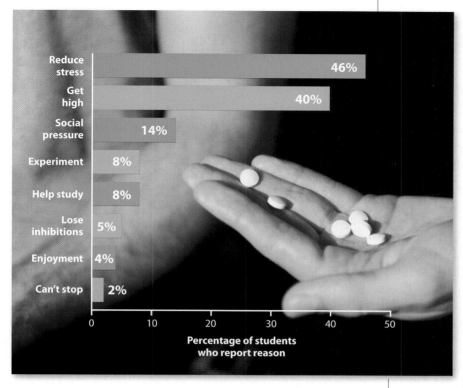

Figure 6.2 Reasons College Students Use Illicit Drugs or Controlled Prescription Drugs
Source: Adapted from *Wasting the Best and the Brightest: Substance Abuse at America's Colleges and Universities* (New York: National Center on Addiction and Substance Abuse at Columbia University, March 2007), 47. Copyright © 2007. Reprinted with permission of The National Center on Addiction and Substance Abuse at Columbia University (CASA Columbia).

Illicit Drugs

The problem of illicit drug use touches us all. We may use illicit substances ourselves, watch someone we love struggle with drug abuse, or become the victim of a drug-related crime. At the very least, we are forced to pay increasing taxes for law enforcement and drug rehabilitation. Illicit drug use spans ages, genders, ethnicities, occupations, and socioeconomic groups.

Use of illicit drugs in the United States increased during the 1970s, peaked between 1979 and 1986, and declined until 1992, from which point it has not changed. In 2009, an estimated 21.8 million Americans were illicit drug users, compared to the 1979 peak of 25 million users. Among youth, however, illicit drug use, notably of marijuana, has been rising in recent years.[35]

Illicit Drug Use on Campus After more than a decade of declining use on American college campuses, illicit drugs have reappeared. In 2008, the number of college students who had tried any drug stood at almost 50 percent; over a third had smoked marijuana in the past year. Daily use of marijuana is at its highest point since 1989.[36] Cocaine use is down sharply, but LSD use has more than doubled.

For many students, our culture's societal mores regarding substance use and abuse on college campuses may make it seem like the norm. The proportion of students who use illicit drugs other than marijuana increased 52 percent—from 5 percent to 8 percent of all students—in the past decade.[37] College staff are concerned about the link between substance abuse and poor academic performance, depression, anxiety, suicide, vandalism, fights, serious medical problems, and death.[38]

Research has identified factors in a student's life that increase the risk of substance abuse. The more of these factors, the greater the risk:

- **Positive expectations.** The most common reason students give to explain why they drink, smoke, or use drugs is to relax, reduce stress, or forget about problems (**Figure 6.2**). Some students take drugs, most notably prescription ADHD drugs and caffeine, in the belief that the drugs will help them study.
- **Genetics and family history.** These play a significant role in risk for addiction.
- **Substance use in high school.** Two-thirds of college students who use illicit drugs began doing so in high school.
- **Mental health problems.** Students who report being diagnosed with depression are more likely to have abused prescription drugs, or to have used marijuana or other illicit drugs.
- **Sorority and fraternity membership.** Being a member of a sorority or fraternity increases the likelihood of using alcohol, marijuana, or cocaine and makes one twice as likely to abuse prescription drugs.
- **Stress.** For some students under academic and social stress, seemingly easy relief comes in the form of drugs or alcohol. Taking a pill to relax or "fit in," may push students to begin to use or abuse drugs they otherwise might avoid.

Many factors influence students to avoid drugs; the most commonly reported include these:[39]

- **Parental attitudes and behavior.** Students who say they are more influenced by their parents' concerns or expectations drink, use marijuana, and smoke significantly less than those less influenced by parents.
- **Religion and spirituality.** The greater students' level of religiosity (hours in prayer, attendance at services), the less likely they are to drink, smoke, or use other drugs.
- **Student engagement.** The more a student is involved in learning and extracurricular activities, the less likely he or she is to binge drink, use marijuana, or abuse prescription drugs.
- **College athletics.** College athletes drink at higher rates than nonathletes but are less likely to use illicit drugs.

129

- **What are recent trends in how college students misuse and abuse drugs?**
- **What factors increase or decrease a college student's risk of substance abuse?**
- **Just because a drug is legal, does that mean it's safe? Explain your answer.**

Common Drugs of Abuse: Stimulants

learning outcomes

- **Identify stimulants that are commonly misused or abused.**
- **Discuss the effects and health risks of stimulants.**

Hundreds of drugs are subject to abuse—some are legal, such as recreational drugs and prescription medications, whereas many others are illegal and classified as "controlled substances." Some of the drugs of most concern are stimulants, marijuana, depressants, hallucinogens, inhalants, and anabolic steroids.

Stimulants

A **stimulant** is a drug that increases activity of the central nervous system. Its effects usually involve increased activity, anxiety, and agitation; users often seem jittery or nervous while high. Commonly used stimulants include cocaine, amphetamines, methamphetamine, and caffeine. Nicotine, the addictive substance in tobacco products, is another common stimulant.

Cocaine A white crystalline powder derived from the leaves of the South American coca shrub (not related to cocoa plants), *cocaine* ("coke") has been described as one of the most powerful naturally occurring stimulants. It binds at receptor sites in the central nervous system, producing an intense high that usually disappears quickly, leaving a powerful craving for more.

Cocaine can be taken in several ways, including snorting, smoking, and injecting. The powdered form is snorted through the nose, which can damage mucous membranes and cause sinusitis. It can destroy the user's sense of smell, and occasionally it even eats a hole through the septum. When snorted, the drug enters the bloodstream through the lungs in less than 1 minute and reaches the brain in less than 3 minutes.

Cocaine alkaloid, or *freebase*, is obtained by removing the hydrochloride salt from cocaine powder. *Freebasing* refers to the smoking of freebase by placing it at the end of a pipe and holding a flame near it to produce a vapor, which is then inhaled. *Crack* is identical pharmacologically to freebase, but the hydrochloride salt is still present and is processed with baking soda and water. It is a

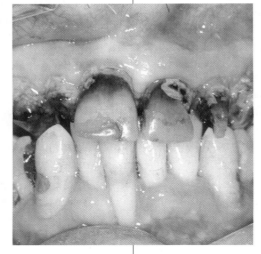

cheap, widely available drug that is smokable and very potent. Crack is commonly smoked in the same manner as freebase. Because crack is such a pure drug, it takes little time to achieve the desired high, and a crack user can become addicted quickly.

Some cocaine users inject the drug intravenously, which introduces large amounts into the body rapidly, creating a brief, intense high and subsequent crash. Injecting users place themselves at risk not only for contracting HIV and hepatitis through shared needles, but also for skin infections, vein damage, inflamed arteries, and infection of the heart lining.

Cocaine is both an anesthetic and a central nervous system stimulant. In tiny doses, it can slow the heart rate. In larger doses, the physical effects are dramatic: increased heart rate and blood pressure, loss of appetite that can lead to dramatic weight loss, convulsions, muscle twitching, irregular heartbeat, and even death resulting from an overdose. Other effects of cocaine include temporary relief of depression, decreased fatigue, talkativeness, increased alertness, and heightened self-confidence. However, as the dose increases, users become irritable and apprehensive, and their behavior may turn paranoid or violent.

Amphetamines The **amphetamines** include a large and varied group of synthetic agents that stimulate the central nervous system. Small doses of amphetamines improve alertness, lessen fatigue, and generally elevate mood. With repeated use, however, physical and psychological dependencies develop. Sleep patterns are affected (insomnia); heart rate, breathing rate, and blood pressure increase; and restlessness, anxiety, appetite suppression, and vision problems are common. High doses over long periods of time can produce hallucinations, delusions, and disorganized behavior.

Certain types of amphetamines or amphetamine-like drugs are used for medicinal purposes. As discussed earlier, drugs prescribed to treat ADHD are stimulants and are increasingly abused on campus.

Methamphetamine An increasingly common form of amphetamine, *methamphetamine* (commonly called simply "meth") is a potent, long-acting, addictive drug that strongly activates the brain's reward center by producing a sense of euphoria. Methamphetamine can be snorted, smoked, injected, or orally ingested. When snorted, the effects can be felt in 3 to 5 minutes; if orally ingested, effects occur within 15 to 20 minutes. The pleasurable effects of methamphetamine are typically an intense rush lasting only a few

Methamphetamine users often damage their teeth beyond repair because of the toxic chemicals in the substance. This condition is commonly referred to as "meth mouth."

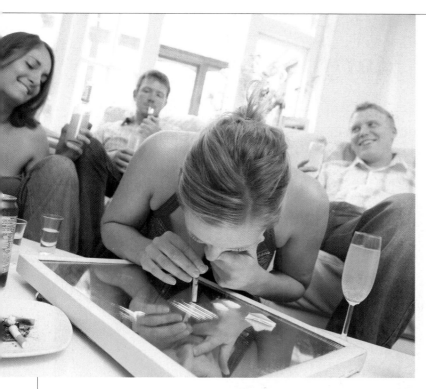

Although cocaine use has declined from its peak in the 1980s, it continues to be a commonly abused illicit drug.

minutes when snorted; in contrast, smoking the drug can produce a high lasting more than 8 hours.

In the short term, methamphetamine produces increased physical activity, alertness, euphoria, rapid breathing, increased body temperature, insomnia, tremors, anxiety, confusion, and decreased appetite; the drug's effects quickly wear off, leaving the user seeking more. Users often experience tolerance after the first use, making methamphetamine a highly addictive drug.

The long-term effects of methamphetamine can include severe weight loss, cardiovascular damage, increased risk of heart attack and stroke, hallucinations, extensive tooth decay and tooth loss, violence, paranoia, psychotic behavior, and even death. Brain damage similar to Parkinson's disease and Alzheimer's disease has been reported in long-term meth users.

Ice is a potent form of methamphetamine that is imported primarily from Asia, particularly South Korea and Taiwan. It is purer and more crystalline than the version manufactured in the United States, and it is odorless when smoked. Its effects can last for more than 12 hours.

Like that of other amphetamines, the downside of methamphetamine is devastating. Prolonged use can cause fatal lung and kidney damage as well as long-lasting psychological damage. In some instances, major psychological dysfunction can persist as long as 2.5 years after last use. Methamphetamine can cause psychosis, increased risk for heart attack and stroke, and brain damage that results in impaired motor skills and cognitive functions.

Methamphetamine abuse is an increasingly serious problem, especially in rural areas of the United States. In 2010, 2.3 percent of high school seniors reported using methamphetamine in their lifetime. Rates among adults are difficult to determine, but it is believed that more than 12 million Americans have tried metham-

phetamine.[40] A possible contributing factor to the increasing rate of methamphetamine use is that it is relatively easy to make using recipes that often include common OTC ingredients such as ephedrine and pseudoephedrine.

Caffeine What is the most popular and widely consumed drug in the United States? Caffeine. Almost half of all Americans drink coffee every day, and many others consume caffeine in some other form, mainly for its well-known "wake-up" effect. Drinking coffee, tea, soft drinks, and other caffeine-containing products is legal, even socially encouraged. Caffeine may seem harmless, but excessive consumption is associated with addiction and certain health problems.

Caffeine is derived from the chemical family called *xanthines*, which are found in plant products from which coffee, tea, and chocolate are made. The xanthines are mild central nervous system stimulants that enhance mental alertness and reduce feelings of fatigue. Other stimulant effects include increased heart muscle contractions, oxygen consumption, metabolism, and urinary output. A person feels these effects within 15 to 45 minutes of ingesting a caffeinated product. It takes 4 to 6 hours for the body to metabolize half of the caffeine ingested, so, depending on the amount of caffeine taken in, it may continue to exert effects for a day or longer.

Side effects of the xanthines include wakefulness, insomnia, irregular heartbeat, dizziness, nausea, indigestion, and sometimes mild delirium. Some people also experience heartburn. As the effects of caffeine wear off, frequent users may feel let down—mentally or physically depressed, exhausted, and weak. To counteract this, they commonly choose to drink another cup of coffee. Habitually engaging in this practice leads to tolerance and psychological dependence. Symptoms of excessive caffeine consumption include chronic insomnia, jitters, irritability, nervousness, anxiety, and involuntary muscle twitches. Withdrawing from caffeine may compound the effects and produce severe headaches, fatigue, and nausea. Because caffeine meets the requirements for addiction—tolerance, psychological dependence, and withdrawal symptoms—it can be classified as addictive.

Long-term caffeine use has been suspected of being linked to several serious health problems. However, no strong evidence exists to suggest that moderate caffeine use (less than 300 mg, or approximately 3 cups or less of regular coffee, a day) produces harmful effects in healthy, nonpregnant people. Caffeine does not appear to cause long-term high blood pressure, has not been linked to strokes, nor is there any evidence of a relationship between caffeine and heart disease.[41] However, people who suffer from irregular heartbeat are cautioned against using caffeine, because the resultant increase in heart rate might be life threatening.

check yourself

■ **What is a stimulant?**

■ **What are the effects and health risks of commonly abused stimulants?**

■ **Compare caffeine to illicit stimulants.**

Common Drugs of Abuse: Marijuana

- **Discuss the effects and health risks of marijuana.**

Although archaeological evidence indicates that **marijuana** ("grass," "weed," "pot") was used as long as 6,000 years ago, the drug did not become popular in the United States until the 1960s. Today, marijuana is the most commonly used illicit drug in the country. Approximately 41 percent of Americans over the age of 12 have tried marijuana at least once,[42] some 29 million have used marijuana in the past year, and more than 16.7 million have done so in the past month. Among young adults, about 5.3 percent of them use marijuana daily, according to a 2010 survey.[43]

Methods of Use and Physical Effects

Marijuana is derived from either the *Cannabis sativa* or *Cannabis indica* (hemp) plant. Most of the time, marijuana is smoked, although it can also be ingested, as in brownies baked with marijuana in them. When marijuana is smoked, it is usually rolled into cigarettes (joints) or placed in a pipe or water pipe (bong).

Tetrahydrocannabinol (THC) is the psychoactive substance in marijuana and the key to determining how powerful a high it will produce. More potent forms of the drug can contain up to 27 percent THC, but most average 10 percent.[44] *Hashish*, a potent cannabis preparation derived mainly from the plant's thick, sticky resin, contains high THC concentrations. Hash oil, a substance produced by percolating a solvent such as ether through dried marijuana to extract the THC, is a tarlike liquid that may contain up to 300 mg of THC in a dose.

The effects of smoking marijuana are generally felt within 10 to 30 minutes and usually wear off within 3 hours. The most noticeable visible effect of THC is dilation of the eyes' blood vessels, which gives the smoker bloodshot eyes. Marijuana smokers also exhibit coughing; dry mouth and throat ("cotton mouth"); increased thirst and appetite; lowered blood pressure; and mild muscular weakness, primarily exhibited in drooping eyelids. Users can also experience severe anxiety, panic, paranoia, and psychosis and may have intensified reactions to various stimuli—colors, sounds, and the speed at which things move may seem altered. High doses of hashish may produce vivid visual hallucinations.

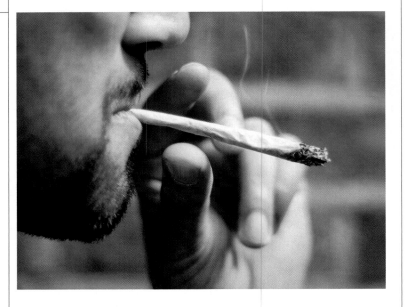

Marijuana and Driving

Marijuana use presents clear hazards for drivers of motor vehicles and others on the road with them. The drug substantially reduces a driver's ability to react and make quick decisions. Perceptual and other performance deficits may persist for some time after the high subsides. Users who attempt to drive, fly, or operate heavy machinery often fail to recognize their impairment. Overall, marijuana is the most prevalent illegal drug detected in impaired drivers, fatally injured drivers, and motor vehicle crash victims.[45] In many of these cases, alcohol is detected as well. Research by the National Highway Traffic Safety Administration indicates that a moderate dose of marijuana alone impairs driving performance; however, the effects of even a low dose combined with alcohol are markedly greater than for either drug alone.[46]

Effects of Chronic Marijuana Use

Because marijuana has been widely used only since the 1960s, long-term studies of its effects have been difficult to conduct. Also, studies conducted in the 1960s involved marijuana with THC levels only a fraction of today's levels; their results may not apply to stronger forms available today.

Numerous studies have shown that marijuana smoke contains 50 to 70 percent more carcinogenic hydrocarbons than does tobacco smoke. Because marijuana smokers typically inhale more deeply and hold their breath longer than tobacco smokers, the lungs are exposed to more carcinogens. As well, effects from irritation (e.g., cough, excessive phlegm, and increased lung infections) similar to those experienced by tobacco smokers can occur.[47] The tar from cannabis also contains higher levels of carcinogens than does tobacco smoke. Lung conditions such as chronic bronchitis, emphysema, and other lung disorders are also associated with smoking marijuana.

Inhaling marijuana smoke introduces carbon monoxide into the bloodstream. Because the blood has a greater affinity for carbon monoxide than it does for oxygen, its oxygen-carrying capacity is diminished; the heart must work harder to pump oxygen to oxygen-starved tissues. Furthermore, the tar from cannabis contains higher levels of carcinogens than does tobacco smoke.

Frequent and/or long-term marijuana use may significantly increase a man's risk of developing testicular cancer; being a marijuana smoker at the time of diagnosis was associated with a 70 percent increased risk of testicular cancer.[48] The risk was particularly elevated for those who used marijuana at least weekly or who had long-term exposure beginning in adolescence. The results also suggested that the association with marijuana use might be limited to *nonseminoma*, an aggressive, fast-growing testicular malignancy that tends to strike early, between ages 20 and 35, and accounts for about 40 percent of all testicular cancer cases.[49]

According to the National Survey on Drug Use and Health, teens and young adults who use marijuana are more likely to develop serious mental health problems. A number of studies have shown an association between marijuana use and increased rates of anxiety, depression, suicidal ideation, and schizophrenia.[50] Some of these studies have shown age at first use as an indicator of vulnerability to later problems. Among individuals 18 and older, those who used marijuana before the age of 12 were twice as likely to have a serious mental illness as those who first used marijuana at age 18 or older.[51]

Other risks associated with marijuana use include suppression of the immune system, blood pressure changes, and impaired memory function. Pregnant women who smoke marijuana are at a higher risk for stillbirth or miscarriage and for delivering low-birth-weight babies and babies with abnormalities of the nervous system.[52]

Medical Marijuana

For years, the use of medical marijuana has been hotly debated. Currently, 31 states and the District of Columbia have laws that recognize marijuana's medical value, and voters in 14 states have chosen to legalize marijuana for medicinal use. These new state laws, however, conflict with federal possession laws and have led to new, as yet unresolved, court battles.[53]

Arguments both for and against legalization have been very strong over the past few decades, and the debate is intense and ongoing.[54] Advocates note that marijuana is a safe and effective treatment for certain complications of dozens of conditions, such as cancer, AIDS, multiple sclerosis, pain, migraines, glaucoma, and epilepsy. It helps control the severe nausea and vomiting produced by chemotherapy. It improves appetite and forestalls the loss of lean muscle mass associated with AIDS-wasting syndrome. In addition, legalizing marijuana and taxing its sale

One common way of smoking marijuana is to use a pipe.

would bring in revenue for the government, and government and U.S. Food and Drug Administration (FDA) oversight would allow for standardization of marijuana growth and production and could promote more responsible cultivation methods.

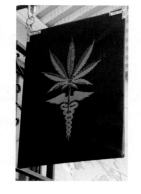

Those who oppose legalization of marijuana say that it is not necessary to legalize marijuana for medical use because there are already FDA-approved drugs that are just as effective in treating the same conditions. They note the dangerous side effects of marijuana use, including lung injury, immune system damage, and interference with fertility, that make it inappropriate for FDA approval. In addition, marijuana is known to be addictive and may lead to harder drug use.

Skills for Behavior Change

RESPONDING TO AN OFFER OF DRUGS

No matter what your experience until now, it is likely that you will be invited to use drugs at some point in your life. Here are some questions to consider *before* you find yourself in a situation in which you have the opportunity or feel pressure to use illicit drugs:

- **Why am I considering trying drugs? Am I trying to fit in or impress my friends? What does this say about my friends if I need to take drugs to impress them? Are my friends really looking out for what is best for me?**
- **Am I using this drug to cope or feel different? Am I depressed?**
- **What could taking drugs cost me? Will this cost me my career if I am caught using? Could using drugs prevent me from getting a job?**
- **What are the long-term consequences of using this drug?**
- **What will this cost me in terms of my friendships and family? How would my close family and friends respond if they knew I was using drugs?**

Even when you make the decision not to use drugs, it can be difficult to say no gracefully. Some good ways to turn down an offer:

- **"Thanks, but I've got a big test (game, meeting) tomorrow morning."**
- **"I've already got a great buzz right now. I really don't need anything more."**
- **"I don't like how (insert drug name here) makes me feel."**
- **"I'm driving tonight. So I'm not using."**
- **"I want to go for a run in the morning."**
- **"No."**

check yourself

- **What are the effects and health risks of marijuana?**
- **How does marijuana affect the ability to drive?**
- **What are the arguments for and against legalization of marijuana?**

Common Drugs of Abuse: Depressants

learning outcomes

- **Identify depressants that are commonly misused or abused.**
- **Discuss the effects and health risks of depressants.**

Whereas central nervous system stimulants increase muscular and nervous system activity, **depressants** have the opposite effect. These drugs slow down neuromuscular activity and cause sleepiness or calmness. If the dose is high enough, brain function can stop, causing death. Alcohol is the most widely used central nervous system depressant; others include opioids, benzodiazepines, and barbiturates.

Opioids

Opioids cause drowsiness, relieve pain, and produce euphoria. Also called *narcotics*, opioids are derived from the parent drug **opium**, a dark, resinous substance made from the milky juice of the opium poppy seedpod. All opioids are highly addictive. Opium and heroin are both illegal in the United States, but some opioids are available by prescription for medical purposes: Morphine is sometimes prescribed for severe pain, and codeine is found in prescription cough syrups and other painkillers. Several prescription drugs, including Vicodin, Percodan, OxyContin, Demerol, and Dilaudid, contain synthetic opioids.

Physical Effects of Opioids Opioids are powerful depressants of the central nervous system. In addition to relieving pain, these drugs lower heart rate, respiration, and blood pressure. Side effects include weakness, dizziness, nausea, vomiting, euphoria, decreased sex drive, visual disturbances, and lack of coordination.

The human body's physiology could be said to make us particularly susceptible to opioid addiction. Opioid-like hormones called **endorphins** are manufactured in the body and have multiple receptor sites, particularly in the central nervous system. When endorphins attach themselves at these sites, they create feelings of painless well-being; medical researchers refer to them as "the body's own opioids." When endorphin levels are high, people feel euphoric. The same euphoria occurs when opioids or

Opium is extracted from opium poppy seedpods like this one.

related chemicals are active at the endorphin receptor sites. Of all the opioids, heroin has the greatest notoriety as an addictive drug. The following section discusses the progression of heroin addiction; addiction to any opioid follows a similar path.

Heroin Use *Heroin* is a white powder derived from morphine. *Black tar heroin* is a sticky, dark brown, foul-smelling form of heroin that is relatively pure and inexpensive. Once considered a cure for morphine dependence, heroin was later discovered to be even more addictive and potent than morphine. Today, heroin has no medical use.

Heroin is a depressant that produces drowsiness and a dreamy, mentally slow feeling. It can cause drastic mood swings, with euphoric highs followed by depressive lows. Heroin slows respiration and urinary output and constricts the pupils of the eyes. Symptoms of tolerance and withdrawal can appear within 3 weeks of first use.

In 2009, 180,000 Americans reported using heroin for the first time, a considerably higher number than in previous years. The average age of first use was 26 years.[55] The most common route of administration for heroin addicts is "mainlining"—intravenous injection of powdered heroin mixed in a solution. Many users describe the "rush" they feel when injecting themselves as intensely pleasurable, whereas others report unpredictable and unpleasant side effects. The temporary nature of the rush contributes to the drug's high potential for addiction—many addicts shoot up four or five times a day. Mainlining can cause veins to scar and eventually collapse. Once a vein has collapsed, it can no longer be used to introduce heroin into the bloodstream. Addicts become expert at locating new veins to use: in the feet, the legs, the temples, under the tongue, or in the groin. Although heroin is usually injected, the contemporary version of heroin is so potent that users can get high by snorting or smoking the drug. This has attracted a more affluent group of users who may not want to inject, for reasons such as the increased risk of contracting diseases such as HIV.

Treatment for Heroin Addiction Heroin addicts experience a distinct pattern of withdrawal. Symptoms of withdrawal include intense desire for the drug, sleep disturbance, dilated pupils, loss of appetite, irritability, goose bumps, and muscle tremors. The most difficult time in the withdrawal process occurs 24 to 72 hours following last use. All of the preceding symptoms continue, along with nausea, abdominal cramps, restlessness, insomnia, vomiting, diarrhea, extreme anxiety, hot and cold flashes, elevated blood pressure, and rapid heartbeat and respiration. Once the peak of withdrawal has passed, all these symptoms begin to subside. Still, the recovering addict has many hurdles to jump.

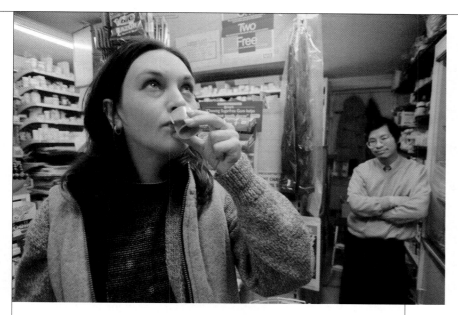

Why is it so hard to **quit** using heroin?

Heroin's effect on the body is similar to the painless well-being created by endorphins. Stopping heroin use causes withdrawal symptoms that are very difficult to withstand or tolerate, which keeps many addicts from attempting to quit. Methadone is a synthetic narcotic that blocks the effects of withdrawal. Although it is still a narcotic and must be administered under the supervision of clinic or pharmacy staff, methadone allows many heroin addicts to lead somewhat normal lives.

Methadone maintenance is one treatment available for people addicted to heroin or other opioids. Methadone is chemically similar enough to opioids to control the tremors, chills, vomiting, diarrhea, and severe abdominal pains of withdrawal. However, methadone maintenance is controversial because of the drug's own potential for addiction. Critics contend that the program merely substitutes one addiction for another. Proponents argue that people on methadone maintenance are less likely to engage in criminal activities to support their habits than heroin addicts are. For this reason, many methadone maintenance programs are financed by state or federal government and available free of charge or at reduced cost.

A number of new drug therapies for opioid dependence are emerging. Naltrexone (Trexan), an opioid antagonist, has been approved as a treatment. While on naltrexone, recovering addicts do not have the compulsion to use heroin, and if they do use it, they don't get high—so there is no point in using the drug. More recently, researchers have reported promising results with buprenorphine (Temgesic), a mild, nonaddicting synthetic opioid that, like heroin and methadone, bonds to certain receptors in the brain, blocks pain messages, and persuades the brain that its cravings for heroin have been satisfied.

Benzodiazepines and Barbiturates

A *sedative* drug promotes mental calmness and reduces anxiety, whereas a *hypnotic* drug promotes sleep or drowsiness. The most common sedative-hypnotic drugs are **benzodiazepines**, more commonly known as *tranquilizers*. These include prescription drugs such as Valium, Ativan, and Xanax. Benzodiazepines are most commonly prescribed for tension, muscular strain, sleep problems, anxiety, panic attacks, and alcohol withdrawal. **Barbiturates** are sedative-hypnotic drugs that include Amytal and Seconal. Today, benzodiazepines have largely replaced barbiturates, which were used medically in the past for relieving tension and inducing relaxation and sleep.

Sedative-hypnotics have a synergistic effect when combined with alcohol, another central nervous system depressant. Taken together, these drugs can lead to respiratory failure and death. All sedative or hypnotic drugs can produce physical and psychological dependence in several weeks. A complication specific to sedatives is cross-tolerance, which occurs when users develop tolerance for one sedative or become dependent on it, and develop tolerance for others as well. Withdrawal from sedative or hypnotic drugs may range from mild discomfort to severe symptoms, depending on the degree of dependence.

Rohypnol One benzodiazepine of concern is Rohypnol, a potent tranquilizer similar in nature to Valium but many times stronger. The drug produces a sedative effect, amnesia, muscle relaxation, and slowed psychomotor responses. The most publicized "date rape" drug, Rohypnol has gained notoriety as a growing problem on college campuses. The drug has been added to punch and other drinks at parties, where it is reportedly given to women in hopes of lowering their inhibitions and facilitating potential sexual conquests.

GHB

Gamma-hydroxybutyrate (GHB) is a central nervous system depressant known to have euphoric, sedative, and anabolic (bodybuilding) effects. It was originally sold over the counter to bodybuilders to help reduce body fat and build muscle. Concerns about GHB led the FDA to ban OTC sales in 1992, and GHB is now a Schedule I controlled substance.[56] GHB is an odorless, tasteless fluid that can be made easily at home or in a chemistry lab. Like Rohypnol, GHB has been slipped into drinks without being detected, resulting in loss of memory, unconsciousness, amnesia, and even death. Other dangerous side effects include nausea, vomiting, seizures, hallucinations, coma, and respiratory distress.

check yourself

- **What is a depressant?**
- **What are the effects and health risks of commonly abused depressants?**

Common Drugs of Abuse: Hallucinogens

- **Identify hallucinogens that are commonly misused or abused.**
- **Discuss the effects and health risks of hallucinogens.**

Hallucinogens, or *psychedelics*, are substances capable of creating auditory or visual hallucinations and unusual changes in mood, thoughts, and feelings.

Major receptor sites for hallucinogens are in the reticular formation (located in the brainstem at the upper end of the spinal cord), which is responsible for interpreting outside stimuli before allowing these signals to travel to other parts of the brain. When a hallucinogen is present at a reticular formation site, messages become scrambled; the user may see wavy walls instead of straight ones or, in a mixing of sensory messages known as *synesthesia*, "smell" colors and "hear" tastes. Users may also become less inhibited or recall events long buried in the subconscious mind.

LSD

First synthesized in the late 1930s, *lysergic acid diethylamide (LSD)* received media attention in the 1960s when young people used it to "turn on and tune out." In 1970, federal authorities placed LSD on the list of controlled substances (Schedule I). Popularity peaked in 1972 then tapered off, primarily because of inability to control dosages accurately.

Today LSD, or "acid," is making a comeback, especially among younger users. Over 9 percent of Americans have tried LSD at least once.[57] A national survey of college students showed that 2.0 percent had used the drug in the past year.[58]

The most popular form is blotter acid—small squares of paper impregnated with LSD and swallowed or chewed. LSD also comes in gelatin squares called *windowpane* and tiny tablets called *microdots*.

One of the most powerful drugs known to science, LSD can produce strong effects in doses as low as 20 micrograms (µg). (A postage stamp weighs 60,000 µg.) The potency of a typical dose currently ranges from 20 to 80 µg, compared to 150 to 300 µg commonly used in the 1960s.

Psychological effects of LSD vary. Euphoria is common, but dysphoria (a sense of evil and foreboding) may also be experienced. LSD also causes distortions of perception and auditory or visual hallucinations. Thoughts may be interposed so the user experiences several thoughts simultaneously. Users become introspective, and suppressed memories may surface. Other possible effects include decreased aggressiveness and enhanced sensory experiences.

Physical effects include increased heart rate, elevated blood pressure, muscle twitches, perspiration, chills, headaches, and mild nausea. Because the drug also stimulates uterine muscle contractions, it can lead to premature labor and miscarriage in pregnant women. Research into long-term effects has been inconclusive.

Although there is no evidence that LSD creates physical dependency, it may well create psychological dependence. Many users become depressed for 1 or 2 days following a trip and turn to the drug to relieve this depression. The result is a cycle of LSD use to relieve post–LSD depression, which can lead to psychological addiction.

Ecstasy

Ecstasy is the most common name for the drug *methylenedioxymethamphetamine (MDMA)*, a synthetic compound with stimulant and mildly hallucinogenic effects. It is one of the most well-known **club drugs** or "designer drugs," synthetic analogs of illicit drugs popular at nightclubs and raves. Ecstasy creates feelings of extreme euphoria, increased willingness to communicate, feelings of warmth and empathy, and heightened appreciation for music. Like other hallucinogenics, Ecstasy can enhance sensory experience and distort perceptions, though it seldom creates visual hallucinations. Effects begin within 20 to 90 minutes and can last for 3 to 5 hours.

Some of the risks associated with Ecstasy use are similar to those of other stimulants. Because of the nature of the drug, Ecstasy users are at greater risk of inappropriate and/or unintended emotional bonding. Physical consequences may include jaw clenching, short-term memory loss or confusion, increased body temperature as a result of dehydration and heat stroke, and increased heart rate and blood pressure. Individuals with high blood pressure, heart disease, or liver trouble are at greatest danger when using this drug. Combined with alcohol, Ecstasy can be extremely dangerous and sometimes fatal. As the effects begin to wear off, the user can experience mild depression, fatigue, and a hangover that can last from days to weeks. Chronic use appears to damage the brain's ability to think and to regulate emotion, memory, sleep, and pain. Some studies indicate that the drug may cause long-lasting neurotoxic effects by damaging brain cells that produce serotonin.[59]

Psilocybe mushrooms produce hallucinogenic effects when ingested.

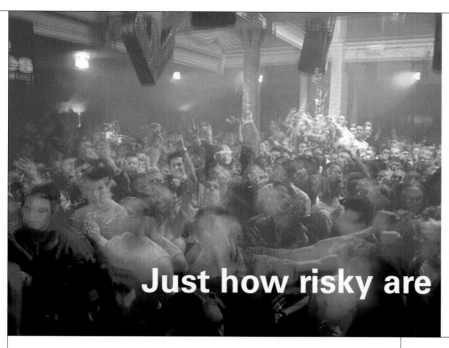

Just how risky are *"club drugs"?*

So-called "club drugs" are a varied group of synthetic drugs, including Ecstasy, GHB, ketamine, Rohypnol, and methamphetamine, that are often abused by teens and young adults at nightclubs, bars, or all-night dances. The sources and chemicals used to make these drugs vary, so dosages are unpredictable and the drugs may not be "pure." Although users may think them relatively harmless, research has shown that club drugs can produce hallucinations, paranoia, amnesia, dangerous increases in heart rate and blood pressure, coma, and, in some cases, death. Some club drugs work on the same brain mechanisms as alcohol and can be particularly dangerous when used in combination with alcohol. In addition, some club drugs can be easily slipped into unsuspecting partygoers' drinks, facilitating sexual assault and other crimes.

Mescaline

Mescaline is both a powerful hallucinogen and a central nervous system stimulant. Products sold on the street as mescaline are likely to be synthetic relatives of the true drug.

Users typically swallow 10 to 12 buttons. They taste bitter and generally induce immediate nausea or vomiting. Those able to keep the drug down feel its effects within 30 to 90 minutes. Effects may persist for up to 9 or 10 hours.

Psilocybin

Psilocybin and *psilocin* are the active chemicals in a group of mushrooms sometimes called "magic mushrooms." Psilocybe mushrooms, which grow throughout the world, can be cultivated from spores or harvested wild. When consumed, they can cause hallucinations. Because many mushrooms resemble the psilocybe variety, people who harvest wild mushrooms for any purpose should be certain of what they are doing. Mushroom varieties can be easily misidentified, and mistakes can be fatal. Psilocybin is similar to LSD in its physical effects, which generally wear off in 4 to 6 hours.

Mescaline comes from the "buttons" of the peyote cactus, like this one.

PCP

Phencyclidine (PCP) was originally developed as a dissociative anesthetic—patients administered it could keep their eyes open, apparently remain conscious, and feel no pain during a medical procedure. Afterward, they would experience amnesia for the time that the drug was in their system. The unpredictability and drastic effects (postoperative delirium, confusion, and agitation) made doctors abandon it, and it was withdrawn from the legal market.

On the illegal market, PCP is a white, crystalline powder that users often sprinkle onto marijuana cigarettes. It is dangerous and unpredictable regardless of method of administration. Effects depend on dosage. A dose as small as 5 mg will produce effects similar to those of strong central nervous system depressants—slurred speech, impaired coordination, reduced sensitivity to pain, and reduced heart and respiratory rate. Doses between 5 and 10 mg cause fever, salivation, nausea, vomiting, and total loss of sensitivity to pain. Doses greater than 10 mg result in a drastic drop in blood pressure, coma, muscular rigidity, violent outbursts, and possible convulsions and death.

Psychologically, PCP may produce either euphoria or dysphoria. It is also known to produce hallucinations, delusions, and overall delirium. Long-term effects of PCP use are unknown.

Ketamine

The liquid form of *ketamine,* or Special K, is used as an anesthetic in hospital and veterinary clinics. After stealing it from hospitals or medical suppliers, dealers typically dry the liquid (usually by cooking it) and grind the residue into powder. Special K inhibits the relay of sensory input, triggering hallucinations as the brain fills the resulting void with visions, memories, and sensory distortions. Effects are similar to those of PCP—confusion, agitation, aggression, and lack of coordination—and less predictable. The aftereffects are less severe than those of Ecstasy, so it has grown in popularity as a club drug among people who must go to work or school the next day.

check yourself

- **What is a hallucinogen?**
- **What are the effects and health risks of commonly abused hallucinogens?**
- **Why do you think some users mistakenly consider hallucinogens to be less harmful than other types of drugs?**

Common Drugs of Abuse: Inhalants

- **Identify products that are commonly misused or abused as inhalants.**
- **Discuss the effects and health risks of inhalants.**

Inhalants are chemicals whose vapors, when inhaled, can cause hallucinations and create intoxicating and euphoric effects. Not commonly recognized as drugs, inhalants are legal to purchase and universally available but dangerous. They generally appeal to young people who can't afford or obtain illicit substances. Some misused products include rubber cement, model glue, paint thinner, aerosol sprays, lighter fluid, varnish, wax, spot removers, and gasoline. Most of these substances are sniffed or "huffed" by users in search of a quick, cheap high.

Because they are inhaled, the volatile chemicals in these products reach the bloodstream and then the brain within seconds. This characteristic, along with the fact that dosages are extremely difficult to control because everyone has unique lung and breathing capacities, makes inhalants particularly dangerous. The effects of inhalants usually last for fewer than 15 minutes and resemble those of central nervous system depressants. Users may experience dizziness, disorientation, impaired coordination, reduced judgment, and slowed reaction times. Combining inhalants with alcohol produces a synergistic effect and can cause severe and sometimes fatal liver damage. An overdose of fumes from inhalants can cause unconsciousness. If the user's oxygen intake is reduced during the inhaling process, death can result within 5 minutes. Sudden sniffing death (SSD) syndrome can be a fatal consequence, whether it's the user's first time or not. This syndrome can occur if a user inhales deeply and then participates in physical activity or is startled.

70%

of first-time users of inhalants in 2008 were under age 18.

Amyl Nitrite

Sometimes called "poppers" or "rush," *amyl nitrite* is packaged in small, cloth-covered glass capsules that can be crushed to release the active chemical for the user to inhale. The drug is often prescribed to alleviate chest pain in heart patients, because it dilates small blood vessels and reduces blood pressure. Dilation of blood vessels in the genital area is thought to enhance sensations or perceptions of orgasm. It also produces fainting, dizziness, warmth, and skin flushing.

Nitrous Oxide

Nitrous oxide is sometimes used as an adjunct to dental anesthesia or minor surgical anesthesia. It is also a propellant chemical in aerosol products such as whipped toppings. Users who inhale nitrous oxide experience a state of euphoria, floating sensations, and illusions. Effects also include pain relief and a silly feeling, demonstrated by laughing and giggling (hence its nickname "laughing gas"). Regulating dosages of this drug can be difficult. Sustained inhalation can lead to unconsciousness, coma, and death.

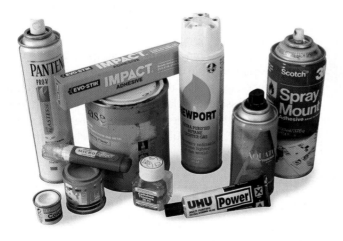

Common household products, such as aerosol sprays, solvents, or glues, can be inhaled for a quick high.

- **What is an inhalant?**
- **What are the effects and health risks of inhalants?**

Common Drugs of Abuse: Anabolic Steroids

learning outcomes

■ **Discuss the effects and health risks of anabolic steroids.**

Anabolic steroids are artificial forms of the male hormone testosterone that promote muscle growth and strength. Steroids are available in two forms: injectable solutions and pills. These **ergogenic drugs** are used primarily by people who believe the drugs will increase their strength, power, bulk (weight), speed, and athletic performance.

It was once estimated that approximately 17 to 20 percent of college athletes used steroids. Now that stricter drug-testing policies have been instituted by the National Collegiate Athletic Association (NCAA), reported use of anabolic steroids among intercollegiate athletes has decreased.[60] Few data exist on the extent of steroid abuse by adults; it has been estimated that approximately 1 million adults have used anabolic steroids.[61] Among both adolescents and adults, steroid abuse is higher among men than it is among women. However, steroid abuse is growing most rapidly among young women.[62]

Physical Effects of Steroids

In both sexes, anabolic steroids produce a state of euphoria, diminished fatigue, and increased bulk and power. These characteristics give steroids an addictive quality. When users stop, they can experience psychological withdrawal and sometimes severe depression, in some cases leading to suicide attempts. If untreated, depression associated with steroid withdrawal has been known to last for a year or more after steroid use stops.

Men and women who use steroids experience a variety of adverse effects, including mood swings (aggression and violence, sometimes known as "'roid rage"); acne; liver tumors; elevated cholesterol levels; hypertension; kidney disease; and immune system disturbances. There is also a danger of transmitting HIV and hepatitis through shared needles. In women, large doses of anabolic steroids may trigger the development of masculine attributes such as lowered voice, increased facial and body hair, and male pattern baldness; they may also result in an enlarged clitoris, smaller breasts, and changes in or absence of menstruation. When taken by healthy males, anabolic steroids shut down the body's production of testosterone, causing men's breasts to grow and testicles to atrophy.

Steroid Use and Society

To combat the growing problem of steroid use, Congress passed the Anabolic Steroids Control Act (ASCA) of 1990. This law makes it a crime to possess, prescribe, or distribute anabolic steroids for any use other than the treatment of specific diseases. Penalties for illegal use include up to 5 years' imprisonment and a $250,000 fine for the first offense and up to 10 years' imprisonment and a $500,000 fine for subsequent offenses.

The use of steroids and related substances among professional athletes periodically makes the news. In recent years, high-profile athletes in sports such as cycling, track and field, swimming, and baseball have all garnered media attention for suspected use of steroids or other banned performance-enhancing drugs. The Mitchell Report released in December 2007 was an investigation into the history of steroid and human growth hormone use by Major League Baseball players, 89 of whom are alleged by the report to have used steroids or other ergogenic drugs.

Olympic sprinter Marion Jones won five medals in the 2000 Summer Olympics in Sydney, Australia, but has since been stripped of them all following her admission of steroid use at the time.

139

check yourself

■ **What are anabolic steroids?**

■ **What are the effects and health risks of anabolic steroids?**

Treatment and Recovery

- **Discuss treatment and recovery options for people with an addiction.**

Recovery from addiction is a lifelong process, starting with treatment—and before that, recognition—of the addiction. This can be difficult because of the power of denial—the inability to see the truth. Denial can be so powerful that intervention is sometimes necessary to break down the addict's defenses against recognizing the problem.

Intervention

Intervention is a planned process of confrontation by people who are important to the addict, including spouses, parents, children, bosses, and friends. Its purpose is to break down denial compassionately so that the person can see the addiction's destructive nature. Getting addicts to admit that they have a problem is not enough; they must come to perceive that the behavior is destructive and requires treatment.

The most difficult step in the recovery process is for the substance abuser to admit that he or she is an addict. An addict's defenses generally crumble when significant others collectively share their observations and concerns about the addict's behavior. Effective interventions include (1) emphasizing care and concern for the addicted person; (2) describing the behavior that is the cause for concern; (3) expressing how the behavior affects the addict, each person taking part in the intervention, and others; and (4) outlining specifically what you would like to see happen.

Participants in the intervention must clarify how they plan to end their enabling. Persons contemplating interventions must also choose consequences they are ready to stick to if the addict refuses treatment—and be ready to give support if the addict is willing to begin a recovery program.

Treatment for Addiction

Treatment and recovery for any addiction generally begin with **abstinence**—refraining from the addictive behavior. Whereas complete abstinence is possible for people addicted to chemicals, it obviously is not feasible for people addicted to behaviors such as work and sex. For these addicts, abstinence means restoring balance to their lives through noncompulsive engagement in the behaviors. An estimated 23.5 million Americans aged 12 or older needed treatment for an illicit drug or alcohol use problem in 2009. Of these, only 2.6 million—approximately 11 percent—received treatment.[63]

Detoxification refers to the early period during which an addict adjusts physically and cognitively to being free from the addiction's influence. It occurs in virtually every recovering addict; while uncomfortable for all addicts, it can be dangerous for some—especially those addicted to alcohol, heroin, and painkillers—who may have withdrawal symptoms requiring medical supervision. Most inpatient programs provide supervised detoxification before further treatment begins.

Abstinence alone does little to change the psychological, biological, and environmental dynamics underlying addictive behavior. Without treatment, an addict is apt to relapse or to change addictions. Treatment involves learning new ways of looking at oneself, others, and the world. It may require exploring a traumatic past so psychological wounds can heal. It also involves learning interdepen-

How can I approach someone who needs help and treatment?

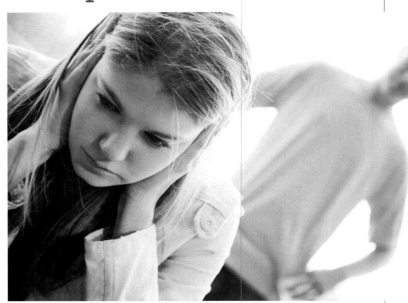

Confronting a person about addiction is a difficult task, and one that usually requires intervention by a group of family members and friends. It is more effective for an addict to be faced with the facts from a group of the people most important to him or her than by one person. In a planned intervention, the goal is to break down the addict's denial compassionately and to get him or her to recognize the addiction's destructive nature. Most addiction treatment centers have specialists who can help plan an intervention.

How do people recover from drug addiction?

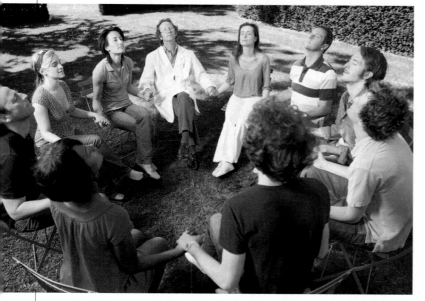

For most addicts, recovery is a long, difficult process—for some people it can be a lifelong journey. Treatment and recovery usually begin with a period of detoxification. Once the person's body has adjusted, the addict usually enters therapy to learn how to cope without the drug and avoid relapse. Therapy often takes the form of group meetings, such as those held by 12-step programs.

dence with significant others and new ways of caring for oneself physically and emotionally.

Finding a Treatment Program

For many addicts, recovery begins with a period of formal treatment. A good treatment program includes the following:

- Staff familiar with the specific addictive disorder for which help is being sought
- Availability of both inpatient and outpatient services
- Medical personnel who can assess the addict's health and treat medical concerns, as needed
- Medical supervision of addicts at risk for complicated detoxification
- Involvement of family members in the treatment process
- A coordinated team approach to treating addictive disorders (e.g., medical personnel, counselors, psychotherapists, clergy, and dietitians)
- Group and individual therapy options
- Peer-led support groups that encourage involvement after treatment ends
- Structured aftercare and relapse-prevention programs
- Accreditation by the Joint Commission (a national organization that accredits and certifies health care organizations and programs) and a license from the state in which it operates

Relapse

Relapse, an isolated occurrence of or full return to addictive behavior, is a defining characteristic of addiction. Addicts are set up to relapse because of their tendency to meet change and other forms of stress with the same kind of denial once used to justify addictive behavior (e.g., "I don't have a problem; I can handle this").

Treatment programs recognize this tendency and teach clients and significant others how to recognize and respond to signs of imminent relapse. Without such a plan, recovering addicts are likely to relapse more frequently, and perhaps permanently.

Relapse should not be interpreted as failure to change or lack of desire to stay well. The appropriate response is to remind addicts that they are addicted and redirect them to strategies that have worked for them. Relapse prevention may involve connecting the recovering person with support groups or counselors.

Treatment Approaches

Outpatient behavioral treatment encompasses a variety of programs for addicts who visit a clinic at regular intervals. Most involve individual or group counseling. *Residential treatment programs* can be effective for those with more severe problems. For example, therapeutic communities (TCs) are highly structured programs in which addicts remain at a residence, typically for 6 to 12 months. The focus is on resocialization to a drug-free lifestyle.

The first *12-step program*, Alcoholics Anonymous (AA), began in 1935. The 12-step program has since become the most widely used approach to dealing with addictive or dysfunctional behaviors. More than 200 recovery programs are based on the program, including Narcotics Anonymous and Crystal Meth Anonymous.

The 12-step program is nonjudgmental and based on the idea that its purpose is to work on personal recovery. Working the 12 steps involves admitting to having a problem, recognizing there is an outside power that could help, consciously relying on that power, admitting and listing character defects, seeking deliverance from defects, apologizing to those one has harmed, and helping others with the same problem. Free meetings, held at a variety of times and locations in almost every city, are open to anyone who wishes to attend. Alternatives such as Rational Recovery and the Secular Organization for Sobriety provide support without the spiritual emphasis of 12-step groups.

For students with substance or behavioral addictions, early intervention increases the likelihood of successful treatment, successful sobriety, and completion of a college education. Depending on the severity of abuse or dependence, students may be required to spend time in a residential drug rehabilitation (rehab) inpatient facility.

check yourself

- **What are the steps in treatment and recovery from addiction?**

Addressing Drug Misuse and Abuse in the U.S.

learning **outcomes**

- **Discuss the financial impact of drug misuse and abuse in the United States.**
- **Identify strategies to address drug misuse and abuse on campus.**

Illegal drug use in the United States costs about $215 billion per year.[64] This includes costs associated with substance abuse treatment and prevention, health care, and consequences such as crime and social welfare.

Also included in this is the annual economic impact of lost productivity due to illicit drug use among workers, which is estimated at $128.6 billion.[65] In addition, roughly half of all expenditures to combat crime are related to illegal drugs. The burden of these costs is absorbed primarily by the government (46%), followed by people who abuse drugs and members of their households (44%).[66]

Preventing Drug Use and Abuse on Campus

College and university campuses should consider multiple strategies to reduce substance use among students:

- Changing student expectations that college is a time to experiment with drugs
- Engaging parents and encouraging them to continue open communication with their children
- Identifying high-risk students through early detection programs
- Providing programs specifically tailored for students needing treatment and recovery support

Most antidrug programs have not been effective, because they have focused on only one aspect of drug abuse rather than examining all factors contributing to the problem. The pressure to take drugs is often tremendous, and reasons for use complex. People who develop drug problems generally believe they can control their use when they start out. Peer influence is also a strong motivator, especially among adolescents.

Drug abuse has been a part of human behavior for thousands of years, and is unlikely to disappear. We must educate ourselves and develop the self-discipline necessary to avoid dangerous drug dependence.

For many years, the most popular antidrug strategy has been total prohibition—an approach that has proved ineffective. Prohibition of alcohol during the 1920s created more problems than it solved, as did prohibition of opioids in 1914. A recent U.S. government campaign, commonly referred to as the "War on Drugs," includes laws and policies intended to reduce illegal drug trade and to diminish and discourage production, distribution, and consumption of illicit substances.

In general, drug education researchers agree that students should be taught the difference between drug use, misuse, and abuse. Factual information that is free of scare tactics must be presented; lecturing and moralizing have proved not to work.

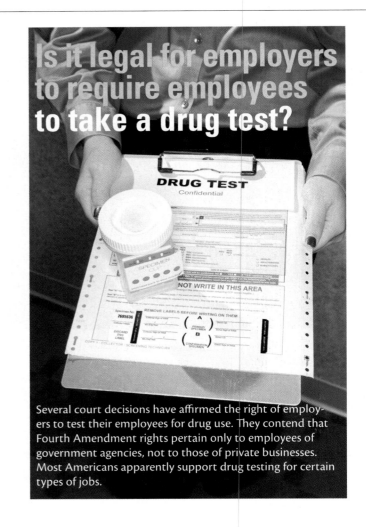

Is it legal for employers to require employees to take a drug test?

Several court decisions have affirmed the right of employers to test their employees for drug use. They contend that Fourth Amendment rights pertain only to employees of government agencies, not to those of private businesses. Most Americans apparently support drug testing for certain types of jobs.

check **yourself**

- **What is the financial impact of drug misuse and abuse? Is this figure higher or lower than you expected?**
- **What are some strategies to address substance abuse on campus? Which, if any, of these are present on your campus?**

Assessyourself

Do You Have a Problem with Drugs?

An interactive version of this assessment is available online. Download it from the Live It! section of www.pearsonhighered.com/donatelle.

1 Are You Controlled by Drugs?

A dependent person can't stop using drugs. This abuse hurts the user and everyone around him or her. The more "yes" checks you make below, the more likely it is that you have a problem.

	Yes	No
1. Do you use drugs to handle stress or escape from life's problems?	◯	◯
2. Have you unsuccessfully tried to cut down on or quit using your drug?	◯	◯
3. Have you ever been in trouble with the law or been arrested because of your drug use?	◯	◯
4. Do you think a party or social gathering isn't fun unless drugs are available?	◯	◯
5. Do you avoid people or places that do not support your usage?	◯	◯
6. Do you neglect your responsibilities because you'd rather use your drug?	◯	◯
7. Have your friends, family, or employer expressed concern about your drug use?	◯	◯
8. Do you do things under the influence of drugs that you would not normally do?	◯	◯
9. Have you seriously thought that you might have a chemical dependency problem?	◯	◯

2 Are You Controlled by a Drug User?

Your love and care may actually be enabling another person to continue chemical abuse, hurting you and others. The more "yes" checks you make below, the more likely there's a problem.

	Yes	No
1. Do you often have to lie or cover up for the chemical abuser?	◯	◯
2. Do you spend time counseling the person about the problem?	◯	◯
3. Have you taken on additional financial or family responsibilities?	◯	◯
4. Do you feel that you have to control the chemical abuser's behavior?	◯	◯
5. At the office, have you done work or attended meetings for the abuser?	◯	◯
6. Do you often put your own needs and desires after the user's?	◯	◯
7. Do you spend time each day worrying about your situation?	◯	◯
8. Do you analyze your behavior to find clues to how it might affect the chemical abuser?	◯	◯
9. Do you feel powerless and at your wit's end about the abuser's problem?	◯	◯

Source: Reprinted by permission of Krames StayWell, LLC.

Your Plan for Change

The Assess Yourself activity describes signs of being controlled by drugs or by a drug user. Depending on your results, you may need to change certain behaviors that may be detrimental to your health.

Today, You Can:

◯ Imagine a situation in which someone offers you a drug and think of several different ways

of refusing. Rehearse these scenarios in your head.

◯ Stop by your campus health center to find out about any drug treatment programs or support groups they may have.

Within the Next 2 Weeks, You Can:

◯ Think about the drug use patterns among your social group. Are you ever

uncomfortable with these people because of their drug use? Is it difficult to avoid using drugs when you are with them? If the answers are yes, begin exploring ways to expand your social circle.

◯ If you are concerned about your own drug use or the drug use of a close friend, make an appointment with a counselor to talk about the issue.

By the End of the Semester, You Can:

◯ Participate in clubs, activities, and social groups that do not rely on substance abuse for their amusement.

◯ If you have a drug problem, make a commitment to enter a treatment program. Acknowledge that you have a problem and that you need the assistance of others to help you overcome it.

Summary

- Addiction is continued use of a substance or activity despite ongoing negative consequences. All addictions share four common symptoms: compulsion, loss of control, negative consequences, and denial.
- Codependents are typically friends or family members who are "addicted to the addict." Enablers are people who protect addicts from consequences of their behavior.
- The biopsychosocial model of addiction takes into account biological (genetic) factors as well as psychological and environmental influences in understanding the addiction process.
- Addictive behaviors include disordered gambling, compulsive buying, compulsive Internet or technology use, work addiction, compulsive exercise, and sexual addiction.
- The six categories of drugs are prescription drugs, over-the-counter (OTC) drugs, recreational drugs, herbal preparations, illicit drugs, and commercial preparations.
- Over-the-counter medications are drugs that do not require a prescription. Some OTC medications can be addictive.
- Prescription drug abuse is at an all-time high, particularly among college students. The most commonly abused prescription drugs are opioids/narcotics, depressants, and stimulants.
- People from all walks of life use illicit drugs. Drug use declined from the mid-1980s to the early 1990s but has remained steady since then. However, among young people, use of drugs has been rising in recent years.
- Controlled substances include cocaine and its derivatives, amphetamines, methamphetamine, marijuana, opioids, depressants, hallucinogens/psychedelics, inhalants, and steroids.
- Treatment begins with abstinence from the drug or addictive behavior, usually instituted through intervention by close family, friends, or other loved ones. Treatment programs may include individual, group, or family therapy, as well as 12-step programs.

Pop Quiz

1. Which of the following is *not* a characteristic of addiction?
   a. Denial
   b. Acknowledgment of self-destructive behavior
   c. Loss of control
   d. Obsession with a substance or behavior

2. Gina is addicted to the Internet. She is so preoccupied with it that she is failing her classes. What symptom of addiction does her preoccupation characterize?
   a. Denial
   b. Compulsion
   c. Loss of control
   d. Negative consequences

3. Chemical dependency *relapse* refers to
   a. a person experiencing a blackout.
   b. a gap in one's drinking or drug-taking patterns.
   c. a full return to addictive behavior.
   d. failure to change one's behavior.

4. An individual who knowingly tries to protect an addict from natural consequences of his or her destructive behaviors is
   a. enabling.
   b. helping the addict to recover.
   c. practicing intervention.
   d. controlling.

5. Cross-tolerance occurs when
   a. drugs work at the same receptor site so that one blocks the action of the other.
   b. the effects of one drug are eliminated or reduced by the presence of another drug at the receptor site.
   c. a person develops a physiological tolerance to one drug and shows a similar tolerance to selected other drugs as a result.
   d. two or more drugs interact so their effects are multiplied.

6. Rebecca takes Prinivil (an antihypertensive drug), insulin (a diabetic medication), and Claritin (an antihistamine). This is an example of
   a. synergism.
   b. illegal drug use.
   c. polydrug use.
   d. antagonism.

7. The most widely used illicit drug in the United States is
   a. alcohol.
   b. heroin.
   c. marijuana.
   d. methamphetamine.

8. Which of the following is classified as a stimulant drug?
   a. Amphetamines
   b. Alcohol
   c. Marijuana
   d. LSD

9. Drugs that depress the central nervous system are called
   a. amphetamines
   b. hallucinogens.
   c. depressants.
   d. psychedelics.

10. The psychoactive drug mescaline is found in what plant?
    a. Mushrooms
    b. Peyote cactus
    c. Marijuana
    d. Belladonna

Answers to these questions can be found on page A-1.

Web Links

1. **Center for Online and Internet Addiction.** Information and assistance for those dealing with Internet addiction. www.netaddiction.com
2. **National Council on Problem Gambling.** Information and help for people with gambling problems and their families. www.ncpgambling.org
3. **Club Drugs.** Science-based information about club drugs. www.clubdrugs.org
4. **Substance Abuse and Mental Health Services Administration (SAMHSA).** An outstanding resource for information about national surveys, ongoing research, and national drug interventions. www.samhsa.gov

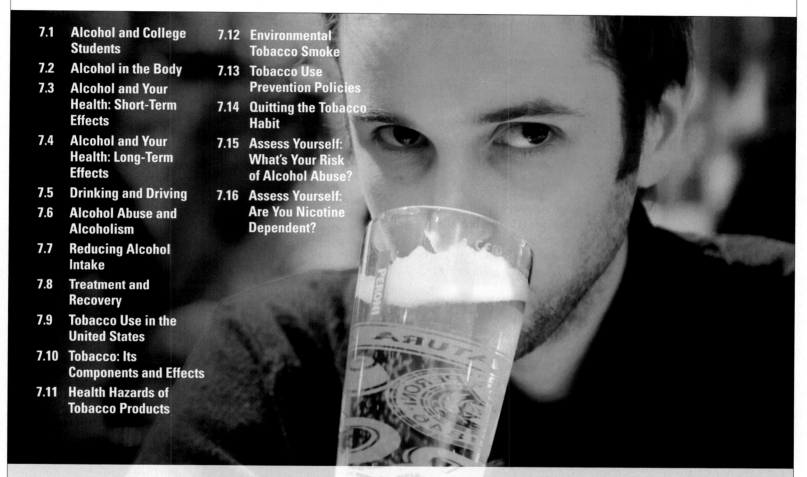

Alcohol and Tobacco

People throughout history have used alcohol. Alcohol consumption is part of many traditions, and moderate use can enhance special times. Although alcohol can play a positive role in some people's lives, it is a drug and, if used irresponsibly, can become dangerous.

Approximately half of all Americans consume alcohol regularly, while 21 percent abstain altogether.[1] Alcohol consumption levels among Americans have declined from 2.64 gallons of pure alcohol per person in 1977 to 2.32 gallons in 2008,[2] a trend tied to growing attention to personal health.

Meanwhile, though the health hazards of tobacco use are well documented, 20 percent of Americans smoke. A 58.2 percent decline in smoking among adults since 1964 has been characterized as one of history's greatest public health achievements.[3] However, tobacco use is still the single most preventable cause of death in the United States;[4] smoking cigarettes kills more Americans than alcohol, car accidents, suicide, AIDS, homicide, and illegal drugs combined.[5] Any contention by the tobacco industry that tobacco use is not dangerous is irresponsible and ignores scientific evidence.

Alcohol and College Students

- **Discuss the alcohol use patterns of college students.**
- **Define heavy episodic (binge) drinking among men and women.**
- **List factors that make college students vulnerable to alcohol-related problems.**

Alcohol is the most popular drug on college campuses, where almost 60 percent of students report having consumed alcoholic beverages in the past 30 days (Figure 7.1).[6]

Almost half of all college students engage in **heavy episodic (binge) drinking**, "a pattern of drinking alcohol that brings blood alcohol concentration (BAC) to 0.08 gram-percent or above . . . . correspond[ing] to consuming 5 or more drinks (male), or 4 or more drinks (female), in about 2 hours."[7] Binge drinking can quickly lead to extreme intoxication, unconsciousness, alcohol poisoning, and even death.

For some students, independence is symbolized by alcohol use. Others drink to "have fun"—which often means drinking simply to get drunk. This may be a way of coping with stress, boredom, anxiety, or academic and social pressures.

In the past 12 months, approximately 50 percent of college students who drank experienced at least one negative consequence of alcohol consumption (**Figure 7.2**).[8] Thirty-two percent reported doing something they regretted after drinking; 29.7 percent forgot where they were or what they did; 15.1 percent physically injured themselves; and 16.1 percent had unprotected sex. Two percent reported having had sex with someone without giving consent, and 0.6 percent reported having sex with someone without getting consent.

On a more positive note, many students reported always or usually practicing protective behaviors when consuming alcohol. Seventy-seven percent reported eating before or during drinking, 84 percent staying with the same friends the entire time they drank, 83 percent using a designated driver, 66 percent keeping track of how many drinks they consumed, and 42 percent determining in advance a set number of drinks they would not exceed.[9]

However, some students don't drink responsibly, and the stakes are high. According to one study, 1,825 college students die each year because of alcohol-related unintentional injuries, including car accidents.[10] Alcohol consumption is the top cause of preventable death among U.S. undergraduates.

Who Drinks?

It's likely that students who enter college will drink at some point, but some groups are more likely to drink more, and more often. For example, students who believe that their parents approve of their drinking are more likely to drink and to report a drinking-related problem.[11] Students who drank heavily in high school are also at risk for heavy drinking in college.[12]

Why Do College Students Drink So Much?

College students seem to be particularly vulnerable to alcohol-related problems. In addition to newfound freedom, several factors encourage drinking during college:

- Many student customs (Greek rush), norms (reputation as party schools), and traditional celebrations (St. Patrick's Day) encourage drinking.
- Alcohol advertising and promotions target students.
- College students are particularly vulnerable to peer influence.
- College women tend to care how much men want them to drink and to overestimate how much men prefer they consume.[13]
- Students believe that alcohol will make them feel better, less stressed, more sociable, and less self-conscious. The primary expectations of students going to bars and nightclubs are becoming intoxicated, socializing with friends, seeking romance or sex, and relieving stress.[14]
- More than 80 percent of college students drink alcohol to celebrate their twenty-first birthdays, and they consume an average of nearly 13 drinks, with estimated blood alcohol concentrations (BACs) of 19 percent and higher.

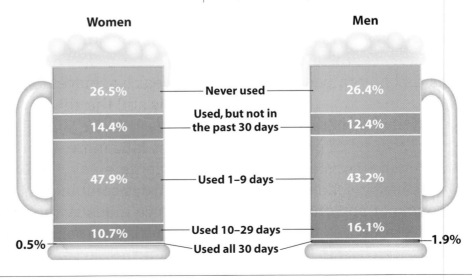

Women / **Men**

- Never used — 26.5% / 26.4%
- Used, but not in the past 30 days — 14.4% / 12.4%
- Used 1–9 days — 47.9% / 43.2%
- Used 10–29 days — 10.7% / 16.1%
- Used all 30 days — 0.5% / 1.9%

Figure 7.1 College Students' Patterns of Alcohol Use in the Past 30 Days

Source: Data are from American College Health Association, *American College Health Association—National College Health Assessment II (ACHA-NCHA II) Reference Group Data Report Fall 2010* (Baltimore: American College Health Association, 2011).

- Students drink as part of hazing rituals, with more than 50 percent of students in Greek and athletic organizations doing so.[15]
- The low price of alcohol is strongly related to higher rates of drinking and binging. In a recent study, students who paid the most money per gram of alcohol consumed the least alcohol.[16]
- Campus communities with more bars and alcohol outlets have a higher rate of binge drinking.[17]

Student Drinking Behavior

College students are more likely than their noncollegiate peers to drink recklessly and to engage in dangerous drinking practices. One such practice, **pre-gaming** (also pre-loading or front-loading), involves planned heavy drinking prior to going out to a bar, nightclub, or sporting event. In a recent study, 55 percent of college men and 60 percent of college women drank before going to a bar or nightclub.[18] Pre-gamers have more negative consequences, such as blackouts, hangovers, passing out, and alcohol poisoning.

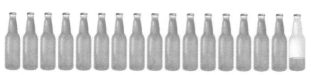
32.4%

Did something they later regretted

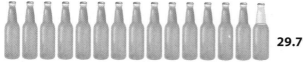
29.7%

Forgot where they were or what they did

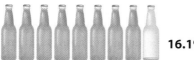
16.1%

Had unprotected sex

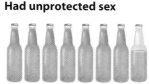
15.1%

Physically injured self

4.3%

Got in trouble with the police

2.7%

Physically injured another person

Figure 7.2 Prevalence of Negative Consequences of Drinking among College Students, Past Year

Source: Data are from American College Health Association, *American College Health Association—National College Health Assessment II (ACHA-NCHA II) Reference Group Executive Summary Fall 2010* (Baltimore: American College Health Association, 2011).

What Is the Impact of Student Drinking?

The more students drink, the more likely they are to miss class, have lower grade point averages (GPAs), and fall behind on schoolwork. Approximately 25 percent of college students report negative academic consequences because of drinking.[19]

One study indicated that over 696,000 students 18 to 24 were assaulted by another student who had been drinking.[20] And an estimated 97,000 students between the ages of 18 and 24 experience alcohol-related sexual assault or date rape each year in the United States.[21] The laws regarding sexual consent are clear: A person who is drunk or passed out cannot consent to sex. If you have sex with someone who is drunk or unconscious, you are committing rape. Claiming you were also drunk does not absolve you of legal and moral responsibility for this crime.

Colleges' Efforts to Reduce Student Drinking

Some colleges are instituting strong policies against drinking; at the same time, schools are making more help available to students with drinking problems. Programs that have proven effective include cognitive-behavioral skills training with *motivational interviewing*, a nonjudgmental approach to behavior change, and e-Interventions, alcohol education interventions via text message.[22] Schools are also trying a *social norms* approach to reducing alcohol consumption. Many students perceive that their peers drink more than they actually do, which may cause them to feel pressured to drink more themselves. In a national survey, for example, college students perceived that 42 percent of students used alcohol 10 to 29 days a month; the actual rate is 12.6 percent.[23] As a result of such campaigns, binge drinking has declined on campuses across the country.

Skills for Behavior Change

TIPS FOR DRINKING RESPONSIBLY

- **Eat before and while you drink.**
- **Don't drink before the party.**
- **Avoid drinking if you are angry, anxious, or depressed.**
- **Drink no more than one alcoholic drink an hour.**
- **Alternate alcoholic and nonalcoholic drinks.**
- **Determine ahead of time how many drinks you'll have.**
- **Avoid drinking games.**
- **Keep track of how much you drink.**
- **Don't drink and drive. Volunteer to be the sober driver.**
- **Avoid parties where you can expect heavy drinking.**

check yourself

- **How does this module's description of college student drinking compare to drinking on your campus?**
- **What is heavy episodic (binge) drinking?**
- **What factors make college students vulnerable to alcohol-related problems? Which of these factors exist on your campus?**

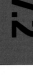
Alcohol in the Body

- **Define a standard drink of alcohol.**
- **Explain the processes by which alcohol is absorbed and metabolized in the human body.**
- **List factors that influence blood alcohol concentration.**

Learning about the metabolism and absorption of alcohol can help you understand how it is possible to drink safely—and how to avoid life-threatening circumstances such as alcohol poisoning. This information can be critical for your safety and that of your friends.

The Chemistry and Potency of Alcohol

The intoxicating substance found in beer, wine, liquor, and liqueurs is **ethyl alcohol**, or **ethanol**. It is produced during **fermentation**, in which yeast organisms break down plant sugars, yielding ethanol and carbon dioxide. Fermentation continues until the solution of plant sugars (*mash*) reaches a concentration of 14 percent alcohol. For beers, ales, and wines, manufacturers then add ingredients that dilute alcohol content. Hard liquor is produced through further processing called **distillation**, in which alcohol vapors are released from the mash at high temperatures, then condensed and mixed with water.

The **proof** of an alcoholic drink is a measure of its percentage of alcohol, and therefore its strength. Alcohol percentage by volume is half of the given proof: 80 proof whiskey is 40 percent alcohol by volume. Lower-proof drinks produce fewer alcohol effects than do the same amount of higher-proof drinks. Most wines are 12 to 15 percent alcohol, and most beers are 2 to 8 percent.

As defined by the National Institute on Alcohol Abuse and Alcoholism (NIAAA), a **standard drink** contains about 14 grams (0.6 fluid ounce or 1.2 tablespoons) of pure alcohol (**Figure 7.3**). A 12-ounce can of beer, a 5-ounce glass of wine, and a 1.5-ounce shot of vodka are each considered one standard drink—each contains the same amount of alcohol. If estimating BAC using standard drinks as a measure, keep in mind both proof and drink size. You may have bought one beer at the ballpark, but if it came in a 22-ounce glass, you actually consumed two standard drinks.

Absorption and Metabolism

Unlike the molecules in most foods and drugs, alcohol molecules are sufficiently small and fat soluble to be absorbed throughout the

entire gastrointestinal system. Approximately 20 percent of ingested alcohol diffuses through the stomach lining into the bloodstream and nearly 80 percent through the lining of the upper third of the small intestine.

Several factors influence how quickly your body will absorb alcohol: the alcohol concentration in your drink; the amount you consume; the amount of food in your stomach; and your metabolism, weight, body mass index, and mood. The higher the concentration of alcohol in your drink, the more rapidly it will be absorbed in your digestive tract. As a rule, wine and beer are absorbed more slowly than distilled beverages. "Fizzy" alcoholic beverages, carbonated beverages, and drinks served with mixers cause the pyloric valve to relax, emptying stomach contents more rapidly into the small intestine and increasing rate of absorption.

Over 28 percent of college students report mixing alcohol and energy drinks, often to mask alcohol's taste or effects.[24] Students who report consuming energy drinks tend to drink more than students who do not (8.3 versus 6.1 drinks).[25] Students who consume alcohol mixed energy drinks (AMEDs) often report not noticing signs of intoxication (e.g., dizziness, fatigue, headache, and trouble walking). Such students are also more likely to be taken advantage of sexually and twice as likely to take advantage of someone sexually, ride with a drunk driver, be hurt or injured, or require medical treatment.[26]

The more alcohol you consume, the longer absorption takes. High concentrations of alcohol can cause irritation of the digestive system or vomiting. Alcohol also takes longer to absorb if there is

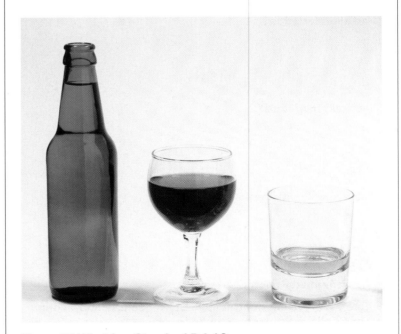

Figure 7.3 What Is a Standard Drink?
One standard drink of beer (12 ounces), wine (5 ounces), or liquor (1 1/2 ounces) contains the same amount of alcohol.

Blood Alcohol Concentration (BAC)	Psychological and Physical Effects
Not Impaired	
<0.01%	Negligible
Sometimes Impaired	
0.01–0.04%	Slight muscle relaxation, mild euphoria, slight body warmth, increased sociability and talkativeness
Usually Impaired	
0.05–0.07%	Lowered alertness, impaired judgment, lowered inhibitions, exaggerated behavior, loss of small muscle control
Always Impaired	
0.08–0.14%	Slowed reaction time, poor muscle coordination, short-term memory loss, judgment impaired, inability to focus
0.15–0.24%	Blurred vision, lack of motor skills, sedation, slowed reactions, difficulty standing and walking, passing out
0.25–0.34%	Impaired consciousness, disorientation, loss of motor function, severely impaired or no reflexes, impaired circulation and respiration, uncontrolled urination, slurred speech, possible death
0.35% and up	Unconsciousness, coma, extremely slow heartbeat and respiration, unresponsiveness, probable death

Figure 7.4 The Psychological and Physical Effects of Alcohol

food in your stomach, because the surface area exposed to alcohol is smaller; a full stomach also retards emptying of alcoholic beverages into the small intestine.

Mood also affects how long it takes for the stomach's contents to empty into the intestine. Alcohol is absorbed much more rapidly when people are tense than when they are relaxed.

Once absorbed into the bloodstream, alcohol circulates throughout the body and is metabolized in the liver, where it is converted to *acetaldehyde* by the enzyme *alcohol dehydrogenase*. It is then rapidly oxidized to *acetate*, converted to carbon dioxide and water, and eventually excreted from the body. Acetaldehyde is a toxic chemical that can cause immediate symptoms such as nausea and vomiting, as well as long-term effects such as liver damage. A very small portion of alcohol is excreted unchanged by the kidneys, lungs, and skin.

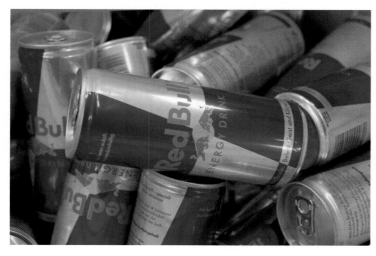

Combining alcohol with energy drinks can have dangerous results.

Alcohol contains 7 calories (kcal) per gram; the average regular beer contains about 150 calories. Mixed drinks may contain more. The body uses the calories in alcohol in the same manner it uses those in carbohydrates: for immediate energy or for storage as fat if not immediately needed.

Breakdown of alcohol occurs at a fairly constant rate of 0.5 ounce (approximately one standard drink) per hour. Unmetabolized alcohol circulates in the bloodstream until enough time passes for the body to break it down.

Blood Alcohol Concentration

Blood alcohol concentration (BAC), the ratio of alcohol to total blood volume, is the primary method used to measure physiological and behavioral effects of alcohol. Despite individual differences, alcohol produces some general effects, depending on BAC (**Figure 7.4**).

At a BAC of 0.02 percent, a person feels relaxed and in a good mood. At 0.05 percent, relaxation increases, and there is some motor impairment and a willingness to talk. At 0.08 percent comes euphoria and further motor impairment. At 0.10 percent, the depressant effects of alcohol become apparent, drowsiness sets in, and motor skills are further impaired, followed by a loss of judgment. A driver may not be able to estimate distance or speed; some drinkers lose their ability to make value-related decisions and may do things they wouldn't do when sober. As BAC increases, the drinker suffers increased negative physiological and psychological effects. Alcohol does not enhance any physical skills or mental functions.

BAC depends on weight and body fat, concentration of alcohol in a beverage, rate of consumption, and volume of alcohol consumed. Heavier people have more body surface through which to diffuse alcohol, so have lower concentrations of blood alcohol than do thin people after drinking the same amount.

Alcohol does not diffuse as rapidly into body fat as into body tissues; BAC is higher in those with more body fat. Because a woman is likely to have proportionately more body fat than a man of the same weight, she will be more intoxicated after drinking the same amount of alcohol.

Breath analysis (breathalyzer tests) and urinalysis are used to determine whether an individual is legally intoxicated, though blood tests are more accurate. An increasing number of states require blood tests for people suspected of driving under the influence of alcohol. In some states, refusal to take a breath or urine test results in immediate driver's license revocation.

check yourself

- **What is a standard drink of alcohol?**
- **How does alcohol enter the bloodstream?**
- **What are some of the factors that increase and decrease blood alcohol concentration?**

Alcohol and Your Health: Short-Term Effects

learning **outcomes**

- **Discuss the short-term health effects of alcohol consumption.**
- **Identify the signs of alcohol poisoning.**
- **Summarize actions to take if someone shows signs of alcohol poisoning.**

Immediate and long-term effects of alcohol consumption can vary greatly (Figure 7.5). The effects you experience depend on you as an individual, how much alcohol you consume, and your circumstances.

The most dramatic effects produced by ethanol occur within the central nervous system (CNS). Alcohol depresses CNS function, which decreases respiratory rate, pulse rate, and blood pressure. As CNS depression deepens, vital functions become affected. In extreme cases, coma and death can result.

Alcohol is a diuretic that increases urinary output. Although this might be expected to lead to **dehydration** (loss of water), the body actually retains water, most of it in the muscles and cerebral tissues. This water is pulled out of the **cerebrospinal fluid** (fluid within the brain and spinal cord), leading to *mitochondrial dehydration* within the nervous system, a state in which the mitochondria—*organelles* within cells that are responsible for cell respiration—cannot carry out their normal functions.

Alcohol irritates the gastrointestinal system and may cause indigestion and heartburn if consumed on an empty stomach. People who consume unusually high amounts of alcohol in a short time also put themselves at risk for irregular heartbeat or even total loss of heart rhythm, which can disrupt blood flow and damage the heart muscle.

Hangover

A **hangover** is often experienced the morning after a drinking spree. Its symptoms are familiar to most people who drink: headache, muscle aches, upset stomach, anxiety, depression, diarrhea, and thirst. **Congeners,** forms of alcohol that are metabolized more slowly than ethanol and are more toxic, are thought to play a role here; the body metabolizes congeners after ethanol is gone from the system, and their toxic byproducts may contribute to hangover. As previously noted, alcohol also upsets the body's water balance, resulting in hangover symptoms including excess urination, dehydration, and thirst. Increased production of hydrochloric acid can irritate the stomach lining and cause nausea. Recovery from a hangover usually takes 12 hours; time is the only cure. Drinking less and drinking slowly and consuming water or other nonalcoholic beverages between drinks will help prevent hangover.

Alcohol and Injuries

Alcohol use plays a significant role in the types of injuries people experience. Annually, more than 658,000 emergency room visits in the United States result from alcohol use, either alone or in combination with one or more other substances.[27] Thirteen percent of emergency room visits by undergraduates are related to alcohol; of these, 34 percent are the result of acute intoxication.[28] A study found that injured patients with a BAC over 0.08 percent who were treated in emergency rooms were 3.2 times more likely to have a violent intentional injury than an unintentional injury.[29] Most people admitted to emergency rooms are men 21 or older, mostly as the result of accidents or fights in which alcohol was involved.[30] Alcohol use is involved in up to half of fatal injuries during leisure activities such as swimming and boating and 40 percent of fatal injuries due to house fires.[31] About two-thirds of all completed suicides involve alcohol, and over 30 percent of rape victims reported that their assailant was under the influence of alcohol.[32]

Alcohol and Sexual Decision Making

Alcohol affects your ability to make good decisions about sex, because it lowers inhibitions; drinkers may do things they might not do when sober. Intoxicated people are less likely to use safer sex practices and more likely to engage in high-risk sexual activity. The chances of sexually transmitted infection and unplanned pregnancy also increase among people who drink more heavily, compared with those who drink moderately or not at all.

Alcohol Poisoning

Alcohol poisoning (*acute alcohol intoxication*) occurs much more frequently than people realize and can be fatal. Drinking large amounts of alcohol in a short period of time can cause one's BAC to quickly reach the lethal range. Alcohol, used either alone or in combination with other drugs, is responsible for more toxic overdose deaths than any other substance.

The amount of alcohol that causes loss of consciousness is dangerously close to the lethal dose. Death from alcohol poisoning can be caused by either CNS and respiratory depression or by inhalation of vomit or fluid into the lungs. Alcohol depresses the nerves that control involuntary actions such as breathing and the gag reflex (which prevents choking). At higher BAC levels, these functions can be completely suppressed. If a drinker becomes unconscious and vomits, there is danger of deadly asphyxiation through choking on one's own vomit. BAC can rise even after a drinker becomes unconscious, because alcohol in the stomach and intestine continues to empty into the bloodstream.

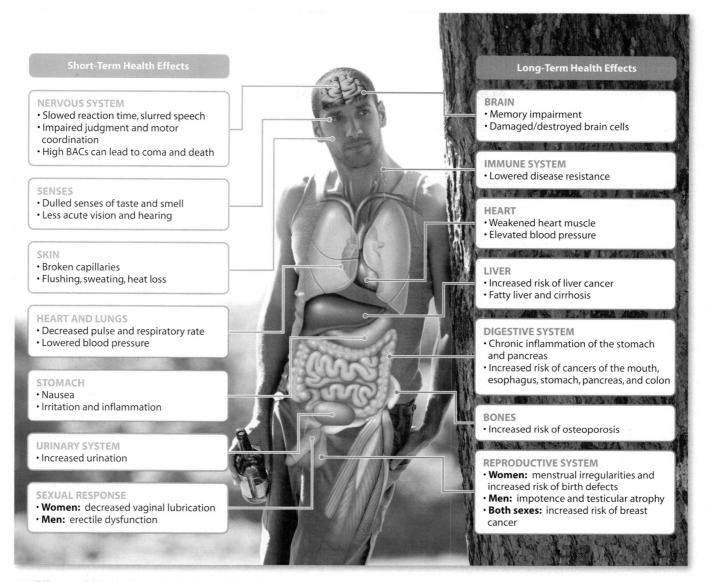

Short-Term Health Effects

NERVOUS SYSTEM
• Slowed reaction time, slurred speech
• Impaired judgment and motor coordination
• High BACs can lead to coma and death

SENSES
• Dulled senses of taste and smell
• Less acute vision and hearing

SKIN
• Broken capillaries
• Flushing, sweating, heat loss

HEART AND LUNGS
• Decreased pulse and respiratory rate
• Lowered blood pressure

STOMACH
• Nausea
• Irritation and inflammation

URINARY SYSTEM
• Increased urination

SEXUAL RESPONSE
• **Women:** decreased vaginal lubrication
• **Men:** erectile dysfunction

Long-Term Health Effects

BRAIN
• Memory impairment
• Damaged/destroyed brain cells

IMMUNE SYSTEM
• Lowered disease resistance

HEART
• Weakened heart muscle
• Elevated blood pressure

LIVER
• Increased risk of liver cancer
• Fatty liver and cirrhosis

DIGESTIVE SYSTEM
• Chronic inflammation of the stomach and pancreas
• Increased risk of cancers of the mouth, esophagus, stomach, pancreas, and colon

BONES
• Increased risk of osteoporosis

REPRODUCTIVE SYSTEM
• **Women:** menstrual irregularities and increased risk of birth defects
• **Men:** impotence and testicular atrophy
• **Both sexes:** increased risk of breast cancer

Figure 7.5 **Effects of Alcohol on the Body and Health**

Skills for **Behavior Change**

DEALING WITH AN ALCOHOL EMERGENCY

Being very drunk can be life threatening. If you think someone has alcohol poisoning, call 9-1-1. Do not leave friends who have passed out to "sleep it off."

Signs of acute alcohol intoxication:

■ Mental confusion, stupor, coma, or inability to be roused
■ Vomiting
■ Seizures
■ Slow breathing (fewer than eight breaths per minute)
■ Rapid or irregular pulse (100 beats or more per minute)
■ Irregular breathing (10 seconds or more between breaths)
■ Cool, clammy skin; bluish skin, fingernails, or lips.

If you suspect alcohol poisoning:

■ Be aware that the person could die.

■ If there's any suspicion of alcohol overdose, call 9-1-1.
■ Roll an unconscious drinker onto his or her side with knees up to minimize the chance of vomit obstructing the airway. With vomiting, position the head lower than the body. If necessary, reach into the mouth and clear the airway.
■ Try to determine if the drinker has taken medications or drugs that may interact with alcohol.
■ Stay with the drinker until medical help arrives.

check yourself

■ **What are the short-term health effects of alcohol consumption?**

■ **What are the signs of alcohol poisoning?**

■ **What actions should you take if you're with someone who shows symptoms of alcohol poisoning?**

- **Discuss the long-term health effects of alcohol consumption.**

Alcohol is distributed throughout most of the body and may affect many organs and tissues. Problems associated with long-term, habitual alcohol abuse include diseases of the nervous system, cardiovascular system, and liver, as well as some cancers.

The nervous system is especially sensitive to alcohol. Even moderate drinkers experience shrinkage in brain size and weight and some loss of intellectual ability. Research also suggests that alcohol damages the frontal areas of the adolescent brain, which are crucial for controlling impulses and thinking through consequences.[33] People who begin drinking at an early age face enormous risk of alcoholism: 47 percent of those who begin drinking alcohol before age 14 become alcohol dependent at some time, compared with 9 percent of those who wait until at least age 21.[34]

Numerous studies have associated light-to-moderate alcohol consumption (no more than two drinks a day) with reduced risk of coronary artery disease, most likely due to an increase in high-density lipoprotein (HDL), or "good" cholesterol. However, alcohol consumption causes many more cardiovascular health hazards than benefits, contributing to high blood pressure and slightly increased heart rate and cardiac output.

One of the most common diseases related to alcohol abuse is **cirrhosis** of the liver (**Figure 7.6**). With heavy drinking, the liver begins to store fat; fat-filled cells stop functioning. Continued drinking can cause *fibrosis*, in which the liver develops fibrous scar tissue. If the person continues to drink, cirrhosis results—the liver cells die and the damage becomes permanent. In **alcoholic hepatitis**, another serious condition, chronic inflammation of the liver develops, which may be fatal in itself or progress to cirrhosis.

Long-term alcohol use has been linked to cancers of the esophagus, stomach, mouth, tongue, and liver. One study discovered a possible link between acetaldehyde and DNA damage that could help explain this connection.[35]

Substantial evidence indicates that women who consume more than three drinks per day have a higher risk of breast cancer than do abstainers.[36] In a recent study, girls and young women who drank 6 or 7 days a week were 5.5 times more likely to have benign breast disease—which itself increases the risk for breast cancer—than those who had less than one drink per week.[37]

The pancreas produces digestive enzymes and insulin. Chronic alcohol abuse reduces enzyme production, inhibiting nutrient absorption. Alcohol may also impair the body's ability to recognize and fight bacteria and viruses. And drinking alcohol can block absorption of calcium—of particular concern to women because of their risk for osteoporosis.

Alcohol and Pregnancy

Teratogenic substances cause birth defects. Of 30 known teratogens, alcohol is one of the most dangerous and common. More than 12 percent of children have been exposed to alcohol *in utero,* and 2 percent of pregnant women reported binge drinking.[38] Consuming four or more drinks a day during pregnancy may significantly increase risk of childhood mental health and learning problems. Alcohol consumed during the first trimester poses the greatest threat to organ development; exposure during the last trimester, when the brain develops rapidly, is most likely to affect the CNS.

Fetal alcohol syndrome (FAS), which is associated with alcohol consumption during pregnancy, is the third most common birth defect and one of the leading causes of mental retardation in the United States, with an estimated incidence of 0.2 to 2 in every 1,000 live births.[39] Symptoms include mental retardation; small head; tremors; abnormalities of the face, limbs, heart, and brain; poor memory; reduced attention span; and impulsive behavior.

Children with some symptoms of FAS may be diagnosed with partial fetal alcohol syndrome (PFAS) or alcohol-related neurodevelopmental disorder (ARND); these, like FAS, are *fetal alcohol spectrum disorders* (FASD).[40] Infants whose mothers habitually consumed more than 3 ounces of alcohol (approximately six drinks) in a short time when pregnant are at high risk for FASD. To avoid any chance of harming her fetus, any woman who is or may become pregnant should not consume alcohol.

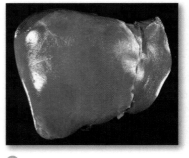 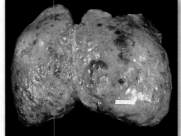

ⓐ A normal liver ⓑ A liver with cirrhosis

Figure 7.6 Comparison of a Healthy Liver with a Cirrhotic Liver

- **What are some long-term health effects of alcohol consumption?**

- **How does awareness of these effects influence your decision whether to consume alcohol?**

Drinking and Driving

learning **outcomes**

- **List effects of alcohol use on the ability to drive safely.**

Traffic accidents are the leading cause of accidental death for all age groups from 5 to 65 years old.[41] Approximately 32 percent of all traffic fatalities in the United States in 2009—10,839 deaths—involved at least one alcohol-impaired driver (a driver having a BAC of 0.08 percent or higher).[42] This number represents an average of one alcohol-related fatality approximately every 48 minutes. Unfortunately, college students are overrepresented in alcohol-related crashes. A recent survey reported that 15.2 percent of college students reported having driven after drinking alcohol sometime in the last 30 days; 2.5 percent of students said that in the past 30 days they had driven after drinking five or more drinks.[43]

Over the past 20 years, the percentage of drivers involved in fatal crashes who were intoxicated (BAC of 0.08 percent or greater) has decreased for all age groups (**Figure 7.7**). Several factors have probably contributed to these reductions in fatalities: laws that increased the drinking age to 21; stricter law enforcement; increased emphasis on zero tolerance (laws prohibiting anyone under 21 from driving with any detectable BAC); and educational programs designed to discourage drinking and driving. The legal limit for BAC in all states is 0.08 percent. Furthermore, all states have zero-tolerance laws for driving while intoxicated, and the penalty is usually suspension of the driver's license.[44]

Despite all these measures, the risk of being involved in an alcohol-related automobile crash remains substantial. Your ability to control a vehicle is affected when you consume even a small amount of alcohol. Among the predictable effects:[45]

- At 0.02 BAC: Your ability to control eye muscles and to perform two tasks at the same time declines.
- At 0.05 BAC: Your coordination declines, as does your ability to track moving objects, to respond to emergency situations, and to steer.
- At 0.08 BAC: Your ability to concentrate, control speed, perceive traffic hazards, and recognize traffic signals and signs diminishes; your reaction time slows; and you experience short-term memory loss.
- At 0.10 BAC: Your ability to maintain lane position and to brake diminishes.
- At 0.15 BAC: Your ability to process information from sight and hearing slows; you experience substantial impairment and the inability to control your vehicle.

Researchers have shown a direct relationship between the amount of alcohol in a driver's bloodstream and the likelihood of a crash. A driver with a BAC level of 0.10 percent is approximately 10 times more likely to be involved in a car accident than a driver who has not been drinking.[46]

Alcohol-related fatal car crashes occur more often at night than during the day; the hours between midnight and 3 AM are the most dangerous. Seventy-two percent of fatally injured drivers involved in nighttime single-vehicle crashes had detectable levels of alcohol in their blood.[47] The risk of being involved in an alcohol-related crash increases not only with the time of day, but also with the day of the week. In 2009, 26 percent of all fatal crashes during the week were alcohol related, compared with 48 percent on weekends.[48] For a driver with a BAC of 0.15 on a weekend night, the likelihood of dying in a single-vehicle crash is more than 382 times higher than that of a nondrinker.

153

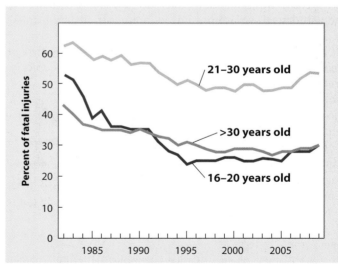

Figure 7.7 Percentage of Fatally Injured Drivers with BACs ≥ 0.08 Percent, by Driver Age, 1982–2009

Source: Insurance Institute for Highway Safety: www.iihs.org, "Fatality Facts 2009: Alcohol," 2011. Used with permission.

check **yourself**

- **How does alcohol impact the ability to drive?**

Alcohol Abuse and Alcoholism

learning outcomes

- **Differentiate between alcohol abuse and alcoholism.**
- **Discuss biological and psychological causes of alcoholism.**
- **Explain effects of alcoholism on family and friends.**

Alcohol use becomes **alcohol abuse** when it interferes with work, school, or social and family relationships or when it entails any violation of the law, including driving under the influence (DUI). **Alcoholism**, or **alcohol dependency**, results when personal and health problems related to alcohol use are severe and stopping alcohol use causes withdrawal symptoms.

Identifying a Problem Drinker

As with other drug addictions, tolerance, psychological dependence, and withdrawal symptoms must be present to qualify a drinker as an addict. Irresponsible and problem drinkers, such as people who get into fights or embarrass themselves or others when they drink, aren't necessarily alcoholics. About 15 percent of people in the United States are problem drinkers; about 5 to 10 percent of male and 3 to 5 percent of female drinkers would be diagnosed as alcohol dependent.[49]

1 in 4

Americans is affected by the alcoholism of a friend or family member.

Nineteen percent of college students meet the criteria for alcohol abuse or dependence (alcoholism).[50] Only 5 percent of these students sought treatment a year prior to the study; 3 percent thought they should seek help, but did not. The heaviest drinkers are the least likely to seek treatment, yet they experience and are responsible for the most alcohol-related problems on campus.[51]

Causes of Alcohol Abuse and Alcoholism

Biological and Family Factors Development of alcoholism among individuals with a family history of alcoholism is four to eight times more common than it is among those with no such history.[52] Children of alcoholics also have higher rates of alcoholism than the general population.[53]

Despite such evidence, scientists do not yet understand the precise role of genes in increased risk for alcoholism, nor have they identified a specific "alcoholism" gene. Adoption studies demonstrate a strong link between individuals' substance use and their biological children's risk for addiction.[54] No single gene causes addiction, though multiple genes can affect the ability to develop addiction.[55]

Social and Cultural Factors Some people begin drinking as a way to dull the pain of an acute loss or an emotional or social problem. Unfortunately, the discomfort that causes many people to turn to alcohol ultimately causes even more discomfort as the drug's depressant effect takes its toll. Eventually, the drinker becomes physically dependent.

Family attitudes also seem to be an influence; people raised in cultures in which alcohol is a part of religious or ceremonial activities or a traditional part of the family meal are less prone to alcohol dependence. In contrast, in societies in which alcohol purchase is carefully controlled and drinking regarded as a rite of passage, the tendency for abuse appears greater. Apparently, some combination of heredity and environment plays a role in development of alcoholism.

How does it affect you to grow up in a family with alcoholism?

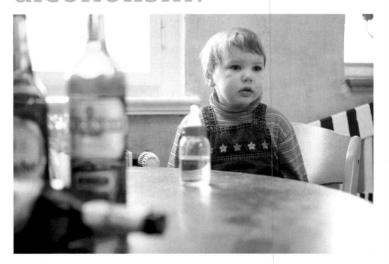

Adult children of alcoholics have unique problems stemming from a lack of parental nurturing during childhood: difficulty developing social attachments, a need to be in control of all emotions and situations, low self-esteem, and depression. Fortunately, not everyone who grows up in an alcoholic family is doomed to lifelong problems. As they mature, many develop resiliency in response to their families' problems and enter adulthood armed with positive strengths and valuable skills.

The amount of alcohol a person consumes seems to be directly related to the drinking habits of that individual's social group. Those whose friends and relatives drink heavily are 50 percent more likely to drink heavily themselves[56]—a finding with importance for individuals who need to sever ties with heavy drinkers to maintain abstinence.

Effects on Family and Friends

An estimated 27.8 million children in the United States are affected or exposed to a family alcohol problem. These children are at increased risk for physical illness, emotional disturbances, behavioral problems, lower educational performance, and susceptibility to alcoholism or other addictions later in life.[57]

In dysfunctional families, children learn certain unspoken rules that allow the family to avoid dealing with real problems—don't talk, don't trust, and don't feel. Unfortunately, these behaviors enable the alcoholic to keep drinking. Children in such families generally assume at least one of the following roles:

- **Family hero** Tries to divert attention from the problem by being too good to be true.
- **Scapegoat.** Draws attention from the family's primary problem through delinquency or misbehavior.
- **Lost child.** Becomes passive and withdraws from upsetting situations.
- **Mascot.** Disrupts tense situations with comic relief.

Children in alcoholic homes have to deal with constant stress, anxiety, and embarrassment. The alcoholic is the center of attention; children's needs are often ignored. It is not uncommon for these children to be victims of violence, abuse, neglect, or incest.

Living with a family member (or friend or roommate) who is an alcoholic can be extremely stressful. People around addicts can find themselves in codependent relationships that enable the addiction. Codependent people often have an exaggerated sense of responsibility for the actions of others, a tendency to always do more than their share, and an extreme need for approval and recognition. Codependents may make excuses or lie to cover for the alcoholic. Eventually, the codependent needs to recognize and stop these behaviors if she or he is to help the alcoholic move toward recovery.

Costs to Society

Alcohol-related costs to society are estimated at well over $185 billion, including health insurance, criminal justice costs, treatment costs, and lost productivity.[58] Alcoholism is directly or indirectly responsible for over 25 percent of the nation's medical expenses and lost earnings.[59]

A 2007 study estimated that underage drinking costs society $68 billion annually,[60] taking into consideration crashes, violence, property crime, suicide, burns, drowning, fetal alcohol syndrome, high-risk sex, poisoning, psychosis, and treatment for alcohol dependence. The largest costs were related to violence ($43.8 billion) and drunk driving accidents ($10 billion). By dividing the cost of underage drinking by the estimated number of underage drinkers, the study estimated that each costs society $2,280 a year.[61]

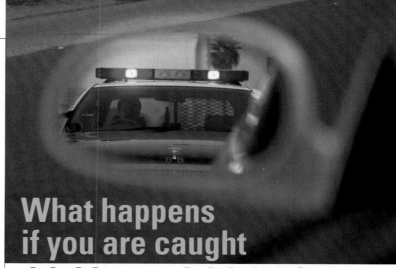

What happens if you are caught drinking and driving?

Getting behind the wheel if you have consumed alcohol is a dangerous choice, with serious legal consequences if you are caught and convicted of driving under the influence (DUI). If you are under age 21 and have any detectable alcohol in your bloodstream, your license can be revoked. Other common penalties for DUI include driver's license restrictions, fines, mandatory counseling, and jail time, even for a first offense. In many states, if you are convicted three times for DUI, you are considered a habitual violator and penalized as a felon, meaning that you lose your right to vote and to own a weapon, among other rights, as well as possibly losing your license permanently. If you are involved in an accident in which someone is injured or killed, the consequences are even more serious. Involvement in such an incident is considered a felony in many states. If a person dies as a result of the accident, the drunk driver may be charged with manslaughter or second-degree murder.

Women and Alcoholism

Women are the fastest growing population of alcohol abusers; there are now almost as many female as male alcoholics. Women get addicted faster with less use and suffer the consequences more profoundly. Women alcoholics have death rates 50 to 100 percent higher than male alcoholics, including deaths from suicide, alcohol-related accidents, heart disease and stroke, and cirrhosis.[62]

Women at highest risk are those who are unmarried but living with a partner, are in their twenties or early thirties, or have a husband or partner who drinks heavily. Risk factors for drinking problems among *all women* include family history, pressure to drink from a peer or spouse, depression, and stress. It is estimated that only 14 percent of women needing treatment for alcohol dependency get it.[63]

check yourself

- **What is the difference between alcohol abuse and alcoholism?**
- **What factors can make a person more likely to abuse alcohol or become an alcoholic?**
- **How does alcoholism affect the family and friends of the alcoholic?**

Reducing Alcohol Intake

- **List practical steps for reducing alcohol intake.**

Alcoholism is characterized by symptoms including craving, loss of control, physical dependence, and tolerance. People who recognize one or more of these behaviors in themselves may wish to seek professional help to determine whether alcohol has become a controlling factor in their lives.

There are some steps that you can take on your own if you are concerned about the amount of alcohol that you consume. Being worried about your consumption is a strong signal that there may be cause for alarm. If a counselor or health care practitioner advises you to reduce or eliminate alcohol intake, you should follow their suggestions and guidance. There are also ways for you to cut down your drinking on your own, depending on their recommendations.

Skills for **Behavior Change**

HOW TO CUT DOWN ON YOUR DRINKING

If you suspect that you drink too much, talk with a counselor or clinician at your student health center. Either of these professionals can tell you whether you should cut down or abstain. If you have a severe drinking problem, alcoholism in your family, or other medical problems, you should stop drinking completely. Your counselor or clinician will advise you about what is right for you.

If you need to cut down on your drinking, these steps can help you:

- **Write your reasons for cutting down or stopping.** There are many reasons you may want to cut down or stop drinking. You may want to improve your health, sleep better, or get along better with your family or friends.
- **Set a drinking goal.** Determine a limit for how much you will drink. You may choose to cut down, or to not drink at all. If you aren't sure what goal is right for you, talk with your counselor. Once you determine your goal, write it down on a piece of paper. Put it someplace you can see it, such as on your refrigerator or bathroom mirror.
- **Keep a diary of your drinking.** Write down every time you have a drink. Try to keep your diary for 3 or 4 weeks. This will show you how much you drink and when. You may be surprised. How different is your goal from the amount you drink now?
- **Keep little or no alcohol at home.** You don't need the temptation.

- **Drink slowly.** When you drink, sip slowly. Take a break of 1 hour between drinks. Drink a nonalcoholic beverage, such as soda, water, or juice, after every alcoholic drink you consume. Do not drink on an empty stomach! Eat food when you are drinking.
- **Take a break from alcohol.** Pick a day or two each week when you will not drink at all. Then try to stop drinking for 1 week. Think about how you feel physically and emotionally on these days. When you succeed and feel better, you may find it easier to cut down for good.
- **Learn how to say no.** You do not have to drink when other people are or take a drink when offered one. Practice ways to say no politely. Stay away from people who give you a hard time about not drinking.
- **Stay active.** Use the time and money once spent on drinking to do something fun with your family or friends. Go out to eat, see a movie, or play sports or a game.
- **Get support.** Cutting down on your drinking may be difficult at times. Ask your family and friends for support to help you reach your goal. Talk to your counselor if you are having trouble cutting down. Get the help you need to reach your goal.

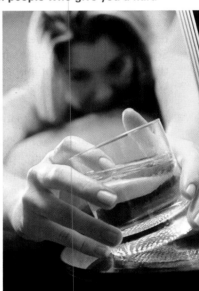

- **Avoid temptations.** Watch out for people, places, or times that lead you to drink, even if you did not want to. Plan ahead of time what you will do to avoid drinking when you are tempted. Do not drink when you are angry, upset, or having a bad day.
- **Remember, don't give up!** Most people don't cut down or give up drinking all at once. As with a diet, it is not easy to change. That's OK. If you don't reach your goal the first time, try again. Remember, get support from people who care about you and want to help.

- **What are some practical steps to cut down on your drinking?**
- **Have you ever decided to reduce the amount of alcohol you consume? If so, what were the steps that you took?**

Treatment and Recovery

- **List factors explaining the low percentage of alcoholics who receive treatment.**
- **Explain treatment options available to alcoholics.**

Despite growing recognition of our national alcohol problem, only 15 percent of alcoholics in the United States receive any care.[64] Contributing factors include inability or unwillingness to admit to a problem, social stigma, failure of medical providers to recognize or diagnose symptoms or follow through with treatments, and failure of rehabilitation facilities to give quality care.

Most problem drinkers who seek help reach a turning point—finally recognizing that alcohol controls their lives. The first steps toward recovery are regaining control and assuming responsibility for one's actions.

An alcoholic's family sometimes takes action before the alcoholic does. An effective method of helping an alcoholic confront the disease is **intervention**, a planned confrontation involving family and friends plus professional counselors.

Treatment Programs

Private Treatment Facilities Private treatment facilities have made concerted efforts to attract patients through advertising. On admission, the patient receives a complete physical exam. Alcoholics who quit drinking experience detoxification, the process by which addicts end their dependence on a drug. Withdrawal symptoms include hyperexcitability, confusion and agitation, sleep disorders, convulsions, tremors, depression, headaches, and seizures. A small percentage of people have **delirium tremens (DTs)**—confusion, delusions, agitation, and hallucinations.

After detoxification, alcoholics begin treatment for psychological addiction. Most treatment facilities keep patients from 3 to 6 weeks and charge several thousand dollars; some insurance programs or employers assume most of the expense.

Therapy Several types of therapy are commonly used in alcoholism recovery. In family therapy, the person and family members examine psychological reasons underlying the addiction. In individual and group therapy with fellow addicts, alcoholics learn positive coping skills for situations that have caused them to turn to alcohol.

On some college campuses, the problems associated with alcohol abuse are so great that student health centers are opening their own treatment programs. At some schools, students in recovery live together in special housing. Programs such as these hope to provide the support and comfortable environment recovering students need.

Pharmacological Treatment Disulfiram (trade name Antabuse), is a drug commonly used for treating alcoholism. If users drink alcohol or consume foods with alcohol content, disulfiram causes acetaldehyde to build up in the liver, triggering nausea, vomiting, headache, bad breath, drowsiness, and impotence. Naltrexone is used to reduce alcohol cravings and decrease the pleasant effects of alcohol, without making the user ill. Acamprosate (Campral) is thought to restore normal brain balance, which has been disturbed in the alcohol dependent, and to reduce the physical and emotional discomfort often associated with staying alcohol free. All pharmacological treatments for alcoholism should be used in conjunction with psychotherapy or support groups.

Group Support Treatments **Alcoholics Anonymous (AA)** is a nonprofit self-help organization with more than 1 million members; it offers group support to help people stop drinking. Related *Al-Anon* and *Alateen* groups help relatives, friends, and children of alcoholics understand the disease and how they can contribute to the recovery process. Other self-help groups include Women for Sobriety, which addresses the specific needs of female alcoholics, and Secular Organizations for Sobriety (SOS), founded to help those uncomfortable with AA's spiritual emphasis.

Relapse

Success with recovery varies. Alcoholics most likely to recover completely are those who developed dependency after age 20, who have intact and supportive families, and who have reached a high level of personal disgust plus strong motivation to recover.

People in recovery must not only confront addictions but also guard against relapse. Over half relapse within the first 3 months of treatment. Many alcoholics refer to themselves as "recovering" throughout their lifetime, never using the word *cured*. Effective recovery programs offer alcoholics ways to increase self-esteem and resume personal growth. A comprehensive approach combining drug therapy, group support, and counseling is most effective. A very small number of recovering alcoholics are able to resume limited drinking without reverting to alcoholic behavior, though abstinence is the safest and sanest path.

- **Why do so few alcoholics receive treatment?**
- **What treatment options are available for alcoholics?**

Tobacco Use in the United States

learning outcomes

- **Discuss advertising tactics used by the tobacco industry.**
- **Examine reasons that people start smoking.**
- **List factors that contribute to tobacco use by college students.**

Approximately 70 million Americans report using tobacco products (cigarettes, cigars, smokeless tobacco, and pipe tobacco) at least once in the past month. In 2009, 25.3 percent of men and 21.4 percent of women were current cigarette smokers. Every day approximately 1,100 people under 18 and 1,900 people over 18 become daily smokers.[65]

Education is closely linked to cigarette use: Adults with a bachelor's degree or higher education are three times *less* likely to smoke than are those with less than a high school education. Cigarette smoking also varies by ethnicity and gender, with the highest rates of smoking found among non-Hispanic black men and American Indian and Alaska Native men.[66]

More than 20 percent of Americans are former smokers; about 60 percent have never smoked. The most commonly used tobacco product is cigarettes, followed by cigars and smokeless tobacco. Approximately 6 percent of Americans smoke cigars, and 7 percent of men and less than 1 percent of women use smokeless tobacco.[67]

Why Do People Use Tobacco?

Nicotine Addiction Beginning smokers usually feel the effects of nicotine with their first puff. These symptoms, called **nicotine poisoning**, can include dizziness, lightheadedness, rapid and erratic pulse, clammy skin, nausea, vomiting, and diarrhea. Symptoms cease as tolerance develops, which happens as quickly as the second or third cigarette. Many regular smokers experience no "buzz," but continue to smoke because stopping is too difficult.

Two studies on twins found genetic factors to be more influential than environmental factors in smoking initiation and nicotine dependence.[68] Two specific genes may influence smoking behavior by affecting the action of the brain chemical dopamine.[69] Understanding the influence of genetics on nicotine addiction could be crucial to developing more effective treatments for smoking cessation.[70]

Behavioral Dependence People who smoke are not just physically but also psychologically dependent. Nicotine "tricks" the brain into creating pleasurable associations with sensory stimuli or environmental cues that may trigger the urge for a cigarette.[71] Some former smokers remain vulnerable to sensory and environmental cues for many years after they quit.

Weight Control Nicotine is an appetite suppressant and slightly increases basal metabolic rate. After smoking a cigarette, one's metabolism quickly increases then returns to normal; heavy smokers have such surges throughout the day. When a smoker quits, the metabolic rate slows down and appetite returns. People tend to eat more, particularly sweets. Fear of gaining weight is one of the biggest reasons smokers are reluctant to quit. To avoid weight gain after quitting smoking, avoid crash diets, keep low-calorie treats handy, and drink plenty of water.

Advertising The tobacco industry spends an estimated $36 million per day on advertising and promotion.[72] Because children and teenagers constitute 90 percent of all new smokers, much of the advertising has been directed toward them. Evidence of product recognition among underage smokers is clear: 86 percent prefer one of the three most heavily advertised brands—

Reason	Percentage
Reduce stress	38%
Social pressure	16%
Can't stop	12%
Social smoker	11%
Experiment	7%
Concentrate	6%
Control appetite	3%

Percentage of students who report reason

Figure 7.8 Reasons for Smoking among College Student Smokers

Source: Adapted from *Wasting the Best and the Brightest: Substance Abuse at America's Colleges and Universities*, March 2007, p. 48. Copyright © 2007 by The National Center on Addiction and Substance Abuse. Reprinted with permission of The National Center on Addiction and Substance Abuse at Columbia University (CASA Columbia).

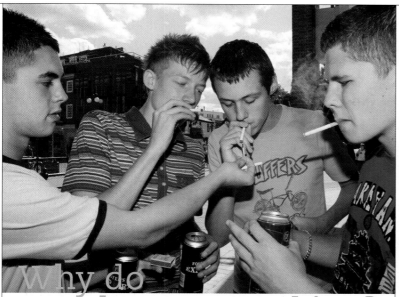

Why do people start smoking?

Peer pressure plays a large role, as do advertising and the portrayal of smoking in films and on TV. Tobacco companies know that once a person starts smoking chances are good that he or she will get hooked and become a long-term customer, so they make a concerted effort to attract kids and teens.

Marlboro, Newport, or Camel.[73] After R. J. Reynolds introduced the popular Joe Camel ad campaign, Camel's market share among underage smokers jumped from 3 to 13.3 percent in 3 years.[74] Tobacco companies have also targeted children and teens with products using candy, fruit, or alcohol flavorings that mask the harshness of tobacco.[75]

In the past several years, the tobacco industry has launched aggressive campaigns aimed at women, depicting cigarette smoking as feminine and fashionable. "Slim" and "light" cigarettes also cash in on women's fear of gaining weight. These ads have apparently been working; from the mid-1970s through the early 2000s, cigarette sales to women increased dramatically. But women are not the only targets of gender-based advertisements. Men in cigarette ads are depicted charging over rugged terrain in off-road vehicles or riding stallions into the sunset, in blatant appeals to stereotypical masculinity. Minorities are also often targeted; for example, studies have shown a higher concentration of tobacco advertising in magazines aimed at African Americans than in similar magazines aimed at broader audiences.

Financial Costs to Society

The economic burden of tobacco use totals more than $96 billion in medical expenditures (costs include hospital, physician, and nursing home expenses; prescription drugs; and home health care expenditures) plus $97 billion in indirect costs (absenteeism, added cost of fire insurance, training costs to replace employees who die prematurely, disability payments, and so on). The economic costs of smoking are estimated to be about $3,391 per smoker per year,[76] far exceeding tax revenues on the sale of tobacco products.[77]

College Students and Tobacco Use

Although college students are the targets of heavy tobacco advertising campaigns, cigarette smoking among U.S. college students has decreased in recent years. In a 2010 study, about 15 percent of college students reported having smoked cigarettes in the past 30 days, down from about 30 percent in 1999.[78] About 11 percent of college students meet the criteria for tobacco dependence.[79]

College men and women have nearly identical rates of cigarette smoking, but men use more cigars and smokeless tobacco.[80] On college campuses, female students who smoke are viewed in a more negative light than male students who smoke.[81]

Why Do College Students Smoke?

In a recent survey, the main reason students gave for smoking was to relax or to reduce stress (38%).[82] Other reasons were to fit in or because of social pressure (16%) and because they cannot stop or are addicted (12%; see **Figure 7.8**). For some students weight control is a motivator. Students diagnosed or treated for depression are 7.5 times more likely to use tobacco.[83]

Many college smokers identify themselves as "social smokers"— those who smoke when they are with people, rather than alone. Social smokers smoke less often and are less dependent on nicotine. However, even occasional smoking is not without risks. Smoking less than a pack of cigarettes a week has been shown to damage blood vessels and increase the risk of heart disease and cancer.[84] Occasional smokers also experience more colds, sore throats, shortness of breath, and fatigue.[85] In women taking birth control pills, even a few cigarettes a week can increase the likelihood of heart disease, blood clots, stroke, liver cancer, and gallbladder disease.[86] Pregnant women who smoke only occasionally still run a risk of giving birth to unhealthy babies.

In one study, over the course of 4 years of college, about half of students who smoked every few days, every few weeks, or every few months quit, as did 13 percent of daily smokers.[87] Unfortunately, almost all daily smokers continue to smoke throughout college.[88]

A recent Harvard University survey found tobacco companies giving away cigarettes at bars and social events on 109 of 119 campuses. The research suggests that tobacco companies are targeting college students, according to study coauthor Henry Wechsler. "These are very important years," says Wechsler. "They're also the earliest years that the tobacco industry can legally try to get new customers." Students exposed to the giveaways were three times more likely to start smoking or use smokeless tobacco by age 19.[89]

159

check yourself

- **The tobacco industry has been accused of targeting college students in its marketing campaigns. Do you agree? If so, give examples of tobacco marketing that target young adults.**

- **What factors make college students more likely to use tobacco?**

Tobacco: Its Components and Effects

- **Examine the addictive nature of tobacco products.**
- **Compare and contrast tobacco products on the market.**

Smoking, the most common form of tobacco use, delivers a strong dose of nicotine directly to the lungs, along with 4,000 other chemical substances, including 250 that are harmful or toxic and 50 known carcinogens (cancer-causing agents).[90] Inhaling hot toxic gases exposes sensitive mucous membranes to irritating chemicals that weaken the tissues and contribute to cancers of the mouth, larynx, and throat. The heat from tobacco smoke, which can reach 1,616°F, is also harmful.

Nicotine

The highly addictive chemical stimulant **nicotine** is the major psychoactive substance in all tobacco products. When tobacco leaves are burned in a cigarette, pipe, or cigar, nicotine is inhaled into the lungs. Sucking or chewing tobacco releases nicotine into the saliva; it is then absorbed through the mucous membranes in the mouth.

Nicotine is a powerful central nervous system stimulant that produces a variety of physiological effects. In the cerebral cortex, it produces an aroused, alert mental state. It stimulates production of adrenaline, increases heart and respiratory rates, constricts blood vessels, and, in turn, increases blood pressure because the heart must work harder to pump blood through narrowed vessels.

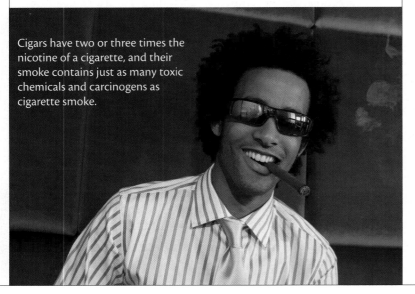

Cigars have two or three times the nicotine of a cigarette, and their smoke contains just as many toxic chemicals and carcinogens as cigarette smoke.

Tar and Carbon Monoxide

Cigarette smoke is a complex mixture of chemicals and gases produced by the burning of tobacco and its additives. Particulate matter condenses in the lungs to form a sludge called **tar** containing carcinogenic agents, such as benzopyrene, and chemical irritants, such as phenol. Phenol has the potential to combine with other chemicals that contribute to developing lung cancer.

In healthy lungs, millions of tiny hairlike projections (*cilia*) on the surfaces lining the upper respiratory passages sweep away foreign matter, which is then expelled from the lungs by coughing. However, in smokers, nicotine paralyzes the cilia for up to 1 hour following a single cigarette, impairing their cleansing function. This allows tars and other solids in tobacco smoke to accumulate and irritate sensitive lung tissue.

Cigarette smoke also contains poisonous gases, the most dangerous of which is **carbon monoxide,** the deadly gas that comes out of exhaust pipes in cars. In the human body, carbon monoxide reduces the oxygen-carrying capacity of red blood cells by binding with the receptor sites for oxygen; this causes oxygen deprivation in many body tissues. It is at least partly responsible for increased risk of heart attacks and strokes in smokers.

Tobacco Products

Cigarettes Cigarettes are the most common form of tobacco available today. Some people purchase loose tobacco and rolling papers to roll their own cigarettes, but most buy manufactured cigarettes. Almost all manufactured cigarettes have filters designed to reduce levels of gases such as hydrogen cyanide and carbon monoxide. However, these filtered products may not be much better than their nonfiltered counterparts. Filters themselves contain chemical substances that may be inhaled. People who smoke filtered products may think they are protected and, therefore, take deeper "drags," inhale more often, or even smoke more cigarettes. The truth is that no cigarette is healthy.

Clove cigarettes contain about 40 percent ground cloves and 60 percent tobacco. Many users mistakenly believe that these products are made entirely of ground cloves and that smoking them eliminates the risks associated with tobacco. In fact, clove cigarettes contain higher levels of tar, nicotine, and carbon monoxide than do regular cigarettes. In addition, the numbing effect of eugenol, an ingredient in cloves, allows smokers to inhale more deeply. The same effect is true of *menthol cigarettes:* The throat-numbing effect of the menthol allows for deeper inhalation. Menthol cigarettes also have higher carbon monoxide concentrations than do regular cigarettes.

Cigars Cigars are nothing more than tobacco fillers wrapped in more tobacco. Cigar sales in the United States increased by nearly 124 percent between 1993 and 2007.[91] The fad, especially popular among young men and women, is fueled in part by the willingness of celebrities to be photographed puffing on a cigar. Cigars also cost much less than cigarettes in most states. Also, among some women, cigar smoking symbolizes being slightly outrageous and liberated. According to a recent national survey, about 11 percent of Americans aged 18 to 25 had smoked a cigar in the past month.[92]

Many people believe that cigars are safer than cigarettes, when in fact the opposite is true. Cigar smoke contains 23 poisons and 43 carcinogens. Most cigars contain as much nicotine as several cigarettes, and when cigar smokers inhale nicotine is absorbed as rapidly as it is with cigarettes. For those who don't inhale, nicotine is still absorbed through the mucous membranes in the mouth.

Pipes and Hookahs Pipes have had a long history of use throughout the world, including ritualistic and ceremonial usage for many cultures. Often thought to be safer than cigarettes or cigars, pipes are not risk-free. According to cumulative research by the National Cancer Institute and the American Cancer Society, pipe smoking carries similar risks to cigar smoking. Of concern in recent years is the increasing prevalence, particularly among college students, of the use of "hookahs," or water pipes. Hookah smoking originated in the Middle East and involves burning flavored tobacco in a water pipe and inhaling the smoke through a long hose. Hookahs are marketed as reducing risks from hazardous chemicals by filtering the smoke through water before you inhale. Water pipes may cool the smoke, but they do not eliminate or filter out nicotine, carbon monoxide, or tar.[93] In addition to the health risks associated with all tobacco products, risks associated with hookah use include hygiene concerns from sharing the pipe.

Bidis Generally made in India or Southeast Asia, **bidis** are small, hand-rolled cigarettes in a variety of flavors, such as vanilla, chocolate, and cherry. They have become increasingly popular with college students. Though often viewed as safer than cigarettes, they are actually far more toxic. Smoke from a bidi contains three times more carbon monoxide and nicotine and five times more tar than cigarettes.[94] The leaf wrappers are nonporous, which means that smokers must suck harder to inhale and must inhale more to keep the bidi lit, resulting in much more exposure to the higher amounts of tar, nicotine, and carbon monoxide. Bidi smoking increases risks of oral cancer, lung cancer, stomach cancer, and esophageal cancer. It is also associated with emphysema and chronic bronchitis.[95]

Smokeless Tobacco An estimated 3.5 percent of adults in the United States use smokeless tobacco products.[96] In the most recent National College Health Assessment, about 8 percent of college men and 1 percent of college women reported having used smokeless tobacco in the past 30 days.[97] Use of chewing tobacco by teenage boys, especially in rural areas, has increased by 30 percent in the past 10 years.[98]

Chewing tobacco comes in three forms—loose leaf, plug, or pouch—and contains tobacco leaves treated with molasses and other flavorings. The user "dips" the tobacco by placing a small amount between the lower lip and teeth to stimulate the flow of saliva and release the nicotine. **Dipping** rapidly releases nicotine into the bloodstream.

Snuff is a finely ground form of tobacco that can be inhaled, chewed, or placed against the gums. It comes in dry or moist powdered form or sachets (tea bag–like pouches). In 2009, "snus" became the latest form of smokeless tobacco to hit the market in the United States. Popular for more than 100 years in Sweden, these small sachets of tobacco are placed inside the cheek and sucked.

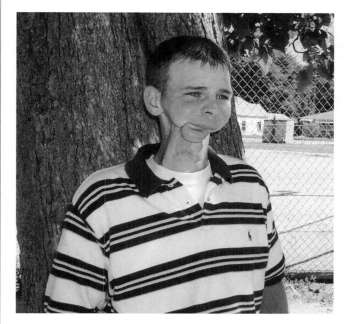

Is chewing tobacco as harmful as smoking cigarettes?

No matter in what form you use it—cigar, pipe, bidi, dip, snuff, or cigarette—tobacco is hazardous to your health. Chewing tobacco and snuff contain *more* nicotine than cigarettes, and just as many toxic and carcinogenic chemicals. This young cancer survivor began using smokeless tobacco at age 13; by age 17, he was diagnosed with squamous cell carcinoma. He has undergone surgery to remove neck muscles, lymph nodes, and his tongue, and he now educates others about the dangers of chewing tobacco.

Smokeless tobacco is just as addictive as cigarettes and actually contains more nicotine—holding an average-sized dip or chew in the mouth for 30 minutes delivers as much nicotine as smoking four cigarettes. A 2-can-a-week snuff user gets as much nicotine as a 10-pack-a-week smoker.

It is time to banish the notion the idea that smokeless tobacco is safe. All forms of oral tobacco have chemicals known to cause cancer. A pinch of smokeless tobacco exposes users to the same amount of dangerous chemicals as the smoke of five cigarettes. Smokeless tobacco causes an increase in heart rate, blood pressure, and epinephrine. Smokeless tobacco also contains strong carcinogens, including nitrosamines, polycyclic aromatic hydrocarbons (PAHs), and radiation-emitting polonium.

check yourself

- **How does nicotine affect the body?**
- **Why do some people mistakenly believe that some tobacco products are less harmful than others?**

Health Hazards of Tobacco Products

■ **Summarize the health risks of tobacco products.**

Cigarette smoking adversely affects the health of every person who smokes, as well as the health of everyone nearby. Each day, cigarettes contribute to more than 1,200 deaths from cancer, cardiovascular disease, and respiratory disorders.[99] In addition, tobacco use can negatively affect the health of almost every system in your body (Figure 7.9).

Cancer

Lung cancer is the leading cause of cancer deaths in the United States. Tobacco smoking causes 85 to 90 percent of all cases of lung cancer and 87 percent of lung cancer deaths.[100] There were an estimated 222,520 *new* cases of lung cancer in the United States in 2010 alone, and an estimated 157,300 Americans died from the disease in 2010.[101]

Lung cancer can take 10 to 30 years to develop, and the outlook for its victims is poor; the 5-year survival rate is only 16 percent.[102] Smokers' risk of developing lung cancer depends on several factors. Someone who smokes two packs a day is 15 to 25 times more likely to develop lung cancer than a nonsmoker. A second factor is when you started smoking; an earlier start greatly increases risk. A third factor is whether you inhale deeply when you smoke.

A major risk of chewing tobacco is **leukoplakia,** leathery white patches inside the mouth produced by contact with irritants in tobacco juice. Three to 17 percent of diagnosed leukoplakia cases develop into oral cancer.[103] Approximately 75 percent of the 36,540 new oral cancer cases in 2010 resulted from either smokeless tobacco or cigarettes.[104] Users of smokeless tobacco are 50 times more likely to develop oral cancers than are nonusers. Warning signs include lumps in the jaw, neck or lips; white, smooth, or scaly patches in the mouth or on the neck, lips, or tongue; mouth sores or bleeding that don't heal in 2 weeks; and difficulty speaking or swallowing. The time between first use and contracting cancer is shorter for smokeless tobacco users than for smokers.

Tobacco is linked to other cancers as well. The rate of pancreatic cancer is more than twice as high for smokers as for nonsmokers, and of cancers of the lip, tongue, salivary glands, and esophagus five times as high. Smokers are also more likely to develop kidney, bladder, and larynx cancers. Long-term smokeless tobacco use increases risk of larynx, esophagus, nasal cavity, pancreas, kidney, and bladder cancers.

Cardiovascular Disease

Smokers have a 70 percent higher death rate from heart disease than nonsmokers, and heavy smokers have a 200 percent higher death rate than moderate smokers. Daily cigar smoking, especially for people who inhale, also increases the risk of heart disease (double the risk of heart attack and stroke compared to nonsmokers) and chronic obstructive pulmonary disease.[105] Smoking and exposure to environmental

30%
of all cancer deaths have smoking as a primary causal factor.

tobacco smoke (ETS) accelerates buildup of fatty deposits (plaque) in the heart and major blood vessels (atherosclerosis). People regularly exposed to ETS can have a 20 percent increase in plaque buildup.[106]

Smoking decreases oxygen supplied to the heart and contributes to irregular heart rhythms, which can trigger a heart attack. Smokers are also twice as likely to suffer strokes as nonsmokers.[107] A stroke occurs when a small blood vessel in the brain bursts or is blocked by a blood clot, denying the brain oxygen and nourishment. Depending on the brain area affected, stroke can result in paralysis, loss of mental functioning, or death. Smoking contributes to strokes by raising blood pressure, which increases stress on vessel walls, and by increasing **platelet adhesiveness**, where red blood cells stick together, making blood clots more likely.

The risk of dying from a heart attack falls by half after only 1 year without smoking, and declines steadily thereafter. After about 15 years, the ex-smoker's risk of cardiovascular disease and stroke is similar to that of people who have never smoked.[108]

Respiratory Disorders

Smokers are more prone to breathlessness, chronic cough, and excess phlegm production than are nonsmokers their age. Ultimately, smokers are up to 18 times more likely to die of lung disease than are nonsmokers.[109]

Chronic bronchitis may develop in smokers, because their inflamed lungs produce more mucus, which they constantly try to expel along with foreign particles. This results in the persistent cough known as "smoker's hack." Smokers are also more prone to respiratory ailments such as influenza, pneumonia, and colds.

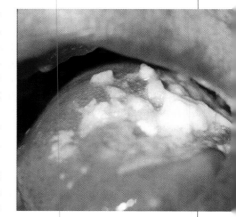

Leukoplakia, which can appear on the tongue or in the mouth as shown here, can be a precursor to oral cancer.

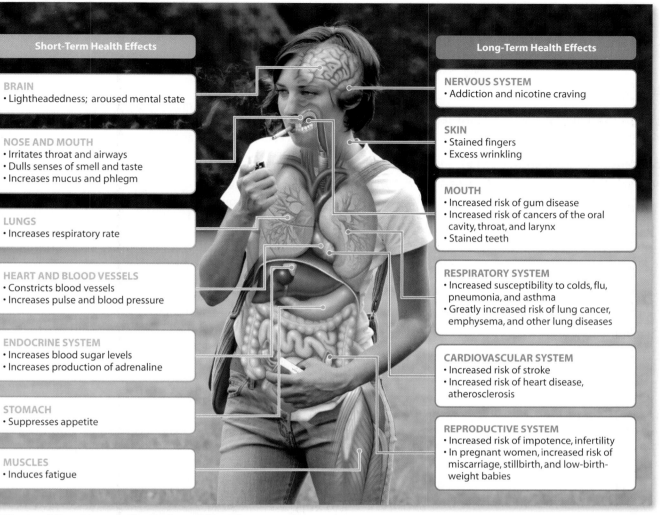

Short-Term Health Effects

BRAIN
• Lightheadedness; aroused mental state

NOSE AND MOUTH
• Irritates throat and airways
• Dulls senses of smell and taste
• Increases mucus and phlegm

LUNGS
• Increases respiratory rate

HEART AND BLOOD VESSELS
• Constricts blood vessels
• Increases pulse and blood pressure

ENDOCRINE SYSTEM
• Increases blood sugar levels
• Increases production of adrenaline

STOMACH
• Suppresses appetite

MUSCLES
• Induces fatigue

Long-Term Health Effects

NERVOUS SYSTEM
• Addiction and nicotine craving

SKIN
• Stained fingers
• Excess wrinkling

MOUTH
• Increased risk of gum disease
• Increased risk of cancers of the oral cavity, throat, and larynx
• Stained teeth

RESPIRATORY SYSTEM
• Increased susceptibility to colds, flu, pneumonia, and asthma
• Greatly increased risk of lung cancer, emphysema, and other lung diseases

CARDIOVASCULAR SYSTEM
• Increased risk of stroke
• Increased risk of heart disease, atherosclerosis

REPRODUCTIVE SYSTEM
• Increased risk of impotence, infertility
• In pregnant women, increased risk of miscarriage, stillbirth, and low-birth-weight babies

Figure 7.9 Effects of Smoking on the Body and Health

Emphysema is a chronic disease in which the alveoli (the tiny air sacs in the lungs) are destroyed, impairing the lungs' ability to obtain oxygen and remove carbon dioxide and making breathing very difficult. Because the heart has to work harder to do even the simplest tasks, it may become enlarged and death from heart damage may result. There is no known cure, and the damage is irreversible. Approximately 80 percent of all cases of emphysema are related to cigarette smoking.[110]

Sexual Dysfunction and Fertility Problems

Despite tobacco advertisers' attempts to make smoking appear sexy, male smokers are about twice as likely as nonsmokers to suffer from some form of impotence.[111] Women who smoke increase their risk for infertility, ectopic pregnancy, spontaneous abortion, and stillbirth. They also increase their baby's risk of sudden infant death syndrome and chances of being born with a cleft lip or palate.[112] Smoking during pregnancy accounts for approximately 30 percent of premature births and increases risk of low birth weight, which, in turn, increases babies' likelihood of illness or death.[113]

Other Health Effects

Dental problems are common among users of both smokeless tobacco and cigarettes. Contact with tobacco juice causes receding gums, tooth decay, bad breath, and discolored teeth. Gum disease is three times more common among smokers than among nonsmokers, and smokers lose significantly more teeth.[114]

Nicotine speeds up the process by which the body uses and eliminates drugs, making medications less effective for smokers. In addition, heavy smokers might be accelerating damage to the brain, which could lead to Alzheimer's disease.[115]

check yourself

- **What do lung cancer and emphysema have in common? How do they differ?**
- **Explain how the use of tobacco products affects the lungs and heart.**
- **Name at least four types of cancer that are linked to the use of tobacco.**

Environmental Tobacco Smoke

- **Describe the risks of environmental tobacco smoke.**

Environmental tobacco smoke (ETS), also known as *secondhand smoke*, is divided into two categories: **mainstream smoke** (smoke exhaled by a smoker) and **sidestream smoke** (smoke from a burning cigarette, pipe, or cigar).[116] Since the 1986 Surgeon General's report *The Health Consequences of Involuntary Smoking*, detectable levels of nicotine exposure in nonsmoking Americans has decreased by 48 percent, due to the growing number of laws banning smoking in work and public places.[117]

Almost 54 percent of U.S. children aged 3 to 11 are exposed to ETS.[118] Disparities in ETS also occur along racial and class lines. African Americans have been found to have higher levels of exposure to ETS than whites and Hispanics; exposure is also higher for low-income persons.[119]

Risks from ETS

Although involuntary smokers breathe less tobacco than active smokers do, secondhand smoke actually contains more carcinogenic substances than the smoke a smoker inhales; it has about 2 times more tar and nicotine, 5 times more carbon monoxide, and 50 times more ammonia. Every year, ETS is estimated to be responsible for 3,400 lung cancer deaths in nonsmoking adults, 46,000 coronary and heart disease deaths in nonsmoking adults who live with smokers, and 430 deaths in newborns from sudden infant death syndrome (SIDS).[120]

The Environmental Protection Agency (EPA) has designated secondhand smoke as a known (group A) carcinogen. According to the Surgeon General, more than 70 cancer-causing agents are found in secondhand smoke.[121] The most likely mechanism whereby secondhand smoke causes lung cancer is continuous exposure to these carcinogens over time. There is also strong evidence that secondhand smoke interferes with functioning of the heart, blood, and vascular systems. Nonsmokers exposed to secondhand smoke are 25 to 30 percent more likely to have coronary heart disease than nonsmokers not exposed to smoke.[122]

Children and ETS

Exposure to ETS increases children's risk of lower respiratory tract infections, leading to an estimated 150,000 to 300,000 new cases of bronchitis and pneumonia in children each year.[123] In addition, children exposed to secondhand smoke have a greater chance of coughing, wheezing, asthma, and chest colds, along with a decrease in lung function. The greatest effects of secondhand smoke are seen in children under 5. Children exposed to secondhand smoke daily in the home miss 33 percent more school days and have 10 percent more colds and acute respiratory infections than those not exposed.[124]

Secondhand smoke also affects children's cognitive abilities. One study found that children exposed to high levels of secondhand smoke had lower standardized test scores in reading, math, and problem solving.[125] In addition, children exposed to secondhand smoke are twice as likely to become smokers during adolescence than children who are not exposed.[126]

ETS and Additional Health Problems

Environmental tobacco smoke can cause allergic reactions such as itchy eyes, difficulty breathing, headaches, nausea, and dizziness. It may also increase risk of breast cancer in women; cancers of the nasal sinus cavity and pharynx in adults; and leukemia, lymphoma, and brain tumors in children.[127] The level of carbon monoxide in cigarette smoke contained in enclosed places is 4,000 times higher than that allowed in the clean-air standard recommended by the EPA.

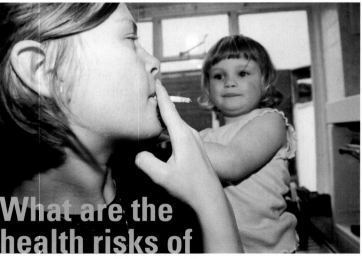

What are the health risks of secondhand smoke?

ETS is linked to deaths from cancer and heart disease in adults and SIDS in infants. Because their bodies and brains are still developing, babies and children are particularly vulnerable to the toxins in secondhand smoke.

- **What are the health risks of exposure to ETS?**
- **Considering the risks of ETS to children, do you think parents should be prohibited from using tobacco?**

Tobacco Use Prevention Policies

- **Describe policy efforts to discourage tobacco use.**

It has been more than 40 years since the U.S. government began warning that tobacco use was hazardous to the nation's health. In an effort to recoup state expenditures on health care costs related to treating smokers, 46 states sued the tobacco industry.[128] In 1998, the tobacco industry reached a master's settlement agreement with 40 states. The agreement requires tobacco companies to pay approximately $206 billion over 25 years nationwide. The agreement also includes a variety of measures to support antismoking education and advertising and to fund research to determine effective smoking-cessation strategies. It also curbs tobacco industry billboard advertising and promotions and advertising that appeals to youth (including merchandise samples and using cartoon characters in ads). Faced with the settlement restrictions and strong opposition from antismoking organizations, the tobacco companies have been struggling to improve their image.

Unfortunately, most of the money designated for tobacco control and prevention at the state level has not been used for this purpose. Facing budget woes, many states have drastically cut spending on antismoking programs. In the few states that have spent the settlement money on smoking-cessation programs, there has been some reported success in decreasing cigarette use.[129]

The Family Smoking Prevention and Tobacco Control Act, signed into law in 2009, allows the U.S. Food and Drug Administration (FDA) to forbid advertising geared toward children, to lower the amount of nicotine in tobacco products, to ban sweetened cigarettes that appeal to young people, and to prohibit labels such as "light" and "low tar."[130]

One of the most significant impacts of the Family Smoking Prevention and Tobacco Control Act is its requirement for more prominent health warnings on advertising of tobacco products. Beginning June 2010, smokeless tobacco ads now must contain a warning

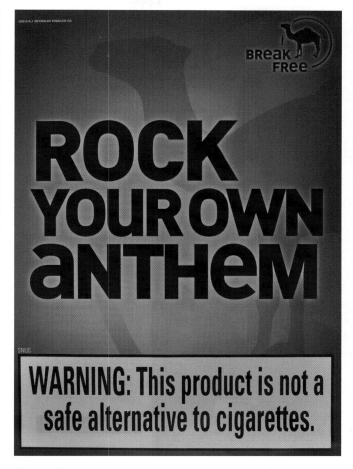

The Family Smoking Prevention and Tobacco Control Act requires that smokeless tobacco ads, such as this full-page magazine ad for Snus, now must contain a warning that fills 20 percent of the advertising space.

that fills 20 percent of the advertising space and, as of June 2011, cigarette packages and advertising are now required to have bigger, stronger warnings. These warnings must cover the top half of the front and back of each package and include "color graphics depicting the negative health consequences of smoking." The graphics are to be modeled on ads in Canada, Australia, and New Zealand that show cancers, lung disease, and other damaging effects of using these products. Even more explicit photos and warnings about the effects of tobacco use will be in place by September 2012.

- **Which policies do you think have been most successful in discouraging tobacco use?**
- **What would you recommend as further steps?**

Quitting the Tobacco Habit

■ **Discuss strategies for quitting tobacco use.**

Approximately 70 percent of adult smokers in the United States want to quit smoking, and up to 44 percent make a serious attempt to quit each year. However, only 4 to 7 percent succeed.[131] Quitting smoking isn't easy, and often involves several unsuccessful attempts before success is finally achieved.

Benefits of Quitting

Many tissues damaged by smoking repair themselves (see **Figure 7.10**). Within 8 hours, carbon monoxide and oxygen levels return to normal, and "smoker's breath" disappears. Within weeks, the mucus that clogs airways is eliminated, and circulation and sense of taste and smell improve. Many ex-smokers have more energy, sleep better, and feel more alert.

After 1 year, risk for lung cancer and stroke decreases. Ex-smokers considerably reduce their chances of developing cancers of the mouth, throat, esophagus, larynx, pancreas, bladder, and cervix, as well as peripheral artery disease, COPD, coronary heart disease,

and ulcers. Women are less likely to bear babies of low birth weight. Within 2 years, the risk for heart attack drops to near normal. After 10 smoke-free years, ex-smokers can expect to live out their normal life span.

Another benefit is money saved. A pack of cigarettes averages $5.28; a pack-a-day smoker burns through $1,921.92 per year. A 40-year-old who quits smoking and puts the savings into a 401(k) earning 9 percent a year would have approximately $250,000 by age 70.

How Can You Quit?

Many people quit "cold turkey"—they simply decide not to smoke again. Others choose programs based on behavior modification and self-reward, treatment centers, or work privately with a physician. Plans that combine several approaches have shown the most promise.

Nicotine addiction may be one of the toughest addictions to overcome. Symptoms of **nicotine withdrawal** include irritability, restlessness, nausea, vomiting, and intense cravings. Pharmacological treatments can help: 25 to 33 percent of people who have used nicotine replacement therapy or smoking-cessation medications continue to abstain from cigarettes for over 6 months.[132]

Nicotine Replacement Products Nontobacco products that replace depleted levels of nicotine in the bloodstream have helped some people stop using tobacco; the dose of nicotine is gradually reduced until the smoker is fully weaned from the drug. Nicotine

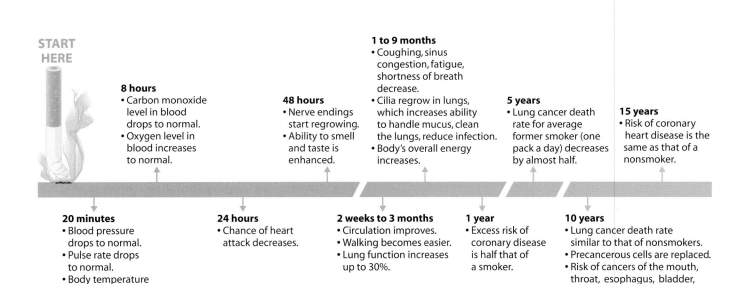

START HERE

8 hours
• Carbon monoxide level in blood drops to normal.
• Oxygen level in blood increases to normal.

48 hours
• Nerve endings start regrowing.
• Ability to smell and taste is enhanced.

1 to 9 months
• Coughing, sinus congestion, fatigue, shortness of breath decrease.
• Cilia regrow in lungs, which increases ability to handle mucus, clean the lungs, reduce infection.
• Body's overall energy increases.

5 years
• Lung cancer death rate for average former smoker (one pack a day) decreases by almost half.

15 years
• Risk of coronary heart disease is the same as that of a nonsmoker.

20 minutes
• Blood pressure drops to normal.
• Pulse rate drops to normal.
• Body temperature of hands and feet increases to normal.

24 hours
• Chance of heart attack decreases.

2 weeks to 3 months
• Circulation improves.
• Walking becomes easier.
• Lung function increases up to 30%.

1 year
• Excess risk of coronary disease is half that of a smoker.

10 years
• Lung cancer death rate similar to that of nonsmokers.
• Precancerous cells are replaced.
• Risk of cancers of the mouth, throat, esophagus, bladder, kidney, and pancreas decreases.

Figure 7.10 When Smokers Quit

Will quitting smoking reverse the damage that's already done?

When you quit using tobacco, your body immediately starts to repair the damage. Over time, the body's repair processes reduce the former smoker's risks of heart disease and cancer; after 10 years, heart disease and lung cancer risks are comparable to those of nonsmokers.

gum delivers about as much nicotine as a cigarette but doesn't produce the same rush. Users experience no withdrawal symptoms and fewer cravings. Nicotine lozenges, like the gum, are available over the counter. The nicotine patch is a small, thin patch placed on the smoker's upper body that delivers a continuous flow of nicotine through the skin, helping relieve cravings. Some insurance plans will pay for the patch.

Nicotine nasal spray, which requires a prescription, is much more powerful. Patients must be careful not to overdose; as little as 40 mg of nicotine at once could be lethal. The spray should be used for no more than 3 months and never for more than 6 months, so smokers don't find themselves dependent on it; also, those with nasal or sinus problems, allergies, or asthma shouldn't use the spray. The nicotine inhaler also requires a prescription. The smoker inhales air saturated with nicotine, which is absorbed through the lining of the mouth, entering the body much more slowly than the nicotine in cigarettes does.

Smoking-Cessation Medications Some smoking-cessation aids are aimed at reducing withdrawal symptoms and decreasing cravings. Zyban (buproprion) is an antidepressant thought to work on dopamine and norepinephrine receptors in the brain. Chantix (varenicline) reduces cravings and the urge to smoke while blocking the effects of nicotine at receptor sites in the brain. NicVAX, a vaccine now in clinical trials, is intended to prevent nicotine from reaching the brain, making smoking less pleasurable and therefore easier to give up. In early trials, twice as many people given the vaccine had quit smoking as those given the placebo.[133]

Therapy For some smokers, the road to quitting includes psychological therapy. Operant conditioning often pairs the act of smoking with an external stimulus; in one technique, smokers carry a timer that sounds a buzzer at intervals. When the buzzer sounds, the patient is required to smoke a cigarette. Once the smoker is conditioned to associate the sound with smoking, the buzzer is eliminated and, one hopes, so is the smoking. Self-control strategies, meanwhile view smoking as a learned habit associated with specific situations such as driving, studying, drinking, or watching TV. Therapy is aimed at identifying these situations and teaching smokers the skills necessary to resist smoking.

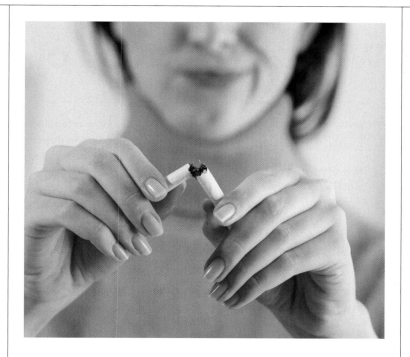

Skills for Behavior Change

TIPS FOR QUITTING SMOKING

If you're a smoker and you're ready to quit, try these tips:

- Use the four Ds: Delay (put off smoking for 10 minutes, then another 10 after that, etc.), Deep breathing, Drink water, Do something else.
- Keep "mouth toys" like hard candy, gum, toothpicks, and carrot sticks handy.
- If you've had trouble stopping before, ask your doctor about nicotine gum, patches, nasal sprays, inhalers, or lozenges.
- Have your teeth cleaned.
- Examine associations that trigger your urge to smoke.
- Tell family and friends that you've stopped so they won't offer you cigarettes.
- Spend time in places that prohibit smoking.
- To shake up your routine and distract you from smoking, take up a new sport, hobby, or organizational commitment.
- Throw out your cigarettes or keep them in a place that makes smoking inconvenient, such as in the freezer or at a friend's house.

check yourself

- **What are the benefits of stopping the use of tobacco products?**
- **Discuss products that can help people stop using tobacco.**
- **Discuss strategies that can help smokers break the habit of smoking.**

What's Your Risk of Alcohol Abuse?

An interactive version of this assessment is available online. Download it from the Live It! section of www.pearsonhighered.com/donatelle.

1. **How often do you have a drink containing alcohol?**
   - ⓪ Never
   - ① Monthly or less
   - ② 2 to 4 times a month
   - ③ 2 to 3 times a week
   - ④ 4 or more times a week

2. **How many alcoholic drinks do you have on a typical day when you are drinking?**
   - ⓪ 1 or 2
   - ① 3 or 4
   - ② 5 or 6
   - ③ 7 to 9
   - ④ 10 or more

3. **How often do you have six drinks or more on one occasion?**
   - ⓪ Never
   - ① Less than monthly
   - ② Monthly
   - ③ Weekly
   - ④ Daily or almost daily

4. **How often during the past year have you been unable to stop drinking once you had started?**
   - ⓪ Never
   - ① Less than monthly
   - ② Monthly
   - ③ Weekly
   - ④ Daily or almost daily

5. **How often during the past year have you failed to do what was normally expected of you because of drinking?**
   - ⓪ Never
   - ① Less than monthly
   - ② Monthly
   - ③ Weekly
   - ④ Daily or almost daily

6. **How often during the past year have you needed a first drink in the morning to get yourself going after a heavy drinking session?**
   - ⓪ Never
   - ① Less than monthly
   - ② Monthly
   - ③ Weekly
   - ④ Daily or almost daily

7. **How often during the past year have you had a feeling of guilt or remorse after drinking?**
   - ⓪ Never
   - ① Less than monthly
   - ② Monthly
   - ③ Weekly
   - ④ Daily or almost daily

8. **How often during the past year have you been unable to remember what happened the night before because you had been drinking?**
   - ⓪ Never
   - ① Less than monthly
   - ② Monthly
   - ③ Weekly
   - ④ Daily or almost daily

9. **Have you or someone else been injured as a result of your drinking?**
   - ⓪ No
   - ① Yes, but not in the past year
   - ② Yes, during the past year

10. **Has a relative, friend, or health care professional been concerned about your drinking or suggested you cut down?**
    - ⓪ No
    - ① Yes, but not in the past year
    - ② Yes, during the past year

Scoring

Scores above 8: Your drinking patterns are putting you at high risk for illness, unsafe sexual situations, or alcohol-related injuries, and may even affect your academic performance.

Source: Taken from the AUDIT Manual, box 4, p. 17, World Health Organization, Division of Mental Health and Prevention of Substance Abuse. http://whqlibdoc.who.int/hq/2001/WHO_MSD_MSB_01.6a.pdf. Copyright © 2001 World Health Organization. Used with permission.

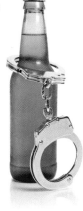

Chapter 7 | Alcohol and Tobacco

Your Plan for Change

The Assess Yourself activity gave you a chance to evaluate your alcohol use. If some of your answers concerned you, consider taking steps to change your behavior.

Today, You Can:

○ Start a diary of your drinking habits—how much you drink, how much money you spend on drinks, and how you feel when you are drinking.

○ Spend some time thinking about the ways your family members use alcohol. Consider whether your current alcohol use is healthy, or whether it is likely to create problems for you in the future.

Within the Next 2 Weeks, You Can:

○ Make your first drink a nonalcoholic beverage the next time you go to a party.

○ Intersperse alcoholic drinks with nonalcoholic beverages to help you pace your consumption.

By the End of the Semester, You Can:

○ Cultivate friendships and explore activities that do not center on alcohol. If your current group of friends drinks heavily, and it is becoming a problem for you, you may need to step back.

Assessyourself

Are You Nicotine Dependent?

An interactive version of this assessment is available online. Download it from the Live It! section of www.pearsonhighered.com/donatelle.

Many social smokers (who often consider themselves nonsmokers) may be more addicted to nicotine than they think. Do you have a dependence on nicotine? Take the following quiz to see.

		Points	
1.	How soon after you wake do you smoke your first cigarette?	0	After 60 min
		1	31–60 min
		2	6–30 min
		3	Within 5 min
2.	Do you find it difficult to refrain from smoking in places where it is forbidden?	0	No
		1	Yes
3.	Which cigarette would you hate most to give up?	0	The first one in the morning
		1	Any other
4.	How many cigarettes a day do you smoke?	0	10 or fewer
		1	11–20
		2	21–30
		3	31 or more
5.	Do you smoke more frequently during the first hours after awakening than during the rest of the day?	0	No
		1	Yes
6.	Do you smoke even if you are so ill that you are in bed most of the day?	0	No
		1	Yes

Interpreting Your Score

0–1 points (20% of smokers): You have a very low dependence, and are likely to experience few and light withdrawal symptoms. You should be able to quit without assistance.

2–3 points (30% of smokers): You have a certain degree of dependence and may experience difficult withdrawal symptoms. Many smokers in this group are able to quit by themselves, but medicines can be of help.

4–5 points (30% of smokers): You have above average dependence and a real risk for smoking-related disorders. Smokers in this group commonly experience withdrawal symptoms and often find medicines very helpful in quitting.

6–7 points (15% of smokers): You have a strong dependence and will likely experience strong withdrawal symptoms. Your risk for smoking-related disorders is high. Both support treatment and medicines (possibly in higher doses and for longer durations) will be important in helping you quit.

8–10 points (5% of smokers): You have extreme dependence and are likely to experience handicapping withdrawal symptoms. Most smokers within this group will already have smoking-related disorders. Support treatment and medications (preferably long term and in high doses) are essential in helping people in this group quit.

Source: T. F. Heatherton, L. T. Kozlowski, R. C. Frecker, and K. O. Fagerstrom, "The Fagerstrom Test for Nicotine Dependence: A Revision of the Fagerstrom Tolerance Questionnaire," *British Journal of Addictions* 86 (1991): 1119–27. Reprinted by permission of Dr. Karl Fagerstrom.

Your Plan for Change

The Assess Yourself activity gave you the chance to evaluate your current smoking habits. Regardless of your current level of nicotine addiction, now is the time to take steps toward kicking the habit.

Today, You Can:

◯ Develop a plan to kick the tobacco habit. The first step in quitting smoking is to identify why you want to quit. Write your reasons down on a sheet of paper.

◯ Think about the times and places you usually smoke. What could you do instead of smoking at those times? Make a list of positive tobacco alternatives.

Within the Next 2 Weeks, You Can:

◯ Say good-bye to your cigarettes. Pick a day to stop smoking, fill out a behavior change contract, and have a family member or friend sign it.

◯ Throw away all your cigarettes, lighters, and ashtrays.

By the End of the Semester, You Can:

◯ Make a list of the good things about not smoking. Carry a copy with you, and look at it whenever you have the urge to smoke.

◯ If you are experiencing difficulty quitting, contact your campus health center or consult with your personal physician to discuss medications or other therapies that may help you quit.

Summary

- Alcohol is a central nervous system (CNS) depressant used by about half of all Americans. Although consumption trends are creeping downward, students are under extreme pressure to consume alcohol.
- Negative consequences associated with alcohol use among college students are academic problems, traffic accidents, dropping out of school, unplanned sex, alcohol poisoning, and injury.
- Alcohol's effect on the body is measured by blood alcohol concentration (BAC), the ratio of alcohol to total blood volume.
- Long-term alcohol overuse can cause nervous system damage, cardiovascular damage, liver disease, and increased cancer risk. Drinking during pregnancy can cause fetal alcohol spectrum disorders (FASDs).
- Alcohol use becomes alcoholism when it interferes with school, work, or relationships or entails legal violations. Causes are biological, social, and cultural.
- Most alcoholics deny having a problem until reaching a major crisis. Treatment options include detoxification at private facilities, therapy, and self-help programs such as Alcoholics Anonymous. Most alcoholics relapse; alcoholism is a behavioral and chemical addiction.
- Tobacco use is widespread in the United States and costs the nation as much as $193 billion per year. Tobacco companies target college students in their marketing campaigns.
- Tobacco is available in smoking and smokeless forms, both of which contain nicotine, an addictive psychoactive substance.
- Hazards of smoking include increased rates of cancer, heart and circulatory disorders, and respiratory and gum diseases. Smoking during pregnancy presents risks for the fetus. Smokeless tobacco dramatically increases oral cancer risk.
- Environmental tobacco smoke (secondhand smoke) puts nonsmokers at risk for cancer and heart disease.
- To quit, smokers must kick a chemical addiction *and* a behavioral habit. Nicotine replacement products or drugs can help wean smokers off nicotine. Therapy methods can also help.

Pop Quiz

1. BAC is the
   a. concentration of plant sugars in the bloodstream.
   b. percentage of alcohol in a beverage.
   c. ratio of alcohol to body weight.
   d. ratio of alcohol to total blood volume.

2. Which of the following statements is *false*?
   a. College students under 21 drink less often than older students but drink more heavily.
   b. College students tend to underestimate the amount their peers drink.
   c. In the past 10 years, the number of female college students reporting being drunk 10 or more times has increased.
   d. Alcohol is involved in at least two-thirds of suicides on campus.

3. The fastest-growing population of alcohol abusers is
   a. older adults.
   b. adolescents.
   c. women.
   d. immigrants.

4. When Amanda goes out with her friends, she usually has four or five beers in a row. This type of high-risk drinking is called
   a. tolerance.
   b. alcoholic addiction.
   c. alcohol overconsumption.
   d. binge drinking.

5. To adapt to his father's alcoholic behavior, Jake played the obedient son. What role did he assume?
   a. Family hero
   b. Mascot
   c. Scapegoat
   d. Lost child

6. What does carbon monoxide do to smokers?
   a. Makes it difficult for a smoker to breathe
   b. Causes dizzy spells and lightheadedness
   c. Reduces the ability of blood hemoglobin to carry oxygen
   d. Impairs the cleaning function of the lung's cilia.

7. What age group is most targeted by tobacco advertisers with free products and social events?
   a. Teenagers 14 to 17
   b. College students 18 to 24
   c. Young adults 25 to 30
   d. Married men 31 to 35

8. What does nicotine do to cilia?
   a. Instantly destroys them
   b. Thickens them
   c. Paralyzes them
   d. Accumulates on them

9. A major health risk of chewing tobacco is
   a. lung cancer.
   b. leukoplakia.
   c. heart disease.
   d. emphysema.

10. Quitting smoking
    a. usually results in minor withdrawal symptoms.
    b. does little to reverse damage to the lungs.
    c. can be aided by nicotine replacement.
    d. is best done by transitioning to "light" cigarettes.

Answers to these questions can be found on page A-1.

Web Links

1. **Alcoholics Anonymous (AA).** General information about AA and the 12-step program. www.aa.org
2. **The Alcohol Calculators.** Calculate the cost of your drinking on a monthly and yearly basis, the calories you consume from alcohol, and your BAC. www.collegedrinkingprevention.gov/CollegeStudents/calculator/default.aspx
3. **American Lung Association.** Information on smoking trends, environmental smoke, and smoking cessation. www.lungusa.org
4. **TIPS (Tobacco Information and Prevention Source).** Information on tobacco use in the United States, with specific information for and about young people. www.cdc.gov/tobacco

Nutrition

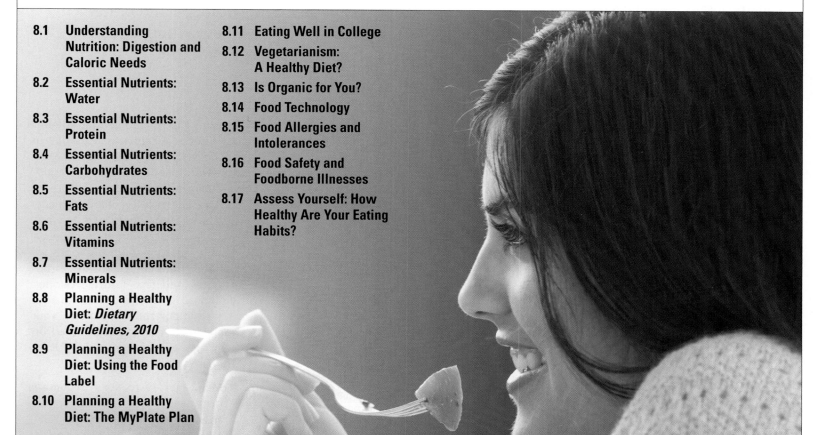

Advice about food can come at us from all directions. Knowing what to eat, how much to eat, and how to choose can be mind-boggling. Why does something so good ultimately end up being a problem for so many? What influences our eating habits and how can we learn to eat more healthfully?

True **hunger** occurs when there is a lack of basic foods. When we're hungry, our brains initiate a physiological response that prompts us to seek food for the energy and **nutrients** our bodies need for proper functioning. Most people in the United States don't know true hunger—most of us eat because of our **appetite,** a learned psychological desire to consume food. Other reasons for eating include cultural and social meanings attached to food, convenience and advertising, habit or custom, emotional eating, perceived nutritional value, social interaction, and financial means.

Nutrition is the science that investigates the relationship between physiological function and the essential elements of the foods we eat. An overwhelming factor in health is on what and how much you eat.

Understanding Nutrition: Digestion and Caloric Needs

- **Describe the digestive process.**
- **Identify daily calorie needs.**

Food provides the chemicals we need for activity and body maintenance. Our bodies cannot synthesize certain *essential nutrients* (or cannot synthesize them in adequate amounts)—we must obtain them from the foods we eat. Before the body can use foods, the digestive system must break down larger food particles into smaller, more usable forms. The sequence of functions by which the body breaks down foods and either absorbs or excretes them is the **digestive process (Figure 8.1)**.

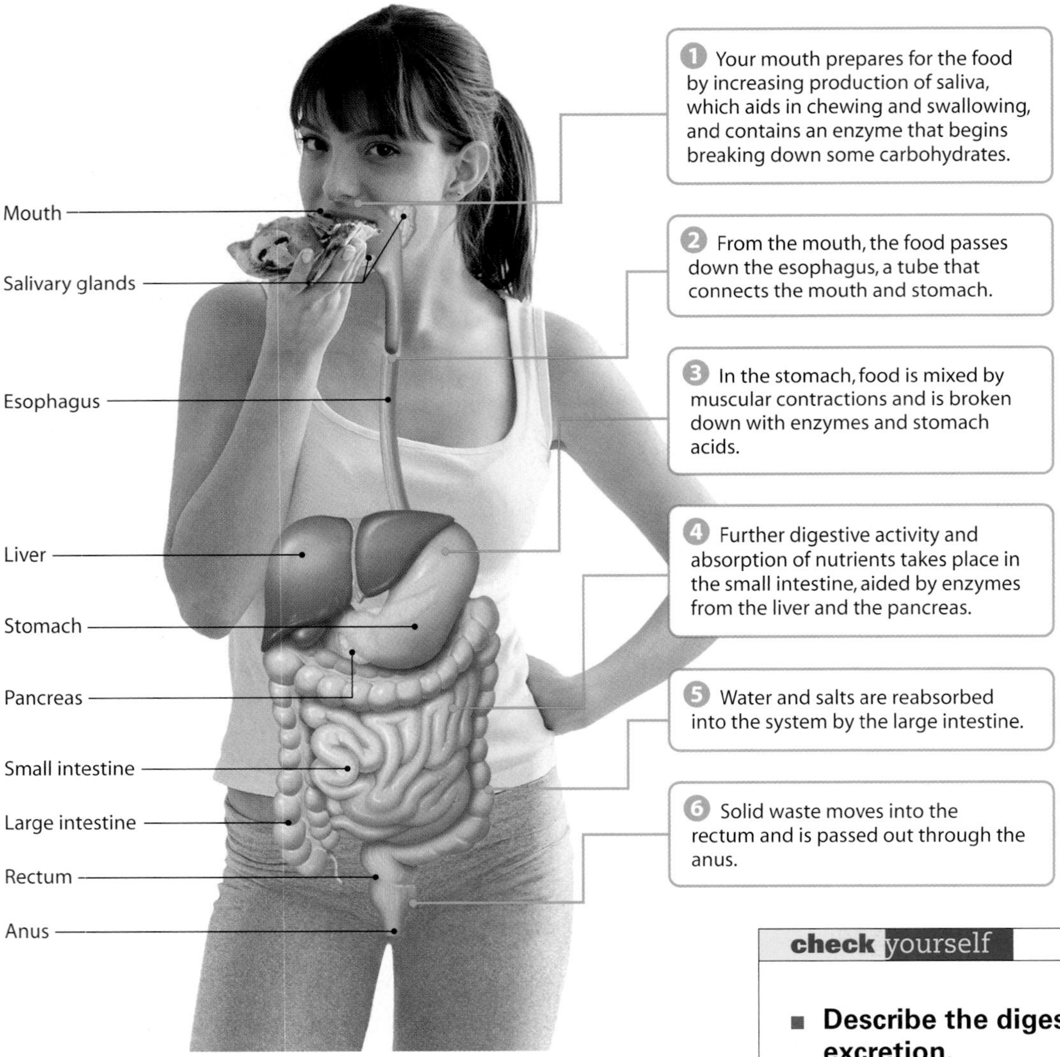

Calories

A kilocalorie is a unit of measure that quantifies the amount of energy in food that the body can use. A **calorie** is also a unit of measure—technically, 1 kilocalorie is equal to 1,000 calories. Most nutrition labels, however, use the word calories to refer to kilocalories. As such, we will use the word calorie throughout this chapter to indicate energy levels of foods. Energy is defined as the capacity to do work. We derive energy from the energy-containing nutrients in the foods we eat. These nutrients—proteins, carbohydrates, and fats—provide calories. Vitamins, minerals, and water do not.

It's important to know your approximate caloric needs, based on your age, gender, and activity level. They are as follows:[1]

- **Men, ages 19 to 30:** A sedentary man needs 2,400 calories per day; an active man requires 3,000.
- **Men, ages 31 to 50:** A sedentary man needs 2,200 calories per day; an active man requires 3,000.
- **Women, ages 19 to 30:** A sedentary woman needs 2,000 calories per day; an active woman requires 2,400.
- **Women, ages 31 to 50:** A sedentary woman needs 1,800 calories per day; an active woman requires 2,200.

(A sedentary person partakes in less than 30 minutes a day of moderate physical activity, whereas an active person partakes in at least an hour a day of physical activity.)

Mouth
Salivary glands
Esophagus
Liver
Stomach
Pancreas
Small intestine
Large intestine
Rectum
Anus

1 Your mouth prepares for the food by increasing production of saliva, which aids in chewing and swallowing, and contains an enzyme that begins breaking down some carbohydrates.

2 From the mouth, the food passes down the esophagus, a tube that connects the mouth and stomach.

3 In the stomach, food is mixed by muscular contractions and is broken down with enzymes and stomach acids.

4 Further digestive activity and absorption of nutrients takes place in the small intestine, aided by enzymes from the liver and the pancreas.

5 Water and salts are reabsorbed into the system by the large intestine.

6 Solid waste moves into the rectum and is passed out through the anus.

Figure 8.1 The Digestive Process
The entire digestive process takes approximately 24 hours.

- **Describe the digestive process, from mouth to excretion.**
- **What are your estimated daily calorie needs?**

Essential Nutrients: Water

learning outcomes

■ **Explain the functions of water in the body.**

The average person can go for weeks without food or certain vitamins and minerals before experiencing serious deficiency symptoms. However, **dehydration**, or abnormal depletion of body fluids, can cause serious problems within a matter of hours and death after a few days. Too much water—*hyponatremia*—can also pose a serious risk.

The human body consists of 50 to 60 percent water by weight. The water in our system bathes cells, aids in fluid and electrolyte balance, maintains pH balance, and transports molecules and cells throughout the body. Water is the major component of blood, which carries oxygen and nutrients to the tissues, removes metabolic wastes, and keeps cells in working order.

Individual needs for water vary according to dietary factors, age, size, overall health, environmental temperature and humidity, and exercise. For the most part, scientists now refute the conventional wisdom that you need to drink eight glasses of water per day;[2] most people can meet their hydration needs simply by eating a healthy diet and drinking in response to thirst. The general recommendations for women are approximately 11 cups of total water from all beverages and foods each day; for men, 16 cups.[3]

About 20 percent of our daily water needs are met through the food we eat. Fruits and vegetables are 80 to 95 percent water, meats more than 50 percent water, and bread and cheese about 35 percent water! Contrary to popular opinion, caffeinated drinks, including coffee, tea, and soda, also count toward total fluid intake for those who regularly consume them. Caffeinated beverages have not been found to dehydrate people whose bodies are used to caffeine.

Of course, there are situations in which a person needs additional fluids to stay properly hydrated. It is important to drink extra fluids when you have a fever or an illness in which there is vomiting or diarrhea. People with kidney problems, diabetes, or cystic fibrosis may need more water, as may the elderly and very young. When the weather heats up or when you sweat profusely, extra water is needed to keep your core temperature within a normal range; see the American College of Sports Medicine guidelines on exercise and fluid replacement at www.acsm.org.[4]

Bottled Water: Who Pays the Price?

Bottled water is now our second most popular drink, right behind soda, with over $100 billion in sales each year. Between 1976 and 2009, annual per person consumption of bottled water went from 1.6 to 27.6 gallons.[5]

We may imagine that bottled water comes from pristine mountain streams, but the fact is that most of the water sold in bottles comes from municipal water supplies. Ordinary tap water in the United States is among the safest in the world, largely because it is subject to legally mandated strict and constant monitoring. Bottled water, meanwhile, is considered a "food" and requires much less frequent monitoring for safety and quality.

The environmental and social consequences of bottled water are significant.[6] Meeting today's demand for bottled water takes approximately 18 million barrels of oil and 130 billion gallons of fresh water each year. When you include the resource cost of transporting bottled water, the total energy required to create and transport every bottle is the equivalent of filling that bottle one-quarter full of oil. And companies taking part in the bottled water boom are buying water supplies throughout the world for financial gain, leaving entire populations vulnerable to water shortages.

The bottles themselves raise other issues. In 2006, more than 900,000 tons of plastic were used to package 8 billion gallons of bottled water. Chemicals found in plastic bottles can leach into the water, particularly bisphenol-A (BPA). Research has suggested links between BPA and negative estrogen-related effects, including breast enlargement in young boys, some forms of cancer, early onset of puberty, and increased risk for type 2 diabetes.[7]

You can help curb the personal and global environmental threats caused by bottled water use. Don't buy bottled water unless absolutely necessary; purchase and reuse a washable stainless steel or glass container. Recycle the plastic you do use. Encourage your campus to install water dispensers rather than selling bottled water; find out about other steps you can take at www.beyondthebottle.org.

It's important to drink adequate amounts of fluid daily. A stainless steel bottle that you can reuse is a better choice than buying plastic bottles every day.

check yourself

■ **Why is water considered an essential nutrient?**

Essential Nutrients: Protein

- **Describe the functions of protein in the body.**
- **List sources of protein.**

Next to water, **proteins** are the most abundant substances in the human body. Proteins are major components of nearly every cell; they've been called the "body builders" because of their role in developing and repairing bone, muscle, skin, and blood cells. They are the key elements of antibodies that protect us from disease, of enzymes that control chemical activities in the body, and of hormones that regulate body functions. Proteins help transport iron, oxygen, and nutrients to all body cells and supply another source of energy to cells when fats and carbohydrates are not available. Adequate amounts of protein in the diet are vital to many body functions and ultimately to survival.

Your body breaks down proteins into smaller nitrogen-containing **amino acids.** Nine of the 20 amino acids are **essential amino acids,** which the body must obtain from the diet; the other 11 can be produced by the body. Dietary protein that supplies all the essential amino acids is called **complete (high-quality) protein.** Typically, protein from animal products is complete. For proteins to be complete, they also must be present in digestible form and in amounts proportional to body requirements. When we consume foods that are deficient in some of the essential amino acids, the total amount of protein that can be synthesized from the other amino acids is decreased.

Proteins from plant sources are often **incomplete proteins** in that they may lack one or two of the essential amino acids. However, nonmeat eaters can easily eat complementary sources of plant protein (**Figure 8.2**). Plant sources of protein fall into three general categories: *legumes* (e.g., beans, peas, peanuts, and soy products), *grains* (e.g., wheat, corn, rice, and oats), and *nuts and seeds.* Certain vegetables, such as leafy green vegetables and broccoli, also contribute valuable plant proteins. Mixing two or more foods from each of these categories will provide all the essential amino acids necessary to ensure adequate protein absorption.

Although protein deficiency poses a threat to the global population, few Americans suffer from protein deficiencies. In fact, the average American consumes more than 78 grams of protein daily, much of this from high-fat animal flesh and dairy products.[8] The recommended daily protein intake for adults is only 0.8 gram (g) per kilogram (kg) of body weight. To calculate your recommended daily protein intake, divide your body weight (in pounds) by 2.2 to get your weight in kilograms, then multiply by 0.8. The typical recommendation is that in a 2,000-calorie diet, 10 to 35 percent of calories should come from lean protein, for a total average of 50 to 175 grams per day. A 6-ounce steak contains 53 grams of protein—more than the daily needs of an average-sized woman!

A person might need extra protein if she is pregnant, fighting off a serious infection, recovering from surgery or blood loss, or recovering from burns. In these instances, proteins that are lost to

78.1
grams of protein is what the average American consumes daily—much more than the recommended amount.

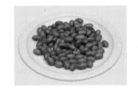
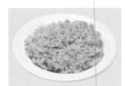

Legumes and grains

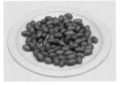
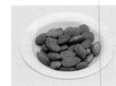

Legumes and nuts and seeds

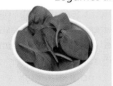
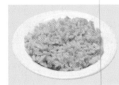

Green leafy vegetables and grains

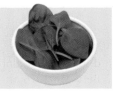
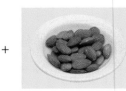

Green leafy vegetables and nuts and seeds

Figure 8.2
Complementary Proteins

Eaten in the right combinations, plant-based foods can provide complementary proteins and all essential amino acids.

BEST CHOICES	GOOD ALTERNATIVES	AVOID
Arctic Char (farmed) Barramundi (US farmed) Catfish (US farmed) Clams (farmed) Cobia (US farmed) Cod: Pacific (US bottom longline) Crab: Dungeness, Stone Halibut: Pacific (US) Lobster: Spiny (US) Mussels (farmed) Oysters (farmed) Sablefish/Black Cod (Alaska and BC) Salmon (Alaska wild) Sardines (US Pacific) Scallops (farmed off-bottom) Shrimp, Pink (OR) Striped Bass (farmed and wild*) Tilapia (US farmed) Trout: Rainbow (US farmed) Tuna: Albacore, Skipjack, Yellowfin (US troll/pole)	Basa/Pangasius/Swai (farmed) Caviar, Sturgeon (US farmed) Clams (wild) Cod: Atlantic (imported) Cod: Pacific (US trawled) Crab: Blue*, King (US), Snow Flounders, Soles (Pacific) Flounder: Summer (US Atlantic)* Grouper: Black, Red (US Gulf of Mexico)* Herring: Atlantic Lobster: American/Maine Mahi Mahi (US) Oysters (wild) Pollock: Alaska Sablefish/Black Cod (CA, OR, WA) Scallops: Sea Shrimp (US, Canada) Squid Swordfish (US)* Tilapia (Central & South America farmed) Tuna: Bigeye, Tongol, Yellowfin (troll/pole)	Caviar, Sturgeon* (imported wild) Chilean Seabass/Toothfish* Cobia (imported farmed) Cod: Atlantic (trawled, Canada and US) Crab: King (imported) Flounders, Halibut, Soles (US Atlantic except Summer Flounder) Groupers (Hawaii, US Atlantic*) Lobster: Spiny (Brazil) Mahi Mahi (imported longline) Marlin: Blue, Striped (Pacific)* Monkfish Orange Roughy* Salmon (farmed, including Atlantic)* Sharks* and Skates Shrimp (imported) Snapper: Red Swordfish (imported)* Tilapia (Asia farmed) Tuna: Albacore*, Bigeye*, Skipjack, Tongol, Yellowfin* (except troll/pole) Tuna: Bluefin* Tuna: Canned (except troll/pole)

Support Ocean-Friendly Seafood

Best Choices are abundant, well-managed and caught or farmed in environmentally friendly ways.

Good Alternatives are an option, but there are concerns with how they're caught or farmed—or with the health of their habitat due to other human impacts.

Avoid for now as these items are caught or farmed in ways that harm other marine life or the environment.

Key
BC = British Columbia   CA = California
OR = Oregon   WA = Washington
*Limit consumption due to concerns about mercury or other contaminants. Visit www.edf.org/seafoodhealth

Contaminant information provided by: ENVIRONMENTAL DEFENSE FUND

Seafood may appear in more than one column

Figure 8.3 Sustainable Seafood Guide
Source: Monterey Bay Aquarium Seafood Watch, *National Sustainable Seafood Guide, July 2011*. Copyright © 2011, Monterey Bay Aquarium. www.montereybayaquarium.org/cr/cr_seafoodwatch/download.aspx. Reprinted with permission.

175

cellular repair and development must be replaced. There is controversy over whether someone in high-level physical training needs additional protein to build and repair muscle fibers or whether normal daily requirements should suffice. In addition, a sedentary person or one who gets little exercise may find it easier to stay in energy balance if more of his calories come from protein and fewer from carbohydrates. Why? Because proteins make a person feel full and satisfied for a longer period of time.

Toward Sustainable Seafood

The U.S. Department of Agriculture recommends consuming fish two or three times per week to reduce saturated fat and cholesterol levels and increase omega-3 fatty acid levels. However, the many environmental concerns surrounding the seafood industry today call into question the sustainability and safety of such consumption. More than 70 percent of the world's natural fishing grounds have been overfished, and whole stretches of the oceans are dead zones where fish and shellfish can no longer live. The 2010 oil spill in the Gulf of Mexico is likely to contribute to seafood shortages and contamination of precious fishing grounds for years to come. In an effort to counteract the loss of wild fish populations, increasing numbers of fish are being farmed, which itself poses additional health risks and environmental concerns. Some farmed fish are laden with antibiotics, while highly concentrated levels of parasites and bacteria from fish farm runoff may enter the ocean and river fish populations through adjacent waterways. And some farmed fish are fed wild fish, resulting in a net loss of fish from the sea.

At the same time, high levels of chemicals, parasites, bacteria, and toxins are also found in many of the fish available on the market. Mercury, a waste product of many industries, binds to proteins and stays in an animal's body, accumulating as it moves up the food chain. In humans, mercury can damage the nervous system and kidneys and cause birth defects and developmental problems. Polychlorinated biphenyls (PCBs), chemicals that can build up in the fatty tissue of fish, are another cause of concern.

Your consumer choices make a difference. Purchasing seafood from regularly inspected, environmentally responsible sources will support fisheries and fish farms that are healthier for you and the environment. Knowing where your fish are caught and the methods by which they are caught is important. Several major environmental groups have developed guides to inform consumers of safe and sustainable seafood choices. **Figure 8.3** lists safe and sustainable seafood choices available for purchase in the United States; this information is also available as a free smartphone or mobile device application at http://mobile.seafoodwatch.org. Another great resource is the FishPhone service: Send a text message to 30644 with the word *FISH* and the type of fish you want to know about, and it will send you information about whether it is safe to eat.

check yourself

- **What are the functions of protein in the body?**
- **What are the best sources of protein?**

Essential Nutrients: Carbohydrates

- **Describe the functions of carbohydrates in the body, including fiber.**
- **List sources of carbohydrates.**

Carbohydrates supply us with the energy needed to sustain normal daily activity. The human body metabolizes carbohydrates more quickly and efficiently than it does proteins for a quick source of energy for the body. Carbohydrates are easily converted to glucose, the fuel for the body's cells. Carbohydrates also play an important role in the functioning of internal organs, the nervous system, and muscles. They are the best fuel for endurance athletics because they provide both an immediate and a time-released energy source; they are digested easily and then consistently metabolized in the bloodstream. There are two major types of carbohydrates: **simple carbohydrates**, or *simple sugars*, which are found naturally in fruits and many vegetables, and **complex carbohydrates**, which are found in grains, cereals, and vegetables.

Simple Carbohydrates

A typical American diet contains large amounts of simple carbohydrates. The most common form is *glucose*. Eventually, the human body converts all types of simple sugars to glucose to provide energy to cells. Another simple sugar is *fructose* (commonly called *fruit sugar*), which is found in fruits and berries. Glucose and fructose are **monosaccharides.**

Disaccharides are combinations of two monosaccharides. Perhaps the best-known example is *sucrose* (granulated table sugar). *Lactose* (milk sugar), found in milk and milk products, and *maltose* (malt sugar) are other common disaccharides. Disaccharides must be broken down into monosaccharides before the body can use them.

Americans typically consume far too many refined carbohydrates (i.e., carbohydrates containing only sugars and starches, discussed below), which have few health benefits and are a major

factor in our growing epidemic of overweight and obesity. Many of the simple sugars in these foods come from *added sugars*, sweeteners put in during processing to flavor foods, make sodas taste good, and ease our craving for sweets. A classic example is the amount of added sugar in one can of soda: more than 10 teaspoons per can! All that refined sugar can cause tooth decay and put on pounds.

Sugar is found in high amounts in a wide range of food products. Such diverse items as ketchup, barbecue sauce, and flavored coffee creamers derive 30 to 65 percent of their calories from sugar. Knowing what foods contain these sugars, considering the amounts you consume each day that are hidden in foods, and then trying to reduce these levels can be a great way to reduce excess weight. Read food labels carefully before purchasing. If *sugar* or one of its aliases (including *high fructose corn syrup* and *cornstarch*) appears near the top of the ingredients list, then that product contains a lot of sugar and is probably not your best nutritional bet. Also, most labels list the amount of sugar as a percentage of total calories.

Complex Carbohydrates

Starches and Glycogen Complex carbohydrates, or **polysaccharides,** are formed by long chains of monosaccharides. Like disaccharides, they must be broken down into simple sugars before the body can use them. *Starches, glycogen,* and *fiber* are the main types of complex carbohydrates.

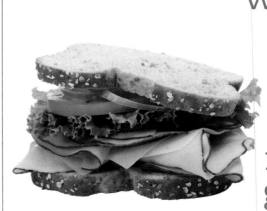

Why are whole grains better than refined grains?

Whole-grain foods contain fiber, a crucial form of carbohydrate that protects against some gastrointestinal disorders and reduces risk for certain cancers. Fiber is also associated with lowered blood cholesterol levels; studies have shown that eating 2.5 servings of whole grains per day can reduce cardiovascular disease risk by as much as 21%. But are people getting the message? One nutrition survey showed that only 8% of U.S. adults consume three or more servings of whole grains each day, and 42% ate no whole grains at all on a given day.

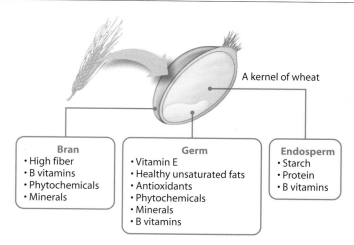

A kernel of wheat

Bran
• High fiber
• B vitamins
• Phytochemicals
• Minerals

Germ
• Vitamin E
• Healthy unsaturated fats
• Antioxidants
• Phytochemicals
• Minerals
• B vitamins

Endosperm
• Starch
• Protein
• B vitamins

Figure 8.4 Anatomy of a Whole Grain
Whole grains are more nutritious than refined grains, because they contain the bran, germ, and endosperm of the seed—sources of fiber, vitamins, minerals, and beneficial phytochemicals (chemical compounds that occur naturally in plants).
Source: Adapted from Joan Salge Blake, Kathy D. Munoz, and Stella Volpe, *Nutrition: From Science to You*, 1st ed., © 2010. Reprinted by permission of Pearson Education, Inc., Upper Saddle River, New Jersey.

Starches, which make up the majority of the complex carbohydrate group, come from flours, breads, pasta, rice, corn, oats, barley, potatoes, and related foods. The body breaks down these complex carbohydrates into the monosaccharide glucose, which can be easily absorbed by cells and used as energy. Polysaccharides can also be stored in body muscles and the liver as **glycogen.** When the body requires a sudden burst of energy, it breaks down glycogen into glucose.

Fiber   **Fiber,** sometimes referred to as "bulk" or "roughage," is the indigestible portion of plant foods that helps move foods through the digestive system, delays absorption of cholesterol and other nutrients, and softens stools by absorbing water. Dietary fiber is found only in plant foods, such as fruits, vegetables, nuts, and grains. The Food and Nutrition Board of the Institute of Medicine makes three fiber distinctions: dietary fiber, functional fiber, and total fiber.[9] *Dietary fiber* comprises the nondigestible parts of plants—the leaves, stems, and seeds. *Functional fiber* consists of nondigestible forms of carbohydrates that may come from plants or may be manufactured in the laboratory and have known health benefits. *Total fiber* is the sum of dietary fiber and functional fiber in a person's diet.

A more user-friendly classification of fiber types divides fibers into *soluble* and *insoluble* fibers. Soluble fibers, such as pectins, gums, and mucilages, dissolve in water, form gel-like substances, and can be digested easily by bacteria in the colon. Major food sources of soluble fiber include citrus fruits, berries, oat bran, dried beans (e.g., kidney, garbanzo, pinto, and navy beans), and some vegetables. Insoluble fibers, such as lignins and cellulose, are those that typically do not dissolve in water and that cannot be fermented by bacteria in the colon. They are found in most fruits and vegetables and in **whole grains,** such as brown rice, wheat, bran, and whole-grain breads and cereals (see **Figure 8.4**).

Despite growing evidence supporting the benefits of whole grains and high-fiber diets, fiber intake among the general public remains low. Most experts believe that Americans should double

their current consumption of dietary fiber—to 20 to 35 grams per day for most people and perhaps to 40 to 50 grams for others. To increase your fiber intake, eat fewer refined or processed carbohydrates in favor of more whole grains, fruits, vegetables, legumes, nuts, and seeds. If you haven't been eating enough fiber, however, make any such change gradually—in this case, too much of a good thing too quickly can pose problems. Sudden increases in dietary fiber may cause flatulence (intestinal gas), cramping, or bloating. Consume plenty of water or other (sugar-free!) liquids to reduce such side effects.

Fiber-rich diets can also help protect against colon and rectal cancer[10] and prevent the development of precancerous growths. Fiber also protects against constipation and diverticulosis (a condition in which tiny bulges form on the large intestinal wall and can become irritated under strain from constipation). Insoluble fiber helps reduce constipation and discomfort by absorbing moisture and producing softer stools. In addition, fiber helps reduce blood cholesterol,[11] primarily by lowering low-density lipoprotein (LDL) or "bad" cholesterol;[12] lower LDL offers protection against heart disease.[13] Soluble fiber also improves control of blood sugar and can reduce the need for insulin or medication in people with type 2 diabetes.[14] And because most high-fiber foods are high in carbohydrates and low in fat, they help control caloric intake for those wishing to lose unhealthy weight. Fiber also stays in the digestive tract longer than other nutrients, making you feel full sooner.

Skills for Behavior Change

BULK UP YOUR FIBER INTAKE!

To increase your intake of dietary fiber:

■ Whenever possible, select whole-grain breads low in fat and sugars, with 3 or more grams of fiber per serving. Read labels—just because bread is brown doesn't mean it's better for you.

■ Eat whole, unpeeled fruits and vegetables rather than drinking their juices. The fiber in whole fruit tends to slow blood sugar increases and helps you feel full longer.

■ Substitute whole-grain pastas, bagels, and pizza crust for the refined, white flour versions.

■ Add wheat crumbs or grains to meat loaf and burgers to increase fiber intake.

■ Toast grains to bring out their nutty flavor and make foods more appealing.

■ Sprinkle ground flaxseed on cereals, yogurt, and salads or add it to casseroles, burgers, and baked goods. Flaxseeds have a mild flavor and are also high in beneficial fatty acids.

check yourself

■ **What are the functions of carbohydrates in the body?**

■ **What are the preferred sources of carbohydrates?**

■ **Why is fiber important in the diet?**

Essential Nutrients: Fats

learning outcomes

■ **Describe the functions of fats in the body.**

■ **List sources of fats.**

Fats are perhaps the most misunderstood required nutrients. This most energy-dense source of calories plays a vital role in maintaining healthy skin and hair, insulating body organs against shock, maintaining body temperature, and promoting healthy cell function. Fats make foods taste better and carry vitamins A, D, E, and K to cells. They provide concentrated energy in the absence of sufficient carbohydrates. So why are we constantly urged to cut back on fats? Because some fats are less healthy than others, and because excessive consumption of fats can lead to weight gain.

Triglycerides, which make up about 95 percent of total body fat, are the most common form of fat circulating in the blood. When we consume too many calories from any source, the liver converts the excess into triglycerides, which are stored throughout our bodies. The remaining 5 percent of body fat is composed of substances such as **cholesterol**. The ratio of total cholesterol to a group of compounds called **high-density lipoproteins (HDLs)** is important in determining risk for heart disease. Lipoproteins facilitate transport of cholesterol in the blood. HDLs can transport more cholesterol than can **low-density lipoproteins (LDLs)**. Whereas LDLs transport cholesterol to the body's cells, HDLs transport circulating cholesterol to the liver for metabolism and elimination. People with a high percentage of HDLs appear to be at lower risk for developing cholesterol-clogged arteries.

Types of Dietary Fats

Fat molecules include *fatty acid* chains of carbon and hydrogen atoms. Fatty acid chains that cannot hold any more hydrogen in their chemical structure are called **saturated fats**. These generally come from animal sources such as meat, dairy, and poultry and are solid at room temperature. **Unsaturated fats** have room for additional hydrogen atoms in their chemical structure and are liquid at room temperature. They come from plants and include most vegetable oils.

The terms *monounsaturated fatty acids (MUFAs)* and *polyunsaturated fatty acids (PUFAs)* refer to the relative number of hydrogen atoms missing in a fatty acid chain. Peanut and olive oils are high in

monounsaturated fats. Corn, sunflower, and safflower oils are high in polyunsaturated fats.

There is currently controversy about which unsaturated fats are most beneficial. Monounsaturated fatty acids, such as olive oil, which seem to lower LDL levels and increase HDL levels, are currently preferred. **Figure 8.5** shows fats in common vegetable oils.

Polyunsaturated fatty acids come in two forms: *omega-3 fatty acids* (in many fatty fish) and *omega-6 fatty acids* (in corn, soybean, and cottonseed oils). Some researchers believe PUFAs may decrease both harmful LDL cholesterol *and* beneficial HDL cholesterol. However, two PUFAs are *essential fatty acids*—we must receive them from our diets. *Linoleic acid*, an omega-6 fatty acid, and *alpha-linolenic acid*, an omega-3 fatty acid, are needed to make hormone-like compounds that control immune function, pain perception, and inflammation and reduce CVD risks.[15]

It is believed that early humans ate a diet of approximately equal portions of omega-6 to omega-3. Today, Americans consume a ratio

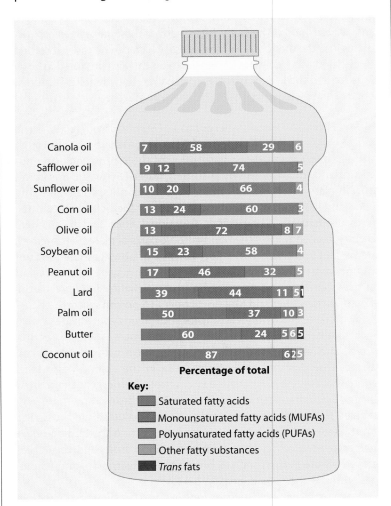

Figure 8.5 Percentages of Saturated, Polyunsaturated, Monounsaturated, and *Trans* Fats in Common Vegetable Oils

of approximately 10:1 omega-6 to omega-3 fats.[16] Recently, an American Heart Association advisory panel stated concern over people reducing omega-6 when instead the focus should be on limiting saturated fat.[17] About 20 to 35 percent of calories should come from fat, with 5 to 10 percent coming from omega-6 fatty acids.

Avoiding *Trans* Fatty Acids

For decades, Americans shunned butter, red meat, and other foods because of their saturated fats. What they didn't know is that foods low in saturated fat, such as margarine, could be just as harmful. As early as the 1990s, Dutch researchers reported that a form of fat known as *trans* fats increased LDL cholesterol levels while decreasing HDL cholesterol levels.[18] In a more recent study, just a 2 percent caloric intake of *trans* fats was associated with a 23 percent increased risk for heart disease and a 47 percent increased chance of sudden cardiac death.[19]

***Trans* fats (*trans* fatty acids)** are produced by adding hydrogen molecules to liquid oil, making "partially hydrogenated" fats that stay solid or semisolid at room temperature. These change into irregular shapes at the molecular level, priming them to clog up arteries. *Trans* fats have been used in margarines, many commercial baked goods, and restaurant deep-fried foods.

In 2006, the U.S. Food and Drug Administration (FDA) began to require *trans* fat labeling on all foods. In July 2008, a California law stipulated that as of January 2010, all oils, margarines, and shortenings used for frying in restaurants must contain less than 0.5 percent *trans* fat per serving.[20] Today, *trans* fats are being removed from most foods; if they *are* present, they must be clearly indicated on food labels as *partially hydrogenated oils, fractionated oils, shortening, lard,* or *hydrogenation.*

Is More Fat Ever Better?

Despite all this, some studies have shown that when comparing low-fat diets to other diets, there are few improvements in weight loss and blood fat measures.[21]

228,000

deaths related to coronary heart disease could be averted each year by reducing Americans' consumption of *trans* fats, according to some estimates.

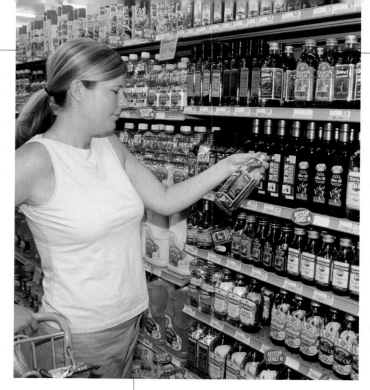

Are all fats bad for me?

All fats are not the same, and your body needs some fat to function healthily. Try to reduce saturated fats, those that come in meat, dairy, and poultry products; avoid *trans* fats, those that can come in stick margarine, commercially baked goods, and deep-fried foods; and replace these with monounsaturated fats, such as those in peanut and olive oils.

The bottom line is that moderation is the key. No more than 7 to 10 percent of total calories should come from saturated fat and no more than 35 percent from all forms of fat. Follow these dietary guidelines to add more healthy fats while reducing less healthy fats:

- Eat sustainable fatty seafood (bluefish, herring, mackerel, salmon, sardines, or tuna) at least twice weekly.
- Substitute olive, soy, and canola oils for corn, safflower, and sunflower oils when you need an oil (remember that each tablespoon of olive oil is 100 calories).
- Add green leafy vegetables, walnuts, walnut oil, and ground flaxseed to your diet.
- Read the Nutrition Facts Panel on foods. No more than 10 percent of your total calories should come from saturated fat, and no more than 30 percent from all fats.
- Chill soups and stews, scrape off any fat that hardens on top, then reheat to serve.
- Fill up on fruits and vegetables.
- Avoid margarine products with *trans* fatty acids. Whenever possible, opt for fresh vegetable spreads, sugar-free jams, fat-free cheese, and other healthy toppings.
- Choose lean meats, fish, or skinless poultry. Broil or bake whenever possible. Drain off fat after cooking.
- Choose fewer cold cuts, bacon, sausages, hot dogs, and organ meats.
- Select nonfat and low-fat dairy products.
- When cooking, use substitutes for butter, margarine, oils, sour cream, mayonnaise, and full-fat salad dressings. Chicken or beef broth, fresh herbs, wine, vinegar, and low-calorie dressings provide flavor with less fat.

check yourself

- **What are the functions of fats in the body?**
- **What are more and less healthful sources of fats?**

Essential Nutrients: Vitamins

learning outcomes

■ **Describe the functions of vitamins in the body.**

■ **List key vitamins and some recommended food sources for each.**

Vitamins are potent and essential organic compounds that promote growth and help maintain life and health. They help maintain nerves and skin, produce blood cells, build bones and teeth, heal wounds, and convert food energy to body energy.

Vitamins can be *fat soluble* (absorbed through the intestinal tract with the help of fats) or *water soluble* (dissolvable in water). See **Table 8.1** for the fat-soluble vitamins and **Table 8.2** for the water-soluble vitamins. Vitamins A, D, E, and K are fat soluble; C and B-complex vitamins are water soluble. Fat-soluble vitamins tend to be stored in the body; over-

accumulation in the liver may cause cirrhosis-like symptoms. Water-soluble vitamins generally are excreted and cause few toxicity problems.

Some people believe that **functional foods** may prevent or cure disease. Many functional foods contain **antioxidants** or other *phytochemicals* (from the Greek "plant"). Among the more commonly cited nutrients touted as providing a protective antioxidant effect are vitamin C, vitamin E, and beta-carotene, a precursor to vitamin A; these appear to protect against cell damage. **Carotenoids** are vegetable pigments such as *lycopene* (in tomatoes, papaya, pink grapefruit, and guava) and *lutein* (in leafy greens and Brussels sprouts). Few clearly established benefits of functional foods have been demonstrated, although researchers are investigating their effects on conditions such as cancer, CVD, and stroke.

TABLE 8.1 A Guide to Fat-Soluble Vitamins

Vitamin Name and Recommended Intake	Reliable Food Sources	Primary Functions	Toxicity/Deficiency Symptoms
VITAMIN A RDA: Men = 900 µg Women = 700 µg UL = 3,000 µg/day	Preformed retinol: beef and chicken liver, egg yolks, milk Carotenoid precursors: spinach, carrots, mango, apricots, cantaloupe, pumpkin, yams	Required for ability of eyes to adjust to changes in light; protects color vision; assists cell differentiation; required for sperm production in men and fertilization in women; contributes to healthy bone and healthy immune system	**Toxicity:** fatigue, bone and joint pain, spontaneous abortion and birth defects of fetuses in pregnant women, nausea and diarrhea, liver damage, nervous system damage, blurred vision, hair loss, skin disorders **Deficiency:** night blindness, xerophthalmia; impaired growth, immunity, and reproductive function
VITAMIN D AI (assumes that person does not get adequate sun exposure): Adult 19–50 = 5 µg/day Adult 50–70 = 10 µg/day Adult > 70 = 15 µg/day UL = 50 µg/day	Canned salmon and mackerel, milk, fortified cereals	Regulates blood calcium levels, maintains bone health, assists cell differentiation	**Toxicity:** hypercalcemia **Deficiency:** rickets in children; osteomalacia and/or osteoporosis in adults
VITAMIN E RDA: Men = 15 mg/day Women = 15 mg/day UL = 1,000 mg/day	Sunflower seeds, almonds, vegetable oils, fortified cereals	As a powerful antioxidant, protects cell membranes, polyunsaturated fatty acids, and vitamin A from oxidation; protects white blood cells; enhances immune function; improves absorption of vitamin A	**Toxicity:** rare **Deficiency:** hemolytic anemia; impairment of nerve, muscle, and immune function
VITAMIN K AI: Men = 120 µg/day Women = 90 µg/day	Kale, spinach, turnip greens, Brussels sprouts	Serves as a coenzyme during production of specific proteins that assist in blood coagulation and bone metabolism	**Toxicity:** none known **Deficiency:** impaired blood clotting; possible effect on bone health

Note: RDA = Recommended Daily Allowance; AI = Adequate Intakes; UL = Tolerable Upper Level Intakes. Values are for all adults aged 19 and older, except as noted. Values increase among women who are pregnant or lactating.

Source: Adapted from Janice Thompson and Melinda Manore, *Nutrition: An Applied Approach,* 2nd ed., © 2009. Reprinted by permission of Pearson Education, Inc., Upper Saddle River, New Jersey.

TABLE

8.2

A Guide to Water-Soluble Vitamins

Vitamin Name and Recommended Intake	Reliable Food Sources	Primary Functions	Toxicity/Deficiency Symptoms
THIAMIN (VITAMIN B₁) RDA: Men = 1.2 mg/day Women = 1.1 mg/day	Pork, fortified cereals, enriched rice and pasta, peas, tuna, legumes	Required as enzyme cofactor for carbohydrate and amino acid metabolism	**Toxicity:** none known **Deficiency:** beriberi, fatigue, apathy, decreased memory, confusion, irritability, muscle weakness
RIBOFLAVIN (VITAMIN B2) RDA: Men = 1.3 mg/day Women = 1.1 mg/day	Beef liver, shrimp, milk and dairy foods, fortified cereals, enriched breads and grains	Required as enzyme cofactor for carbohydrate and fat metabolism	**Toxicity:** none known **Deficiency:** ariboflavinosis, swollen mouth and throat, seborrheic dermatitis, anemia
NIACIN, NICOTINAMIDE, NICOTINIC ACID RDA: Men = 16 mg/day Women = 14 mg/day UL = 35 mg/day	Beef liver, most cuts of meat/fish/poultry, fortified cereals, enriched breads and grains, canned tomato products	Required for carbohydrate and fat metabolism; plays role in DNA replication and repair and cell differentiation	**Toxicity:** flushing, liver damage, glucose intolerance, blurred vision differentiation **Deficiency:** pellagra; vomiting, constipation, or diarrhea; apathy
VITAMIN B6 (PYRIDOXINE, PYRIDOXAL, PYRIDOXAMINE) RDA: Men and women 19–50 = 1.3 mg/day Men > 50 = 1.7 mg/day Women > 50 = 1.5 mg/day UL = 100 mg/day	Chickpeas (garbanzo beans), most cuts of meat/fish/poultry, fortified cereals, white potatoes	Required as enzyme cofactor for carbohydrate and amino acid metabolism; assists synthesis of blood cells	**Toxicity:** nerve damage, skin lesions **Deficiency:** anemia; seborrheic dermatitis; depression, confusion, and convulsions
FOLATE (FOLIC ACID) RDA: Men = 400 µg/day Women = 400 µg/day UL = 1,000 µg/day	Fortified cereals, enriched breads and grains, spinach, legumes (lentils, chickpeas, pinto beans), greens (spinach, romaine lettuce), liver	Required as enzyme cofactor for amino acid metabolism; required for DNA synthesis; involved in metabolism of homocysteine	**Toxicity:** masks symptoms of vitamin B₁₂ deficiency, specifically signs of nerve damage **Deficiency:** macrocytic anemia; neural tube defects in a developing fetus; elevated homocysteine levels
VITAMIN B12 (COBALAMIN) RDA: Men = 2.4 µg/day Women = 2.4 µg/day	Shellfish, all cuts of meat/fish/poultry, milk and dairy foods, fortified cereals	Assists with formation of blood; required for healthy nervous system function; involved as enzyme cofactor in metabolism of homocysteine	**Toxicity:** none known **Deficiency:** pernicious anemia; tingling and numbness of extremities; nerve damage; memory loss, disorientation, and dementia
PANTOTHENIC ACID AI: Men = 5 mg/day Women = 5 mg/day	Meat/fish/poultry, shiitake mushrooms, fortified cereals, egg yolks	Assists with fat metabolism	**Toxicity:** none known **Deficiency:** rare
BIOTIN RDA: Men = 30 µg/day Women = 30 µg/day	Nuts, egg yolks	Involved as enzyme cofactor in carbohydrate, fat, and protein metabolism	**Toxicity:** none known **Deficiency:** rare
VITAMIN C (ASCORBIC ACID) RDA: Men = 90 mg/day Women = 75 mg/day Smokers = 35 mg more per day than RDA UL = 2,000 mg	Sweet peppers, citrus fruits and juices, broccoli, strawberries, kiwi	Antioxidant in extracellular fluid and lungs; regenerates oxidized vitamin E; assists with collagen synthesis; enhances immune function; assists in synthesis of hormones, neurotransmitters, and DNA; enhances iron absorption	**Toxicity:** nausea and diarrhea, nosebleeds, increased oxidative damage, increased formation of kidney stones in people with kidney disease **Deficiency:** scurvy, bone pain and fractures, depression, and anemia

Note: RDA = Recommended Daily Allowance; AI = Adequate Intakes; UL = Tolerable Upper Level Intakes. Values are for all adults aged 19 and older, except as noted. Values increase among women who are pregnant or lactating.
Source: Adapted from Janice Thompson and Melinda Manore, *Nutrition: An Applied Approach,* 2d ed., © 2009. Reprinted by permission of Pearson Education, Inc., Upper Saddle River, New Jersey.

check yourself

- What are some functions of vitamins in the body?
- What are key vitamins and some recommended food sources for them? Are there any that are difficult for you to eat in the recommended quantity?

Essential Nutrients: Minerals

learning outcomes

- **Describe the functions of minerals in the body.**
- **List key minerals and identify some recommended food sources for them.**

Minerals are the inorganic, indestructible elements that aid physiological processes within the body. Without minerals, vitamins could not be absorbed.

Minerals are readily excreted and, with a few exceptions, are usually not toxic. **Macrominerals** are the minerals that the body needs in fairly large amounts: sodium, calcium, phosphorus, magnesium, potassium, sulfur, and chloride. Trace minerals include iron, zinc, manganese, copper, and iodine. Only very small amounts of **trace minerals** are needed by the body; serious problems may result if excesses or deficiencies of trace minerals occur. Sodium and calcium are two minerals of particular concern. Americans consume much more sodium than our bodies need, about 150% of the recommended amount. Processed foods are the main source of sodium;

TABLE
8.3 A Guide to Selected Major Minerals

Mineral Name and Recommended Intake	Reliable Food Sources	Primary Functions	Toxicity/Deficiency Symptoms
SODIUM AI: Adults = 1.5 g/day (1,500 mg/day)	Table salt, pickles, most canned soups, snack foods, cured luncheon meats, canned tomato products	Fluid balance; acid–base balance; transmission of nerve impulses; muscle contraction	**Toxicity:** water retention, high blood pressure, loss of calcium **Deficiency:** muscle cramps, dizziness, fatigue, nausea, vomiting, mental confusion
POTASSIUM AI: Adults = 4.7 g/day (4,700 mg/day)	Most fresh fruits and vegetables: potato, banana, tomato juice, orange juice, melon	Fluid balance; transmission of nerve impulses; muscle contraction	**Toxicity:** muscle weakness, vomiting, irregular heartbeat **Deficiency:** muscle weakness, paralysis, mental confusion, irregular heartbeat
PHOSPHORUS RDA: Adults = 700 mg/day	Milk/cheese/yogurt, soymilk and tofu, legumes (lentils, black beans), nuts (almonds, peanuts), poultry	Fluid balance; bone formation; component of ATP, which provides energy for our bodies	**Toxicity:** muscle spasms, convulsions, low blood calcium **Deficiency:** muscle weakness, muscle damage, bone pain, dizziness
CALCIUM AI: Adults 19–50 = 1,000 mg/day Adults > 50 = 1,200 mg/day UL = 2,500 mg	Milk/yogurt/cheese (best absorbed form of calcium), sardines, collard greens and spinach, calcium-fortified juices	Primary component of bone; acid–base balance; transmission of nerve impulses; muscle contraction	**Toxicity:** mineral imbalances, shock, kidney failure, fatigue, mental confusion **Deficiency:** osteoporosis, convulsions, heart failure
MAGNESIUM RDA: Men 19–30 = 400 mg/day Men > 30 = 420 mg/day Women 19–30 = 310 mg/day Women > 30 = 320 mg/day UL = 350 mg/day	Greens (spinach, kale, collards), whole grains, seeds, nuts, legumes (navy and black beans)	Component of bone; muscle contraction; assists more than 300 enzyme systems	**Toxicity:** none known **Deficiency:** low blood calcium; muscle spasms or seizures; nausea; weakness; increased risk of chronic diseases such as heart disease, hypertension, osteoporosis, and type 2 diabetes

Note: RDA = Recommended Daily Allowance; AI = Adequate Intakes; UL = Tolerable Upper Level Intake. Values are for all adults aged 19 and older, except as noted.
Source: Adapted from Janice Thompson and Manore, Melinda, *Nutrition: An Applied Approach*, 2nd ed., © 2009. Reprinted by permission of Pearson Education, Inc., Upper Saddle River, New Jersey.

TABLE 8.4 A Guide to Selected Trace Minerals

Mineral Name and Recommended Intake	Reliable Food Sources	Primary Functions	Toxicity/Deficiency Symptoms
SELENIUM RDA: Adults = 55 µg/day UL = 400 µg/day	Nuts, shellfish, meat/fish/poultry, whole grains	Required for carbohydrate and fat metabolism	**Toxicity:** brittle hair and nails, skin rashes, nausea and vomiting, weakness, liver disease **Deficiency:** specific forms of heart disease and arthritis, impaired immune function, muscle pain and wasting, depression, hostility
FLUORIDE AI: Men = 4 mg/day Women = 3 mg/day UL = 2.2 mg/day for children 4–8 years; children > 8 years = 10 mg/day	Fluoridated water and other beverages made with this water	Development and maintenance of healthy teeth and bones	**Toxicity:** fluorosis of teeth and bones **Deficiency:** dental caries, low bone density
IODINE RDA: Adults = 150 µg/day UL = 1,100 µg/day	Iodized salt and foods processed with iodized salt	Synthesis of thyroid hormones; temperature regulation; reproduction and growth	**Toxicity:** goiter **Deficiency:** goiter, hypothyroidism, cretinism in infant of mother who is iodine deficient
CHROMIUM AI: Men 19–50 = 35 µg/day Men > 50 = 30 µg/day Women 19–50 = 25 µg/day Women > 50 = 20 µg/day	Grains, meat/fish/poultry, some fruits and vegetables	Glucose transport; metabolism of DNA and RNA; immune function and growth	**Toxicity:** none known *Deficiency:* elevated blood glucose and blood lipids, damage to brain and nervous system
IRON RDA: Men = 8 mg/day Women 19–50 = 18 mg/day Women > 50 = 8 mg/day UL = 45 mg/day	Meat/fish/poultry (best absorbed form of iron), fortified cereals, legumes, spinach	Component of hemoglobin in blood cells; component of myoglobin in muscle cells; assists many enzyme systems	**Toxicity:** nausea, vomiting, and diarrhea; dizziness, confusion; rapid heartbeat; organ damage; death **Deficiency:** iron-deficiency microcytic anemia, hypochromic anemia
ZINC RDA: Men 11 mg/day Women = 8 mg/day UL = 40 mg/day	Meat/fish/poultry (best absorbed form of zinc), fortified cereals, legumes	Assists more than 100 enzyme systems; immune system function; growth and sexual maturation; gene regulation	**Toxicity:** nausea, vomiting, and diarrhea; headaches; depressed immune function; reduced absorption of copper **Deficiency:** growth retardation, delayed sexual maturation, eye and skin lesions, hair loss, increased incidence of illness and infection

Note: RDA = Recommended Daily Allowance; AI = Adequate Intakes; UL = Tolerable Upper Intake Level. Values are for all adults aged 19 and older, except as noted.
Source: Adapted from Janice Thompson and Melinda Manore, *Nutrition: An Applied Approach*, 2d ed., © 2009. Reprinted by permission of Pearson Education, Inc., Upper Saddle River, New Jersey.

researchers recommend that Americans cut back on sodium intake to reduce their risk of cardiovascular disorders. The issue of calcium consumption has gained attention with the rising incidence of osteoporosis. To prevent bone loss later in life, young adults, particular women, must obtain adequate amounts of calcium.

Tables 8.3 and 8.4 provide information on mineral requirements.

check yourself

■ **What are some functions of minerals in the body?**

■ **What are key minerals and some recommended food sources for them? Are there any that are difficult for you to eat in the recommended quantity?**

Planning a Healthy Diet: *Dietary Guidelines, 2010*

- **Explain how to use the *Dietary Guidelines, 2010*.**

Now that you have some idea of your nutritional needs, let's discuss what a healthy diet looks like, how you can begin to meet your needs, and how you can meet the challenge of getting the foods you need on campus. This section gives you some practical advice for meeting your goals and for dealing with issues specific to eating in college.

Generally speaking, a healthful diet provides the combination of energy and nutrients needed to sustain proper functioning. A healthful diet should be:

- **Adequate.** It provides enough energy, nutrients, and fiber to maintain health and essential body functions. Everyone's nutritional needs differ. For example, a small woman with a sedentary lifestyle may need only 1,700 calories of energy daily to support her body's functions, whereas a competitive bicyclist may need several thousand calories of energy to be fit for a race.
- **Moderate.** It often isn't what you eat that causes nutrition imbalance or weight gain—it's the amount you consume. Moderate caloric consumption, portion control, and awareness of the total amount of nutrients in the foods you eat are key aspects of dietary health.
- **Balanced.** Your diet should contain the proper combination of foods from different groups. Following the recommendations for the MyPlate plan described later in this chapter should help you achieve balance.
- **Varied.** Eat many different foods each day. Variety keeps you interested and makes it less likely that your diet will contain nutrient deficiencies.
- **Nutrient dense.** *Nutrient density* refers to the proportion of vitamins, minerals, and other nutrients compared to the number of calories. The foods you eat should have the biggest nutritional bang possible for the calories consumed.

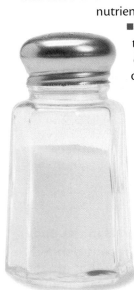

Trends indicate that Americans today overall eat more food than ever before. From 1970 to 2008, average calorie consumption increased from 2,157 to 2,673 calories per day.[22] In general, it isn't the actual amounts of food but the number of calories in the foods we choose to eat that has increased. When these trends

Even if you never use table salt, you still may be getting excess sodium in your diet.

are combined with our increasingly sedentary lifestyle, it is not surprising that we have seen a dramatic rise in obesity.

Highlights

The following guidelines for healthy eating are adapted from the USDA's *Dietary Guidelines for Americans, 2010*. Complete guidelines and more information are available at http://health.gov/dietaryguidelines.

- Eat a moderate number of calories to maintain a healthy weight. If you are overweight or obese, this means consuming fewer calories.
- Get moving—increase physical activity and reduce time spent in sedentary behaviors.
- Keep your daily sodium intake under 2,300 milligrams (mg)—1,500 if you're over 50, African American, or have hypertension, diabetes, or chronic kidney disease.
- Get less than 10 percent of your daily calories from saturated fatty acids; replace them with monounsaturated and polyunsaturated fatty acids. Keep *trans* fatty acids as low as possible. Limit solid fats (especially butter, meat fat, coconut and palm oils, shortening, and most margarines) and foods that contain synthetic *trans* fats.
- Consume less than 300 mg of dietary cholesterol daily.
- Eat more whole grains and fewer refined grains—at least half should be whole grains.
- If you drink alcohol, do so in moderation—no more than one drink per day for women and two for men.
- Eat more fruits and vegetables. Get a variety of vegetables, especially dark-green and red and orange vegetables and beans and peas.
- Get calcium from fat-free or low-fat milk, yogurt, cheese, soy milk, and leafy greens.
- Choose a variety of protein foods, including seafood, lean meat and poultry, eggs, beans and peas, soy products, and unsalted nuts and seeds.
- Woman capable of becoming pregnant should choose foods that supply iron and vitamin C–rich foods. They should also consume 400 micrograms (mg) per day of synthetic folic acid, in addition to getting folate in a varied diet.
- Women who are pregnant or breastfeeding should try to consume 8 to 12 ounces of a variety of seafood weekly, but limit white (albacore) tuna to 6 ounces or less weekly and avoid tilefish, shark, swordfish, and king mackerel due to their high methyl mercury content. Take an iron supplement as recommended by a health care provider.
- Individuals older than age 50 should consume foods fortified with vitamin B_{12}.

- **How would following the *Dietary Guidelines, 2010* improve your diet?**

Planning a Healthy Diet: Using the Food Label

- **Understand each component of the food label.**

Food labels provide valuable information that you can use to make healthy choices, including serving size, calories, calories from fat per serving, and percentage of *trans* fats in a food.

Labels also include percentages listed as "% Daily Value." This is derived from the **Daily Values (DVs),** a number calculated from the Reference Daily Intakes (RDIs) and Daily Reference Values (DRVs). The RDIs indicate recommended daily amounts of vitamins and minerals; the DRVs indicate recommended amounts of macronutrients such as total fat, saturated fat, total carbohydrates, dietary fiber, sodium, potassium, and protein. **Figure 8.6** walks you through a typical food label.

Start here. The size of the serving on the food package influences the number of calories and all the nutrient amounts listed on the top part of the label. Pay attention to the serving size, especially how many servings there are in the food package. Then ask yourself, "How many servings am I consuming?"

Limit these nutrients. The nutrients listed first are the ones Americans generally eat in adequate amounts, or even too much of. Eating too much fat, saturated fat, *trans* fat, cholesterol, or sodium may increase your risk of certain chronic diseases, such as heart disease, some cancers, or high blood pressure.

Get enough of these nutrients. Most Americans don't get enough dietary fiber, vitamin A, vitamin C, calcium, and iron in their diets. Eating enough of these nutrients can improve your health and help reduce the risk of some diseases and conditions.

The footnote is not specific to the product. It shows recommended dietary advice for all Americans. The Percent Daily Values are based on a 2,000-calorie diet, but the footnote lists daily values for both a 2,000- and 2,500-calorie diet.

Pay attention to calories (and calories from fat). Many Americans consume more calories than they need. Remember: The number of servings you consume determines the number of calories you actually eat (your portion amount). Dietary guidelines recommend that no more than 30% of your daily calories consumed come from fat.

5% DV or less is low and 20% DV or more is high. The % DV helps you determine if a serving of food is high or low in a nutrient, whether or not you consume the 2,000-calorie diet it is based on. It also helps you make easy comparisons between products (just make sure the serving sizes are similar).

Note that a few nutrients—*trans* fats, sugars, and protein—do not have a % DV. Experts could not provide a reference value for *trans* fat, but it is recommended that you keep your intake as low as possible. There are no recommendations for the total amount of sugar to eat in one day, but check the ingredient list to see information on added sugars, such as high fructose corn syrup. A % DV for protein is required to be listed if a claim is made (such as "high in protein") or if the food is meant for infants and children under 4 years old. Otherwise, none is needed.

Sample Label for Macaroni and Cheese

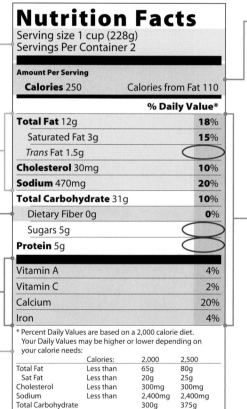

Nutrition Facts

Serving size 1 cup (228g)
Servings Per Container 2

Amount Per Serving

Calories 250	Calories from Fat 110

	% Daily Value*
Total Fat 12g	**18%**
Saturated Fat 3g	**15%**
Trans Fat 1.5g	
Cholesterol 30mg	**10%**
Sodium 470mg	**20%**
Total Carbohydrate 31g	**10%**
Dietary Fiber 0g	**0%**
Sugars 5g	
Protein 5g	

Vitamin A	4%
Vitamin C	2%
Calcium	20%
Iron	4%

* Percent Daily Values are based on a 2,000 calorie diet. Your Daily Values may be higher or lower depending on your calorie needs:

		Calories:	2,000	2,500
Total Fat	Less than		65g	80g
Sat Fat	Less than		20g	25g
Cholesterol	Less than		300mg	300mg
Sodium	Less than		2,400mg	2,400mg
Total Carbohydrate			300g	375g
Dietary Fiber			25g	30g

Figure 8.6 Reading a Food Label

Source: Center for Food Safety and Applied Nutrition, "A Key to Choosing Healthful Foods: Using the Nutrition Facts on the Food Label," Updated May 2009, www.fda.gov/Food/ResourcesForYou/Consumers/ucm079449.htm.

- **What are the key components of a food label? How can they help you make better food choices?**

Planning a Healthy Diet: The MyPlate Plan

- **Explain the principles for a healthy diet contained in the MyPlate plan.**

Federal agencies continue to strive to help Americans make healthy eating choices, offering a variety of food guidance systems.

Food Guidance Systems

In 2005, the former Food Guide Pyramid created and promoted by the USDA underwent an overhaul to account more completely for the variety of nutritional needs in the U.S. population. The 2000 pyramid emphasized variety in daily intake, but did not reflect what we now know about restricting fats, eating more fruits and vegetables, and consuming whole grains. The 2005 MyPyramid Plan took into consideration the dietary and caloric needs for a wider variety of individuals, such as people over age 65, children, and adults with different activity levels. However, it was criticized for being difficult to understand and for requiring consumers to go online to develop their customized eating plan.

Dietary Guidelines and the My-Plate Plan

As described previously, the *Dietary Guidelines for Americans* are a set of recommendations for healthy eating created by the U.S. Department of Health and Human Services and the USDA. These guidelines are revised every 5 years, and have undergone major changes, both in 2005, with much more focus on aspects of choosing healthy foods from within each of the pyramid's categories, and now again, in 2010, with a focus on physical activity, personalization, and customizability.[23]

The *Dietary Guidelines for Americans, 2010* are designed to help bridge the gap between the standard American diet and the key recommendations that aim to combat the growing obesity epidemic by balancing calories with adequate physical activity.[24] The dietary recommendations are transformed into an easy-to-follow graphic and guidance system called MyPlate, which can be found at www.choosemyplate.gov and is illustrated in **Figure 8.7**.

The MyPlate Plan

The MyPlate plan takes into consideration the dietary and caloric needs for a wide variety of individuals, such as pregnant or breastfeeding women, those trying to lose weight, and adults with different activity levels. At the www.choosemyplate.gov website you can create personalized dietary and exercise recommendations based on the individual information you enter.

MyPlate also encourages consumers to eat for health through three general areas of recommendation as follows:[25]

1. **Balance calories.** Find out how many calories you need for a day is a first step in managing your weight. Go to www.choosemyplate.gov to find your calorie level. Being physically active also helps you balance calories.

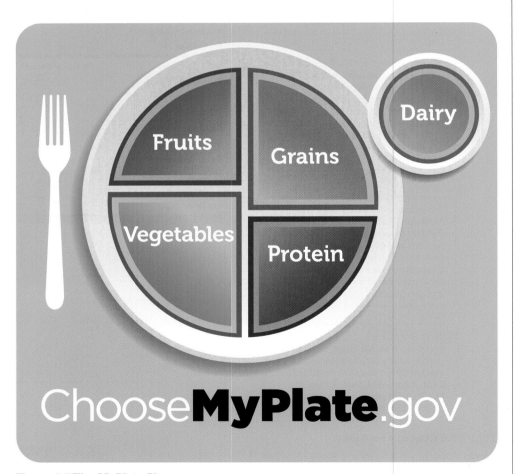

Figure 8.7 The MyPlate Plan

The USDA MyPlate plan takes a new approach to dietary and exercise recommendations. Each colored section of the plate represents a food group. An interactive tool on www.choosemyplate.gov can provide individualized recommendations for users.

Source: U.S. Department of Agriculture, 2011, www.choosemyplate.gov.

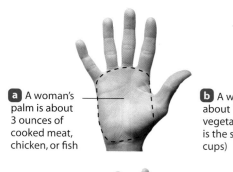

a A woman's palm is about 3 ounces of cooked meat, chicken, or fish

b A woman's fist is about 1 cup of pasta or vegetables (a man's fist is the size of about 2 cups)

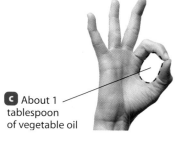

c About 1 tablespoon of vegetable oil

Your hands can guide you in estimating portion sizes.

Figure 8.8 What's a Serving?

- Enjoy your food, but eat less. Take time to fully enjoy your food as you eat it. Eating too fast or when your attention is elsewhere may lead to eating too many calories. Pay attention to hunger cues before, during, and after meals. Use them to recognize when to eat and when you've had enough.
- Avoid oversized portions. Use a smaller plate, bowl, and glass. Portion out food before you eat. When eating out, choose a smaller size option, share a dish, or take home part of your meal.

2. **Increase some foods.** Eat more vegetables, fruits, whole grains, and fat-free or 1% milk and dairy products, These foods have the nutrients you need for health—including potassium, calcium, vitamin D, and fiber. Make them the basis for meals and snacks.

   - Make half your plate fruits and vegetables. Choose red, orange, and dark-green vegetables like tomatoes, sweet potatoes, and broccoli. Add fruit to meals as part of main or side dishes or as dessert.
   - Make at least half your grains whole grains. Substitute whole-wheat bread for white bread or brown rice for white rice.
   - Switch to fat-free or 1% milk. They have the same amount of calcium and other essential nutrients as whole milk, but fewer calories and less saturated fat.

3. **Reduce some foods.** Cut back on foods high in solid fats, added sugars, and salt. They include cakes, cookies, ice cream, candies, sweetened drinks, pizza, and fatty meats like ribs, sausages, bacon, and hot dogs. Enjoy these foods as occasional treats, not everyday foods.

   - Compare sodium in foods like soup, bread, and frozen meals—and choose the foods with lower numbers. Use the food label to choose lower sodium versions of foods like soup, bread, and frozen meals. Look for "low sodium," "reduced sodium," or "no salt added" on the label.

- Drink water instead of sugary drinks. Cut calories by drinking water or unsweetened beverages. Soda, energy drinks, and sports drinks are a major source of added sugar and calories in American diets.

Understand Serving Sizes MyPlate presents personalized dietary recommendations in terms of numbers of servings of particular nutrients. But how much is one serving? Is it different from a portion? Although these two terms are often used interchangeably, they actually mean very different things. A *serving* is the recommended amount you should consume, whereas a *portion* is the amount you choose to eat at any one time. Most of us select portions that are much bigger than recommended servings. In a survey conducted by the American Institute for Cancer Research, respondents were asked to estimate the standard servings for eight different foods. Only 1 percent of those surveyed correctly answered all serving size questions, and nearly 65 percent answered five or more of them incorrectly.[26] See **Figure 8.8** for an easy way to recognize serving sizes.

Unfortunately, we don't always get a clear picture from food producers and advertisers about what a serving really is. Consider a bottle of soda: The food label may list one serving size as 8 fluid ounces and 100 calories. However, note the size of the entire bottle; if the bottle holds 20 ounces, drinking the whole thing serves up 250 calories.

Eat Nutrient-Dense Foods Although eating the proper number of servings from MyPlate is important, it is also important to recognize that there are large caloric, fat, and energy differences among foods within a given food group. For example, fish and hot dogs provide vastly different nutrient levels per ounce. If you had a portion of fish and a portion of hot dog, both containing the same amount of calories, the fish will provide less fat and more nutritional value than the hot dog, making it more nutrient dense. It is important to eat foods that have a high nutritional value for their caloric content. Avoid "empty calories"; that is, high-calorie foods that have little nutritional value. Also remember that many nutrient-dense sports bars pack a lot of calories into a small package.

Physical Activity Strive to be physically active for at least 30 minutes per day, preferably with moderate to vigorous activity levels on most days. Physical activity does not mean you have to go to the gym, jog 3 miles a day, or hire a personal trainer. Any activity that gets your heart pumping (e.g., gardening, playing basketball, heavy yard work, or dancing) is a good way to get moving. In addition to personalized recommendations on diet, MyPlate personalized plans will also offer recommendations for weekly physical activity.

check yourself

- **What are the main guidelines of the MyPlate plan?**
- **Which parts of MyPlate can you most easily adopt in your diet? Which are the most challenging? Why?**

Eating Well in College

- **Describe the unique challenges college students face when trying to eat healthfully.**
- **Provide examples of what college students can do to eat more healthfully.**

College students often face a challenge when trying to eat healthy foods. Some students live in dorms and do not have their own cooking or refrigeration facilities. Others live in crowded apartments where everyone forages in the refrigerator for everyone else's food. Still others eat at university food services where food choices may be overwhelming. Nearly all have financial and time constraints that make buying, preparing, and eating healthy food a difficult task. What's a student to do?

Many college students may find it hard to fit a well-balanced meal into the day, but eating breakfast and lunch are important if you are to keep energy levels up and get the most out of your classes. If your campus is like many others, you've probably noticed a distinct move toward fast-food restaurants in your student unions. However, eating a complete breakfast that includes complex carbohydrates, protein, and healthy, unsaturated fat (such as a banana, peanut butter and whole-grain bread sandwich, or a dry fruit and nut mix without added sugar or salt) is key. If you are short

on time you can bring these items to class to ensure that your meals fit into your day. Generally speaking, you can eat more healthfully and for less money if you bring food from home or your campus dining hall. If you must eat fast food, follow the tips below to get more nutritional bang for your buck:

- Ask for nutritional analyses of items. Most fast-food chains now have them.
- Order salads, but be careful about what you add to them. Taco salads and Cobb salads are often high in fat, calories, and sodium. Ask for dressing on the side, and use it sparingly. Try the vinaigrette or low-fat dressings. Stay away from eggs and other high-fat add-ons, such as bacon bits, croutons, and crispy noodles.
- If you must have fries, check to see what type of oil is used to cook them. Avoid lard-based or other saturated-fat products and *trans* fats. Some fast-food restaurants offer baked "fries," which may be lower in fat.
- Avoid giant sizes, and refrain from ordering extra sauce, bacon, cheese, dressings, and other extras that add additional calories, sodium, carbohydrates, and fat.
- Limit beverages and foods that are high in added sugars. Common forms of added sugars include sucrose, glucose, fructose, maltose, dextrose, corn syrups, concentrated fruit juices, and honey.
- At least once per week, substitute a vegetable-based meat substitute into your fast-food choices. Most places now offer Gardenburgers, Boca Burgers, or similar products, which provide excellent sources of protein and often have considerably less fat and fewer calories.

In the dining hall, try these ideas:

- Choose lean meats, grilled chicken, fish, or vegetable dishes. Avoid fried chicken, fatty cuts of red meat, or meat dishes smothered in creamy or oily sauce.

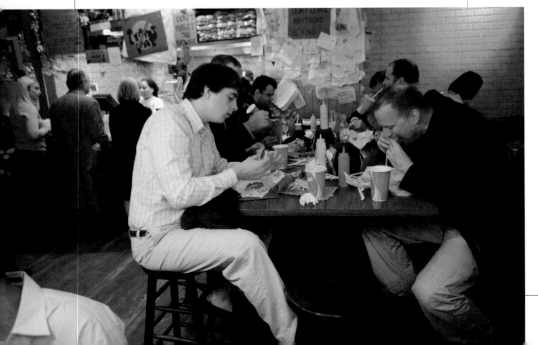

How can I eat well when I'm in a hurry?

Meals like this one may be convenient, but they are high in fat, calories, sodium, and refined carbohydrates. Even when you are short on time and money, it is possible—and worthwhile—to make healthier choices. If you are ordering fast food, opt for foods prepared by baking, roasting, or steaming; ask for the leanest meat option; and request that sauces, dressings, and gravies be served on the side.

- Hit the salad bar and load up on leafy greens, beans, tuna, or tofu. Choose items such as avocado or nuts for a little "good" fat, and go easy on the dressing.
- Get creative: Choose items such as a baked potato with salsa or add grilled chicken to your salad. Top toast with veggies, hummus, or grilled chicken or tuna.
- When choosing items from a made-to-order food station, ask the preparer to hold the butter, oil, mayonnaise, sour cream, or cheese- or cream-based sauces.
- Avoid going back for seconds and consuming large portions.
- If there is something you'd like but don't see in your dining hall, or if you are vegetarian and feel like your food choices are limited, speak to your food services manager and provide suggestions.
- Pass on high-calorie, low-nutrient foods such as sugary cereals, ice cream, and other sweet treats. Choose fruit or low-fat yogurt to satisfy your sweet tooth.

Maintaining a nutritious diet within the confines of student life can be challenging. However, if you take the time to plan healthy meals, you will find that you are eating better, enjoying it more, and actually saving money.

What's Healthy on the Menu?

No matter what type of cuisine you enjoy, there will always be healthier and less healthy options on the menu. To help you order wisely, here are lighter options and high-fat pitfalls. "Best" choices contain fewer than 30 grams of fat, a generous meal's worth for an active, medium-sized woman. "Worst" choices have up to 100 grams of fat.

Breakfast
- Best: Hot or cold cereal with 2 percent milk; pancakes or French toast with syrup; scrambled eggs with hash browns and plain toast
- Worst: Belgian waffle with sausage; sausage and eggs with biscuits and gravy; ham-and-cheese omelet with hash browns and toast
- Tips: Ask for whole-grain cereal or shredded wheat with 2 percent milk or whole wheat toast without butter or margarine. Order omelets without cheese, and order fried eggs without bacon or sausage.

Sandwiches
- Best: Ham and Swiss cheese; roast beef; turkey
- Worst: Tuna salad; Reuben; submarine
- Tips: Ask for mustard; hold the mayonnaise and high-fat cheese. See if turkey-ham is available.

Seafood
- Best: Broiled bass, halibut, or snapper; grilled scallops; steamed crab or lobster
- Worst: Fried seafood platter; blackened catfish
- Tips: Order fish broiled, baked, grilled, or steamed—not pan fried or sautéed. Ask for lemon instead of tartar sauce. Avoid creamy and buttery sauces.

Italian
- Best: Pasta with red or white clam sauce; spaghetti with marinara or tomato-and-meat sauce
- Worst: Eggplant parmigiana; fettuccine Alfredo; fried calamari; lasagna
- Tips: Stick with plain bread instead of garlic bread made with butter or oil. Ask for the waiter's help in avoiding cream- or egg-based sauces. Try vegetarian pizza, and don't ask for extra cheese.

Mexican
- Best: Bean burrito (no cheese); chicken fajitas
- Worst: Beef chimichanga; quesadilla; chile relleno; refried beans
- Tips: Choose soft tortillas (not fried) with fresh salsa, not guacamole. Special-order grilled shrimp, fish, or chicken. Ask for beans made without lard or fat, and have cheeses and sour cream provided on the side or left out altogether.

Skills for Behavior Change

HEALTHY EATING SIMPLIFIED

Messages from nutrition experts, marketing campaigns, and media blitzes may leave you scratching your head about how to eat healthfully. When it all starts to feel too complicated to be worthwhile, here are some simple tips to follow for health-conscious eating:

- You don't need foods from fancy packages to improve your health. Fruits, vegetables, and whole grains should make up the bulk of your diet. Shop the perimeter of the store and the bulk foods aisle.
- Let the plate method guide you. Your plate should be half vegetables, a quarter lean protein, and a quarter whole grains/bread. Have a serving of fruit for dessert.
- Limit processed and packaged foods. This will assist you in limiting added sodium, sugar, and fat. If you can't make sense of the ingredients, don't eat it.
- Eat natural "snacks" such as dried fruit, nuts, fresh fruits, string cheese, yogurt without added sugar, hard-boiled eggs, and vegetables.
- Be mindful of your eating. Eat until you are satisfied but not overfull.
- Bring healthful foods with you when you head out the door. Whether going to class, to work, or on a road trip, you *can* control the foods that are available. Don't put yourself in a position where you're forced to buy from a vending machine or convenience store.

Source: M. Pollan, *Food Rules: An Eater's Manual* (New York: Penguin Books, 2010).

check yourself

- **What challenges do you face when trying to eat more healthfully?**
- **What are some steps that you can take to eat more healthfully?**

Vegetarianism: A Healthy Diet?

- **Describe the benefits and drawbacks of a vegetarian diet.**

According to a 2009 poll by the Vegetarian Resource Group, more than 3 percent of U.S. adults, approximately 6 to 8 million people, are vegetarians.[27] Other surveys have shown that nearly 23 million Americans are "vegetarian inclined," or "flexitarians"—omnivores reducing meat consumption in favor of other forms of protein.[28] The word **vegetarian** can mean different things to different people—*vegans* eat no animal products at all, while many vegetarians eat dairy or other animal products but not animal flesh, and some eat seafood but not beef, pork, or poultry.

Common reasons for such eating choices include concern for animal welfare, improving health, environmental concerns, natural approaches to wellness, food safety, and weight loss or maintenance. Generally, people who follow a balanced vegetarian diet weigh less and have better cholesterol levels, less constipation and diarrhea, and a lower risk of heart disease than do nonvegetarians. The benefits of vegetarianism also include a reduced risk of some cancers, particularly colon cancer, and a reduced risk of kidney disease.[29]

With proper information and food choices, vegetarianism provides a superb alternative to a high-fat, high-calorie, meat-based cuisine. Although in the past vegetarians often suffered from vitamin deficiencies, most today are adept at combining foods and eating a variety of foods to ensure proper nutrient intake. Purely vegan diets may be deficient in some important vitamins and minerals, though these can be obtained from supplements. Pregnant women, older adults, sick people, and children who are vegans or vegetarians need to take special care to ensure that their diets are adequate. In all cases, seek advice from a health care professional if you have questions.

Do Vegetarians Need to Take Supplements?

Dietary supplements are products intended to supplement existing diets. Ingredients range from vitamins, minerals, and herbs to enzymes, amino acids, fatty acids, and organ tissues. Supplement sales have skyrocketed in the last few decades. The FDA does not evaluate the safety and efficacy of supplements prior to their marketing; it can take action to remove a supplement from the market only after it has been proved harmful.

But, do you really need any dietary supplements? That's a matter of some debate. A 2001 article in the *Journal of the American Medical Association* (JAMA) recommended that "a vitamin/mineral supplement a day just might be important in keeping the doctor away, particularly for some groups of people."[30] Although the article acknowledged a possible risk of overdosing on fat-soluble vitamins, it noted that preliminary research has linked inadequate amounts of vitamins B_6, B_{12}, D, and E and lycopene to coronary heart disease, cancer, and osteoporosis. A 2006 National Institutes of Health report, however, concluded that "the present evidence is insufficient to recommend either for or against the use of multivitamins and minerals . . . to prevent chronic diseases."[31] More recently, Canadian researchers argued that vitamins A, E, D, folic acid, and niacin should be categorized as over-the-counter medications.[32]

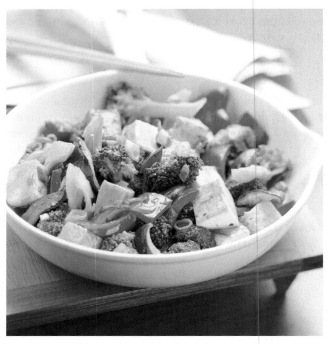

Are vegetarian diets healthy?

Adopting a vegan or vegetarian diet can be a very healthy way to eat. Take care to prepare your food healthfully by limiting the use of oils and avoiding added sugars and sodium. Make sure you get all the essential amino acids by eating meals like this tofu and vegetable stir fry. To further enhance it, add a whole grain such as brown rice.

- **What are some of the benefits and drawbacks of a vegetarian diet?**
- **Should vegetarians supplement their diet in any way?**

Is Organic for You?

■ **Explain the nature of organic foods.**

Concerns about food safety, genetically modified foods, and the health impacts of chemicals used in the growth and production of food have led many people to turn to foods that are **organic**—foods and beverages developed, grown, or raised without the use of synthetic pesticides, chemicals, or hormones. As of 2002, any food sold in the United States as organic has to meet criteria set by the USDA under the National Organic Rule and can carry a USDA seal verifying products as "certified organic."

Under this rule, a product that is certified may carry one of the following terms: "100 percent Organic" (100% compliance with organic criteria), "Organic" (must contain at least 95% organic materials), "Made with Organic Ingredients" (must contain at least 70% organic ingredients), or "Some Organic Ingredients" (contains less than 70% organic ingredients—usually listed individually). To be labeled with any of the above terms, the foods must be produced without hormones, antibiotics, herbicides, insecticides, chemical fertilizers, genetic modification, or germ-killing radiation. However, reliable monitoring systems to ensure credibility are still under development, especially for foods labeled as organic produced outside the United States, and several organic farmers' groups have questioned the stringency of the USDA guidelines regarding organics.

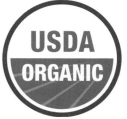

USDA label for certified organic foods.

Is buying organic really better for you? It is almost impossible to assess the health impact of organic versus nonorganic foods. Nevertheless, the market for organics has been increasing by more than 20 percent per year—five times faster than food sales in general. Where only a small subset of the population once bought organic, nearly all U.S. consumers now occasionally reach for something labeled organic. In 2010, annual organic food sales were estimated to be $25 billion.[33] Proponents of organic foods state that, beyond the compelling health issues, organic farming produces foods that simply taste better.

In 2007, several reports by consumer groups questioned the nutrient value of organic foods. Some sources say that smaller organic farmers may have trouble getting their produce to market in the proper climate-controlled vehicles. As such, their foods might lose valuable nutrients while sitting in warm trucks or at a roadside stand compared to the refrigerated section of a local supermarket, or, as important, increased bacterial growth may occur. Certainly, both organic and nonorganic foods are subject to issues of food safety. All farmers and food producers can fall prey to dangerous food safety issues without proper monitoring and safety measures. For example, factory meat farming and slaughterhouses present more opportunities for food safety problems than do smaller farms producing grass-fed cows, for reasons of scale, and also (in the case of meat and poultry producers) because such megaproducers tend to use antibiotics and artificial hormones to control disease, which itself may lead to health problems for the animals and those who eat them.

Issues also arise around long-distance transportation of foods, whether organic or not. Today, the word **locavore** has been coined to describe people who eat only food grown or produced locally, usually within close proximity to their homes. Farmers' markets or homegrown foods or those grown by independent farmers are thought to be fresher and to require far fewer resources to get them to market and keep them fresh for longer periods of time. Locavores believe that locally grown organic food is preferable to foods produced by large corporations or supermarket-based organic foods, because they have a smaller impact on the environment and are believed to retain more of their nutritive value. Although there are many reasons organic farming is better for the environment, the fact that pesticides, herbicides, and other products are not used is perhaps the greatest benefit.

check yourself

■ **What are organic foods?**

■ **What are your reasons for buying or for not buying organic foods?**

Food Technology

- **Identify technologies being used in food production today.**

Food Irradiation

Food irradiation involves treating foods with low doses of radiation, or ionizing energy, which breaks chemical bonds in the DNA of harmful bacteria, damaging pathogens and keeping them from replicating. Essentially, the rays pass through the food without leaving any radioactive residue.[34]

Irradiation lengthens food products' shelf life and prevents spread of deadly microorganisms, particularly in high-risk foods such as ground beef and pork. Use of food irradiation is limited because of consumer concerns about safety and because irradiation facilities are expensive to build. Still, food irradiation is now common in over 40 countries. Irradiated foods are marked with the "radura" logo.

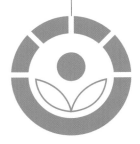

U.S. FDA label for irradiated foods.

Food Additives

Additives are substances added to food to reduce the risk of foodborne illness, to prevent spoilage, and to enhance look and taste. Additives can also enhance nutrient value, as with the fortification of milk with vitamin D and of grain products with folate. Beyond this, however, as a general rule, the fewer chemicals, colorants, and preservatives the better. Common additives include antimicrobial agents (substances that make foods less hospitable for microbes); antioxidants (substances that reduce loss of color and flavor due to oxygen exposure); artificial colors, nutrient additives, and flavor enhancers, such as MSG (monosodium glutamate); and sulfites (used to preserve vegetable color).

Genetically Modified Food Crops

Genetic modification involves insertion or deletion of genes into the DNA of an organism. In the case of **genetically modified (GM) foods**, this is usually done to enhance production by making disease- or insect-resistant plants, improving yield, or controlling weeds. GM foods are sometimes created to improve foods' appearance or enhance nutrients; GM technology has been used to create rice containing vitamin A and iron, designed to help reduce disease in developing countries.

The first genetically modified food crop was the FlavrSavr tomato, developed in 1996 to ripen without getting soft, increasing shipping capacity and shelf life. Since then, U.S. farmers have widely accepted GM crops.[35] Now 93 percent of soy and between 63 and 70 percent of corn grown in the U.S. is genetically modified.[36] Many consumers are also accepting of GM foods. However, in a recent report in *New Scientist*, three strains of maize (corn) showed signs of causing liver and kidney toxicity.[37] These claims are refuted by producers, but it does leave others questioning the safety of these foods.

Some scientists and food producers believe that GM crops could help address worldwide hunger and malnutrition. But many researchers and health advocates believe GM foods carry serious risks to humans and the ecosystem. Others are concerned about seeds being controlled by large corporations, while organic farmers are concerned about genetically modified seeds drifting into their fields. GM foods may also lead to an increase in allergens and antibiotic resistance.[38] According to the World Health Organization, no effects on human health have been shown from consumption of GM foods in countries that have approved their use.[39] However, many organizations would like to see greater regulation of GM foods; several lawsuits are pending.

Arguments for the Development of GM Foods

- People have been manipulating food crops through selective breeding since the beginning of agriculture.
- Genetically modified seeds and products are tested for safety, and there has never been a substantiated claim for human illness resulting from their consumption.
- Insect- and weed-resistant GM crops will allow farmers to use fewer chemical insecticides and herbicides.
- GM crops can be created to grow more quickly than conventional crops, increasing food yield. Nutrient-enhanced crops can address malnutrition.

Arguments Against the Development of GM Foods

- Genetic modification is fundamentally different from and more problematic than selective breeding.
- There haven't been enough independent studies of GM products to confirm their safety. There are potential health risks if GM products approved for other uses are mistakenly or inadvertently used in production of food for human consumption.
- Inadvertent cross-pollination could lead to "super weeds." Insect-resistant crops could harm insect species that are not pests, and insect- and disease-resistant crops could prompt evolution of even more virulent species, which would then require aggressive control measures.
- Because corporations create and patent GM seeds, they control the market, forcing farmers worldwide to become reliant on these corporations.

- **What are two technologies being used in our food?**
- **Are you more or less likely to buy foods that have been modified or irradiated? Why?**

Food Allergies and Intolerances

learning **outcomes**

- **Define food allergies and intolerances.**
- **Distinguish between a food allergy and an intolerance.**

About 33 percent of people today think they have an allergy or avoid a certain food because they think they are allergic to it; however, only 4 to 8 percent of children and 2 percent of adults have a true food allergy. Still, there may be reason to be concerned. From 1997 through 2007 the prevalence of reported food allergies rose 18 percent.[40]

Food Allergies

A **food allergy**, or hypersensitivity, is an abnormal response to a food that is triggered by the immune system. Symptoms of an allergic reaction vary in severity and may include a tingling sensation in the mouth; swelling of the lips, tongue, and throat; difficulty breathing; hives; vomiting; abdominal cramps; diarrhea; drop in blood pressure; loss of consciousness; and death. Approximately 200 deaths per year occur from the anaphylaxis (the acute systemic immune and inflammatory response) that occurs with allergic reactions. These symptoms may appear within seconds to hours after eating the foods to which one is allergic.[41]

In 2004, Congress passed the Food Allergen Labeling and Consumer Protection Act (FALCPA), which requires food manufacturers to label foods clearly to indicate the presence of (or possible contamination by) any of the eight major food allergens: milk, eggs, peanuts, wheat, soy, tree nuts (walnuts, pecans, etc.), fish, and shellfish. Although over 160 foods have been identified as allergy triggers, these 8 foods account for 90 percent of all food allergies in the United States.[42]

If you suspect that you have an actual allergic reaction to food, see an allergist to be tested to determine the source of the problem. Because there are several diseases that share symptoms with food allergies (ulcers and cancers of the gastrointestinal tract can cause vomiting, bloating, diarrhea, nausea, and pain), you should have persistent symptoms checked out as soon as possible. If particular foods seem to bother you consistently, look for alternatives or modify your diet. In true allergic instances, you may not be able to consume even the smallest amount of a substance safely.

Food Intolerance

In contrast to allergies, **food intolerance** can cause symptoms of gastric upset, but the upset is not the result of an immune system response. Probably the best example of a food intolerance is *lactose intolerance*, a problem that affects about 1 in every 10 adults. Lactase is an enzyme in the lining of the gut that degrades lactose, which is in dairy products. If you don't have enough lactase, you cannot digest lactose, and it remains in the gut to be used by bacteria. Gas is formed, causing bloating, abdominal pain, and sometimes diarrhea. Food intolerance also occurs in response to some food additives, such as the flavor enhancer MSG, certain dyes, sulfites, gluten, and other substances. In some cases, the food intolerance may have psychological triggers.

Celiac Disease

Celiac disease is an inherited autoimmune disorder that affects digestive activity in the small intestine. Affecting over 3 million Americans, most of whom are undiagnosed, it is a growing problem, particularly for those younger than age of 20.[43] When a person with celiac disease consumes gluten, a protein found in wheat, rye, and barley, the person's immune system attacks the small intestine and stops nutrient absorption. Pain, cramping, and other symptoms often follow in the short term. Untreated, celiac disease can lead to other health problems, such as osteoporosis, nutritional deficiencies, and cancer. Once a person is diagnosed with celiac disease, the best treatment is to avoid breads, pastas, and other foods containing gluten.

A gluten-free diet can be difficult to achieve and maintain. There are increasing numbers of products available, however, such as specially formulated gluten-free breads, pasta, and cereal products, that allow people with celiac disease to enjoy meals similar to those without the disease. Reading food labels is particularly important, because many foods that seem safe may have hidden sources of gluten. Bouillon cubes, cold cuts, and soups are three examples of processed foods that may contain wheat, barley, or rye.

Peanuts are among the eight most common food allergens: 0.6% of the general population is allergic to them, with slightly higher rates in children.

check yourself

- **What causes food allergies and intolerances?**
- **What is the difference between a food allergy and an intolerance?**

Food Safety and Foodborne Illnesses

learning outcomes

- **Provide examples of food safety concerns.**
- **Provide tips for reducing exposure to unsafe food.**

Eating unhealthy food is one thing. Eating food that has been contaminated with a pathogen, toxin, or other harmful substance is quite another. As outbreaks of salmonella in chicken and vegetables or *Escherichia coli* (*E. coli*, a potentially lethal bacterial pathogen) in spinach or beef periodically make the news, the food industry has come under fire. To convince us that their products are safe, some manufacturers have come up with "new and improved" ways of protecting our foods. What are the dangers of contaminated foods, and how well do food manufacturers' new strategies work?

Are you concerned that the chicken you are buying doesn't look pleasingly pink or that your "fresh" fish smells a little *too* fishy? You may have good reason to be worried. In increasing numbers, Americans are becoming sick from what they eat, and many of these illnesses are life threatening. Based on several studies conducted over the past 10 years, scientists estimate that foodborne pathogens sicken over 48 million people and cause some 128,000 hospitalizations and 3,000 deaths in the United States annually.[44] These numbers have declined in the last 5 years, perhaps because of increased attention to prevention in the United States.[45] Still, because most of us don't go to the doctor every time we feel ill, we may not make a connection between what we eat and later symptoms.

Most foodborne infections and illnesses are caused by several common types of bacteria and viruses.[46] The most common:[47]

- **Salmonella.** Often found in meats and poultry.
- **Campylobacter.** Found in undercooked chicken or food contaminated with fluids from raw chicken.
- **Shigella.** Bacterium commonly found in human stool, most likely transmitted via improper hand washing.
- **Cryptosporidium.** A microscopic parasite that lives in the small intestine of humans and animals; transmitted via the fecal–oral route.
- **E. coli.** Lives in the intestines of cattle and other livestock.
- **Listeria.** Bacterium in soil and in water that can contaminate raw or processed foods.

Foodborne illnesses can also be caused by a toxin in food originally produced by a bacterium or other microbe in the food. These toxins can produce illness even if the microbes that produced them are no longer there. For example, botulism is caused by a deadly neurotoxin produced by the bacterium *Clostridium botulinum*. This bacterium is widespread in soil, water, plants, and intestinal tracts, but it can grow only in environments with limited or no oxygen. Potential food sources include improperly canned food and vacuum-packed or tightly wrapped foods. Though rare, this illness is fatal if untreated, because the powerful neurotoxin causes paralysis and can lead to the cessation of breathing.

Signs of foodborne illnesses vary tremendously and usually include one or several symptoms: diarrhea, nausea, cramping, and vomiting. Depending on the amount and virulence of the pathogen, symptoms may appear as early as 30 minutes after eating contaminated food or as long as several days or weeks later. Most of the time, symptoms occur 5 to 8 hours after eating and last only a day or two. For certain populations, such as the very young; older adults; or people with severe illnesses such as cancer, diabetes, kidney disease, or AIDS, foodborne diseases can be fatal.

Several factors may contribute to the increase in foodborne illnesses. The movement away from a traditional meat-and-potato American diet to "heart-healthy" eating—increasing consumption of fruits, vegetables, and grains—has spurred demand for fresh foods that are not in season most of the year. This means that we must import many fresh fruits and vegetables, thus putting

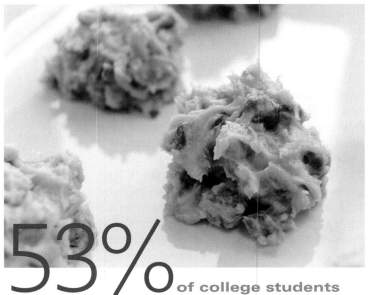

53% of college students admitted to eating raw homemade cookie dough (which contains uncooked eggs, a potential source of salmonella), and 33% ate fried eggs with soft or runny yolks.

ourselves at risk for ingesting exotic pathogens or even pesticides that have been banned in the United States for safety reasons. Depending on the season, up to 70 percent of the fruits and vegetables consumed in the United States come from Mexico. Although we are told when we travel to developing countries to "boil it, peel it, or don't eat it," we bring these foods into our kitchens at home and eat them, often without even washing them. Food can become contaminated by being watered with tainted water, fertilized with animal manure, picked by people who have not washed their hands properly after using the toilet, or by not being subjected to the same rigorous pesticide regulations as American-raised produce. To give you an idea of the implications, studies have shown that *E. coli* can survive in cow manure for up to 70 days and can multiply in foods grown with manure unless heat or additives such as salt or preservatives are used to kill the microbes.[48] No regulations prohibit farmers from using animal manure to fertilize crops. In addition, *E. coli* actually increases in summer months as factory-farmed cows await slaughter in crowded, overheated pens. This increases the chances of meat coming to market already contaminated.

Other key factors associated with the increasing spread of foodborne diseases include the inadvertent introduction of pathogens into new geographic regions and insufficient education about food safety. Globalization of the food supply, climate change, and global warming are also factors that may influence increasing spread.

Avoiding Risks in the Home

Part of the responsibility for preventing foodborne illness lies with consumers—more than 30 percent of all such illnesses result from unsafe handling of food at home. Fortunately, consumers can take several steps to reduce the likelihood of contaminating their food (see **Figure 8.9**). Among the most basic precautions: wash your hands and wash all produce before eating it. Also, avoid cross-contamination in the kitchen by using separate cutting boards and utensils for meats and produce.

Temperature control is also important—refrigerators must be set at 40 degrees or less. Be sure to cook meats to the recommended temperature to kill contaminants before eating. Hot foods must be kept hot and cold foods kept cold in order to avoid unchecked bacterial growth. Eat leftovers within 3 days; if you're unsure how long something has been sitting in the fridge, don't take chances. When in doubt, throw it out. See the Skills for Behavior Change below for more tips about reducing risk of foodborne illness when shopping for and preparing food.

Skills for Behavior Change

REDUCE YOUR RISK FOR FOODBORNE ILLNESS

- When shopping for fish, buy from markets that get their supplies from state-approved sources.
- Check for cleanliness at the salad bar and at the meat and fish counters.
- Keep most cuts of meat, fish, and poultry in the refrigerator no more than 1 or 2 days. Check the shelf life of all products before buying. Use the sniff test—if fish smells really fishy, or meat too pungent, don't eat it.
- Use a meat thermometer to ensure that meats are completely cooked. Beef and lamb steaks and roasts should be cooked to at least 145°F; ground meat, pork chops, ribs, and egg dishes to 160°F; ground poultry and hot dogs to 165°F; chicken and turkey breasts to 170°F; and chicken and turkey legs, thighs, and whole birds to 180°F. Fish is done when the thickest part becomes opaque and the fish flakes easily when poked with a fork.
- Never leave cooked food standing on the stove or table for more than 2 hours.
- Never thaw frozen foods at room temperature. Put them in the refrigerator for a day to thaw or thaw in cold water, changing the water every 30 minutes.
- Wash your hands, countertop, and cutting boards with soap and water when preparing food, particularly after handling meat, fish, or poultry.
- When freezing chicken or other raw meats, make sure "juices" can't spill over into ice cubes or into other areas of the refrigerator.

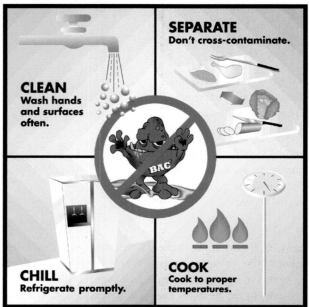

Keep Food Safe From Bacteria™

Figure 8.9 The USDA's Fight BAC!
This logo reminds consumers how to prevent foodborne illness.

check yourself

- **What are some current food safety concerns?**
- **Have you ever experienced a foodborne illness? If so, what were possible causes and how could you have avoided it?**

Assessyourself

How Healthy Are Your Eating Habits?

An interactive version of this assessment is available online. Download it from the Live It section of www.pearsonhighered.com/donatelle.

1 Keep Track of Your Food Intake

Keep a food diary for 5 days, writing down everything you eat or drink. Be sure to include the approximate amount or portion size. Add up the number of servings from each of the major food groups on each day and enter them into the chart below.

Number of Servings of:

	Day 1	Day 2	Day 3	Day 4	Day 5	Average
Fruits						
Vegetables						
Grains						
Protein foods						
Dairy						
Fats and oils						
Sweets						

2A Does Your Diet Have Proportionality?

	Yes	No
1. Are grains the main food choice at all your meals?	○	○
2. Do you often forget to eat vegetables?	○	○
3. Do you typically eat fewer than three pieces of fruit daily?	○	○
4. Do you often have fewer than 3 cups of milk daily?	○	○
5. Is the portion of meat, chicken, or fish the largest item on your dinner plate?	○	○

Scoring 2A

If you answered yes to three or more of these questions, your diet probably lacks proportionality. Review the recommendations in this chapter, particularly the MyPlate guidelines, to learn how to balance your diet.

2 Evaluate Your Food Intake

Now compare your consumption patterns to the MyPlate recommendations. Visit www.choosemyplate.gov/myplate/index.aspx to evaluate your daily caloric needs and the recommended consumption rates for the different food groups. How does your diet match up?

	Less than the recommended amount	About equal to the recommended amount	More than the recommended amount
1. How does your daily fruit consumption compare to the recommendation for your age and activity level?	○	○	○
2. How does your daily vegetable consumption compare to the recommendation for your age and activity level?	○	○	○
3. How does your daily grain consumption compare to the recommendation for your age and activity level?	○	○	○
4. How does your daily protein food consumption compare to the recommendation for your age and activity level?	○	○	○
5. How does your daily fats and oils consumption compare to the recommendation for your age and activity level?	○	○	○

Scoring

If you found that your food intake is consistent with the MyPlate recommendations, congratulations! If, however, you are falling short in a major food group or overdoing it in certain categories, consider taking steps described in this chapter to adopt healthier eating habits.

2B Are You Getting Enough Fat-Soluble Vitamins in Your Diet?

	Yes	No
1. Do you eat at least 1 cup of deep yellow or orange vegetables, such as carrots and sweet potatoes, or dark green vegetables, such as spinach, every day?	◯	◯
2. Do you consume at least two glasses (8 ounces each) of milk daily?	◯	◯
3. Do you eat a tablespoon of vegetable oil, such as corn or olive oil, daily? (Tip: Salad dressings, unless they are fat free, count.)	◯	◯
4. Do you eat at least 1 cup of leafy green vegetables in your salad and/or put lettuce in your sandwich every day?	◯	◯

Scoring 2B

If you answered yes to all four questions, you are on your way to acing your fat-soluble vitamin needs! If you answered no to any of the questions, your diet needs some fine-tuning. Deep orange and dark green vegetables are excellent sources of vitamin A, and milk is an excellent choice for vitamin D. Vegetable oils provide vitamin E; if you put them on top of your vitamin K–rich leafy green salad, you'll hit the vitamin jackpot.

2C Are You Getting Enough Water-Soluble Vitamins in Your Diet?

	Yes	No
1. Do you consume at least 1/2 cup of rice or pasta daily?	◯	◯
2. Do you eat at least 1 cup of a ready-to-eat cereal or hot cereal every day?	◯	◯
3. Do you have at least one slice of bread, a bagel, or a muffin daily?	◯	◯
4. Do you enjoy a citrus fruit or fruit juice, such as an orange, a grapefruit, or orange juice every day?	◯	◯
5. Do you have at least 1 cup of vegetables throughout your day?	◯	◯

Scoring 2C

If you answered yes to all of these questions, you are a vitamin B and C superstar! If you answered no to any of the questions, your diet could use some refinement. Rice, pasta, cereals, bread, and bread products are all excellent sources of B vitamins. Citrus fruits are a ringer for vitamin C. In fact, all vegetables can contribute to meeting your vitamin C needs daily.

Source: Adapted from J. Blake, *Nutrition and You*, 2nd ed. (San Francisco: Benjamin Cummings, 2011).

Your Plan for Change

The Assess Yourself activity gave you the chance to evaluate your current nutritional habits. Now that you have considered these results, you can decide whether you need to make changes in your daily eating for long-term health.

Today, you can:

◯ Start keeping a more detailed food log. Take note of the nutritional information of the various foods you eat and write down particulars about the number of calories, grams of fat, grams of sugar, milligrams of sodium, and so on of each food. Try to find specific weak spots: Are you consuming too many calories or too much salt or sugar? Do you eat too little calcium or iron?

◯ Take a field trip to the grocery store. Forgo your fast-food dinner and instead spend some time in the produce section of the supermarket. Purchase your favorite fruits and vegetables, and try something new to expand your tastes.

Within the next 2 weeks, you can:

◯ Plan at least three meals that you can make at home or in your dorm room, and purchase the ingredients you'll need ahead of time. Something as simple as a chicken sandwich on whole-grain bread will be more nutritious, and probably cheaper, than heading out for a fast-food meal.

◯ Start reading labels. Be aware of the amount of calories, sodium, sugars, and fats in prepared foods; aim to buy and consume those that are lower in all of these and are higher in calcium and fiber.

By the end of the semester, you can:

◯ Get in the habit of eating a healthy breakfast every morning. Combine whole grains, proteins, and fruit in your breakfast—for example, eat a bowl of cereal with milk and bananas or a cup of yogurt combined with granola and berries. Eating a healthy breakfast will jump-start your metabolism, prevent drops in blood glucose levels, and keep your brain and body performing at their best through those morning classes.

◯ Commit to one or two healthful changes to your eating patterns for the rest of the semester. You might resolve to eat five servings of fruits and vegetables every day, to switch to low-fat or nonfat dairy products, to stop drinking soft drinks, or to use only olive oil in your cooking. Use your food diary to help you spot places where you can make healthier choices on a daily basis.

Summary

- Recognizing that we eat for more reasons than just survival is the first step toward improving our nutritional habits.
- The essential nutrients include water, proteins, carbohydrates, fats, vitamins, and minerals. Water makes up 50 to 60 percent of our body weight and is necessary for nearly all life processes. Proteins are major components of our cells and are key elements of antibodies, enzymes, and hormones. Carbohydrates are our primary sources of energy. Fats play important roles in maintaining body temperature and cushioning and protecting organs. Vitamins are organic compounds, and minerals are inorganic compounds. We need both in relatively small amounts to maintain healthy body function.
- Food labels provide information on serving size and number of calories in a food, as well as the amounts of various nutrients and the percentage of recommended daily values those amounts represent.
- A healthful diet is adequate, moderate, balanced, varied, and nutrient dense. The *Dietary Guidelines for Americans* and the MyPlate plan provide guidelines for healthy eating. These recommendations, developed by the USDA, place emphasis on balancing calories and making appropriate food choices. Vegetarianism can provide a healthy alternative for people wishing to eat less or no meat.
- College students face unique challenges in eating healthfully. Learning to make better choices at restaurants, to eat healthfully on a budget, and to eat nutritionally in the dorm are all possible when you use the information in this chapter.
- Organic foods are grown and produced without the use of synthetic pesticides, chemicals, or hormones. The USDA offers certification of organics. These foods have become increasingly available and popular, as people take a greater interest in eating healthfully and sustainably.
- Foodborne illnesses, food irradiation, food additives, food allergies, food intolerances, GM foods, and other food safety

and health concerns are becoming increasingly important to health-wise consumers. Recognizing potential risks and taking steps to prevent problems are part of a sound nutritional plan.

Pop Quiz

1. Triglycerides make up about _____ percent of total body fat.
   a. 5
   b. 35
   c. 55
   d. 95

2. Which of the following foods would be considered a healthy, *nutrient-dense* food?
   a. Nonfat milk
   b. Celery
   c. Soft drink
   d. Potato chips

3. What is the most crucial nutrient for life?
   a. Water
   b. Fiber
   c. Minerals
   d. Protein

4. Which of the following nutrients moves food through the digestive tract?
   a. Water
   b. Fiber
   c. Minerals
   d. Starch

5. Which of the following nutrients is required for the repair and growth of body tissue?
   a. Carbohydrates
   b. Proteins
   c. Vitamins
   d. Fats

6. What substance plays a vital role in maintaining healthy skin and hair, insulating body organs against shock, maintaining body temperature, and promoting healthy cell function?
   a. Fats
   b. Fibers
   c. Proteins
   d. Carbohydrates

7. Which vitamin maintains bone health?
   a. B_{12}
   b. D
   c. B_6
   d. Niacin

8. What is the most common nutrient deficiency worldwide?
   a. Protein deficiency
   b. Iron deficiency
   c. Fiber deficiency
   d. Calcium deficiency

9. Which of the following is NOT a recommendation of the MyPlate plan:
   a. Half of your plate should be fruits and vegetables.
   b. Milk and dairy products should be 1% or fat-free.
   c. Sweets should be eaten once a week or less.
   d. Half of your grains should be whole grains.

10. Which of the following is a healthier fat to include in the diet?
    a. *Trans* fat
    b. Saturated fat
    c. Unsaturated fat
    d. Hydrogenated fat

Answers to these questions can be found on page A-1.

Web Links

1. **American Dietetic Association (ADA).** The ADA provides information on a range of dietary topics, including sports nutrition, healthful cooking, and nutritional eating. www.eatright.org

2. **U.S. Food and Drug Administration (FDA).** The FDA provides information for consumers and professionals in the areas of food safety, supplements, and medical devices. www.fda.gov

3. **Food and Nutrition Information Center.** This site offers a wide variety of information related to food and nutrition. http://fnic.nal.usda.gov

4. **U.S. Department of Agriculture (USDA).** The USDA offers a full discussion of the USDA's Dietary Guidelines for Americans. www.usda.gov

5. **Linus Pauling Institute.** This is a key U.S. research center for studies on macro- and micronutrients and antioxidants. http://lpi.oregonstate.edu

Weight Management and Body Image

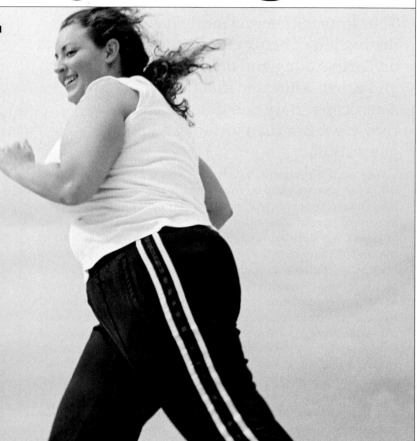

"The surge in obesity in this country is nothing short of a public health crisis . . . the health consequences are so severe that medical experts have warned that our children could be on track to live shorter lives than their parents."

—*First Lady Michelle Obama, Introduction of New Plan to Combat Overweight and Obesity, January 28, 2010*

In a landmark report, the U.S. Surgeon General stated it plainly: "Overweight and obesity result from an energy imbalance. This means eating too many calories and not getting enough exercise."[1] But if all it took were eating less and exercising more, Americans would merely reevaluate their diets, cut calories, and exercise. Unfortunately, it's not that easy. And the problem goes beyond body weight to increasingly common issues of self-perception and disordered eating, among both men and women.

What factors predispose us to problems with weight? Although diet and exercise are clearly major contributors, genetics and physiology are also important. And the environment you live, eat, and work in has a significant influence on what, how much, and when you eat.[2]

Obesity in the United States and Worldwide

learning outcomes

- **Examine obesity trends in the United States.**

The United States currently has the dubious distinction of being among the fattest nations on Earth. Young and old, rich and poor, rural and urban, educated and uneducated Americans share one thing in common— they are fatter than virtually all previous generations.

The word **obesogenic**, which the Centers for Disease Control defines as "characterized by environments that promote increased food intake, nonhealthful foods and physical inactivity," has increasingly become an apt descriptor of our society.[3] The maps in **Figure 9.1** illustrate the rapidly increasing levels of obesity in the United States over the last 20 years. Indeed, the prevalence of obesity has tripled among children and doubled among adults in recent decades.[4] Research indicates that the rate of increase in obesity began to slow between 1999 and 2008 for many populations.[5] However, although the rate of increase has slowed, current rates are still extremely high, with more than 68 percent of U.S. adults overall (72.3% of men and 64.1% of women) considered to be *overweight* (having a body mass index [BMI] of 25.0–29.9) or *obese* (having a BMI of 30.0 or higher).[6]

This translates into over 72 million adults—32.2 percent of men and 35.5 percent of women—who are classified as obese. This has staggering implications for increased risks from heart disease, diabetes, and other health complications associated with obesity.[7] Research suggests that the prospect is even more bleak for certain populations within the United States. A recent study of American preschool children showed obesity rates of nearly 19 percent among children younger than age 4.[8] The rates are even more troubling when broken down by ethnicity: In the under-4 age group, nearly 32 percent of Native Americans/Native Alaskans, 22 percent of Hispanics, and nearly 21 percent of non-Hispanic blacks were found to be obese. Rates among non-Hispanic whites and Asian Americans were 16 percent and 13 percent, respectively. Other research points to higher obesity risks among adults of different ethnicities—most notably African American women, who have been found to have rates of overweight/obesity as high as 80 percent.[9] Similar racial disparities exist for both children and adolescents.[10]

The United States is not alone in its increasing weight problem. During the past 20 years, the world's population has grown progressively heavier. Today, more than 1.5 billion adults worldwide are overweight, and approximately 500 million of them are obese. Add to that the 155 million children worldwide—43 million under age 5—who are overweight or obese and the scope of the problem,

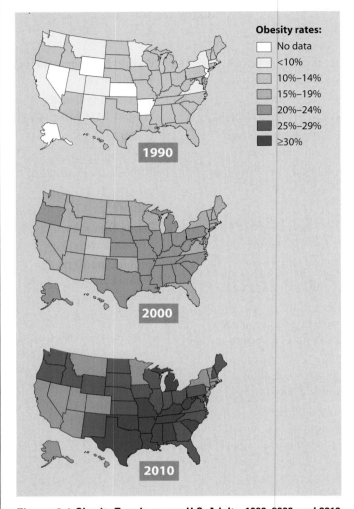

Figure 9.1 Obesity Trends among U.S. Adults, 1990, 2000, and 2010
These maps indicate the percentage of population in each state considered obese, based on a body mass index of 30 or higher, or about 30 pounds overweight for a person 5 feet 4 inches tall.
Source: Centers for Disease Control and Prevention, "U.S. Obesity Trends: 1985–2010," 2011, www.cdc.gov/obesity/data/trends.html#State.

sometimes called *globesity*, is clear. The World Health Organization (WHO) projects that by 2015 approximately 2.3 billion adults will be overweight and more than 700 million will be obese.[11]

check yourself

- **How have levels of obesity changed in the United States over the last 20 years?**
- **Why do you think disparities in obesity levels exist among certain populations in the United States?**

Health Effects of Overweight and Obesity

learning outcomes

- **List health effects associated with overweight and obesity.**

Obesity is the second greatest preventable cause of death in the United States, after smoking. Obesity and inactivity increase the risks from three of our leading killers: heart disease, cancer, and cerebrovascular ailments, including strokes.[12] In addition, some experts predict that the number of Americans diagnosed with diabetes, another major obesity-associated problem, will soon increase from 15 million in 2005 to as much as 50 million in 2050.[13] Other health risks associated with obesity include gallstones, sleep apnea, osteoarthritis, and several cancers.

Figure 9.2 summarizes these and other potential health consequences of obesity.

Short- and long-term health consequences of obesity are not our only concern: The estimated annual financial cost of obesity in the United States exceeds $147 billion in medical expenses and lost productivity.[14] Overall, obese individuals average $1,500 more per year in medical costs, about 41 percent more than individuals of average weight.[15] Of course, it is impossible to place a dollar value on a life lost prematurely due to diabetes, stroke, or heart attack or to assess the cost of the social isolation of and discrimination against overweight individuals. Of growing importance is the recognition that obese individuals suffer

significant disability during their lives, in terms of both mobility and activities of daily living.[16]

Other effects of overweight and obesity can be more subtle. Consequences can include: depression, anxiety, low self-esteem, poor body image, and suicidal acts and thoughts; binge eating and unhealthy weight-control practices; lack of adequate health care due to doctors spending less time with and doing fewer interventions on overweight patients, and doctor reluctance to perform preventive health screenings; and reluctance to visit the doctor and get necessary preventive health care services.

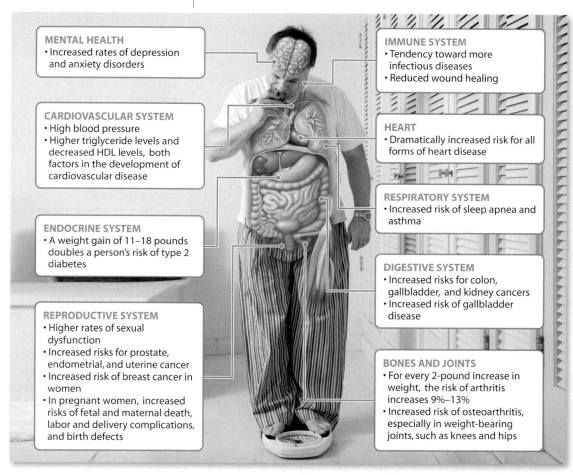

Figure 9.2 **Potential Negative Health Effects of Overweight and Obesity**

check yourself

- **What are some potential effects on the body of overweight and obesity?**

- **Do you consider the most significant consequences of overweight and obesity to be physical, financial, emotional, or other?**

Factors Contributing to Overweight and Obesity: Genetics, Physiology, and the Environment

learning outcomes

- **Explain the impact of genetics and physiology on body weight.**
- **Explain the impact of environment on body weight.**

Several factors appear to influence why one person becomes obese and another remains thin.

Body Type and Genes

In spite of decades of research, the exact role of genes in one's predisposition toward obesity remains in question. Family history of obesity has long been thought to increase one's chances of becoming obese.[17] However, newer meta-analyses of twin studies indicate that both genetics and environment play a substantial role in body composition.[18]

Researchers continue to explore whether and how genes might set metabolic rates, influence how the body balances calories and energy, or lead us to crave certain foods.[19] Some researchers focus on areas of the brain that may contribute to the desire to eat and **satiety**—the feeling of fullness when nutritional needs are satisfied and the stomach signals "no more."[20] Genetic variation, along with environmental influences, may increase risks of obesity—though a growing number of experts believe genes may play less of a role than originally believed.[21]

Thrifty Gene Theory

Researchers have noted higher body fat and obesity levels in certain Indian and African tribes than in the general population.[22] The theory: Their ancestors struggled through centuries of famine and survived by adapting with slowed metabolism. If this "thrifty gene" hypothesis is true, certain people may be genetically programmed to burn fewer calories. Nevertheless, only 2 to 5 percent of childhood obesity cases are caused by a defect that impairs function in a gene. Most childhood obesity seems to result primarily from obesogenic behaviors in an obesogenic environment.[23]

Physiological Factors

Metabolic Rates Although number of calories consumed is important, metabolism also helps determine weight. The **basal metabolic rate (BMR)** is the minimum rate at which the body uses energy when working to maintain basic vital functions. BMR for the average healthy adult is 1,200 to 1,800 calories per day.

The **resting metabolic rate (RMR)** includes the BMR plus any energy expended through daily sedentary activities such as food digestion, sitting, studying, or standing. The **exercise metabolic rate (EMR)** accounts for all remaining daily calorie expenditures. For most of us, these calories come from activities such as walking, climbing stairs, and mowing the lawn.

In general, the younger you are, the higher your BMR. Growth consumes a good deal of energy, and BMR is highest during infancy, puberty, and pregnancy. After age 30, a person's BMR slows down by 1 to 2 percent a year. Less activity, shifting priorities (family and career become more important than fitness), and loss in muscle mass also contribute to weight gain in many middle-aged people.

Theories abound concerning mechanisms regulating metabolism and food intake. Some sources indicate that the hypothalamus (the part of the brain that regulates appetite) closely monitors levels of certain nutrients in the blood; when they fall, the brain signals us to eat. According to one theory, the monitoring system in obese people makes cues to eat more frequent and intense than in others. Another theory, **adaptive thermogenesis**, suggests that in thin people the appetite center of the brain speeds up metabolic activity to compensate for increased food consumption.

On the other side of the BMR equation is the **set point theory**, which suggests that our bodies fight to maintain our weight around a narrow range or at a set point. If we go on a drastic diet, our bodies slow our BMR to conserve energy. The good news is that set points can be changed, slowly and steadily, via healthy diet, steady weight loss, and exercise.

Do my genes have any effect on my weight?

Many factors help determine weight and body type, including heredity and genetic makeup, environment, and learned eating patterns, which are often connected to family habits.

Yo-yo diets, in which people repeatedly gain weight then lose it quickly, are doomed to fail. When such dieters resume eating, their BMR is set lower, making them almost certain to regain lost pounds. After repeated gains and losses, such people find it increasingly hard to lose weight and easy to regain it.

Hormonal Influences: Ghrelin and Leptin Obese people may be more likely than thin people to eat for reasons other than nutrition.[24] Many people have attributed obesity to problems with the thyroid gland and resultant hormone imbalances that impede the ability to burn calories. Although less than 2 percent of the obese population have a thyroid problem and can trace their weight problems to a metabolic or hormone imbalance,[25] hormones may still affect one's weight.

Ghrelin,[26] "the hunger hormone," plays a key role in appetite regulation, food intake control, gastrointestinal motility, gastric acid secretion, endocrine and exocrine pancreatic secretions, glucose and lipid metabolism, and cardiovascular and immunologic processes.[27] Another hormone, *leptin,* is produced by fat cells; its levels in the blood increase as fat tissue increases. Scientists believe leptin serves as a satiety signal.[28] When levels of leptin in the blood rise, appetite levels drop. Although obese people have adequate leptin and leptin receptors, the receptors do not seem to work properly—though why remains a mystery. It may be simply that environmental cues are stronger than our hunger pangs.

Fat Cells and Predisposition to Fatness Some obese people may have excessive numbers of fat cells. An average-weight adult has approximately 25 to 35 billion fat cells, a moderately obese adult 60 to 100 billion, and an extremely obese adult as many as 200 billion.[29] This type of obesity, **hyperplasia**, usually appears in early childhood and perhaps, due to the mother's dietary habits, even prior to birth. Critical periods for development of hyperplasia seem to be the last 2 to 3 months of fetal development, the first year of life, and from ages 9 to 13. Central to this theory is the belief that the number of fat cells in a body does not increase appreciably during adulthood. However, the ability of each cell to swell (**hypertrophy**) and shrink does carry over into adulthood. Weight gain may be tied to both the number of fat cells and the capacity of individual cells to enlarge.

Environmental Factors

Automobiles, remote controls, desk jobs, and computer use all lead us to sit more and move less. Our culture also urges us to eat more. Many environmental factors can trigger our "eat" responses:[30]

- We are bombarded with advertising for high-calorie foods at a low price and marketing of super-sized portions. Standard portions have increased dramatically in the past 20 years (**Figure 9.3**).

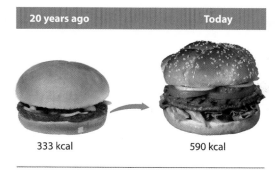

20 years ago	Today
333 kcal	590 kcal

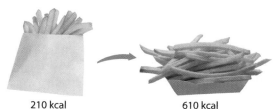

210 kcal	610 kcal

Figure 9.3 Today's Bloated Portions
The increase in average portion sizes has made it tougher than ever to manage your weight.
Source: Data are from the National Institutes of Health/ National Heart, Lung, and Blood Institute (NHLBI), "Portion Distortion," Accessed June 2011, Available at http:// hp2010.nhlbihin.net/portion.

- Prepackaged, high-fat meals; fast food; and sugar-laden soft drinks are increasingly widespread, as are high-calorie coffee drinks and energy drinks.
- As society eats out more, higher-calorie, high-fat foods become the norm.
- Bottle-feeding infants may increase energy intake relative to breastfeeding.
- Misleading food labels confuse consumers about portion and serving sizes.
- Fast-food restaurants, cafes, vending machines, and quick-stop markets offer easy access to high-calorie foods and beverages.
- Larger dishes mask serving sizes and lead to increased calorie and fat intake.

A Youthful Start on Obesity Children have always loved junk food. However, today's youth tend to eat larger portions and exercise less than any previous generation,[31] and children are subject to the same environmental, social, and cultural factors that influence obesity in their elders. Maternal undernutrition, obesity, and diabetes during gestation and lactation are also strong predictors of obesity in children.[32] Race and ethnicity also seem intricately interwoven with environmental factors in increasing risks to young people by as much as three times in Native Americans/Alaska Natives, Hispanics, and African Americans.[33]

Psychosocial and Economic Factors

The relationship of weight problems to emotional needs and wants remains uncertain. Food often is used as a reward for good behavior in childhood. For adults facing economic and interpersonal stress, the bright spot in the day is often "what's for dinner." Again, the research here is controversial. What is certain is that eating is a social ritual associated with companionship, celebration, and enjoyment.

Socioeconomic factors can also affect weight control. When economic times are tough, people tend to eat more inexpensive, high-calorie processed foods.[34] Unsafe neighborhoods and lack of recreational areas make it difficult for less affluent people to exercise.[35] And the more educated you are, the lower your body mass index and overall obesity profile are likely to be. Highly educated men and, in particular, highly educated women in the United States and Europe have a lower average BMI than their less educated counterparts.[36]

check yourself

- **What are the influences of genetics, physiology, and environment on body weight? Which do you consider most important?**
- **How does the importance of genetics and physiology affect strategies for weight management?**

Factors Contributing to Overweight and Obesity: Lifestyle

learning **outcomes**

■ **Explain the impact of lifestyle on body weight.**

Of all the factors affecting obesity, perhaps the most critical is the relationship between activity level and calorie intake. Determining activity levels using surveys, however, is difficult. One big problem in that people surveyed overestimate their daily exercise level and intensity. It is also difficult to determine which measures of fitness were actually used and how indicative of overall health these may ultimately be. Four in 10 adults in the United States *never* engage in any exercise, sports, or physically active hobbies in their leisure time.[37] Based on the most recent data, using leisure-time activity as a measure, only 35 percent of adults aged 18 and over reported regular activity.[38]

Do you know people who seemingly can eat whatever they want without gaining weight? With few exceptions, if you were to monitor the level and intensity of their activity, you would discover why. Even if their schedule does not include intense exercise, it probably includes a high level of activity.

15 or more hours each day is the average amount of time that Americans spend sitting.

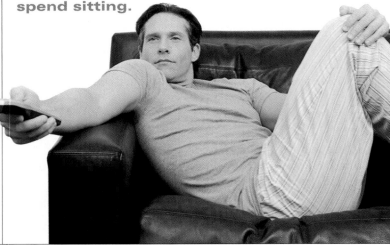

Rather than focusing only on how much formal exercise we get in each day, health and fitness experts have begun to focus on how much time we spend sitting. How many of us exercise, then go into "slo-mo" mode for much of the day? If the body isn't moving, it's not burning many calories.

New research indicates a dose-response association between sitting time and mortality from all causes and from cardiovascular disease, independent of leisure-time activity; that is, the more time you spend sitting, the worse your health is likely to be, regardless of whether you exercise or not. Because muscle activity burns energy, passive sitting is one of the worst things you can do if you are trying to burn calories. If you stood up while reading this chapter, the large and small muscle groups in your legs would be constantly working to keep you from falling over—and burning more calories.

Recent research suggests that we should make an effort to balance light-intensity activities and sedentary behaviors throughout our days.[39] What if instead of spending all of our effort on getting in 30 minutes of exercise each day, we focused more on the little things we can do to burn calories 24/7? What if workplaces were designed to get people up and moving at intervals throughout the day? How about standing to use your computer rather than sitting, or riding a stationary bike at a comfortable speed while watching TV or reading your textbooks? What if you didn't let yourself sit anywhere other than in classes for the first 5 or 6 hours of the day? These little extra bouts of movement may make a big difference in daily calories burned, weight management, and overall health.

Skills for **Behavior Change**

FINDING THE FUN IN HEALTHY EATING AND EXERCISE

With a little creativity, you can make weight management a fun, positive part of your life. Try these tips:

■ Cook and eat with friends. Share the responsibility for making the meal while you spend time with people you like.

■ Experiment with new foods to add variety to your meals.

■ Vary your exercise routine—change the exercise or your location, join a team for the social aspects in addition to exercise, decide to run a long foot race for the challenge, or learn how to skateboard for fun.

check yourself

■ **What are some lifestyles changes that can contribute to weight management?**

Assessing Body Weight and Body Composition

learning outcomes

- **Distinguish among overweight, obesity, and underweight.**

Everyone has his or her own ideal weight, based on individual variables such as body structure, height, and fat distribution. Traditionally, experts used measurement techniques such as height–weight charts to determine whether an individual fell into the ideal weight, overweight, or obese category. However, these charts can be misleading because they don't take body composition (i.e., a person's ratio of fat to lean muscle) or fat distribution into account.

In fact, weight can be a deceptive indicator. Many extremely muscular athletes would be considered overweight based on traditional height–weight charts, whereas many young women might think their weight is normal based on charts, only to be shocked to discover that 35 to 40 percent of their weight is body fat!

More accurate measures of evaluating healthy weight and disease risk focus on a person's percentage of body fat and how that fat is distributed in his or her body.

Many people worry about becoming fat, but some fat is essential for healthy body functioning. Fat regulates body temperature, cushions and insulates organs and tissues, and is the body's main source of stored energy. Body fat is composed of two types of fat: essential and storage. *Essential fat* is that fat necessary for maintenance of life and reproductive functions. *Storage fat*, the nonessential fat that many of us try to shed, makes up the remainder of our fat reserves.

Overweight and Obesity

In general, **overweight** is increased body weight due to excess fat that exceeds healthy recommendations, whereas **obesity** refers to body weight that greatly exceeds health recommendations. Traditionally, *overweight* was defined as being 1 to 19 percent above one's ideal weight, based on a standard height–weight chart, and

obesity was defined as being 20 percent or more above one's ideal weight. **Morbidly obese** people are 100 percent or more above their ideal weight. Experts now usually define *overweight* and *obesity* in terms of BMI, a measure discussed later, or percentage of body fat, as determined by some of the methods we'll discuss shortly. Although opinion varies somewhat, most experts agree that men's bodies should contain between 8 and 20 percent total body fat, and women should be within the range of 20 to 30 percent. At various ages and stages of life, these ranges also vary, but generally, men who exceed 22 percent body fat and women who exceed 35 percent are considered overweight (see **Table 9.1**).

Underweight

There are percentages of body fat below which a person is considered **underweight**, and health is compromised. In men, this lower limit is approximately 3 to 7 percent of total body weight; in women, it is approximately 8 to 15 percent. Extremely low body fat can cause hair loss, visual disturbances, skin problems, a tendency to fracture bones easily, digestive system disturbances, heart irregularities, gastrointestinal problems, difficulties in maintaining body temperature, and amenorrhea (in women).

TABLE 9.1 Selected Percent Body Fat Norms for Men and Women*

	Men Age 20–29	Men Age 30–39	Women Age 20–29	Women Age 30–39
Very Lean	6% or lower	10% or lower	13% or lower	14% or lower
Excellent	7%–10%	11%–14%	14%–16%	15%–17%
Good	11%–15%	15%–18%	17%–19%	18%–21%
Fair	16%–19%	19%–21%	20%–23%	22%–25%
Poor	20%–23%	22%–25%	24%–27%	26%–29%
Very Poor	24% or higher	26% or higher	28% or higher	30% or higher

*Assumes nonathletes.
Source: American College of Sports Medicine, *ACSM's Guidelines for Exercise Testing and Prescription*, 8th ed. (Baltimore, MD: Lippincott Williams & Wilkins, 2009). Copyright © 2009 by Lippincott Williams & Wilkins. Reprinted with permission.

check yourself

- **What are the differences between overweight and obesity?**

Assessing Body Weight and Body Composition: BMI and Other Methods

learning outcomes

■ **Compare and contrast different methods of body composition assessment.**

Although people have a general sense that BMI is an indicator of how "fat" a person is, most do not really know what it assesses. **Body mass index (BMI)** is a description of body weight relative to height, numbers highly correlated with total body fat. BMI is not gender specific, and it does not directly measure percentage of body fat, but it provides a more accurate measure than weight alone.[40] Find your BMI in inches and pounds in **Figure 9.4**, or you can calculate your BMI by dividing your weight in kilograms by height in meters squared:

$$BMI = weight(kg)/height\ squared\ (m^2)$$

A BMI calculator is also available at http://nhlbisupport.com/bmi/bmicalc.htm.

Desirable BMI levels may vary with age and by sex; however, most BMI tables for adults do not account for such variables. *Healthy weights* are defined as those with BMIs of 18.5 to 24.9, the range of lowest statistical health risk.[41] A BMI of 25 to 29.9 indicates overweight and potentially significant health risks. A BMI of 30 or above is classified as obese, whereas a BMI of 40 or higher is morbidly obese.[42] Nearly 3 percent of obese men and almost 7 percent of obese women are morbidly obese.[43]

Although useful, BMI levels don't account for the fact that muscle weighs more than fat; a well-muscled person could weigh enough to be classified as obese according to his or her BMI. Nor are bone mass and water weight considered in BMI calculations. For people who are less than 5 feet tall, are highly muscled, or are older and have little muscle mass, BMI levels can be inaccurate. More precise methods of determining body fat, described below, should be used for these individuals.

Youth and BMI The labels *obese* and *morbidly obese* have been used for years for

adults, though there is growing concern about the consequences of pinning these potentially stigmatizing labels on children.[44] BMI ranges above normal weight for children and teens are often labeled as "at risk of overweight" and "overweight." After BMI is calculated, the number is plotted on the Centers for Disease Control and Prevention (CDC) BMI-for-age growth charts to obtain a percentile ranking. Percentiles are the most commonly used indicator to assess size and growth patterns of individual children in the United States. The percentile indicates the relative position of the child's BMI number among children of the same sex and age.[45]

Waist Circumference and Ratio Measurements

Knowing where your fat is carried may be more important than knowing how much you carry. Men and postmenopausal women tend to store fat in the abdominal area. Premenopausal women usually store fat in the hips, buttocks, and thighs. Waist circumference measurement is increasingly recognized as a useful tool in assessing abdominal fat, which is considered more threatening to health than fat in other regions. In particular, as waist circumference increases, the risk for diabetes, cardiovascular disease, and stroke increases. A waistline greater than 40 inches (102 centimeters) in men and 35 inches (88 centimeters) in women may be particularly indicative of greater health risk.[46] If a person is less than 5 feet tall or has a BMI of 35 or above, waist circumference standards used for the general population might not apply.

The **waist-to-hip ratio** measures regional fat distribution. A waist-to-hip ratio greater than 1 in men and 0.8 in women indicates increased health risks.[47] Although used

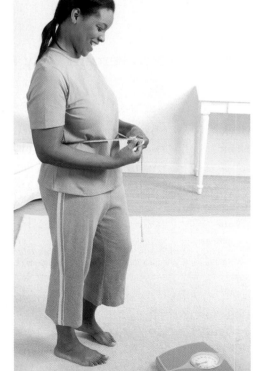

How can I tell if I am **overweight or overfat?**

Observing the way you look and how your clothes fit can give you a general idea of whether you weigh more or less than in the past. But for evaluating your weight and body fat levels in terms of potential health risks, it's best to use more scientific measures, such as BMI, waist circumference, waist-to-hip ratio, or a technician-administered body composition test.

extensively in the past, waist-to-hip ratios are used less often today, with BMI and waist circumference the preferred measures of health risk.

Measures of Body Fat

There are many other ways to assess body fat levels. One low-tech way is simply to look in the mirror or consider how your clothes fit now compared with how they fit in the past. For those who wish to take a more precise measurement of their percentage of body fat, more accurate techniques are available, including caliper measurement, underwater weighing, and various body scans. These methods usually involve the help of a skilled professional and typically must be done in a lab or clinical setting.

BMI	19	20	21	22	23	24	25	26	27	28	29	30	31	32	33	34	35	36	37	38	39	40	41	42
Height											**Weight in pounds**													
4'10"	91	96	100	105	110	115	119	124	129	134	138	143	148	153	158	162	167	172	177	181	186	191	196	201
4'11"	94	99	104	109	114	119	124	128	133	138	143	148	153	158	163	168	173	178	183	188	193	198	203	208
5'	97	102	107	112	118	123	128	133	138	143	148	153	158	163	168	174	179	184	189	194	199	204	209	215
5'1"	100	106	111	116	122	127	132	137	143	148	153	158	164	169	174	180	185	190	195	201	206	211	217	222
5'2"	104	109	115	120	126	131	136	142	147	153	158	164	169	175	180	186	191	196	202	207	213	218	224	229
5'3"	107	113	118	124	130	135	141	146	152	158	163	169	175	180	186	191	197	203	208	214	220	225	231	237
5'4"	110	116	122	128	134	140	145	151	157	163	169	175	180	186	192	197	204	209	215	221	227	232	238	244
5'5"	114	120	126	132	138	144	150	156	162	168	174	180	186	192	198	204	210	216	222	228	234	240	246	252
5'6"	118	124	130	136	142	148	155	161	167	173	179	186	192	198	204	210	216	223	229	235	241	247	253	260
5'7"	121	127	134	140	146	153	159	166	172	178	185	191	198	204	211	217	223	230	236	242	249	255	261	268
5'8"	125	131	138	144	151	158	164	171	177	184	190	197	204	210	216	223	230	236	243	249	256	262	269	276
5'9"	128	135	142	149	155	162	169	176	182	189	196	203	210	216	223	230	236	243	250	257	263	270	277	284
5'10"	132	139	146	153	160	167	174	181	188	195	202	209	216	222	229	236	243	250	257	264	271	278	285	292
5'11"	136	143	150	157	165	172	179	186	193	200	208	215	222	229	236	243	250	257	265	272	279	286	293	301
6'	140	147	154	162	169	177	184	191	199	206	213	221	228	235	242	250	258	265	272	279	287	294	302	309
6'1"	144	151	159	166	174	182	189	197	204	212	219	227	235	242	250	257	265	275	280	288	295	302	310	318
6'2"	148	155	163	171	179	186	194	202	210	218	225	233	241	249	256	264	272	280	287	295	303	311	319	326
6'3"	152	160	168	176	184	193	200	208	216	224	232	240	248	256	264	272	279	287	295	303	311	319	327	335
6'4"	156	164	172	180	189	197	205	213	221	230	238	246	254	263	271	279	287	295	304	312	320	328	336	344

Healthy weight BMI 18.5–24.9	Overweight BMI 25–29.9	Obese BMI 30–39.9	Morbidly obese BMI ≥40

Figure 9.4 Body Mass Index (BMI)

Locate your height, read across to find your weight, and then read up to determine your BMI. Any weight less than those listed for a given height would yield a BMI of less than 18.5, classified as underweight.

Source: National Institutes of Health/National Heart, Lung, and Blood Institute (NHLBI). *Evidence Report of Clinical Guidelines on the Identification, Evaluation, and Treatment of Overweight and Obesity in Adults*, 1998, www.nhlbi.nih.gov/guidelines/obesity/ob_gdlns.htm.

check yourself

- **Which of the various assessment methods do you consider the most accurate? Which is the most accessible to the average person?**

Weight Management: Understanding Energy Balance and Improving Eating Habits

- **Explain how energy expenditure and energy intake affect weight management.**
- **List ways to change eating habits in order to successfully manage your weight.**

At some point in our lives, almost all of us will decide to lose weight or modify our diet. Many will have mixed success. Failure is often related to thinking about losing weight in terms of short-term "dieting" rather than carefully analyzing individual risks for obesity and adjusting long-term eating behaviors (such as developing the habit of healthy snacking).

Low-calorie diets produce only temporary losses and may actually lead to disordered binge eating or related problems.[48] Repeated bouts of restrictive dieting may be physiologically harmful; moreover, the sense of failure we experience each time we don't meet our goal can exact far-reaching psychological costs. Drugs and intensive counseling can contribute to positive weight loss, but, even then, many people regain weight after treatment. Maintaining a healthful body takes constant attention and nurturing over the course of your lifetime.

Understanding Calories and Energy Balance

A *calorie* is a unit of measure that indicates the amount of energy gained from food or expended through activity. Each time you consume 3,500 calories more than your body needs to maintain weight, you gain a pound of storage fat. Conversely, each time your body expends an extra 3,500 calories, you lose a pound of fat. If you consume 140 calories (the amount in one can of regular soda) more than you need every single day and make no other changes in diet or activity, you would gain 1 pound in 25 days (3,500 calories ÷ 140 calories ÷ day = 25 days). Even when you think you are watching fat intake by ordering your Starbucks vanilla latte with skim milk, you are still consuming a whopping 230 calories with every 16 ounces.

Assuming you start having the same drink every day and do nothing else differently, you'll gain 1 pound every 15 days because of your positive caloric balance. Conversely, if you walk for 30 minutes each day at a pace of 15 minutes per mile (172 calories burned) in addition to your regular activities, you would lose 1 pound in 20 days (3,500 calories ÷ 172 calories ÷ day = 20.3 days) due to the negative caloric balance. This is an example of the concept of energy balance described in **Figure 9.5**. Of course, these are generic formulas. If you weigh more, you will burn more calories moving your body through the same exercise routine than someone who is thinner.

The Importance of Exercise

Increasing BMR, RMR, or EMR levels will help burn calories. Any increase in the intensity, frequency, and duration of daily exercise levels can have a significant impact on total calorie expenditure.

Physical activity makes a greater contribution to metabolic rate when large muscle groups are used. The energy spent on physical activity is the energy used to move the body's muscles and the extra energy used to speed up heartbeat and respiration rate. The number of calories spent depends on three factors:

1. The number and proportion of muscles used
2. The amount of weight moved
3. The length of time the activity takes

An activity involving both the arms and legs burns more calories than one involving only the legs. An activity performed by a heavy

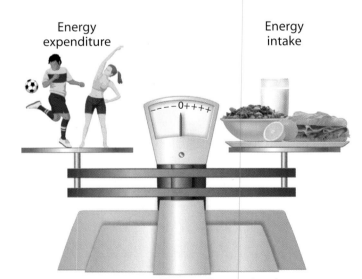

Energy expenditure = Energy intake

Figure 9.5 The Concept of Energy Balance

If you consume more calories than you burn, you will gain weight. If you burn more than you consume, you will lose weight. If both are equal, your weight will not change, according to this concept.

person burns more calories than the same activity performed by a lighter person. And an activity performed for 40 minutes requires twice as much energy as the same activity performed for only 20 minutes. Thus, an obese person walking for 1 mile burns more calories than does a slim person walking the same distance. It also may take overweight people longer to walk the mile, which means that they are burning energy for a longer time and therefore expending more overall calories than the thin walkers.

Improving Your Eating Habits

Before you can change a behavior, such as unhealthy eating habits, you must first determine what causes (or "triggers") it. Many people find it helpful to keep a chart of their eating patterns: when they feel like eating, where they are when they decide to eat, the amount of time they spend eating, other activities they engage in during the meal (watching television or reading), whether they eat alone or with others, what and how much they consume, and how they felt before they took their first bite. If you keep a detailed daily log of eating triggers for at least a week, you will discover useful clues about what in your environment or your emotional makeup causes you to want food. Typically, these dietary triggers center on patterns and problems in everyday living rather than on real hunger pangs. Many people eat compulsively when stressed; however, for other people, the same circumstances diminish their appetite, causing them to lose weight.

Once you've evaluated your behaviors and determined your triggers, you can begin to devise a plan for improved eating. If you are unsure of where to start, seek assistance from reputable sources in selecting a dietary plan that is nutritious and easy to follow. Registered dietitians, some physicians (not all doctors have a strong background in nutrition), health educators and exercise physiologists with nutritional training, and other health professionals can provide reliable information. Beware of people who call themselves nutritionists; there is no such official designation. Avoid weight-loss programs that promise quick, "miracle" results or those run by "trainees," often people with short courses on nutrition and exercise that are designed to sell products or services.

Before engaging in any weight-loss program, ask about the credentials of the adviser; assess the nutrient value of the prescribed diet; verify that dietary guidelines are consistent with reliable nutrition research; and analyze the suitability of the diet to your tastes, budget, and lifestyle. Any diet that requires radical behavior changes or sets up artificial dietary programs through prepackaged products that don't teach you how to eat healthfully is likely to fail. Supplements and fad diets that claim fast weight loss will invariably mean fast weight regain. The most successful plans allow you to make food choices in real-world settings and do not ask you to sacrifice everything you enjoy.

You will also need to address some of the triggers that you may have for eating that are unrelated to hunger. For example, if you tend to eat in stressful situations, try to acknowledge the feelings of stress and anxiety and develop stress management techniques to practice daily. If you find yourself eating when you are bored or tired, identify the times when you feel low energy, and fill them with activities other than eating, such as exercise breaks, or cultivate a

new interest or hobby that keeps your mind and hands busy. If your trigger is feeling angry or upset, analyze your emotions and look for a noneating activity to deal with them, such as taking a quick walk or calling a friend. If it is the sight and smell of food, stop buying high-calorie foods that tempt you, or store them in an inconvenient place, out of sight. Avoid walking past or sitting or standing near the table of tempting treats at a meeting, party, or other gathering.

Skills for Behavior Change

TIPS FOR SENSIBLE SNACKING

- **Keep healthy munchies around.** Buy 100-percent whole-wheat breads. If you need to spice up your snack, use low-fat or soy cheese, low-fat cream cheese, peanut butter, hummus, or other healthy favorites. Some baked crackers or chips are low in fat and calories and high in fiber. Look for these on your grocery shelves.

- **Keep "crunchies" on hand.** Apples, pears, red or green pepper sticks, popcorn, carrots, and celery all are good choices. Wash the fruits and vegetables and cut them up to carry with you; eat them when a snack attack comes on.

- **Quench your thirst with hot drinks.** Hot tea, heated milk, plain or decaffeinated coffee, hot chocolate made with nonfat milk or water, or soup broths will help keep you satisfied.

- **Choose natural beverages.** Drink plain water, 100 percent juice in small quantities, or other low-sugar choices to satisfy your thirst. Avoid certain juices, energy drinks, and soft drinks that have added sugars, low fiber, and no protein. Usually, they are high in calories and low in longer-term satisfaction.

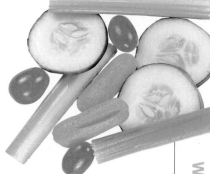

- **Eat nuts instead of candy.** Although nuts are relatively high in calories, they are also loaded with healthy fats and make a healthy snack when consumed in moderation.

- **If you must have a piece of chocolate, keep it small.** Note that dark chocolate is better than milk chocolate or white chocolate because of its antioxidant content.

- **Avoid high-calorie energy bars.** Eat these only if you are exercising hard and don't have an opportunity to eat a regular meal. If you buy energy bars, look for ones with a good mixture of fiber and protein and that are low in fat and calories.

---

check yourself

- **How do changes in energy expenditure and energy intake affect weight?**

- **How important is snacking to a sensible weight management program? Why?**

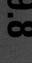

Weight Management: Assessing Diet Books

learning outcomes

■ **Identify typical strengths and weaknesses of popular diet books.**

People looking to lose weight and improve eating habits often turn to diet books for advice and guidance. Without guidance, finding a diet book that is both medically sound and that fits your individual needs can seem daunting.

Table 9.2 describes and evaluates a sample of popular diet books. For information on other books, check out the regularly updated list of the diet book reviews on the American Dietetic Association website at www.eatright.org.

TABLE 9.2 Analyzing Popular Diet Books

Diet Book	Author Credentials	Claims	What You Eat	Science Validity	Cautions
The Best Life Diet, revised and updated	Bob Greene (Oprah Winfrey's personal fitness trainer)	• Prepares "festive foods" • Watch weight go away • Emphasis on lifestyle change	Three phases: 1. Adopt healthy habits and increase activity 2. Weekly weigh-ins and eliminate emotional eating 3. Rest of life	• Sensible multipronged approach • Sticks to good science • No quick weight loss	None evident
The Complete Beck Diet for Life: The Five-Stage Program for Permanent Weight Loss	Judith S. Beck, PhD	• Teaches self-motivation • Teaches how to handle cravings and hunger	• Five-stage program • Meal plans • 1,600–2,400 daily calories • Recipes	• Sensible approach • Well-balanced meals • Flexible "bonus" calories • Behavior based	None evident
The Flexitarian Diet: The Mostly Vegetarian Way to Lose Weight, Be Healthier, Prevent Disease, and Add Years to Your Life	Dawn Jackson Blatner, RD, LDN	• Be healthier • Prevent disease; add years to your life	• 5 × 5 Flex Plan • Vegetarian • Occasional meat, poultry, fish	• In the beginning, small amounts of meat allowed	• No direction on how to wean self off meat • No step-by-step instruction on how to include meat in a mostly vegetarian diet
You: On a Diet: The Owner's Manual for Waist Management	Michael F. Roizen, MD, and Mehmet C. Oz, MD	• Shave inches off your waistline: 2 inches in 2 weeks	• 14-Day Rebooting Plan • Focus on whole grains, nuts, lean meat, fish	• Simplified science • Daily exercise • Strength training • Describes how emotions and hormones affect eating behaviors	• 2 inches in 2 weeks are mostly water • Inch mentality not as relevant as BMI and health
Your Big Fat Boyfriend: How to Stay Thin When Dating a Diet Disaster	Jenna Bergen	• How to eat healthfully when dining at not-so-healthy places • Healthy recipes	• Humorous solutions to unhealthy situations • Simple formulas	• Lacking nutrition and scientific research	• Only for target audience, i.e., young women with no medical conditions
The All-New Atkins Advantage: The 12-Week Low-Carb Program to Lose Weight, Achieve Peak Fitness and Health, and Maximize Your Willpower to Reach Life Goals	Stuart L. Trager, MD, with Colette Heimowitz, MSc	• Achieve peak fitness and health • Maximize willpower	• 12-week meal plan • 20–80 grams of net carbohydrates • Multivitamin supplement recommended	• Vague approach	• Unproven claims to control cravings • Misleading regarding intake of saturated fats • Eating fewer whole grains, fruits, and vegetables reduces natural vitamins and minerals • Emphasis on carbohydrate cuts is questionable

Source: Adapted from American Dietetic Association's Diet and Lifestyle Book Reviews, Available at www.eatright.org/Media/content.aspx?id=6442452236#E-H.

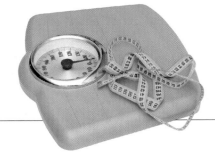

check yourself

■ **What are important factors to consider when evaluating current diet books?**

Weight Management: In Perspective

- **List steps to successful weight management.**

Weight loss may require supportive friends, relatives, and community resources. People can have large differences in RMR. Other factors, such as depression, stress, culture, and available foods, can also affect one's ability to lose weight. Being overweight does not mean people are weak willed or lazy.

To reach and maintain the weight at which you will be healthy and feel your best, develop a program of exercise and healthy eating that will work for you now and over the long term. It is unrealistic and potentially dangerous to try to lose weight in a short period of time. Instead, try to lose a healthy 1 to 2 pounds during the first week, then stay with this slow-and-easy regimen. Making permanent changes to your lifestyle by adding exercise and cutting back on calories to expend about 500 calories more than you consume each day will help you lose weight at a rate of 1 pound per week.

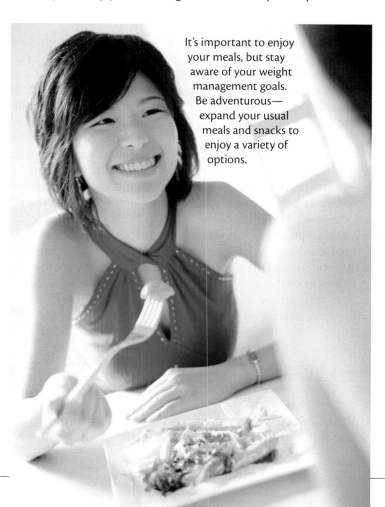

It's important to enjoy your meals, but stay aware of your weight management goals. Be adventurous—expand your usual meals and snacks to enjoy a variety of options.

Skills for **Behavior Change**

KEYS TO SUCCESSFUL WEIGHT MANAGEMENT

The key to successful weight management is finding a sustainable way to control what you eat and to make exercise a priority.

- Write down the things you find positive about your diet and exercise behaviors. Then write down things that need to be changed. For each change you need to make, list three or four small things you could change right now.
- Ask yourself some key questions. Why do you want to make this change right now? What are your ultimate goals?
- What resources on campus or in your community could help? Out of your friends and family members, who will help you?
- Keep a food and exercise log for 2 or 3 days. Note the good things you are doing, the things that need improvement, and the triggers you need to address.

Make a Plan

- Set realistic short- and long-term goals.
- Establish a plan. What diet and exercise changes can you make this week? Once you do 1 week, plot a course for 2 weeks, and so on.
- Look for balance. Remember that it is calories taken in and burned over time that make the difference.

Change Your Habits

- Notice whether you're hungry before starting a meal. Eat slowly, noting when you start to feel full. Stop before you are full.
- Eat breakfast. This will prevent you from being too hungry and overeating at lunch.
- Keep healthful snacks on hand for when you get hungry.
- Don't constantly deprive yourself or set unrealistic guidelines.

Incorporate Exercise

- Be active; slowly increase your time, speed, distance, or resistance levels.
- Vary your physical activity. Find activities you love; try things you haven't tried before.
- Find an exercise partner to help you stay motivated.
- Make it a fun break. Go for a walk in a place that interests you.

- **What are the key components of a successful weight management plan?**

Considering Drastic Weight-Loss Measures

- **Explain measures that may be taken when body weight poses an extreme threat to health.**

In certain limited instances, extreme measures may be considered to reduce weight. In severe cases of obesity, patients may be given powdered formulas with daily values of 400 to 700 calories plus vitamin and mineral supplements. Such **very-low-calorie diets (VLCDs)** should never be undertaken without strict medical supervision.

One dangerous potential complication of VLCDs or starvation diets is *ketoacidosis,* in which a patient's blood becomes more acidic, causing severe damage to body tissues.[49] Risk is greatest for those with untreated type 1 diabetes, anorexia nervosa, or bulimia nervosa. If fasting continues, the body turns to its last resort—protein—for energy, breaking down essential muscle and organ tissue to stay alive. Within about 10 days after the typical adult begins a complete fast, the body will have depleted its energy stores, and death may occur.

Dieters often turn to commercially marketed weight-loss supplements. U.S. Food and Drug Administration (FDA) approval is not required for over-the-counter "diet aids" or supplements, whose effectiveness is largely untested and unproven. Virtually all persons who use diet pills eventually regain their weight.[50]

In 2007, the FDA approved the first over-the-counter weight loss pill—a half-strength version of the drug orlistat (Xenical), marketed as Alli. This drug inhibits the action of lipase, an enzyme that helps the body digest fats, causing about 30 percent of fats consumed to pass through the digestive system. Side effects include gas with watery fecal discharge; frequent, often unexpected, bowel movements; and possible deficiencies of fat-soluble vitamins.

So far, no prescription diet drug has been proven usable over time without adverse effects or

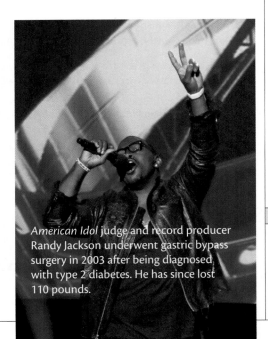

American Idol judge and record producer Randy Jackson underwent gastric bypass surgery in 2003 after being diagnosed with type 2 diabetes. He has since lost 110 pounds.

abuse. The drugs Pondimin and Redux, known as *fen-phen* (from their chemical names fenfluramine and phentermine), were thought to be safe.[51] When they were found to damage heart valves and contribute to pulmonary hypertension, a massive recall and lawsuit ensued.

View all diet drugs and supplements with caution, including these:

- **Sibutramine (Meridia).** This prescription medication suppresses appetite by inhibiting serotonin uptake in the brain. Side effects include dry mouth, headache, and high blood pressure. The FDA has issued warnings about Meridia for people with hypertension or heart disease.[52]
- **Hoodia gordonii.** This cactus-like plant native to Africa is a purported appetite suppressant. To date, it is not FDA approved and has not been tested in clinical trials.[53]
- **Herbal weight-loss aids.** Products containing *Ephedra* can cause rapid heart rate, seizures, insomnia, and raised blood pressure, all without significant effects on weight. *St. John's wort* and other herbs reported to suppress appetite have not been shown effective.

A few people who are severely overweight and have diabetes or hypertension may be candidates for surgical options. In *gastric banding,* an inflatable band partitions off the stomach, leaving only a small opening between its two parts. The upper part of the stomach is smaller, so the person feels full more quickly; digestion slows, making the person feel full longer.

Gastric bypass is designed to drastically decrease how much food a person can eat and absorb. Results are fast and dramatic, but there are many risks, including blood clots in the legs, a leak in a staple line in the stomach, pneumonia, infection, and death. Because the stomach pouch that remains after surgery is so small (about the size of a lime), the person can eat or drink only a tiny amount at a time. Possible side effects include nausea and vomiting, vitamin and mineral deficiencies, and dehydration. Patients must learn to eat healthy foods and exercise, or they could gain back the weight.

Research has shown unexpected results from gastric surgeries: complete remission of type 2 diabetes in the majority of cases, with drastic reductions in blood glucose levels in others.[54] Researchers are exploring surgical options for diabetes prevention in other populations.[55]

Liposuction is a surgical procedure in which fat cells are removed from specific areas of the body; it is cosmetic rather than weight-loss surgery. Liposuction is not without risk: Infections, severe scarring, and even death have resulted. In many cases, people who have liposuction regain fat or require multiple surgeries to repair lumpy, irregular surfaces.

- **What measures can be taken when body weight poses a risk to health? What are their risks?**

Trying to Gain Weight

learning outcomes

- **Describe healthy strategies for trying to gain weight.**

For some people, trying to gain weight is a challenge for a variety of metabolic, hereditary, psychological, and other reasons. If you are one of these individuals, the first priority is to determine why you cannot gain weight.

Perhaps you're an athlete and you burn more calories than you manage to eat. Perhaps you're stressed out and skipping meals to increase study time. Or stress, depression, or other emotional issues may make it difficult to focus on food and taking good care of your body. Among older adults, the senses of taste and smell may decline, which makes food taste different and therefore less pleasurable to eat. Visual problems and other disabilities may make meals more difficult to prepare, and dental problems may make eating more difficult.

People who engage in extreme energy-burning sports and exercise routines may be at risk for caloric and nutritional deficiencies, which can lead not only to weight loss, but to immune system problems and organ dysfunction; weakness, which leads to falls and fractures; slower recovery from diseases; and a host of other problems as well.

People who are too thin need to take the same kind of steps as those who are overweight or obese to find out what their healthy weight is and attain that weight.

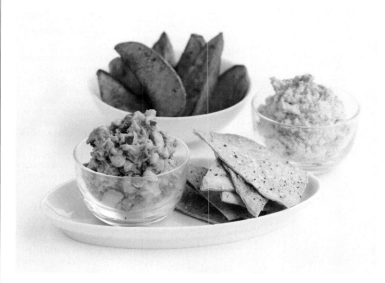

A snack of guacamole and whole-grain tortilla chips or hummus and baked potatoes is a healthy, nutrient-dense way to increase calorie intake.

The Skills for Behavior Change section gives ideas and tips for gaining weight. Depending on your situation, you may aim to gain as much as a pound per week, which would mean adding up to 500 calories a day to your diet. It is important that these calories be added in the form of energy-dense, nutritious choices from a variety of foods. For example, you could choose to eat a waffle instead of a slice of toast for breakfast, or add coleslaw to your lunch at the salad bar instead of plain cabbage. One cup of whole-wheat flakes provides 128 calories, while a cup of granola is 464 calories. Similarly, plain low-fat yogurt is 154 calories per cup, while strawberry low-fat yogurt offers 238 calories per cup. Just be sure that the calories you add are coming from high quality sources, not high-fat junk food.[56]

Skills for Behavior Change

TIPS FOR GAINING WEIGHT

- Eat at regularly scheduled times.
- Eat more frequently, spend more time eating, eat high-calorie foods first if you fill up fast, and always start with the main course.
- Take time to shop, to cook, and to eat slowly.
- Put extra spreads such as peanut butter, cream cheese, or cheese on your foods. Make your sandwiches with extra-thick slices of bread and add more filling. Take seconds whenever possible, and eat high-calorie, nutrient-dense snacks such as nuts and cheese during the day.
- Supplement your diet. Add high-calorie drinks that have a healthy balance of nutrients, such as whole milk.
- Try to eat with people you are comfortable with. Avoid people who you feel are analyzing what you eat or make you feel as if you should eat less.
- If you are sedentary, be aware that moderate exercise can increase appetite. If you are exercising, or exercising to extremes, moderate your activities until you've gained some weight.
- Avoid diuretics, laxatives, and other medications that cause you to lose body fluids and nutrients.
- Relax. Many people who are underweight operate in high gear most of the time. Slow down, get more rest, and take steps to control stress and anxiety.

check yourself

- **What are some steps to be taken when weight needs to be gained? Do you think this is as difficult a task as trying to lose weight?**

Understanding and Improving Body Image

learning **outcomes**

- **Identify the elements of the body image continuum.**
- **List steps that can be taken to build a more positive body image.**

When you look in the mirror, do you like what you see? If you feel disappointed, frustrated, or even angry, you're not alone. A majority of adults are dissatisfied with their bodies.[57] Negative feelings about one's body can contribute to behaviors that can threaten your health—and your life. In contrast, a healthy body image can contribute to reduced stress, an increased sense of personal empowerment, and more joyful living.

The National Eating Disorders Association (NEDA) identifies several components of **body image**:[58]

- How you see yourself in your mind
- What you believe about your appearance
- How you feel about your body
- How you sense and control your body as you move

NEDA identifies a *negative body image* as either distorted perception of your shape or feelings of discomfort, shame, or anxiety about your body. A *positive body image* is a true perception of your appearance. You understand that everyone is different, and you celebrate your uniqueness. **Figure 9.6** will help you identify whether your body image is positive, negative, or somewhere in between.

Factors Influencing Body Image

Media images of celebrities media set the standard for what we find attractive, leading some people to go to dangerous extremes to have the biggest biceps or fit into size 2 jeans. Though most of us

Body hate/ dissociation	Distorted body image	Body preoccupied/ obsessed	Body acceptance	Body ownership
I often feel separated and distant from my body—as if it belongs to someone else.	I spend a significant amount of time exercising and dieting to change my body.	I spend a significant amount of time viewing my body in the mirror.	I base my body image equally on social norms and my own self-concept.	My body is beautiful to me.
I don't see anything positive or even neutral about my body shape and size.	My body shape and size keep me from dating or finding someone who will treat me the way I want to be treated.	I spend a significant amount of time comparing my body to others.	I pay attention to my body and my appearance because it is important to me, but it only occupies a small part of my day.	My feelings about my body are not influenced by society's concept of an ideal body shape.
I don't believe others when they tell me I look OK.	I have considered changing or have changed my body shape and size through surgical means so I can accept myself.	I have days when I feel fat.	I nourish my body so it has the strength and energy to achieve my physical goals.	I know that the significant others in my life will always find me attractive.
I hate the way I look in the mirror and often isolate myself from others.		I am preoccupied with my body.		
		I accept society's ideal body shape and size as the best body shape and size.		

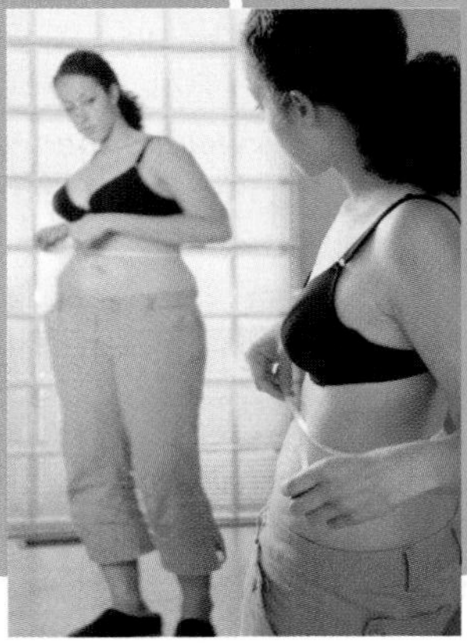

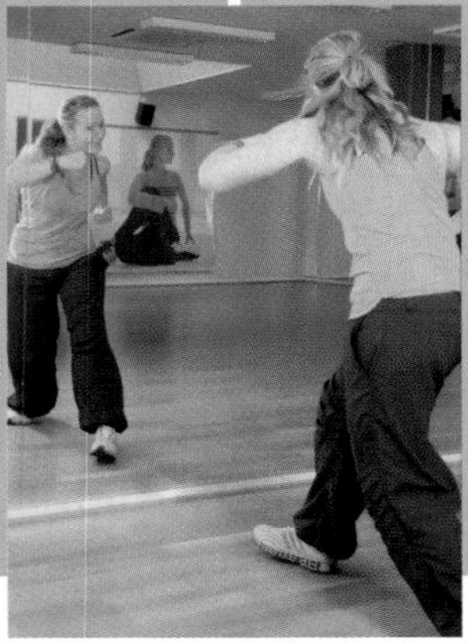

Figure 9.6 Body Image Continuum
This is part of a two-part continuum, the second part of which is shown in **Figure 9.7**. Individuals whose responses fall to the far left side of the continuum have a highly negative body image, whereas responses to the right indicate a positive body image.
Source: Adapted from Smiley/King/Avery, Campus Health Service. Original continuum, C. Schislak, *Preventive Medicine and Public Health*. Copyright © 1997 Arizona Board of Regents. Used with permission.

think of this obsession with appearance as a recent phenomenon, it has long been part of American culture; the ideals may change, but the pressure is the same.

Today, more than 66 percent of Americans are overweight or obese; a significant disconnect exists between idealized images of male and female bodies and the typical American body.[59] At the same time, the media is more powerful and pervasive than ever before. In fact, one study of more than 4,000 television commercials revealed that approximately 1 out of every 4 sends some sort of "attractiveness message."[60]

Others strongly influence how we see ourselves. Parents are especially influential in body image development. For instance, fathers who validate the acceptability of their daughters' appearance throughout puberty and mothers who model body acceptance can help their daughters maintain a positive body image.

Interactions with others outside the family—for instance, teasing and bullying from peers—can contribute to negative body image. Moreover, associations within one's cultural group appear to influence body image. For example, European American females experience the highest rates of body dissatisfaction; as a minority group becomes more acculturated into the mainstream, the body dissatisfaction levels of women in that group increase.[61]

People diagnosed with a body image disorder show differences in the brain's ability to regulate *neurotransmitters* linked to mood,[62] in a way similar to those of depression and anxiety disorders, including obsessive-compulsive disorder. One MRI imaging study linked distortions in body image to malfunctions in the brain's visual processing region.[63]

Building a Positive Body Image

If you want to develop a more positive body image, your first step might be to bust some toxic myths and challenge some commonly held attitudes in contemporary society:[64]

- **Myth 1: How you look is more important than who you are.** Is your weight important in defining who you are? How much does it matter to you to have friends who are thin? How important do you think being thin is in attracting a partner?
- **Myth 2: Anyone can be slender and attractive if they work at it.** When you see someone who is thin, or obese, what assumptions do you make? Have you ever berated yourself for not having the "willpower" to change some aspect of your body?
- **Myth 3: Extreme dieting is an effective weight-loss strategy.** Do you believe in fad diets or "quick-weight-loss" products? How far would you go to attain the "perfect" body?
- **Myth 4: Appearance is more important than health.** How do you evaluate whether a person is healthy? Is your desire to change your body motivated by health or appearance?

Body Image Disorders

Although most Americans are dissatisfied with some aspect of their appearance, only a few have a true body image disorder. Approximately 1 percent of people in the United States suffer from **body dysmorphic disorder (BDD)**.[65] Persons with BDD are obsessively concerned with their appearance and have a distorted view of their

own body shape, body size, and so on. Although the precise cause of BDD isn't known, an anxiety disorder such as obsessive-compulsive disorder is often present. Contributing factors may include genetic susceptibility, childhood teasing, physical or sexual abuse, low self-esteem, and rigid sociocultural expectations of beauty.[66]

People with BDD may try to fix their perceived flaws through excessive bodybuilding, repeated cosmetic surgeries, or other appearance-altering behaviors. It is estimated that 10 percent of people seeking dermatology or cosmetic treatments have BDD.[67] Psychotherapy and/or antidepressant medications are often successful in treating BBD.

In **social physique anxiety (SPA)**, the desire to "look good" is so strong that it has a destructive effect on one's ability to function effectively in interactions with others. People suffering from SPA may spend a disproportionate amount of time fixating on their bodies, working out, and performing tasks that are ego centered and self-directed.[68] Experts speculate that this anxiety may contribute to disordered eating behaviors.

Skills for Behavior Change

STEPS TO A POSITIVE BODY IMAGE

One list cannot create a positive body image, but it can help you think about new ways of looking more healthfully and happily at yourself and your body.

- **Step 1.** Celebrate all of the amazing things your body does for you—running, dancing, breathing, laughing, dreaming.
- **Step 2.** Keep a list of things you like about yourself—things unrelated to how much you weigh or how you look. Read your list often, and add to it regularly.
- **Step 3.** Remind yourself that true beauty is not simply skin deep. When you feel good about who you are, you carry yourself with confidence, self-acceptance, and openness that makes you beautiful.
- **Step 4.** Surround yourself with people who are supportive and who recognize the importance of liking yourself as you are.
- **Step 5.** Shut down voices in your head that tell you your body is not "right" or that you are a "bad" person. You can overpower those negative thoughts with positive ones.
- **Step 6.** Become a critical viewer of social and media messages. Identify and resist images, slogans, or attitudes that make you feel bad about yourself or your body.
- **Step 7.** Do something that lets your body know you appreciate it. Take a bubble bath, make time for a nap, or find a peaceful place outside to relax.
- **Step 8.** Use the time and energy you might have spent worrying about your appearance to do something to help others.

Source: Adapted with permission from the National Eating Disorders Association, www.nationaleatingdisorders.org.

check yourself

- **Where do you place yourself on the body image continuum?**
- **Are there steps that you may take to improve your body image?**

What Is Disordered Eating?

learning **outcomes**

- **Identify the elements of the eating issues continuum.**

The eating issues continuum in **Figure 9.7** identifies thoughts and behaviors associated with **disordered eating**.

Some people who exhibit disordered eating patterns progress to a clinical **eating disorder**—a diagnosis that can be applied only by a physician to a patient who exhibits severe disturbances in thoughts, behavior, and body functioning.

The American Psychiatric Association (APA) has defined several eating disorders: *anorexia nervosa, bulimia nervosa, binge-eating disorder*, and a cluster of conditions referred to as **eating disorders not otherwise specified (EDNOS)**.

In the United States, as many as 24 million people meet the criteria for an eating disorder.[69] In 2010, 1.9 percent of college students reported dealing with either anorexia or bulimia.[70] Disordered eating and eating disorders affect up to 62 percent of college athletes in sports such as gymnastics, wrestling, swimming, and figure skating.[71] Eating disorders are on the rise among men, who represent up to 25 percent of anorexia and bulimia patients and almost 40 percent of binge eaters (a category within EDNOS).[72]

Many people with these disorders feel disenfranchised in other aspects of their lives and try to gain a sense of control through food. Many are clinically depressed, suffer from obsessive-compulsive disorder, or have other psychiatric problems. Individuals with low self-esteem, negative body image, and a high tendency for perfectionism are most at risk.[73]

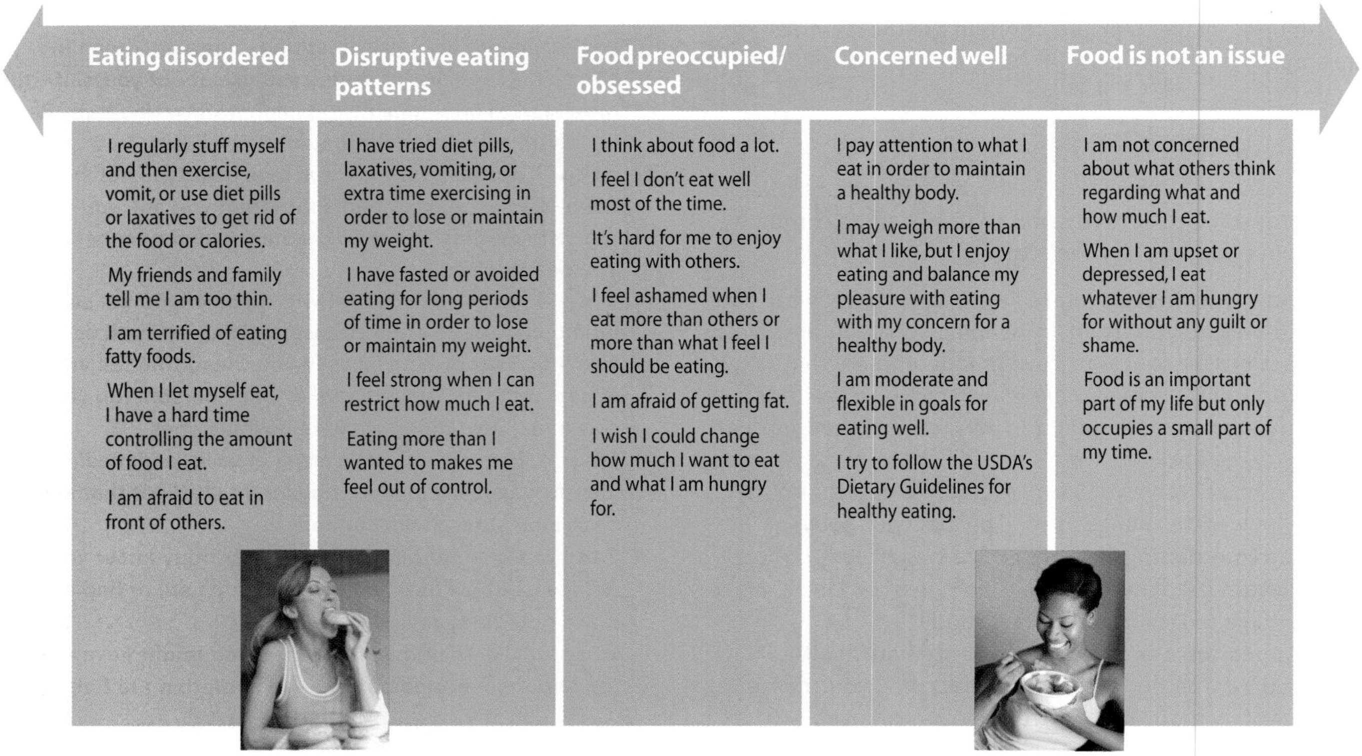

Eating disordered	Disruptive eating patterns	Food preoccupied/ obsessed	Concerned well	Food is not an issue
I regularly stuff myself and then exercise, vomit, or use diet pills or laxatives to get rid of the food or calories.	I have tried diet pills, laxatives, vomiting, or extra time exercising in order to lose or maintain my weight.	I think about food a lot.	I pay attention to what I eat in order to maintain a healthy body.	I am not concerned about what others think regarding what and how much I eat.
My friends and family tell me I am too thin.	I have fasted or avoided eating for long periods of time in order to lose or maintain my weight.	I feel I don't eat well most of the time.	I may weigh more than what I like, but I enjoy eating and balance my pleasure with eating with my concern for a healthy body.	When I am upset or depressed, I eat whatever I am hungry for without any guilt or shame.
I am terrified of eating fatty foods.	I feel strong when I can restrict how much I eat.	It's hard for me to enjoy eating with others.	I am moderate and flexible in goals for eating well.	Food is an important part of my life but only occupies a small part of my time.
When I let myself eat, I have a hard time controlling the amount of food I eat.	Eating more than I wanted to makes me feel out of control.	I feel ashamed when I eat more than others or more than what I feel I should be eating.	I try to follow the USDA's Dietary Guidelines for healthy eating.	
I am afraid to eat in front of others.		I am afraid of getting fat.		
		I wish I could change how much I want to eat and what I am hungry for.		

Figure 9.7 Eating Issues Continuum
This second part of the continuum shown in Figure 9.6 suggests that the progression from normal eating to eating disorders occurs on a continuum.
Source: Adapted from Smiley/King/Avery, Campus Health Service. Original continuum, C. Schislak, *Preventive Medicine and Public Health*. Copyright © 1997 Arizona Board of Regents. Used with permission.

check yourself

- **Where do you place yourself on the eating issues continuum?**

Eating Disorders: Anorexia Nervosa

- **List the criteria, effects, and treatment of anorexia nervosa.**

Anorexia nervosa is a persistent, chronic eating disorder characterized by deliberate food restriction and severe, life-threatening weight loss. It involves self-starvation motivated by an intense fear of gaining weight along with an extremely distorted body image. Initially, most people with anorexia nervosa lose weight by reducing total food intake, particularly of high-calorie foods. Eventually, they progress to restricting their intake of almost all foods. The little they do eat, they may purge through vomiting or use of laxatives. Although they lose weight, people with anorexia nervosa never seem to feel thin enough and constantly identify body parts that are "too fat."

It is estimated that between 0.5 and 3.7 percent of females suffer from anorexia nervosa in their lifetime.[74] The revised APA criteria for anorexia nervosa are as follows:[75]

- Refusal to maintain body weight at or above a minimally normal weight for age and height
- Intense fear of gaining weight or becoming fat, even though considered underweight by all medical criteria
- Disturbance in the way in which one's body weight or shape is experienced, undue influence of body weight or shape on self-evaluation, or denial of the seriousness of the current low body weight

Physical symptoms and negative health consequences associated with anorexia nervosa are illustrated in **Figure 9.8**. Because it involves starvation and can lead to heart attacks and seizures, anorexia nervosa has the highest death rate (20%) of any psychological illness.

The causes of anorexia nervosa are complex and variable. Many people with anorexia have other coexisting psychiatric problems, including low self-esteem, depression, an anxiety disorder such as obsessive-compulsive disorder, and substance abuse. Some people with anorexia nervosa have a history of being physically or sexually abused, and others have troubled interpersonal relationships with family members. Cultural norms that value people on the basis of their appearance and glorify thinness are of course a factor, as is weight-based teasing and weight bias.[76] Physical factors are thought to include an imbalance of neurotransmitters and genetic susceptibility.[77]

Treatment involves long-term therapy, usually after emergency intervention.

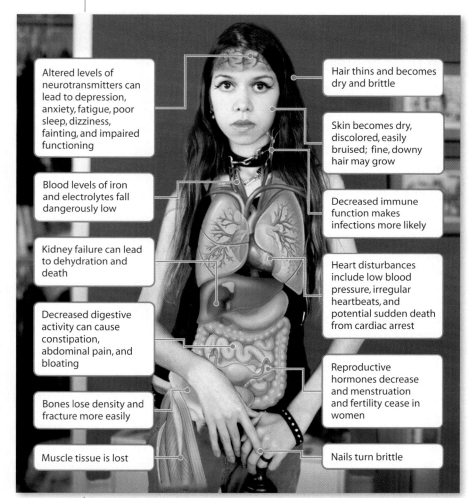

Altered levels of neurotransmitters can lead to depression, anxiety, fatigue, poor sleep, dizziness, fainting, and impaired functioning

Blood levels of iron and electrolytes fall dangerously low

Kidney failure can lead to dehydration and death

Decreased digestive activity can cause constipation, abdominal pain, and bloating

Bones lose density and fracture more easily

Muscle tissue is lost

Hair thins and becomes dry and brittle

Skin becomes dry, discolored, easily bruised; fine, downy hair may grow

Decreased immune function makes infections more likely

Heart disturbances include low blood pressure, irregular heartbeats, and potential sudden death from cardiac arrest

Reproductive hormones decrease and menstruation and fertility cease in women

Nails turn brittle

Figure 9.8 What Anorexia Nervosa Can Do to the Body

check yourself

- **What are the criteria, effects, and treatment for anorexia nervosa?**

Eating Disorders: Bulimia Nervosa and Binge Eating

- **List the criteria, effects, and treatments for bulimia nervosa and binge eating.**

Individuals with **bulimia nervosa** often binge on huge amounts of food and then engage in some kind of purging or "compensatory behavior," such as vomiting, taking laxatives, or exercising excessively, to lose the calories they have just consumed. People with bulimia are obsessed with their bodies, weight gain, and appearance, although their problem is often "hidden" from the public eye because their weight may fall within a normal range or they may be over-weight.

Up to 3 percent of adolescents and young women are bulimic; rates among men are about 10 percent of the rate among women.[78] The revised APA diagnostic criteria include recurrent episodes of binge eating and recurrent inappropriate compensatory behavior such as self-induced vomiting, use of laxatives or diuretics, fasting, or excessive exercise. The behavior must occur at least once a week for 3 months.[79]

Physical symptoms and negative health consequences associated with bulimia nervosa are shown in **Figure 9.9**.

A combination of genetic and environmental factors is thought to cause bulimia nervosa.[80] A family history of obesity, an underlying anxiety disorder, and an imbalance in neurotransmitters are all possible contributing factors.[81]

Individuals with **binge-eating disorder** gorge, but do not take excessive measures to lose the weight they gain; they are often clinically obese. As in bulimia, binge-eating episodes are characterized by eating large amounts of food rapidly, even when not feeling hungry, and feeling guilty or depressed after overeating.[82]

Binge-eating disorder is experienced by 3.5 percent of women and 2 percent of men.[83] The APA criteria for binge-eating disorder are similar to those for bulimia nervosa, without compensatory behavior.[84] Those diagnosed with the condition also show three or more of the following behaviors: (1) eating much more rapidly than normal; (2) eating until uncomfortably full; (3) eating large amounts when not physically hungry; (4) eating alone because of embarrassment over how much one is eating; (5) feeling disgusted, depressed, or very guilty after overeating.

Without treatment, approximately 20 percent of people with a serious eating disorder will die from it; with treatment, long-term full recovery rates range from 44 to 76 percent.[85] Treatment often focuses first on reducing the threat to life; long-term therapy then allows the patient to work on adopting new eating behaviors, building self-confidence, and finding other ways to deal with life's problems.

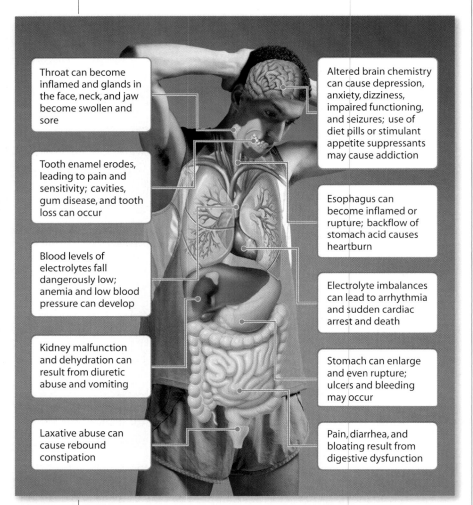

Throat can become inflamed and glands in the face, neck, and jaw become swollen and sore

Tooth enamel erodes, leading to pain and sensitivity; cavities, gum disease, and tooth loss can occur

Blood levels of electrolytes fall dangerously low; anemia and low blood pressure can develop

Kidney malfunction and dehydration can result from diuretic abuse and vomiting

Laxative abuse can cause rebound constipation

Altered brain chemistry can cause depression, anxiety, dizziness, impaired functioning, and seizures; use of diet pills or stimulant appetite suppressants may cause addiction

Esophagus can become inflamed or rupture; backflow of stomach acid causes heartburn

Electrolyte imbalances can lead to arrhythmia and sudden cardiac arrest and death

Stomach can enlarge and even rupture; ulcers and bleeding may occur

Pain, diarrhea, and bloating result from digestive dysfunction

Figure 9.9 What Bulimia Nervosa Can Do to the Body

check yourself

- **What are the criteria, effects, and treatment for bulimia nervosa and binge eating?**

Exercise Disorders

learning outcomes

■ **List the criteria, effects, and treatment for exercise disorders.**

Although exercise is generally beneficial to health, in excess it can be a problem. In addition to being a common compensatory behavior used by people with anorexia or bulimia, exercise can become a compulsion or contribute to muscle dysmorphia and the female athlete triad.

A recent study of almost 600 college students revealed that 18 percent met the criteria for **compulsive exercise**.[86] Also called *anorexia athletica*, it is characterized not by a *desire* to exercise but a *compulsion* to do so, with guilt and anxiety if the person doesn't work out.

Compulsive exercise can contribute to injuries to joints and bones. It can also put significant stress on the heart, especially if combined with disordered eating. Psychologically, people who engage in compulsive exercise are often plagued by anxiety and/or depression.

Muscle Dysmorphia

Muscle dysmorphia appears to be a relatively new form of body image disturbance and exercise disorder in which a man believes that his body is insufficiently lean or muscular.[87] Men with muscle dysmorphia believe that they look "puny," when in reality they look normal or may even be unusually muscular. Behaviors characteristic of muscle dysmorphia include comparing oneself unfavorably to others, checking one's appearance in the mirror, and camouflaging one's appearance. Men with muscle dysmorphia also have higher rates of substance abuse and suicide than other men.[88]

Men with muscle dysmorphia may have unusually muscular bodies but suffer from very low self-esteem.

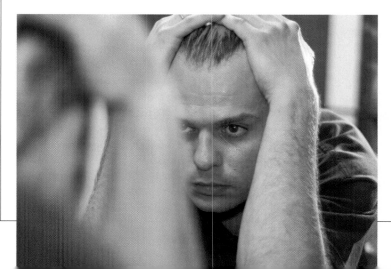

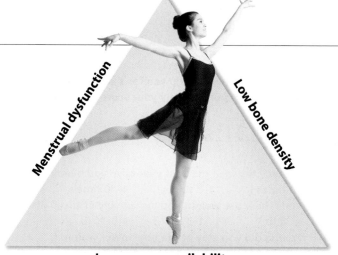

Figure 9.10 The Female Athlete Triad
The female athlete triad is a cluster of three interrelated health problems.

The Female Athlete Triad

Female athletes in competitive sports often strive for perfection. In an effort to be the best, they may put themselves at risk for a syndrome called the **female athlete triad**, with three interrelated problems (**Figure 9.10**): low energy intake, typically prompted by disordered eating; menstrual dysfunction such as amenorrhea; and poor bone density.[89]

How does the female athlete triad develop? First, a chronic pattern of low food intake and intensive exercise depletes nutrients essential to health. The body begins to burn stores of fat tissue for energy, reducing levels of the female reproductive hormone *estrogen*, and so stopping menstruation. Depletion of fat-soluble vitamins, calcium, and estrogen weakens the athlete's bones, leaving her at high risk for fracture.

The triad is particularly prevalent in athletes in highly competitive individual sports that emphasize leanness—gymnasts, figure skaters, cross-country runners, and ballet dancers.

Warning signs include dry skin; light-headedness/fainting; fine, downy hair covering the body; multiple injuries; and changes in endurance, strength, or speed. Associated behaviors include preoccupation with food and weight, compulsive exercising, use of weight-loss products or laxatives, self-criticism, anxiety, and depression. Treatment requires a multidisciplinary approach involving the athlete's coach or trainer, a psychologist, and family members and friends.

219

check yourself

■ **What are the criteria, effects, and treatment for exercise disorders? How might these differ for men and women?**

WEIGHT MANAGEMENT AND BODY IMAGE

Assessyourself

Are You Ready for Weight Loss?

An interactive version of this assessment is available online. Download it from the Live It! section of www.pearsonhighered.com/donatelle.

How well do your attitudes equip you for a weight-loss program? For each question, circle the answer that best describes your attitude. As you complete sections 2–5, tally your score and analyze it according to the scoring guide.

1 Diet History

A. How many times in the past year have you been on a diet?

    0 times   1–3 times   4–10 times   11–20 times   More than 20

B. What is the most weight you lost on any of these diets?

    0 lb   1–5 lb   6–10 lb   11–20 lb   More than 20 lb

C. How long did you stay at the new lower weight?

    Less than 1 mo   2–3 mo   4–6 mo   6–12 mo   Over 1 yr

D. Put a check mark by each dieting method you have tried:

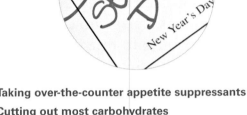

____Skipping breakfast   ____Skipping lunch or dinner   ____Taking over-the-counter appetite suppressants

____Counting calories   ____Cutting out most fats   ____Cutting out most carbohydrates

____Increasing regular exercise   ____Taking weight-loss supplements   ____Cutting out all snacks

____Using meal replacements such as Slim Fast   ____Taking prescription appetite suppressants   ____Taking laxatives

____Inducing vomiting   ____ Other

2 Readiness to Start a Weight-Loss Program

If you are thinking about starting a weight-loss program, answer questions A–F.

A. How motivated are you to lose weight?

1	2	3	4	5
Not at all	Slightly motivated	Somewhat motivated	Quite motivated	Extremely motivated

B. How certain are you that you will stay committed to a weight-loss program long enough to reach your goal?

1	2	3	4	5
Not at all certain	Slightly certain	Somewhat certain	Quite certain	Extremely certain

C. Taking into account other stresses in your life (school, work, and relationships), to what extent can you tolerate the effort required to stick to your diet plan?

1	2	3	4	5
Cannot tolerate	Can tolerate somewhat	Uncertain	Can tolerate well	Can tolerate easily

D. Assuming you should lose no more than 1 to 2 pounds per week, have you allotted a realistic amount of time for weight loss?

1	2	3	4	5
Very unrealistic	Somewhat unrealistic	Moderately realistic	Somewhat realistic	Very realistic

E. While dieting, do you fantasize about eating your favorite foods?

1	2	3	4	5
Always	Frequently	Occasionally	Rarely	Never

F. While dieting, do you feel deprived, angry, upset?

1	2	3	4	5
Always	Frequently	Occasionally	Rarely	Never

3 Total your scores

from questions A–F and circle your score category.

6 to 16: This may not be a good time for you to start a diet. Inadequate motivation and commitment and unrealistic goals could block your progress. Think about what contributes to your unreadiness. What are some of the factors? Consider changing these factors before undertaking a diet.

17 to 23: You may be nearly ready to begin a program but should think about ways to boost your readiness.

24 to 30: The path is clear—you can decide how to lose weight in a safe, effective way.

3 Hunger, Appetite, and Eating

Think about your hunger and the cues that stimulate your appetite or eating, and then answer questions A–C.

A. When food comes up in conversation or in something you read, do you want to eat, even if you are not hungry?

1	2	3	4	5
Never	Rarely	Occasionally	Frequently	Always

B. How often do you eat for a reason other than physical hunger?

1	2	3	4	5
Never	Rarely	Occasionally	Frequently	Always

C. When your favorite foods are around the house, do you succumb to eating them between meals?

1	2	3	4	5
Never	Rarely	Occasionally	Frequently	Always

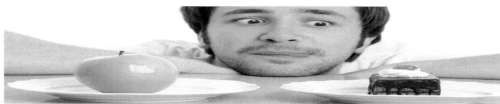

Total your scores

from questions A–C and circle your score category.

3 to 6: You might occasionally eat more than you should, but it is due more to your own attitudes than to temptation and other environmental cues. Controlling your own attitudes toward hunger and eating may help you.

7 to 9: You may have a moderate tendency to eat just because food is available. Losing weight may be easier for you if you try to resist external cues and eat only when you are physically hungry.

10 to 15: Some or much of your eating may be in response to thinking about food or exposing yourself to temptations to eat. Think of ways to minimize your exposure to temptations so you eat only in response to physical hunger.

4 Controlling Overeating

How good are you at controlling overeating when you are on a diet? Answer questions A–C.

A. A friend talks you into going out to a restaurant for a midday meal instead of eating a brown-bag lunch. As a result, for the rest of the day, you:

1	2	3	4	5
Would eat much less	Would eat somewhat less	Would make no difference	Would eat somewhat more	Would eat much more

B. You "break" your diet by eating a fattening, "forbidden" food. As a result, for the rest of the day, you:

1	2	3	4	5
Would eat much less	Would eat somewhat less	Would make no difference	Would eat somewhat more	Would eat much more

C. You have been following your diet faithfully and decide to test yourself by taking a bite of something you consider a treat. As a result, for the rest of the day, you:

1	2	3	4	5
Would eat much less	Would eat somewhat less	Would make no difference	Would eat somewhat more	Would eat much more

Total your scores

from questions A–C and circle your score category.

3 to 7: You recover rapidly from mistakes. However, if you frequently alternate between out-of-control eating and very strict dieting, you may have a serious eating problem and should get professional help.

8 to 11: You do not seem to let unplanned eating disrupt your program. This is a flexible, balanced approach.

12 to 15: You may be prone to overeating after an event breaks your control or throws you off track. Your reaction to these problem-causing events could use improvement.

5 Emotional Eating

Consider the effects of your emotions on your eating behaviors, and answer questions A–C.

A. Do you eat more than you would like to when you have negative feelings such as anxiety, depression, anger, or loneliness?

1	2	3	4	5
Never	Rarely	Occasionally	Frequently	Always

B. Do you have trouble controlling your eating when you have positive feelings (i.e., do you celebrate feeling good by eating)?

1	2	3	4	5
Never	Rarely	Occasionally	Frequently	Always

C. When you have unpleasant interactions with others in your life or after a difficult day at work, do you eat more than you'd like?

1	2	3	4	5
Never	Rarely	Occasionally	Frequently	Always

Total your scores

from questions A–C and circle your score category.

3 to 8: You do not appear to let your emotions affect your eating.

9 to 11: You sometimes eat in response to emotional highs and lows. Monitor this behavior to learn when and why it occurs, and be prepared to find alternative activities to respond to your emotions.

12 to 15: Emotional ups and downs can stimulate your eating. Try to deal with the feelings that trigger the eating and find other ways to express them.

6 Exercise Patterns and Attitudes

Exercise is key for weight loss. Think about your attitudes toward it, and answer questions A–D.

A. How often do you exercise?

1	2	3	4	5
Never	Rarely	Occasionally	Somewhat frequently	Frequently

B. How confident are you that you can exercise regularly?

1	2	3	4	5
Not at all confident	Slightly confident	Somewhat confident	Highly confident	Completely confident

C. When you think about exercise, do you develop a positive or negative picture in your mind?

1	2	3	4	5
Completely negative	Somewhat negative	Neutral	Somewhat positive	Completely positive

D. How certain are you that you can work regular exercise into your daily schedule?

1	2	3	4	5
Not at all certain	Slightly certain	Somewhat certain	Quite certain	Extremely certain

Total your scores

from questions A–D and circle your score category.

4 to 10: You're probably not exercising as regularly as you should. Determine whether it is your attitude about exercise or your lifestyle that is blocking your way, then change what you must and put on those walking shoes!

11 to 16: You need to feel more positive about exercise so you can do it more often. Think of ways to be more active that are fun and fit your lifestyle.

17 to 20: The path is clear for you to be active. Now think of ways to get motivated.

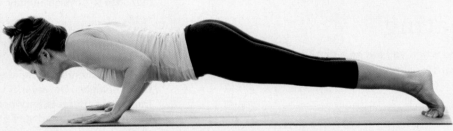

Source: Adapted from "The Diet Readiness Test," from "When and How to Diet" by Kelly D. Brownell, from *Psychology Today*, June 1989. Copyright © by Kelly D. Brownell. Reprinted with permission.

Your Plan for Change

The Assess Yourself activity identifies six areas of importance in determining your readiness for weight loss. If you wish to lose weight to improve your health, understanding your attitudes about food and exercise will help you succeed in your plan.

Today, You Can:

◯ Set "SMART" goals for weight loss and give them a reality check: Are they specific, measurable, achievable, relevant, and time-oriented? For example, rather than aiming to lose 15 pounds this month (which probably wouldn't be healthy or achievable), set a comfortable goal to lose 5 pounds. Realistic goals will encourage weight-loss success by boosting your confidence in your ability to make lifelong healthy changes.

◯ Begin keeping a food log and identifying the triggers that influence your eating habits. Think about what you can do to eliminate or reduce the influence of your two most common food triggers.

Within the Next 2 Weeks, You Can:

◯ Get in the habit of incorporating more fruits, vegetables, and whole grains in your diet and eating less fat. The next time you make dinner, look at the proportions on your plate. If vegetables and whole grains do not take up most of the space, substitute 1 cup of the meat, pasta, or cheese in your meal with 1 cup of legumes, salad greens, or a favorite vegetable. You'll reduce the number of calories while eating the same amount of food!

◯ Aim to incorporate more exercise into your daily routine. Visit your campus rec center or a local gym, and familiarize yourself with the equipment and facilities that are available. Try a new machine or sports activity, and experiment until you find a form of exercise you really enjoy.

By the End of the Semester, You Can:

◯ Get in the habit of grocery shopping every week and buying healthy, nutritious foods while avoiding high-fat, high-sugar, or overly processed foods. As you make healthy foods more available and unhealthy foods less available, you'll find it easier to eat better.

◯ Chart your progress and reward yourself as you meet your goals. If your goal is to lose weight and you successfully take off 10 pounds, reward yourself with a new pair of jeans or other article of clothing (which will likely fit better than before!).

Assessyourself

How Sensible Are Your Efforts to Be Thin?

An interactive version of this assessment is available online. Download it from the Live It! section of www.pearsonhighered.com/donatelle.

On one hand, just because you weigh yourself, count calories, or work out every day, don't jump to the conclusion that you have any of the health concerns discussed in this chapter. On the other hand, efforts to lose a few pounds can spiral out of control. To find out whether your efforts to be thin are harmful to you, take the following quiz from the National Eating Disorders Association (NEDA).

1. I constantly calculate numbers of fat grams and calories.   T   F

2. I weigh myself often and find myself obsessed with the number on the scale.   T   F

3. I exercise to burn calories and not for health or enjoyment.   T   F

4. I sometimes feel out of control while eating.   T   F

5. I often go on extreme diets.   T   F

6. I engage in rituals to get me through mealtimes and/or secretly binge.   T   F

7. Weight loss, dieting, and controlling my food intake have become my major concerns.   T   F

8. I feel ashamed, disgusted, or guilty after eating.   T   F

9. I constantly worry about the weight, shape, and/or size of my body.   T   F

10. I feel my identity and value are based on how I look or how much I weigh.   T   F

If any of these statements is true for you, you could be dealing with disordered eating. If so, talk about it! Tell a friend, parent, teacher, coach, youth group leader, doctor, counselor, or nutritionist what you're going through. Check out the NEDA's Sharing with EEEase handout at www .nationaleatingdisorders.org/ nedaDir/files/documents/handouts/ ShEEEase.pdf for help planning what to say the first time you talk to someone about your eating and exercise habits.

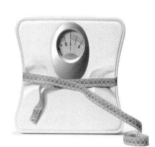

Source: Reprinted with permission from the National Eating Disorders Association, www.nationaleatingdisorders.org.

9.18 | Assess Yourself:
How Sensible Are Your Efforts to Be Thin?

223

Your Plan for Change

The Assess Yourself activity gave you the chance to evaluate your feelings about your body, and to determine whether or not you might be engaging in eating or exercise behaviors that could undermine your health and happiness. Here are some steps you can take to improve your body image, starting today.

Today, You Can:

◯ Talk back to the media. Write letters to advertisers and magazines that depict unhealthy and unrealistic body types. Boycott their products or start a blog commenting on harmful body image messages in the media.

◯ Visit www.choosemyplate .gov and create a personalized food plan. Just for today, eat the recommended number of servings from every food group at every meal, and don't count calories!

Within the Next 2 Weeks, You Can:

◯ Find a photograph of a person you admire *not* for his or her appearance, but for his or her contribution to humanity. Paste it up next to your mirror to remind yourself that true beauty comes from within and benefits others.

◯ Start a diary. Each day, record one thing you are grateful for that has nothing to do with your appearance. At the end of each day, record one small thing you did to make someone's world a little brighter.

By the End of the Semester, You Can:

◯ Establish a group of friends who support you for who you are, not what you look like, and who get the same support from you. Form a group on a favorite social-networking site, and keep in touch, especially when you start to feel troubled by self-defeating thoughts or have the urge to engage in unhealthy eating or exercise behaviors.

◯ Borrow from the library or purchase one of the many books on body image now available, and read it!

Summary

- Overweight, obesity, and weight-related health problems have reached epidemic levels in the United States, largely due to obesogenic behaviors in an obesogenic environment.
- Societal costs from obesity include increased health care costs, lowered worker productivity, low self-esteem, and obesity-related stigma. Individual health risks from overweight and obesity include a variety of chronic diseases.
- Many factors contribute to risk for obesity, including environmental factors, poverty, education level, genetics, developmental factors, endocrine influences, psychosocial factors, eating cues, metabolic changes, and lifestyle.
- Percentage of body fat is a reliable indicator for levels of overweight and obesity. Body mass index (BMI) is one of the most commonly accepted measures of assessing body fat. *Overweight* is most commonly defined as a BMI of 25 to 29, and *obesity* as a BMI of 30 or greater. Waist circumference is believed to be related to risk for several chronic diseases, particularly type 2 diabetes.
- Exercise, dieting, diet pills, surgery, and other strategies are used to maintain or lose weight. However, sensible eating and exercise offer the best options for weight loss and maintenance.
- Negative feelings about one's body can contribute to behaviors that can threaten health. In contrast, a healthy body image can contribute to reduced stress and personal empowerment.
- Body image disorders affect men and women of all ages. Body image can be affected by culture, media, and individual physiological and psychological factors.
- Disordered eating and eating disorders such as anorexia nervosa, bulimia nervosa, and binge-eating disorder can lead to serious health problems and even death.
- Although exercise is healthy in moderation, if it becomes a compulsion it can lead to disorders such as muscle dysmorphia and the female athlete triad.

Pop Quiz

1. Which of the following statements is FALSE?
   a. A slowing basal metabolic rate may contribute to weight gain after age 30.
   b. Hormones are implicated in hunger impulses and eating behavior.
   c. The more muscles you have, the fewer calories you'll burn.
   d. Overweight and obesity can have serious health consequences, even before middle age.

2. Which of the following statements about BMI is FALSE?
   a. BMI is based on height and weight measurements.
   b. BMI is accurate for everyone, including people with high muscle mass.
   c. Children's BMIs are used to determine a percentile ranking among their age peers.
   d. BMI stands for "body mass index."

3. Which of the following BMI ratings is considered overweight?
   a. 20.
   b. 25.
   c. 30.
   d. 35.

4. Which of the following body circumferences is most strongly associated with risk of heart disease and diabetes?
   a. Hip circumference
   b. Chest circumference
   c. Waist circumference
   d. Thigh circumference

5. One pound of additional body fat is created through consuming how many extra calories?
   a. 1,500 calories
   b. 3,500 calories
   c. 5,000 calories
   d. 7,000 calories

6. To lose weight, you must establish a(n):
   a. negative caloric balance.
   b. energy balance.
   c. positive caloric balance.
   d. set point.

7. The rate at which your body consumes food energy to sustain basic functions is your:
   a. basal metabolic rate.
   b. resting metabolic rate.
   c. body mass index.
   d. set point.

8. Successful, healthy weight loss is characterized by:
   a. a lifelong pattern of healthful eating and exercise.
   b. cutting out fats and carbohydrates.
   c. never eating foods considered bad for you.
   d. a pattern of repeatedly losing and regaining weight.

9. Which of the following is NOT a contributor to negative body image?
   a. Idealized media images of celebrities
   b. Increases in portion sizes
   c. Cultural attitudes about body ideals
   d. Neurotransmitter regulation in the brain

10. Which of the following eating disorders includes compensatory behavior in its definition?
    a. Anorexia nervosa
    b. Bulimia nervosa
    c. Binge-eating disorder
    d. Muscle dysmorphia

Answers to these questions can be found on page A-1.

Web Links

1. **American Dietetic Association**. Recommended dietary guidelines and other current information about weight control. www.eatright.org
2. **Duke University Diet and Fitness Center**. Information helping people live healthier lives through weight control and lifestyle change. www.dukedietcenter.org
3. **The Rudd Center for Foods Policy and Obesity**. The latest in obesity research, public policy, and ways to stop obesity at the community level. www.yaleruddcenter.org
4. **National Eating Disorders Association**. Information for eating disorder sufferers and those wishing to help others with eating and body image issues. www.nationaleatingdisorders.org

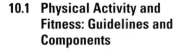

Fitness · 10

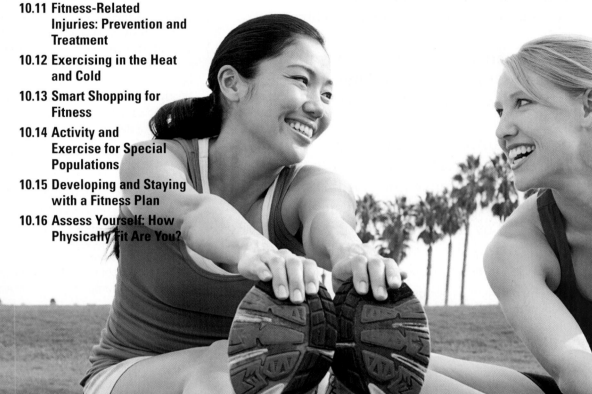

Most Americans are aware of the benefits of physical activity. Physiological changes resulting from regular physical activity reduce the likelihood of coronary artery disease, high blood pressure, type 2 diabetes, obesity, and other chronic diseases. Engaging in physical activity regularly also helps to control stress and increase self-esteem.[1]

Despite these benefits, however, 25.4 percent of American adults engage in no leisure-time physical activity[2]—a situation linked to current high incidences of obesity, type 2 diabetes, and other chronic and mental health diseases.[3]

In general, college students are more physically active than are older adults, but a recent survey indicated that 56 percent of college women and 48 percent of college men do not meet recommended guidelines for engaging in moderate or vigorous physical activities.[4] And in a related survey, only 45.4 percent of college students surveyed had performed any strength training exercises in the past 7 days.[5]

College is a great time to develop attitudes and behaviors that can increase the quality and quantity of your life. This chapter offers knowledge and strategies to help you get moving.

Physical Activity and Fitness: Guidelines and Components

learning outcomes

- **Distinguish among physical activity for health, for fitness, and for performance.**
- **Differentiate exercise from physical activity.**
- **List the core components of physical fitness.**

Physical activity refers to all body movements produced by skeletal muscles resulting in substantial increases in energy expenditure.[6] Physical activities can vary by intensity. For example, walking to class typically requires little effort, while walking to class uphill is more intense and harder to do. The three general categories of physical activity are defined by their purpose: physical activity for health, physical activity for physical fitness, and physical activity for performance.

Exercise is defined as planned, structured, and repetitive bodily movement done to improve or maintain one or more components of physical fitness, such as cardiorespiratory endurance, muscular strength or endurance, or flexibility.[7] Although all exercise is physical activity, not all physical activity would be considered exercise. For example, walking from your car to class is physical activity, whereas going for a brisk 30-minute walk is considered exercise.

Physical Activity for Health

Researchers have found that "there is irrefutable evidence of the effectiveness of regular physical activity in the primary and secondary prevention of several chronic diseases (e.g., cardiovascular disease, diabetes, cancer, hypertension, obesity, depression, and osteoporosis, and premature death)."[8] Adding more physical activity to your day can benefit your health. In fact, if all Americans followed the 2008 Physical Activity Guidelines (**Table 10.1**), an estimated one-third of deaths related to coronary heart disease; one-quarter of deaths related to stroke and osteoporosis; one-fifth of deaths related to colon cancer, high blood pressure, and type 2 diabetes; and one-seventh of deaths related to breast cancer could be prevented.[9]

Physical Activity for Physical Fitness

Physical fitness refers to a set of health- and performance- related attributes. The health-related attributes—cardiorespiratory fitness, muscular strength and endurance, flexibility, and body composition—allow one to perform moderate-to vigorous-intensity physical activities on a regular basis without getting too tired and having energy left over to handle physical or mental emergencies. **Figure 10.1** identifies the major health-related components of physical fitness.

Cardiorespiratory Fitness **Cardiorespiratory fitness** refers to the ability of the heart, lungs, and blood vessels to function efficiently. The primary category of physical activity known to improve cardiorespiratory fitness is **aerobic exercise**. The word *aerobic* means "with oxygen" and describes any exercise that increases

TABLE 10.1 2008 Physical Activity Guidelines for Adult Americans

Key Guidelines for Health*	For Additional Fitness or Weight Loss Benefits*	PLUS
150 min/week moderate-intensity OR 75 min/week of vigorous-intensity OR Equivalent combination of moderate-and vigorous-intensity (i.e., 100 min moderate-intensity + 25 min vigorous-intensity)	300 min/week moderate-intensity OR 150 min/week of vigorous-intensity OR Equivalent combination of moderate-and vigorous-intensity (i.e., 200 min moderate-intensity + 50 min vigorous-intensity) OR More than the previously described amounts	Muscle strengthening activities for ALL the major muscle groups at least 2 days/week

*Accumulate this physical activity in sessions of 10 minutes or more at one time.
Source: Office of Disease Prevention and Health Promotion, U.S. Department of Health and Human Services, *2008 Physical Activity Guidelines for Americans: Be Active, Healthy, and Happy!* ODPHP Publication no. U0036 (Washington, DC: U.S. Department of Health and Human Services, 2008), Available at www.health.gov/paguidelines.

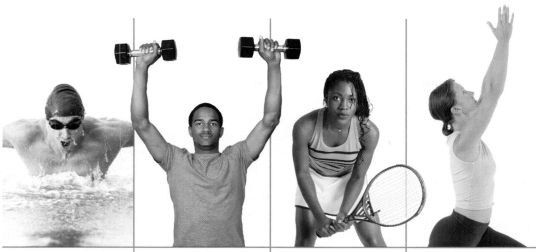

Cardiorespiratory fitness	Muscular strength	Muscular endurance	Flexibility	Body composition
Ability to sustain aerobic whole-body activity for a prolonged period of time	Maximum force able to be exerted by single contraction of a muscle or muscle group	Ability to perform high-intensity muscle contractions repeatedly without fatiguing	Ability to move joints freely through their full range of motion	The amount and relative proportions and distribution of fat mass and fat-free mass in the body

Figure 10.1 Components of Physical Fitness

heart rate. Aerobic activities such as swimming, cycling, and jogging are among the best exercises for improving or maintaining cardiorespiratory fitness.

The fitness of one's cardiorespiratory system is assessed by measuring **aerobic capacity** (or **power**), the volume of oxygen the muscles consume during exercise. Maximal aerobic power (VO_{2max}) is defined as the maximal volume of oxygen that the muscles consume during exercise. The most common measure of maximal aerobic capacity is a walk or run test on a treadmill. For greatest accuracy, this is done in a lab and requires special equipment and technicians to measure the precise amount of oxygen entering and exiting the body during the exercise session. Submaximal tests can be used to get a more general sense of cardiorespiratory fitness; one such test, the 1-mile run test, is described in the **Assess Yourself** module at the end of this chapter.

Muscular Strength **Muscular strength** refers to the amount of force a muscle or group of muscles is capable of exerting in one contraction. A common way to assess the strength of a particular muscle group is to measure the maximum amount of weight you can move one time (and no more), or your one repetition maximum (1 RM).

Muscular Endurance **Muscular endurance** is the ability of a muscle or group of muscles to exert force repeatedly without fatigue or the ability to sustain a muscular contraction. The more repetitions of an endurance activity (e.g., push-ups) you can perform successfully, or the longer you can hold a certain position (e.g., flexed arm hang), the greater your muscular endurance. General muscular endurance is often measured using the number of curl-ups an individual can do; this test is described in the **Assess Yourself** module at the end of this chapter.

Flexibility **Flexibility** refers to the range of motion, or the amount of movement possible, at a particular joint or series of joints: the greater the range of motion, the greater the flexibility. One of the most common measures of general flexibility is the sit-and-reach test, described in the **Assess Yourself** module at the end of this chapter.

Body Composition **Body composition**, the fifth and final component of a comprehensive fitness program, describes the relative proportions and distribution of fat and lean (muscle, bone, water, organs) tissues in the body.

Physical Activity for Performance

People who participate in athletics undertake specific exercises to increase speed, power, agility, coordination, and other performance-related attributes of physical fitness. Although many recreational exercisers use interval training to improve their speed, power, and cardiorespiratory fitness, performance training is safest for those individuals who already have a high physical fitness level.

check yourself

- **What are the differences between physical activity for health, for fitness, and for performance?**
- **What is the difference between exercise and physical activity?**
- **What are the core components of physical fitness?**

Health Benefits of Physical Activity

- **List the health benefits of physical activity.**

The first step in starting a physical fitness program is identifying your goals for that program. You should next consider the things that might get in the way of your achieving those goals. Once you have contemplated these factors, you are ready to create an individual exercise program to meet your physical fitness goals. Before we start, and to help you get motivated, let's take a look at the many physical and psychological benefits of physical activity.

What Are the Health Benefits of Regular Physical Activity?

Regular participation in physical activity improves more than 50 different physiological, metabolic, and psychological aspects of human life. **Figure 10.2** summarizes some of these major health-related benefits.

Reduced Risk of Cardiovascular Diseases Aerobic exercise is good for the heart and lungs and reduces risk for heart-related diseases. It improves blood flow and eases performance of everyday tasks. Regular exercise makes the cardiovascular and respiratory systems more efficient by strengthening the heart muscle, enabling more blood to be pumped with each stroke, and increasing the number of *capillaries* (small blood vessels that allow gas exchange between blood and surrounding tissues) in trained skeletal muscles, which supply more blood to working muscles. Exercise also improves the respiratory system by increasing the amount of oxygen inhaled and distributed to body tissues.[10]

Regular physical activity can reduce hypertension, or chronic high blood pressure—a form of cardiovascular disease and a significant risk factor for coronary heart disease and stroke.[11] Regular aerobic exercise also reduces low-density lipoproteins (LDLs, or "bad" cholesterol), total cholesterol, and triglycerides (a blood fat), thus reducing plaque buildup in the arteries while increasing high-density lipoproteins (HDLs, or "good" cholesterol), which are associated with lower risk for coronary artery disease.[12]

Reduced Risk of Metabolic Syndrome and Type 2 Diabetes Regular physical activity reduces the risk of metabolic syndrome, a combination of heart disease and diabetes risk factors that produces a synergistic increase in risk.[13] Specifically, metabolic syndrome includes high blood pressure, abdominal obesity, low levels of HDLs, high levels of triglycerides, and impaired glucose tolerance.[14] Regular participation in moderate-intensity physical activities reduces risk for these factors both individually and collectively.[15]

Research indicates that a healthy dietary intake combined with sufficient physical activity could prevent many current cases of type 2 diabetes.[16] In a major national clinical trial, researchers found that exercising 150 minutes per week while eating fewer calories and less fat could prevent or delay the onset of type 2 diabetes.[17]

Reduced Cancer Risk After decades of research, most cancer epidemiologists believe that the majority of cancers are preventable and can be avoided by healthier lifestyle and environmental choices.[18] In fact, a report recently released by the World Cancer Research Fund in conjunction with the American Institute for Cancer Research stated that two-thirds of all cancers could be prevented based on lifestyle changes.[19] Specific to a physically active lifestyle, one-third of cancers could be prevented by being physically active and eating well.

30 minutes **of physical activity a day—all at once or in three 10-minute sessions—provides health benefits.**

Regular physical activity appears to lower the risk for some specific types of cancer, particularly breast cancer. Research on exercise and breast cancer risk has found that the earlier in life a woman starts to exercise, the lower her breast cancer risk.[20] Further, regular exercise is also associated with lower risk for colon and rectal cancers.[21] One must keep in mind that just as there may be multiple causes of cancer, there are also many possible factors involved in its prevention.

Improved Bone Mass and Reduced Risk of Osteoporosis A common affliction for older people is *osteoporosis*, a disease characterized by low bone mass and deterioration of bone tissue, which increases fracture risk. Regular weight-bearing and strength-building physical activities are recommended to maintain bone health and prevent osteoporotic fractures. Although both men and women can be affected by osteoporosis, it is more common in women. Women (like men) have much to gain by remaining physically active as they age—bone mass levels are significantly higher among active women than among sedentary women.[22] However, it appears that the full bone-related benefits of physical activity can be achieved only with sufficient hormone levels (estrogen in women; testosterone in men) and adequate calcium, vitamin D, and total caloric intakes.[23]

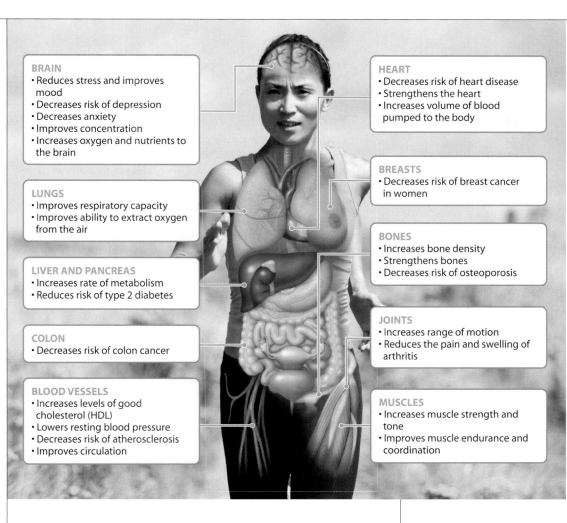

BRAIN
• Reduces stress and improves mood
• Decreases risk of depression
• Decreases anxiety
• Improves concentration
• Increases oxygen and nutrients to the brain

LUNGS
• Improves respiratory capacity
• Improves ability to extract oxygen from the air

LIVER AND PANCREAS
• Increases rate of metabolism
• Reduces risk of type 2 diabetes

COLON
• Decreases risk of colon cancer

BLOOD VESSELS
• Increases levels of good cholesterol (HDL)
• Lowers resting blood pressure
• Decreases risk of atherosclerosis
• Improves circulation

HEART
• Decreases risk of heart disease
• Strengthens the heart
• Increases volume of blood pumped to the body

BREASTS
• Decreases risk of breast cancer in women

BONES
• Increases bone density
• Strengthens bones
• Decreases risk of osteoporosis

JOINTS
• Increases range of motion
• Reduces the pain and swelling of arthritis

MUSCLES
• Increases muscle strength and tone
• Improves muscle endurance and coordination

Figure 10.2 Some Health Benefits of Regular Exercise

Although these mental health benefits are difficult to quantify, they are frequently mentioned as reasons for continuing to be physically active.

Physical activity contributes to mental health in several ways. Regular physical activity tones and develops muscles and can reduce or maintain body fat, thus improving a person's physical appearance, which itself often results in increased self-esteem. Learning new skills, developing increased ability and capacity in recreational activities, and sticking with a physical activity plan also improve self-esteem.

Improved Stress Management Regular vigorous exercise has been shown to "burn off" the chemical by-products of the stress response and increase endorphins, giving mood a natural boost. Elimination of stress hormones reduces the stress response by accelerating the neurological system's return to a balanced state.[28] For this reason, regular physical activity of moderate to vigorous intensity should be an integral component of any stress management plan.

Improved Immunity Research shows that regular moderate-intensity physical activity reduces individual susceptibility to disease.[24] Just how physical activity alters immunity is not well understood. We do know that moderate-intensity physical activity temporarily increases the number of white blood cells (WBCs), which are responsible for fighting infection.[25] Often the relationship of physical activity to immunity, or more specifically to disease susceptibility, is described as a J-shaped curve. In other words, susceptibility to disease decreases with moderate activity, but then increases as you move to more extreme levels of physical activity or exercise or if you continue to exercise without adequate recovery time.[26] Athletes engaging in marathon-type events or very intense physical training programs have been shown to be at greater risk for upper respiratory tract infections (colds and flu).[27]

Improved Back Strength Regular whole-body exercise, as well as exercises targeting the specific muscles of the back (and the rest of the core), create a strong platform for the entire body. A strong and healthy back helps you maintain proper posture and avoid posture-related stress in the neck, shoulders, hips, knees, and ankles. It also gives you a good foundation for a range of exercise and reduces the likelihood of injury.

Improved Mental Health Most people who engage in regular physical activity are likely to notice the psychological benefits, such as feeling better about oneself and an overall sense of well-being.

Longer Life Span Experts have long debated the relationship between physical activity and longevity. In one study of over 5,000 middle-aged and older Americans, researchers found that those who engaged in moderate to high levels of activity lived 1.3 to 3.7 years longer than those who did less.[29] Furthermore, individuals who were physically active at a more intense level outlived sedentary subjects by 3.5 to 3.7 years.

Improved Weight Management Physical activity contributes to weight management by increasing the number of calories burned by the body. In addition, physical activity increases metabolic rate, keeping it elevated for several hours following vigorous physical activities. This increase in rate can reduce body fat and increase lean muscle mass. Lean muscle mass is more metabolically active than fat tissue, so its increase in turn enhances calorie burning. Increased physical activity also improves your chances of maintaining the weight loss.[30]

check yourself

■ **What are five health benefits of physical activity?**

Getting Motivated for Physical Activity

learning **outcomes**

- **List several obstacles people face when deciding to be more physically active.**

- **Explain factors to consider when choosing an exercise activity.**

There are many reasons for wanting to be more physically active and physically fit, including the many health benefits discussed earlier in this chapter. Taking some time to reflect on your personal circumstances, goals, and desires regarding physical fitness will probably make it easier for you to come up with a plan you can stick to. Are you interested in becoming more physically active to be better at sports? To feel better about your body? To manage your stress? Or is it to improve your health and reduce your risk of chronic diseases? Perhaps your most vital goal will be to commit to your physical fitness for the long haul—to establish a realistic schedule of diverse physical activities that you can maintain and enjoy throughout your life.

For many people, the desire to lose weight is the main reason for their physical activity. On the most basic level, physical activity requires your body to generate energy through calorie expenditure; if calories expended exceeds calories consumed over a span of time, the net result will be weight loss. Some activities are more intense or vigorous than others and result in more calories used; **Figure 10.3** shows the caloric cost of various activities when done for 30 minutes.

Overcoming Common Obstacles to Physical Activity

People offer a variety of excuses to explain why they do not exercise, ranging from personal ("I don't have time") to environmental ("I don't have a safe place to be active"). Some people may be reluctant to exercise if they are overweight, are embarrassed to work out with their more "fit" friends, or feel they lack the knowledge and skills required.

What keeps you from being more physically active? Is it time? Do you lack a support group? Is the fitness center location inconvenient, or do you lack money for a membership or equipment? Perhaps you are ready to begin but do not know how to start. Think about your obstacles and write them down. Once you honestly evaluate why you are not as physically active as you want to be, review **Table 10.2** for suggestions on overcoming your hurdles.

Incorporating Fitness into Your Life

When designing your program, you should consider several factors in order to boost your chances of achieving your physical fitness goals. First, choose activities that are appropriate for you, that you genuinely like doing, and that are convenient. For example, you might choose jogging because you like to run and there are beautiful trails nearby, rather than swimming, since you do not really like the water and the pool is difficult to get to. Likewise, choose activities suitable for your current fitness level. If you are overweight or obese

Figure 10.3 Calories Burned by Different Activities
The harder you exercise, the more energy you expend. Estimated calories burned for various moderate and vigorous activities are listed for a 30-minute bout of activity.

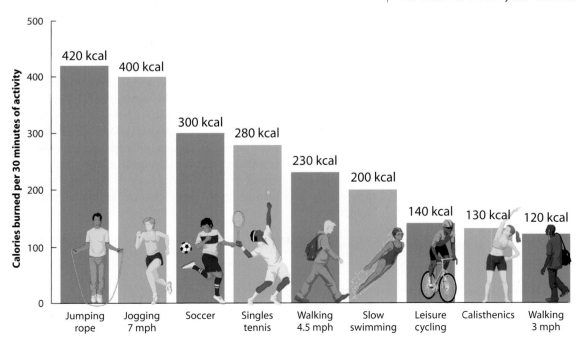

420 kcal	400 kcal	300 kcal	280 kcal	230 kcal	200 kcal	140 kcal	130 kcal	120 kcal
Jumping rope	Jogging 7 mph	Soccer	Singles tennis	Walking 4.5 mph	Slow swimming	Leisure cycling	Calisthenics	Walking 3 mph

Calories burned per 30 minutes of activity

TABLE 10.2 Overcoming Obstacles to Physical Activity

Obstacle	Possible Solution
LACK OF TIME	• Look at your schedule. Where can you find 30-minute time slots? Perhaps you need to focus on shorter times (10 minutes or more) throughout the day. • Multitask. Read while riding an exercise bike or listen to lecture tapes while walking. • Be physically active during your lunch and study breaks as well as between classes. Skip rope or throw a Frisbee with a friend. • Select activities that require less time, such as brisk walking or jogging. • Ride your bike to class, or park (or get off the bus) farther from your destination.
SOCIAL INFLUENCE	• Invite family and friends to be active with you. • Join a class to meet new people. • Explain the importance of exercise and your commitment to physical activity to people who may not support your efforts. • Find a role model to support your efforts. • Plan for physically active dates—go dancing or bowling.
LACK OF MOTIVATION, WILLPOWER, OR ENERGY	• Schedule your workout time just as you would any other important commitment. • Enlist the help of an exercise partner to make you accountable for working out. • Give yourself an incentive. • Schedule your workouts when you feel most energetic. • Remind yourself that exercise gives you more energy. • Get things ready for your workout; for example, if you choose to walk in the morning, set out your walking clothes the night before, or pack your gym bag before going to bed.
LACK OF RESOURCES	• Select an activity that requires minimal equipment, such as walking, jogging, jumping rope, or calisthenics. • Identify inexpensive resources on campus or in the community. • Use active forms of transportation. • Take advantage of no-cost opportunities, such as playing catch in the park/green space on campus.

Source: Adapted from National Center for Chronic Disease Prevention and Health Promotion, "How Can I Overcome Barriers to Physical Activity?" Updated May 2010, Available at www.cdc.gov/physicalactivity/everyone/getactive/barriers.html.

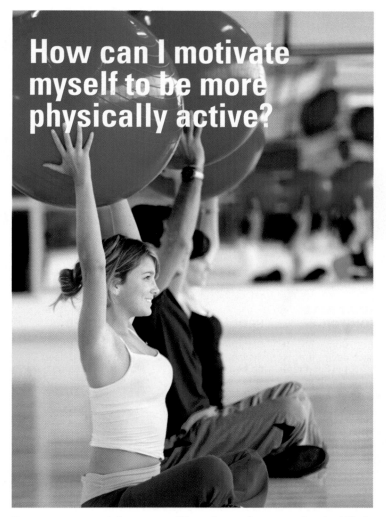

How can I motivate myself to be more physically active?

One great way to motivate yourself is to sign up for an exercise class. Find something that interests you—dance, yoga, aerobics, martial arts, acrobatics—and get yourself involved. The structure, schedule, social interaction, and challenge of learning a new skill can be terrific motivators that make exercising and being physically active exciting and fun.

and have not exercised in months, do not sign up for the advanced aerobics classes. Start slow, plan fun activities, and progress to more challenging activities as your physical fitness improves. You may choose to simply walk more in an attempt to achieve the recommended goal of 10,000 steps per day; keep track with a pedometer (or step counter; see Table 10.3 for more on this handy gadget and other fitness equipment you may consider purchasing or using at a health club). Try to make exercise a part of your routine by incorporating it into something you already have to do—such as getting to class or work.

check yourself

■ **What are some common obstacles people face when deciding to be more physically active? How can these obstacles be overcome?**

■ **What factors should you consider when choosing an exercise activity?**

Some Popular Fitness Gadgets and Equipment

learning **outcomes**

■ **Identify common types of fitness equipment and their uses.**

TABLE

10.3 Some Popular Fitness Gadgets and Equipment

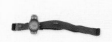   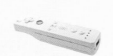

HEART RATE MONITOR	PEDOMETER	STABILITY BALL	WII FIT	RESISTANCE BAND	MEDICINE BALL
Chest strap with watch device that measures heart rate during training. • Instant feedback about intensity of your workout. • Strap can be cumbersome. Cost: $50–$200	Battery-operated device, usually worn on belt, that measures steps taken. Some models also monitor calories, distance, and speed. • Great motivation and feedback. • Must be calibrated for height, weight, and stride length. Cost: $25–$50	Ball made of burst-resistant vinyl used for strengthening core muscles or improving flexibility. • Balls must be inflated correctly to be most effective. Cost: $25–$50	"Active" video-game system in which players move their bodies to play onscreen games. • Opportunities for entertainment and social activity • Can be used indoors in bad weather Cost: $150–$200 for basic system plus $70–$100 for Wii Fit bundle	Rubber or elastic material, sometimes with handles, used to build muscular strength and endurance or for flexibility. • Lightweight, durable, and portable. Cost: $5–$15	Heavy ball, about 14" in diameter, used in rehabilitation and strength training. Weight varies from 2–25 lb. • Can be used in plyometric training and to develop core strength. • If used incorrectly, risk of lower back injuries. Cost: $10–$150

   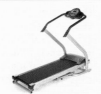

FREE WEIGHTS	ELLIPTICAL TRAINER	STAIR CLIMBER	STATIONARY BIKE	TREADMILL
Dumbbells or barbells, often with adjustable weight. • Build muscular strength and endurance. • Potential for injury with incorrect form; concentrate on alignment and core strength. Cost: $10–$300	Stationary exercise machine that simulates walking or running without impact on bones and joints. Some include arm movements. • Nonimpact; less wear and tear on the joints and risk of shin splints. Cost: $300–$4,000	Stationary exercise machine that provides low-impact lower-body workout via stair climbing. • Nonimpact; less wear and tear on the joints and risk of shin splints. • Various programs are available. Cost: $200–$3,000	Lower-body exercise machine designed to simulate bike riding. • Generally easy to use; does not require balance. • Comes with varied resistance programs. • Recumbent styles offer less strain on back and knees. Cost: $200–$2,000	Exercise machine for walking or running on a moving platform. • Generally easy to use; comes with emergency shutoff. • Lower impact on joints than running on most pavements. Cost: $500–$4,000

check yourself

■ **What are five types of fitness equipment? Which would you be likely to use and why?**

Fitness Program Components and the FITT Principle

learning outcomes

- **List the four parts of the FITT principle.**

A comprehensive workout includes three elements: warm-up, cardiorespiratory and/or resistance training, and cool-down.

Warm-up involves 5 to 15 minutes of large body movements followed by light stretching. This slowly increases heart rate, blood pressure, breathing rate, and body temperature; improves joint lubrication; and increases muscles' and tendons' elasticity and flexibility.

The main part of your workout is 20 minutes or more of cardio-respiratory and/or resistance training You may use an aerobic training device(s) or follow a program of strength and endurance training.

Cool-down includes 5 to 10 minutes of low-intensity activity and 5 to 10 minutes of stretching. This gradually reduces heart rate, blood pressure, and body temperature; reduces the risk of blood pooling in the extremities; and helps speed recovery between exercise sessions.

Creating Your Fitness Program: The FITT Principle

The **FITT (Frequency, Intensity, Time, and Type)** principle shown in **Figure 10.4** can be used to devise a workout plan for health- or performance-related physical fitness. To achieve the desired level of fitness:

- **Frequency** refers to how often you must engage in a given exercise.
- **Intensity** refers to how hard your workout must be.
- **Time,** or *duration*, refers to how many minutes or repetitions of an exercise are required per session.
- **Type** refers to the kind of exercises performed.

	Cardiorespiratory endurance	**Muscular strength and endurance**	**Flexibility**
Frequency	3–5 days per week	2–4 days per week	Minimally 2–3 days per week; optimally daily
Intensity	70%–90% of maximum heart rate	*Strength*: >60% of 1RM *Endurance*: <60% of 1RM	To the point of tension
Time	20–30+ minutes	*Strength*: 2–6 reps, 1–3 sets *Endurance*: 10–15 reps, 2–6 sets	10–30 seconds per stretch, 2–3 repetitions
Type	Any rhythmic, continuous, vigorous activity	Resistance training (with body weight and/or external resistance)	Stretching, dance, yoga, gymnastics

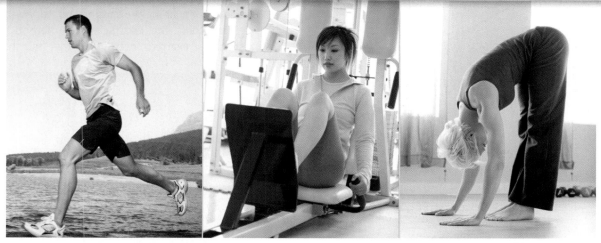

Figure 10.4 The FITT Principle Applied to Cardiorespiratory Fitness, Muscular Strength and Endurance, and Flexibility

check yourself

- **What are the four parts of the FITT principle?**

The FITT Principle for Cardiorespiratory Fitness

- **List the FITT requirements for cardiorespiratory fitness.**

The most effective aerobic exercises for building cardiorespiratory fitness are total-body activities involving the large muscle groups of your body. The FITT prescription for cardiorespiratory fitness includes 3 to 5 days per week of vigorous, rhythmic, continuous activity, at 70 to 90 percent of maximal heart rate, for 20 to 30 minutes.[31]

Frequency

To improve your cardiorespiratory fitness, you must exercise vigorously at least three times a week. If you are a newcomer to exercise, you can still make improvements by doing less intense exercise but doing it more days a week, following the recommendations from the Centers for Disease Control and Prevention (CDC) and the American College of Sports Medicine (ACSM) for moderate physical activity 5 days a week (refer to **Table 10.1**).

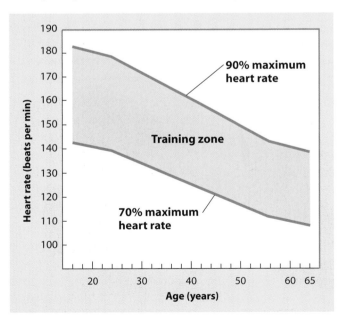

Figure 10.5 Target Heart Rate Ranges
These ranges are based on calculating the maximum heart rate as 220 minus age and the training zone as 70% to 90% of maximum heart rate. Individuals with low fitness levels should start below or at the low end of these ranges.

Intensity

The most common methods used to determine the intensity of cardiorespiratory endurance exercises are target heart rate, rating of perceived exertion, and the talk test. The exercise intensity required to improve cardiorespiratory endurance is a heart rate between 70 and 90 percent of your maximum heart rate. To calculate this **target heart rate,** subtract your age from 220 (males) or 226 (females). This results in your maximum heart rate. Your target heart rate would be 70 to 90 percent of your maximum heart rate. For example, if you are a 20-year-old male, your estimated maximum heart rate is 200 (220 × 20 = 200). Your target heart rate would be somewhere between 140 (200 − 0.70 = 140) and 180 (200 × 0.90 = 180) beats per minute. **Figure 10.5** shows a range of target heart rates.

Take your pulse during your workout to determine how close you are to your target heart rate. Lightly place your index and middle fingers (not your thumb) over one of the major arteries in your neck, or on the artery on the inside of your wrist (**Figure 10.6**). Start counting your pulse immediately after you stop exercising, as your heart rate decreases rapidly. Using a watch or a clock, take your pulse for 6 seconds (the first pulse is "0") and multiply this number by 10 (add a zero to your count) to get the number of beats per minute.

Another way of determining the intensity of cardiorespiratory exercise is to use Borg's rating of perceived exertion (RPE) scale. Perceived exertion refers to how hard you feel you are working, which you might base on your heart rate, breathing rate, sweating, and level of fatigue. This scale uses a rating from 6 (no exertion at all) to 20 (maximal exertion). An RPE of 12 to 16 is generally recommended for training the cardiorespiratory system.

The easiest, but least scientific, method of measuring cardiorespiratory exercise intensity is the "talk test." A heart rate of

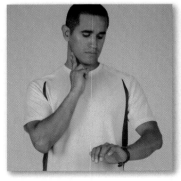
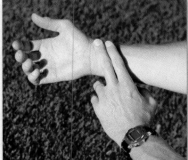

ⓐ Carotid pulse   ⓑ Radial pulse

Figure 10.6 Taking a Pulse
Palpation of the carotid (neck) or radial (wrist) artery is a simple way of determining heart rate.

70 percent of maximum is also called the "conversational" level of exercise, because you are able to talk with a partner while exercising.[32] If you are breathing so hard that talking is difficult, the intensity of your exercise is too high. Conversely, if you are able to sing or laugh heartily while exercising, the intensity of your exercise is insufficient for maintaining and/or improving cardiorespiratory fitness.

Time

For cardiorespiratory fitness benefits, the ACSM recommends that vigorous activities (70% to 90% of heart rate maximum) be performed for at least 20 minutes at a time, and moderate activities (50% to 70% of heart rate maximum) for at least 30 minutes.[33]

Type

Any sort of rhythmic, continuous, and vigorous physical activity that can be done for 20 or more minutes will improve cardiorespiratory fitness. Examples include walking briskly, cycling, jogging, fitness classes, and swimming.

Incorporating Cardiorespiratory Fitness into Daily Life

Before we became a car culture, much of our transportation was human powered. Bicycling and walking historically were important means of transportation and recreation in the United States. These modes not only helped keep people in good physical shape, but they also had little or no impact on the environment. Even in the first few decades after the automobile started to be popularized, people continued to get around under their own power. Since World War II, however, the development of automobile-oriented communities has led to a steady decline of bicycling and walking. Currently, only about 10 percent of trips are made by foot or bike.

The more we use our cars to get around, the more congested our roads, the more polluted our air, and the more sedentary our lives become. That is why many people are now embracing a movement toward more active transportation. *Active transportation* means getting out of your car and using your own power to get from place to place—whether walking, riding a bike, skateboarding, or roller skating. Each of these activities can also be incorporated into your life as a form of exercise that contributes to cardiorespiratory fitness.

The following are just a few of the many reasons to make active transportation a bigger part of your life:

- **You will be adding more exercise into your daily routine.** People who walk, bike, or use other active forms of transportation to complete errands are physically active.
- **Walking or biking can save you money.** With rising gas prices and parking fees, in addition to increasing car maintenance and insurance costs, fewer automobile trips could add up to considerable savings. During the course of a year, regular bicycle commuters who ride 5 miles to work can save about $500 on fuel and more than $1,000 on other expenses related to driving.

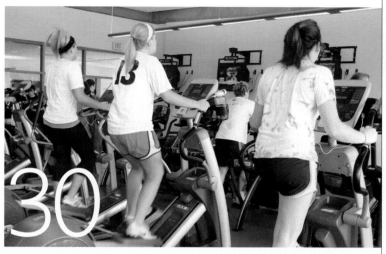

minutes on a cardiorespiratory device generates 50 watt hours of electricity—enough to operate a laptop for an hour. These machines have been retrofitted to help power the student fitness center.

- **Walking or biking may save you time!** Cycling is usually the fastest mode of travel door to door for distances up to 5 or 6 miles in city centers. Walking is simpler and faster for distances of about a mile.
- **You will enjoy being outdoors.** Research is emerging on the physical and mental health benefits of nature and being outdoors. So much of what we do is inside, with recirculated air and artificial lighting, that our bodies are deficient in fresh air and sunlight.
- **You will be making a significant contribution to the reduction of air pollution.** Driving less means fewer pollutants being emitted into the air. Leaving your car at home just two days a week will reduce greenhouse gas emissions by an average of 1,600 pounds per year.
- **You will help reduce traffic.** The average traveler now wastes the equivalent of a full work week stuck in traffic every year. Having more active commuters means fewer cars on the roads and less traffic congestion.
- **You will contribute to global health.** Annually, personal transportation accounts for the consumption of approximately 136 billion gallons of gasoline, or the production of 1.2 billion tons of carbon dioxide. Reducing vehicle trips will help reduce overall greenhouse gas emissions and reduce the need to source more fossil fuel.

check yourself

- **What are the FITT requirements for cardiorespiratory fitness?**

The FITT Principle for Muscular Strength and Endurance

- **List the FITT requirements for muscular strength and endurance.**

The FITT prescription for muscular strength and endurance includes 2 to 4 days per week of exercises that train the major muscle groups, using enough sets and repetitions and enough resistance to maintain or improve muscular strength and endurance.[34]

Frequency

For frequency, the FITT principle recommends performing 8 to 10 exercises that train the major muscle groups 2 to 4 days a week. It is believed that overloading the muscles, a normal part of resistance training (described below), causes microscopic tears in muscle fibers. The rebuilding process that increases the muscle's size and capacity takes about 24 to 48 hours. Thus, resistance-training exercise programs should include at least 1 day of rest between workouts before the same muscles are overloaded again. But don't wait too long between workouts—one of the important principles of strength training is the idea of *reversibility*. Reversibility means that if you stop exercising, the body responds by deconditioning. Even after as little as 4 days without training, muscles begin to revert to their untrained state.[35] The saying "use it or lose it" applies here!

Intensity

To determine the intensity of exercise needed to improve muscular strength and endurance, you need to know the maximum amount of weight you can lift (or move) in one contraction. This value is called your **one repetition maximum (1 RM)** and can be individually determined or predicted from a 10 RM test. Once your 1 RM is determined, it is used as the basis for intensity recommendations for improving muscular strength and endurance. Muscular strength is improved when resistance loads are greater than 60 percent of your 1 RM, whereas muscular endurance is improved using loads of less than 60 percent of your 1 RM.

Everyone begins a resistance-training program at an initial level of strength. To become stronger, you must *overload* your muscles; that is, regularly create a degree of tension in your muscles greater than that which you are accustomed to. Overloading your muscles forces them to adapt by getting larger, stronger, and capable of producing more tension. If you "underload" your muscles, you will not increase strength. If you create too great an overload, you may experience muscle injury, muscle fatigue, and potentially a loss in strength. Once your strength goal is reached, no further overload is necessary; your challenge at that point is to maintain your level of strength by engaging in a regular (once or twice per week) total-body resistance exercise program.

Time

The time recommended for muscular strength and endurance exercises is measured not in minutes of exercise, but rather in repetitions and sets. The types of demands that you put on your body will result in the kind of adaptation that will follow:

Sets and Repetitions. To increase muscular strength, you need higher intensity and fewer repetitions and sets: Use a resistance of at least 60 percent of your 1RM, performing two to six repetitions per set, with one to three sets performed overall. If improving muscular endurance is your goal, use less resistance and more repetitions and sets. The recommendations for improving muscular endurance are to perform two to six sets of 10 to 15 repetitions using a resistance that is less than 60 percent of your 1 RM.

Rest Periods. The amount of rest between exercises is key to an effective strength-training workout. Resting between exercises can reduce fatigue and help with performance and safety in subsequent sets. A rest period of 2 to 3 minutes is recommended for multiple-joint exercises that use large-muscle groups (e.g., squats with overhead presses); a rest period of 1 to 2 minutes is best for single-joint exercises or for strength exercises using machines. It should be pointed out that this "rest period" refers specifically to the muscle group being exercised; it is possible to alternate muscle groups, thus taking advantage of your time available to train. For example, you can

Resistance training to improve muscular strength and endurance can be done with free weights, machines, or even your own body weight.

TABLE 10.4

Methods of Providing Exercise Resistance

Body Weight Resistance (Calisthenics)	Fixed Resistance	Variable Resistance	Accommodating Resistance
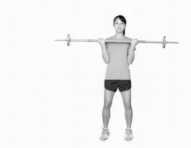		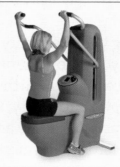	
• Using your own body weight to develop muscular strength, endurance. • Improves overall muscular fitness—in particular core strength and overall muscle tone.	• Provides constant resistance throughout full range of movement. • Requires balance and coordination; promotes development of core strength.	• Resistance is altered so the muscle's effort is consistent throughout full range of motion. • Provides more controlled motion and isolates certain muscle groups.	• Sometimes called isokinetic machines; they maintain constant speed throughout range of motion. • Requires maximal effort, because machine controls speed of exercise. • Often used for rehabilitation after injury.
Examples: Push-ups, pull-ups, curl-ups, dips, leg raises, chair sits.	**Examples:** Free weights such as barbells and dumbbells.	**Examples:** Specific machines in gyms; some home models (such as Nautilus and Bowflex) available.	**Examples:** Specific machines in rehabilitation facilities and gyms.

237

alternate a set of push-ups with a set of curl-ups; the muscle groups worked in one set can rest while you are working the other muscle groups.

Type

To improve muscular strength or endurance, resistance training is most often recommended using either your own body weight or devices that provide a fixed, variable, or accommodating load or resistance (see **Table 10.4**). Some cardiorespiratory training activities also enhance muscular endurance: thousands of repetitions are performed during a 20-minute (or longer) workout using relatively low resistance when jogging or when training on an exercise device such as a stationary bicycle, rowing machine, or stair-climbing machine.

When selecting the type of strength-training exercises to do, keep several important principles in mind. The first of these is *specificity*. According to the specificity principle, the effects of resistance-exercise training are specific to the muscles exercised; only the muscle or muscle group that is overloaded responds to the demands placed upon it. For example, if you regularly do curls, the muscles involved—your biceps—will become larger and stronger, but the other muscles in your body do not change. This sort of training may put opposing muscle groups—in this case the triceps—at increased risk for injury.

To improve total body strength, you must include exercises for all the major muscle groups. You must also ensure that your overload is sufficient to increase strength and not only endurance.

Another important concept to consider is *exercise selection*. Exercises that work a single joint (e.g., chest presses) are effective for building specific muscle strength, whereas multiple-joint exercises (e.g., a squat coupled with an overhead press) are more effective for increasing overall muscle strength. The ACSM recommends that both exercise types be included in a strength-training program, with an emphasis on multiple-joint exercises for maximizing muscle strength.[36]

Finally, for optimal training effects, it is important to pay attention to *exercise order*. When training all major muscle groups in a single workout, complete large-muscle group exercises before small-muscle group exercises, multiple-joint exercises before single-joint exercises, and high-intensity exercises before lower-intensity exercises.

check yourself

- **What are the FITT requirements for muscular strength and endurance?**

The FITT Principle for Flexibility

learning **outcomes**

■ **List the FITT requirements for flexibility.**

Improving your flexibility enhances the efficiency of your movements, increases well-being, and reduces stress. Further, inflexible muscles are susceptible to injury; flexibility training helps reduce incidence and severity of lower back problems and muscle or tendon injuries[37] and reduces joint pain and deterioration.[38]

Frequency

The FITT principle calls for a minimum of 2 to 3 days per week for flexibility training; daily training is even better.

Intensity

Hold static (still) stretching positions at an individually determined "point of tension." You should feel tension or mild discomfort in the muscle(s) stretched, though not pain.[39]

Time

Hold each stretch at the "point of tension" for 10 to 30 seconds for each stretch; repeat two or three times in close succession.[40]

Type

The most effective exercises for building flexibility involve stretching of major muscle groups when the body is already warm, such as after cardiorespiratory activities. The safest such exercises involve **static stretching**, which slowly and gradually lengthens a muscle or group of muscles and their attached tendons.[41] With each repetition, your range of motion improves temporarily due to the slightly lessened sensitivity of tension receptors in the stretched muscles; when done regularly, range of motion increases.[42] **Figure 10.7** shows some basic stretching exercises.

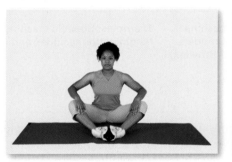

ⓐ Stretching the inside of the thighs

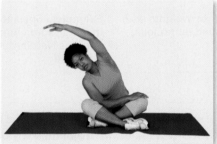

ⓑ Stretching the upper arm and the side of the trunk

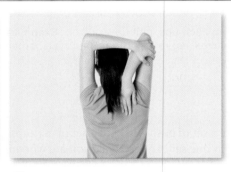

ⓒ Stretching the triceps

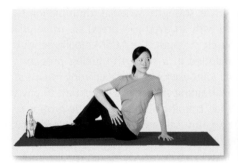

ⓓ Stretching the trunk and the hip

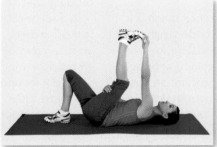

ⓔ Stretching the hip, back of the thigh, and the calf

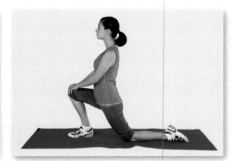

ⓕ Stretching the front of the thigh and the hip flexor

Figure 10.7 Stretching Exercises to Improve Flexibility and Prevent Injury
Use these stretches as part of your warm-up and cool-down. Hold each stretch for 10 to 30 seconds, and repeat two to three times for each limb.

check yourself

■ **What are the FITT requirements for flexibility?**

Developing Core Strength

- **Explain the benefits of a strong core.**
- **List three types of exercise that increase core strength.**

Yoga, tai chi, and Pilates have become increasingly popular in the United States. All three forms of exercise have the potential to improve **core strength**, flexibility, balance, coordination, and agility.

Core Strength Training

The body's core muscles, including deep back and abdominal muscles that attach to the spine and pelvis, are the foundation for all movement.[43] Contraction of these muscles provides the basis of support for movements of the upper and lower body and powerful movements of the extremities. A weak core generally results in poor posture, low back pain, and muscle injuries. A strong core provides a stable center of gravity and so a more stable platform for movements, thus reducing the chance of injury.

You can develop core strength using exercises such as calisthenics, yoga, and Pilates. Core strength does not happen from one single exercise, but rather from a structured regime of postures and exercises.[44] Holding yourself in a front or reverse plank ("up" and reverse of a push-up position) and holding or doing abdominal curl-ups are examples of exercises that increase core strength. The use of instability devices (stability ball, wobble boards, etc.) and exercises to train the core have also become popular.[45]

Yoga

Yoga originated in India about 5,000 years ago. It blends the mental and physical aspects of exercise, a union of mind and body that participants often find relaxing and satisfying. If done regularly, yoga improves flexibility, vitality, posture, agility, balance, coordination, and muscular strength and endurance. Many people report an improved sense of general well-being, too.

The practice of hatha yoga (the physical aspect of yoga) focuses attention on controlled breathing as well as physical exercise and incorporates a complex array of static stretching exercises expressed as postures (asanas).

Some forms of hatha yoga are more meditative in their practice, whereas others are more athletic. Ashtanga yoga, also called "power yoga," focuses on a series of poses done in a continuous, repeated flow, with controlled breathing. Bikram yoga, also known as hot yoga, is unique in that classes are held in rooms heated to 105°F, which practitioners claim helps the potential for increasing flexibility.

Tai Chi

Tai chi is an ancient Chinese form of exercise that combines stretching, balance, muscular endurance, coordination, and meditation. It increases range of motion and flexibility while reducing muscular tension. Tai chi involves a series of positions called forms that are performed continuously. Tai chi is often described as "meditation in motion" because it promotes serenity through gentle movements, connecting the mind and body.

Pilates

Pilates was developed by Joseph Pilates in 1926 as an exercise style that combines stretching with movement against resistance, frequently aided by devices such as tension springs or heavy rubber bands. It teaches body awareness, good posture, and easy, graceful body movements while improving flexibility, coordination, core strength, muscle tone, and economy of motion.

Pilates differs from yoga and tai chi in that it includes sequences of movements specifically designed to increase strength. Some Pilates exercises are carried out on specially designed equipment, whereas others can be performed on mats.

Strengthening core body muscles can also enhance flexibility and help lower stress levels.

- **What are some benefits of having a strong core?**
- **What types of exercise increase core strength?**

Nutrition and Exercise

- **Identify nutritional habits that support healthy exercise.**
- **Explain how hydration affects exercise.**

To make the most of your workouts, follow the recommendations from the MyPlate plan and make sure that you eat sufficient carbohydrates, the body's main source of fuel. Your body stores carbohydrates as glycogen primarily in the muscles and liver and then uses this stored glycogen for energy when you are physically active. Fats are also an important source of energy, packing more than double the energy per gram of carbohydrates. Protein plays a role in muscle repair and growth, but is not normally a source of energy. Another important nutrient to consider is water (or fluids containing water).

Timing Your Food Intake

When you eat is almost as important as what you eat. Eating a large meal before exercising can cause upset stomach, cramping, and diarrhea, because your muscles have to compete with your digestive system for energy. Eat larger meals at least 4 hours before you begin exercising. Smaller meals (snacks) can be eaten about an hour before activity. Not eating at all before a workout can cause low blood sugar levels that, in turn, cause weakness and slower reaction times. It is also important to refuel after your workout. Help your muscles recover and prepare for the next bout of activity by eating a snack or meal that contains plenty of carbohydrates plus a bit of protein.

Staying Hydrated

In addition to eating well, staying hydrated is crucial for active individuals wanting to maintain a healthy, fully functional body. How much fluid

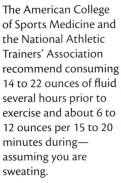

For hydration, electrolytes, carbohydrates, and protein, low-fat chocolate milk may be the ideal post-workout drink.

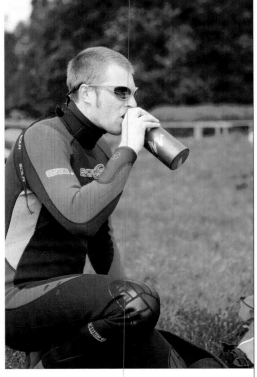

The American College of Sports Medicine and the National Athletic Trainers' Association recommend consuming 14 to 22 ounces of fluid several hours prior to exercise and about 6 to 12 ounces per 15 to 20 minutes during—assuming you are sweating.

How much do I need to drink **before, during, and after** physical activity?

do you need to stay well hydrated? Keep in mind that the goal of fluid replacement is to prevent excessive dehydration (greater than 2% loss of body weight). The ACSM and the National Athletic Trainers Association recommend consuming 5 to 7 mL per kg of body weight (approximately 0.7 to 1.07 oz per 10 pounds of body weight), 4 hours prior to exercise.[46] Drinking fluids during exercise is also important, though it is difficult to provide guidelines for how much or when, because intake should be based on time, intensity, and type of activity performed. A good way to monitor how much fluid you need to replace is to weigh yourself before and after your workout. The difference in weight is how much you should drink. So, for example, if you lost 2 pounds during a training session, you should drink 32 ounces of fluid.[47]

What are the best fluids to drink? For exercise sessions lasting less than 1 hour, plain water is sufficient for rehydration. If your exercise session exceeds 1 hour—and you sweat profusely—consider a sports drink containing electrolytes. The electrolytes in

TABLE

10.5

Performance-Enhancing Dietary Supplements and Drugs—Their Uses and Effects

Substance	Primary Uses	Side Effects
CREATINE Naturally occurring compound that helps supply energy to muscle	• To improve postworkout recovery • To increase muscle mass • To increase strength • To increase power	• Weight gain, nausea, muscle cramps • Large doses have a negative effect on the kidneys
EPHEDRA AND EPHEDRINE Stimulant that constricts blood vessels and increases blood pressure and heart rate	• Weight loss • Increased performance	• Nausea, vomiting • Anxiety and mood changes • Hyperactivity • In rare cases, seizures, heart attack, stroke, psychotic episodes
ANABOLIC STEROIDS Synthetic versions of the hormone testosterone	• To improve strength, power, and speed • To increase muscle mass	• In adolescents, stops bone growth; therefore reduces adult height • Masculinization of females; feminization of males • Mood swings • Severe acne, particularly on the back • Sexual dysfunction • Aggressive behavior • Potential heart and liver damage

STEROID PRECURSORS
Substances that the body converts into anabolic steroids, e.g., androstenedione (andro), dehydroepiandrosterone (DHEA)
	• Converted in the body to anabolic steroids to increase muscle mass	• Same side effects as noted with anabolic steroids:
		  • Body hair growth
		  • Increased risk of pancreatic cancer

HUMAN GROWTH HORMONE Naturally occurring hormone secreted by the pituitary gland that is essential for body growth	• Anti-aging agent • To improve performance • To increase muscle mass	• Structural changes to the face • Increased risk of high blood pressure • Potential for congestive heart failure

Sources: Mayo Clinic Staff, "Performance-Enhancing Drugs and Your Teen Athlete," MayoClinic.com, January 2009, www.mayoclinic.com/health/performance-enhancing-drugs/SM00045; Office of Diversion Control, Drug and Chemical Evaluation Section, "Drugs and Chemicals of Concern: Human Growth Hormone," August 2009, www.deadiversion.usdoj.gov/drugs_concern/hgh.htm; Office of Dietary Supplements, National Institutes of Health, "Ephedra and Ephedrine Alkaloids for Weight Loss and Athletic Performance," Updated July 2004, http://ods.od.nih.gov/factsheets/EphedraandEphedrine.

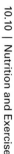

these products are minerals and ions such as sodium and potassium needed for proper functioning of your nervous and muscular systems. Replacing electrolytes is particularly important for endurance athletes engaging in long bouts of exercise or competition. In endurance events lasting more than 4 hours, an athlete's overconsumption of plain water can dilute the sodium concentration in the blood with potentially fatal results, an effect called **hyponatremia** or **water intoxication**.

Dietary Supplements

Today there is a burgeoning market for dietary supplements that claim to deliver the nutrients needed for muscle recovery, as well as some that include additional "performance-enhancing" ingredients. See Table 10.5 for a list of some of the most popular performance-enhancing drugs and supplements, their purported benefits, and associated risks.

check yourself

■ **What are some of the most important nutritional aspects of fitness?**

■ **How does hydration affect exercise?**

Fitness-Related Injuries: Prevention and Treatment

- **Distinguish between traumatic injuries and overuse injuries.**
- **Explain how to prevent and treat common fitness-related injuries.**

The two basic types of fitness-related injuries are traumatic and overuse injuries. **Traumatic injuries** occur suddenly and violently, typically by accident. Typical traumatic injuries are broken bones, torn ligaments and muscles, contusions, and lacerations.

Many traumatic injuries are unavoidable—for example, spraining your ankle by landing on another person's foot after jumping up for a rebound in basketball. Others are preventable through proper training, appropriate equipment and clothing, and common sense. If your traumatic injury causes a noticeable loss of function and immediate pain or pain that does not go away after 30 minutes, consult a physician.

Overtraining is the most frequent cause of injuries related to physical fitness training. Doing too much intense exercise, too much exercise without variation, or not allowing for sufficient rest and recovery time can increase the likelihood of **overuse injuries**. Overuse injuries occur because of the cumulative, day-after-day stresses placed on tendons, muscles, and joints.

Common Overuse Injuries

Common sites of overuse injuries are the hip, knee, shoulder, and elbow joints. Three of the most common overuse injuries are plantar fasciitis, shin splints, and runner's knee.

Plantar Fasciitis *Plantar fasciitis* is an inflammation of the plantar fascia, a broad band of dense, inelastic tissue (fascia) that runs from the heel to the toes on the bottom of your foot. The main function of the plantar fascia is to protect the nerves, blood vessels, and muscles of the foot from injury. In repetitive weight-bearing physical activities such as walking and running, the plantar fascia may become inflamed. Common symptoms are pain and tenderness under the ball of the foot, at the heel, or at both locations.[48] The pain of plantar fasciitis is particularly noticeable during your first steps in the morning. If not treated properly, this injury may progress to the point that weight-bearing activities are too painful to endure.

Shin Splints *Shin splints* is a general term for any pain that occurs on the front part of

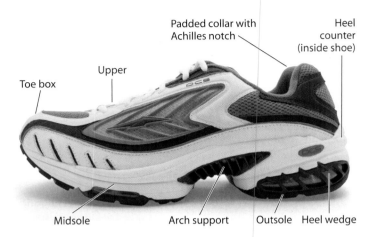

Figure 10.8 Anatomy of a Running Shoe
A good running shoe should fit comfortably; allow room for your toes to move; have a firm, but flexible, midsole; and have a firm grip on your heel to prevent slipping.

Padded collar with Achilles notch · Heel counter (inside shoe) · Upper · Toe box · Midsole · Arch support · Outsole · Heel wedge

the lower legs—the term is used to describe more than 20 different medical conditions. The most common type of shin splints occurs along the inner side of the tibia and is usually a combination of muscle irritation and irritation of the tissues attaching the muscles to the bone. Specific pain on the tibia or on the fibula (the adjacent smaller bone) should be evaluated for a possible stress fracture.

Sedentary people who start a new weight-bearing physical activity program are at the greatest risk for shin splints, although well-conditioned aerobic exercisers who rapidly increase their distance or pace may also be at risk.[49] Running and exercise classes are the most frequent cause of shin splints, but those who do a great deal of walking (such as postal carriers and restaurant workers) may also develop them.

Runner's Knee *Runner's knee* describes a series of problems involving the muscles, tendons, and ligaments of the knee. The most common cause is abnormal movements of the patella (kneecap).[50] Women are more commonly affected because their wider pelvis results in a lateral pull on the patella by the muscles that act on the knee. In women (and some men), this causes irritation to cartilage on the back of the patella and to nearby tendons and ligaments. The main symptom is pain experienced when downward pressure is applied to the kneecap after the knee is straightened fully. Additional symptoms include pain, swelling, redness, and tenderness around the patella, and a dull aching pain in the center of the knee.[51]

Applying ice to an injury such as a sprain can help relieve pain and reduce swelling, but never apply the ice directly to the skin, as that could lead to frostbite.

Treatment of Fitness-Training Related Injuries

First-aid treatment for virtually all fitness-training related injuries involves **RICE**: rest, ice, compression, and elevation. *Rest* is required to avoid further irritation of the injured body part. *Ice* is applied to relieve pain and constrict the blood vessels to reduce internal or external bleeding. To prevent frostbite, wrap the ice or cold pack in a layer of wet toweling or elastic bandage before applying to your skin. A new injury should be iced for approximately 20 minutes every hour for the first 24 to 72 hours. *Compression* of the injured body part can be accomplished with a 4- or 6-inch-wide elastic bandage; this applies indirect pressure to damaged blood vessels to help stop bleeding. Be careful, though, that the compression wrap does not interfere with normal blood flow. Throbbing or pain indicates that a compression wrap should be loosened. *Elevation* of an injured extremity above heart level also helps control internal or external bleeding by forcing the blood to flow upward to reach the injured area.

Preventing Injuries

Using common sense and identifying and using proper gear and equipment can help you avoid an injury. Varying your physical activities and setting appropriate and realistic short- and long-term goals will also help. It is important to listen to your body when working out. Warning signs include muscle stiffness and soreness, bone and joint pains, and whole-body fatigue that simply does not go away.

Appropriate Footwear Proper footwear decreases the likelihood of foot, knee, and back injuries. Biomechanics research has revealed that running is a collision sport—with each stride, a runner's foot collides with the ground with a force three to five times the runner's body weight.[52] Force not absorbed by a shoe is transmitted upward into the foot, leg, thigh, and back. Although our bodies can absorb forces such as these, they may be injured by the cumulative effect of repetitive impact. A shoes' ability to absorb shock is therefore critical—not just for runners, but for anyone engaged in weight-bearing activities.

In addition to providing shock absorption, an athletic shoe should provide a good fit for maximum comfort and performance (see **Figure 10.8**). To get the best fit, shop at a sports or fitness specialty store where there is a large selection to choose from and there are salespeople available who are trained in properly fitting athletic shoes. Because different activities place different stresses on your feet and joints, you should choose shoes specifically designed for your sport or activity. Shoes of any type should be replaced once they lose their cushioning.

Protective Equipment It is essential to use well-fitted, appropriate protective equipment for your physical activities. For some activities, that means choosing what is best for you and your body. For example, use of the "right" racquet with the "right" tension helps prevent the general inflammatory condition known as "tennis elbow." Other activities require specialized protective equipment to reduce your chances of injuries. As many as 90 percent of the eye

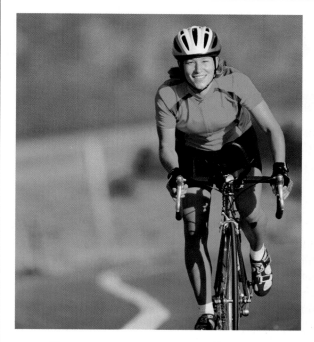

What can I do to avoid injury when I am physically active?

Reducing risk for exercise-related injuries requires common sense and some preventative measures. Wear protective gear, such as helmets, knee pads, elbow pads, eyewear, and supportive footwear, that is appropriate for your activity. Vary your activities to avoid overuse injuries. Dress for the weather, try to avoid exercising in extreme conditions, and always stay properly hydrated. Finally, respect your personal physical limitations, listen to your body, and respond effectively to it.

243

injuries resulting from racquetball and squash, for example, could be prevented by appropriate eye protection; that is, goggles with polycarbonate lenses.[53]

Wearing a helmet while bicycle riding is an important safety precaution. An estimated 45 to 88 percent of head injuries among cyclists can be prevented by wearing a helmet. Sixty-six percent of college students who rode a bike in the past 12 months reported never wearing a helmet (42%) or wearing one only rarely (24%).[54] The direct medical costs from cyclists' failure to wear helmets is an estimated $81 million a year.[55] Cyclists aren't the only ones who should be wearing helmets—so should people who skateboard, use kick-scooters, ski, in-line skate, play contact sports, and snowboard. Look for helmets that meet standards established by the American National Standards Institute or the Snell Memorial Foundation.

check yourself

- **What is the difference between traumatic injuries and overuse injuries?**
- **How can you prevent and treat fitness-related injuries?**

Exercising in the Heat and Cold

- **Describe signs and treatment of heat cramps, heat exhaustion, and heatstroke.**
- **Explain how to prevent hypothermia.**

Exercising in the Heat

Exercising in hot or humid weather increases risk of a heat-related injury, in which the body's rate of heat production can exceed its ability to cool. The three heat stress illnesses, by increasing severity, are heat cramps, heat exhaustion, and heatstroke.

Heat cramps, heat-related involuntary and forcible muscle contractions that cannot be relaxed, can usually be prevented by intake of fluid and electrolytes lost during sweating. **Heat exhaustion** is a mild form of shock, in which blood pools in the arms and legs away from the brain and major organs, caused by excessive water loss because of intense or prolonged exercise or work in a hot and/or humid environment. Symptoms include nausea, headache, fatigue, dizziness and faintness, and, paradoxically, "goose bumps" and chills. In sufferers from heat exhaustion, the skin is cool and moist. **Heatstroke**, or *sunstroke*, is a life-threatening emergency condition with a 20 to 70 percent death rate.[56] Heatstroke occurs when the body's heat production significantly exceeds its cooling capacities. Core body temperature can rise from normal (98.6°F) to 105°F to 110°F; this rapid increase can cause brain damage, permanent disability, or death. Common signs of heatstroke are dry, hot, and usually red skin; very high body temperature; and rapid heart rate. If you experience any of these symptoms, stop exercising immediately, move to the shade or a cool spot to rest, and drink plenty of cool fluids.

To prevent heat stress, follow certain precautions. If possible, acclimatize yourself to hot or humid climates through 10 to 14 days of gradually increased activity in the hot environment. Replace fluids before, during, and after exercise. Wear light, breathable clothing appropriate for the activity and environment. Use common sense—for example, when the temperature is 85°F and the humidity 80 percent, postpone a lunchtime run until evening when it is cooler.

Heat stress illnesses may also occur when the danger is not so obvious. Serious or fatal heat stroke may result from prolonged immersion in a sauna, hot tub, or steam bath or from exercising in a "sauna suit." Similarly, exercising in the heat with heavy clothing and equipment, such as a football uniform, puts one at risk.[57]

Exercising in the Cold

When you exercise in cool weather, especially in windy conditions, your body's rate of heat loss is frequently greater than its rate of heat production. This may lead to **hypothermia**—a potentially fatal condition resulting from abnormally low body core temperature. Hypothermia doesn't require frigid temperatures; it can result from prolonged, vigorous exercise in 40°F to 50°F temperatures, particularly if there is rain, snow, or strong wind.

As body core temperature drops from the normal 98.6°F to about 93.2°F, shivering begins, increasing body temperature using the heat given off by muscle activity. You may also experience cold hands and feet, poor judgment, apathy, and amnesia. Shivering ceases as core temperatures drop to between 87°F and 90°F, a sign the body has lost its ability to generate heat. Death usually occurs at body core temperatures between 75°F and 80°F.[58]

To prevent hypothermia, analyze weather conditions, including wind and humidity, before engaging in outdoor activity. Have a friend join you for cold-weather outdoor activities and wear appropriate clothing (polypropylene or woolen undergarments, a windproof outer garment, and a wool hat and gloves). Keep your head, hands, and feet warm. Do not allow yourself to become dehydrated.[59]

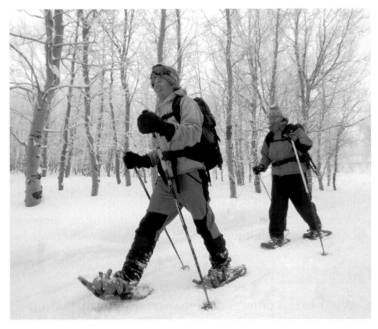

Staying with a friend and dressing in layers are two key tips for making cold weather exercise both safe and fun.

check yourself

- **What are the signs and treatment of heat cramps, heat exhaustion, and heatstroke?**
- **How can you prevent hypothermia?**

Smart Shopping for Fitness

learning **outcomes**

- **List important factors to keep in mind when choosing fitness equipment and facilities.**

Do you really need to belong to the best gym in town or have the latest equipment and fashionable clothing to meet your physical fitness goals? The short answer is no. You can achieve your personal physical fitness goals without becoming a member of a fitness or wellness center, without buying equipment, and without spending lots of money on the latest fitness fashions. All you need is a good pair of shoes, comfortable clothing to suit the environment you will be physically active in, your own body to use as resistance, and a safe place for activity. However, you may enjoy the outing or experience created by going to a fitness or wellness center or prefer to have some exercise equipment in your home. The following will help guide your selections.

Choosing Facilities

Consider the following tips for choosing an exercise facility:

- Visit several facilities before making a decision—and if possible during the time when you intend to use them (so you can see how busy or crowded they are at that time).
- Determine the hours of operation. Are they convenient for you?
- Consider the exercise classes offered. What is the schedule? Can you try one out?
- Consider the equipment. What do they have? Is it sufficient to cover your training needs (i.e., aerobic exercise machines; resistance-training equipment, including both free weights and machines; mats; and other items to assist with stretching)?
- Consider the location. How convenient is it (i.e., on your way to or from work or school, close to your home)?
- Consider the personnel (including their training in first aid and CPR), options for working with a personal trainer, and how friendly and approachable staff members are.
- Consider the financial implications. What membership benefits, student rates, or other discounts are available? Steer clear of clubs

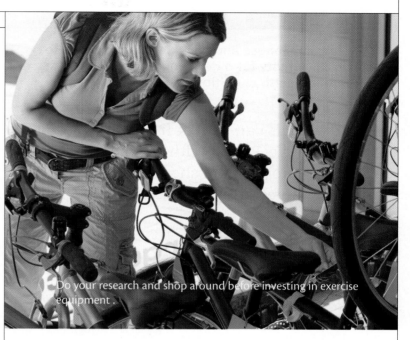

Do your research and shop around before investing in exercise equipment.

that pressure you for a long-term commitment and do not offer trial memberships or grace periods that allow you to get a refund.

Buying Equipment

Keep the following in mind when buying exercise equipment:

- Ignore claims that an exercise device provides lasting "no-sweat" results in a short time.
- Question claims that an exercise device can target or burn fat.
- Read the fine print. Advertised results may be based on more than just using a machine; they may also involve caloric restriction.
- Be skeptical of testimonials and before-and-after pictures of satisfied customers.
- Calculate the cost including shipping and handling fees, sales tax, delivery and setup charges, or long-term commitments.
- Obtain details on warranties, guarantees, and return policies.
- If you can, try the equipment at a gym or borrow it from someone.
- Consider how this piece of equipment will fit in your home. Where will you store it? Will you be able to get to it easily?
- Check out consumer reports or online resources for the best product ratings and reviews.

check yourself

- **What should you keep in mind when choosing fitness equipment and facilities?**

Activity and Exercise for Special Populations

- **Explain challenges and considerations related to physical activity for older people and those with common health conditions.**

All individuals can benefit from a physically active lifestyle. People with the considerations mentioned here should consult a physician before beginning an exercise program.

Asthma

For individuals with asthma, regular physical activity strengthens respiratory muscles, improves immune system functioning, and helps in weight maintenance.

If you have asthma, talk to your physician before you begin your exercise plan. Prior to engaging in exercise, ensure that your asthma is under control—if not, exercise could be dangerous. Ask about adjusting medications. When exercising, keep your inhaler nearby. Warm up and cool down properly; it is particularly important that you allow your lungs and breathing rate to adjust slowly. Protect yourself from asthma triggers when exercising. Finally, if you have symptoms while exercising, stop and use your inhaler; if an asthma attack persists, call 9-1-1.[60]

Obesity

Limitations such as heat intolerance, shortness of breath during physical activity, lack of flexibility, frequent musculoskeletal injuries, and difficulty with balance in weight-bearing activities need to be addressed. Programs for individuals who are obese should emphasize physical activities that can be sustained for 30 minutes or more, such as walking, swimming, or bicycling, with caution recommended in heat or humidity. Start slow (5 to 10 minutes of activity at 55% to 65% of maximal heart rate), then work up to at least 30 minutes per session. Obese individuals can improve health with cardiorespiratory and resistance training activities.[61]

Athletes like Jay Cutler, an NFL quarterback and a type 1 diabetic, are living proof that chronic conditions needn't prevent you from achieving your physical activity goals.

Coronary Heart Disease and Hypertension

Although regular physical activity reduces risk of coronary heart disease, vigorous activity acutely increases risk of sudden cardiac death and heart attack. Cardiorespiratory exercises can improve functional capacity and reduce symptoms. However, given the variation in individuals with coronary heart disease, it is not possible to provide a generic exercise prescription. Individuals must consult their physicians.[62]

Physical activity is an integral component for the prevention and treatment of hypertension. Using the FITT prescription, individuals who are hypertensive should engage in physical activity on most, if not all, days at moderate intensity for 30 minutes or more.[63]

Diabetes

Physical activity benefits individuals with diabetes by controlling blood glucose (for type 2 diabetics) by improving insulin transport into cells, controlling body weight, and reducing risk of heart disease.

Before individuals with type 1 diabetes engage in physical activity, they must learn how to manage their resting blood glucose levels. Recommendations for physical activity are then similar to those for people without diabetes; however, physical activity should be daily to more easily manage blood glucose. Individuals with type 1 diabetes should have an exercise partner; eat 1 to 3 hours before exercise; eat complex carbohydrates after exercise; avoid late-evening physical activities; and monitor blood glucose before, during, and after exercise.

The most important factor for individuals with type 2 diabetes is length of physical activity. Because a critical objective of management of type 2 diabetes is reduction of body fat (obesity), time recommendations are longer—reaching 60 minutes per session at 40 to 60 percent of maximal heart rate.

Older Adults

A physically active lifestyle increases life expectancy by limiting development and progression of chronic diseases and disabling conditions; the general recommendation for older adults is to engage in regular physical activity. For individuals with arthritis, osteoarthritis, and other musculoskeletal problems, non–weight-bearing activities, such as cycling and swimming or other water exercises, are recommended.[64]

- **What should older people and those with health conditions be aware of when choosing a program of physical exercise?**

- **Have you had to make any accommodations in your fitness program due to an existing health condition?**

Developing and Staying with a Fitness Plan

learning **outcomes**

■ **Describe how to stay with and adjust your fitness program over time.**

As your physical fitness improves, in order to continue to improve and/or maintain your level of fitness you will need to adjust your frequency, intensity, time, and type of exercise.

Begin an exercise regimen by picking an exercise and gradually increasing workout frequency. In week 1, you may exercise 3 days, moving to 4 days in week 3 or 4, and so on. Once you are working out 5 or more days per week and that seems comfortable, then increase the length of each workout by 10 percent.[65] For example, for your cardiorespiratory training, if you are accustomed to walking for 20 minutes, then you would add 2 minutes to your time (20 min × 0.10 = 2 min) so you walk for a total of 22 minutes. Continue adding 10 percent until you reach the recommended amount of 30 minutes.

If you have been physically inactive for the past few months or longer, the frequency, intensity, and time of your exercise sessions should begin at the lower end of the recommendations. This is known as *preconditioning,* and it can ease individuals into a workout regime with a minimum of soreness. For example, you might start your cardiorespiratory exercises with a target heart rate between 40 and 50 percent of maximum. You might focus your resistance-training program first on muscular endurance training or training with little or no resistance with an emphasis on developing proper technique and proper body alignment. And, you should start at the lower range of time. Once you have adjusted to these changes and are working out 5 days per week, then increase the intensity of your workout. Do so gradually, using a 10-percent increase as your guideline. So, if you start with a target heart rate of 70 percent of your heart rate maximum (e.g., 140 beats per minute for a 20-year-old male), then increase that by 1 to 2 beats per minute (140 beats/min × 0.10 = 1.4 beats per min). Repeat as you become more fit, but don't rush—move slowly and steadily toward your goal.

Be sure to vary your type of exercise—variety is a fundamental strength training principle also relevant to cardiorespiratory fitness and flexibility training. Changes in one or more parts of your workout not only produce a higher level of physical fitness (because different muscle groups are used), but also keep you motivated and interested.

It's also important to reevaluate your overall goals and plans every month or so. Too often, people deciding to become more physically active (or make any other behavior change) work hard on getting started, then lose steam as they go on. To keep yourself motivated, review your progress, make changes when necessary, and continue to reevaluate regularly.

Skills for **Behavior Change**

PLAN IT, START IT, STICK WITH IT!

The most successful physical activity program is one that is realistic and appropriate for your skill level and needs.

■ **Start slow.** If you have been physically inactive for a while or are a first-time exerciser, any type and amount of physical activity is a step in the right direction. Keep in mind that it is an achievement to get to the fitness center or to put your sneakers on for a walk! Make sure you start slowly—in fact, 5 minutes of walking or exercise may be plenty—and let your body adapt so that your new physical activity or exercise does not cause excess pain the next day (a real reaction to using muscles you have not used much or as intensely before). Do not be discouraged; you will be able to increase your activity each week, and soon you will be on your way to meeting the physical activity recommendations and your personal physical fitness goals!

■ **Make only one lifestyle change at a time.** It is not realistic to change everything at once. Plus, success with one behavioral change will increase your belief in yourself and encourage you to make other positive changes.

■ **Set reasonable expectations for yourself and your physical fitness program.** You will not become "fit" overnight. It takes several months to really feel the benefits of your physical activity. Be patient; there will be a day soon when you will think, "Wow, I feel and look great!"

■ **Choose a specific time to exercise and stick with it.** Learning to establish priorities and keeping to a schedule are vital steps toward improved fitness. Try exercising at different times of the day to learn what schedule works best for you. Yet you should also try to be flexible—if something comes up that you cannot work around, you can find time later that day or evening to do some physical activity. Be careful of an all-or-nothing attitude.

■ **Keep a record of your progress.** Include the intensity, time, type of physical activities, and your emotions and personal achievements.

■ **Take lapses in stride.** Sometimes life gets in the way. Learn how to start again. Don't despair; your commitment to physical fitness will have ebbs and flows like most everything else in life.

check yourself

■ **What are strategies for staying with and adjusting your fitness program over time?**

Assessyourself

How Physically Fit Are You?

An interactive version of this assessment is available online. Download it from the Live It! section of www.pearsonhighered.com/donatelle.

1 Evaluating Your Muscular Strength and Endurance (the 1-Minute Curl-Up Test)

Your abdominal muscles are important for core stability and back support; this test will assess their muscular endurance.

Description/Procedure:

Lie on a mat with your arms by your sides, palms flat on the mat, elbows straight, and fingers extended. Bend your knees at a 90-degree angle. Your instructor or partner will mark your starting finger position with a piece of masking tape aligned with the tip of each middle finger. He or she will also mark with tape your ending position, 10 cm or 3 inches away from the first piece of tape, with one ending position tape for each hand.

Set a metronome to 50 beats per minute and curl up at this slow, controlled pace: one curl-up every two beats (25 curl-ups per minute). Curl your head and upper back upward, lifting your shoulder blades off the mat (your trunk should make a 30-degree angle with the mat) and reaching your arms forward along the mat to touch the ending tape. Then curl back down so that your upper back and shoulders touch the floor. During the entire curl-up, your fingers, feet, and buttocks should stay on the mat. Your partner will count the number of correct repetitions you complete. Perform as many curl-ups as you can in 1 minute without pausing, to a maximum of 25.

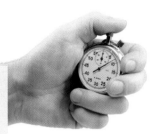

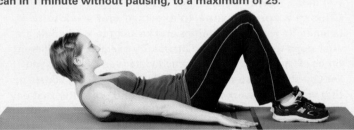

Healthy Musculoskeletal Fitness: Norms and Health Benefit Zones: Curl-Ups

Men	Excellent	Very Good	Good	Fair	Needs Improvement
Ages 20–29	25	21–24	16–20	11–15	≤ 10
Ages 30–39	25	18–24	15–17	11–14	≤ 10
Ages 40–49	25	18–24	13–17	6–12	≤ 5
Ages 50–59	25	17–24	11–16	8–10	≤ 7
Ages 60–69	25	16–24	11–15	6–10	≤ 5
Women	Excellent	Very Good	Good	Fair	Needs Improvement
Ages 20–29	25	18–24	14–17	5–13	≤ 4
Ages 30–39	25	19–24	10–18	6–9	≤ 5
Ages 40–49	25	19–24	11–18	4–10	≤ 3
Ages 50–59	25	19–24	10–18	6–9	≤ 5
Ages 60–69	25	17–24	8–16	3–7	≤ 2

Source: Adapted from *Canadian Physical Activity, Fitness & Lifestyle Approach: CSEP-Health & Fitness Program's Appraisal and Counselling Strategy*, 3rd edition, © 2003. Reprinted with permission from the Canadian Society for Exercise Physiology.

2 Evaluating Your Flexibility (the Sit-and-Reach Test)

This test measures the general flexibility of your lower back, hips, and hamstring muscles.

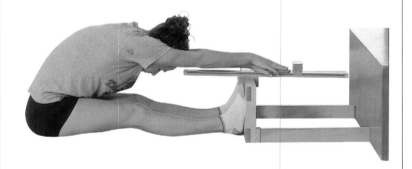

Description/Procedure:

Warm up with some light activity that involves the total body and range-of-motion exercises and stretches for the lower back and hamstrings. For the test, start by sitting upright, straight-legged on a mat with your shoes removed and soles of the feet flat against the flexometer (sit-and-reach box) at the 26-cm mark. Inner edges of the soles are placed within 2 cm of the measuring scale.

Have a partner on hand to record your measurements. Stretch your arms out in front of you and, keeping the hands parallel to each other, slowly reach forward with both hands as far as possible, holding the position for approximately 2 seconds. Your fingertips should be in contact with the measuring portion (meter stick) of the sit-and-reach box. To facilitate a longer reach, exhale and drop your head between your arms while reaching forward. Keep your knees extended the whole time and breathe normally.

Your score is the most distant point (in centimeters) reached with the fingertips; have your partner make note of this number for you. Perform the test twice, record your best score, and compare it with the norms presented in the tables.

Healthy Musculoskeletal Fitness: Norms and Health Benefit Zones: Sit-and-Reach Test*

Men	Excellent	Very Good	Good	Fair	Needs Improvement	Women	Excellent	Very Good	Good	Fair	Needs Improvement
Ages 20–29	≥ 40 cm	34–39 cm	30–33 cm	25–29 cm	≤ 24 cm	Ages 20–29	≥ 41 cm	37–40 cm	33–36 cm	28–32 cm	≤ 27 cm
Ages 30–39	≥ 38 cm	33–37 cm	28–32 cm	23–27 cm	≤ 22 cm	Ages 30–39	≥ 41 cm	36–40 cm	32–35 cm	27–31 cm	≤ 26 cm
Ages 40–49	≥ 35 cm	29–34 cm	24–28 cm	18–23 cm	≤ 17 cm	Ages 40–49	≥ 38 cm	34–37 cm	30–33 cm	25–29 cm	≤ 24 cm
Ages 50–59	≥ 35 cm	28–34 cm	24–27 cm	16–23 cm	≤ 15 cm	Ages 50–59	≥ 39 cm	33–38 cm	30–32 cm	25–29 cm	≤ 24 cm
Ages 60–69	≥ 33 cm	25–32 cm	20–24 cm	15–19 cm	≤ 14 cm	Ages 60–69	≥ 35 cm	31–34 cm	27–30 cm	23–26 cm	≤ 22 cm

*Note: These norms are based on a sit-and-reach box in which the zero point is set at 26 cm. When using a box in which the zero point is set at 23 cm, subtract 3 cm from each value in this table.

Source: Adapted from *Canadian Physical Activity, Fitness & Lifestyle Approach: CSEP-Health & Fitness Program's Appraisal and Counselling Strategy*, 3rd edition, © 2003. Reprinted with permission from the Canadian Society for Exercise Physiology.

3 Evaluating Your Cardiorespiratory Fitness (the 1-Mile Run Test)

The 1-mile run test assesses your cardiorespiratory fitness level.

Description/Procedure:

The objective of this test is to walk 1 mile as quickly as possible. This walk can be completed on an oval track or any properly measured course using a stopwatch to measure the time used. Do not eat a heavy meal for at least 2 to 3 hours prior to the test. Be sure to warm-up for 5 to 10 minutes before the test. It is best to pace yourself on this test and choose a pace/speed you think you can continue for the entire test. If you become extremely fatigued during the test, slow your pace—do not overstress yourself! If you feel faint or nauseated or experience any unusual pains in your upper body, stop and notify your instructor. Upon completion of the test, cool down and record your time and fitness category from the table below.

Cardiorespiratory Fitness Categories: 1-Mile Run Test

Men	Very Poor	Poor	Average	Good	Excellent	Women	Very Poor	Poor	Average	Good	Excellent
		Fitness Category						**Fitness Category**			
Ages 13–19	>17:30	16:01–17:30	14:01–16:00	12:30–14:00	<12:30	Ages 13–19	>18:01	16:31–18:00	14:31–16:30	13:31–14:30	<13:30
Ages 20–29	>18:01	16:31–18:00	14:31–16:30	13:00–14:30	<13:00	Ages 20–29	>18:31	17:01–18:30	15:01–17:00	13:31–15:00	<13:30
Ages 30–39	>19:00	17:31–19:00	15:31–17:30	13:30–15:30	<13:30	Ages 30–39	>19:31	18:01–19:30	16:01–18:00	14:01–16:00	<14:00
Ages 40+	>21:30	18:31–21:30	16:01–18:30	14:00–16:00	<14:00	Ages 40+	>20:01	19:31–20:00	18:01–19:30	14:31–18:00	<14:30

Source: Adapted from Rockport Walking Fitness Test. Copyright © 1993 by The Rockport Company, LLC. Reprinted with permission.

Your Plan for Change

The Assess Yourself activity helped you determine your current level of physical fitness. Based on your results, you may decide to improve one or more components of your physical fitness.

Today, you can:

◯ Visit your campus fitness facility and familiarize yourself with the equipment and resources.

◯ Walk between your classes; make an extra effort to take the long way to get from building to building. Use the stairs instead of the elevator.

◯ Take a stretch break. Spend 5 to 10 minutes in between homework projects doing some stretches to release tension.

Within the next 2 weeks, you can:

◯ Shop for comfortable workout clothes and appropriate athletic footwear.

◯ Ask a friend to join you in your workout once a week. Agree on a date and time in advance so you'll both be committed to following through.

◯ Plan for a physically active outing with a friend or date; go dancing or bowling. Use active transportation (i.e., walk or cycle) to get to a movie.

By the end of the semester, you can:

◯ Establish a regular routine of engaging in physical activity or exercise at least three times a week. Mark your exercise times on your calendar and keep a log to track your progress.

◯ Take your workouts to the next level. If you are walking, perhaps try intermittent jogging or sign up for a fitness event such as a charity 5K.

Summary

- Benefits of regular physical activity include reduced risk of heart attack, some cancers, hypertension, and type 2 diabetes and improved blood profile, bone mass, weight control, immunity, mental health and stress management, and physical fitness. Regular physical activity can also increase life span.
- Planning to improve fitness involves setting goals and designing a program to achieve them. A regular comprehensive workout should include a warm-up with light stretching, strength-development exercises, aerobic activities, and a cool-down period with a heavier emphasis on stretching. The FITT principle can be used to develop a progressive program of physical fitness.
- For general health benefits, every adult should participate in moderate-intensity activities for 30 minutes at least 5 days a week. To improve cardiorespiratory fitness, engage in vigorous, continuous, and rhythmic activities 3 to 5 days per week at an exercise intensity of 70 to 90 percent of your maximum heart rate for 20 to 30 minutes.
- Three key principles for developing muscular strength and endurance are overload, specificity of training, and variation. Muscular strength is improved via resistance training exercises two to four times per week, using an intensity of greater than 60 percent of 1 RM and completing one to three sets of two to six reps. Muscular endurance is improved via resistance training exercises two to four times per week, using an intensity of less than 60 percent of 1 RM and completing two to six sets of 10 to 15 reps.
- Flexibility is improved by engaging in two to three repetitions of static stretching exercises at least 2 to 3 days a week (preferably daily), with each stretch held for 10 to 30 seconds.
- Core strength training is important for maintaining full mobility and stability and for preventing back injury. Yoga, tai chi, and Pilates develop core strength, flexibility, and endurance.
- Fitness training injuries are generally caused by overuse or trauma; the most common are plantar fasciitis, shin splints, and runner's knee. Proper footwear and equipment can help prevent injuries. Exercise in the heat or cold requires special precautions.

Pop Quiz

1. The maximum volume of oxygen consumed by the muscles during exercise defines:
   a. target heart rate.
   b. muscular strength.
   c. aerobic capacity.
   d. muscular endurance.

2. What is physical fitness?
   a. The ability to respond to routine physical demands
   b. Having enough reserves after working out to cope with a sudden challenge
   c. Both aerobic and muscular strength
   d. All of the above

3. People with type 2 diabetes:
   a. should not engage in physical activity.
   b. should concentrate on improving flexibility.
   c. should limit physical activity to 30 minutes a day or less.
   d. can improve blood glucose levels through physical activity.

4. Flexibility is the range of motion around:
   a. specific bones.
   b. a joint or series of joints.
   c. the tendons.
   d. the muscles.

5. The "talk test" measures:
   a. exercise intensity.
   b. exercise time.
   c. exercise frequency.
   d. exercise duration.

6. An example of aerobic exercise is:
   a. brisk walking.
   b. bench-pressing weights.
   c. stretching exercises.
   d. holding yoga poses.

7. Theresa wants to lower her ratio of fat to her total body weight. She wants to work on her:
   a. flexibility.
   b. muscular endurance.
   c. muscular strength.
   d. body composition.

8. Miguel is a runner able to sustain moderate-intensity, whole-body activity for an extended time. This ability relates to what component of physical fitness?
   a. Flexibility
   b. Body composition
   c. Cardiorespiratory fitness
   d. Muscular strength and endurance

9. Janice has been lifting 95 pounds while doing leg curls. To become stronger, she began lifting 105 pounds while doing leg curls. What principle of strength development does this represent?
   a. Reversibility
   b. Overload
   c. Strain increase
   d. Specificity of training

10. Overuse injuries can be prevented by:
    a. monitoring quantity and quality of workouts.
    b. engaging in only one type of aerobic training.
    c. working out daily.
    d. working out with a friend.

Answers to these questions can be found on page A-1.

Web Links

1. **ACSM Online**. The American College of Sports Medicine and all its resources. www.acsm.org
2. **American Council on Exercise**. Information on exercise and disease prevention. www.acefitness.org
3. **CDC Division of Nutrition and Physical Activity**. A great resource for current information on exercise and health. www.cdc.gov/nccdphp/dnpa

CVD, Cancer, and Diabetes

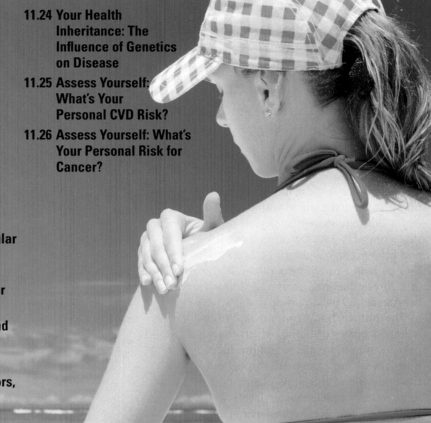

251

An overwhelming percentage of deaths in the United States are due to three major causes: cardiovascular disease, diabetes, and cancer. Over 82 million Americans—1 of every 3 adults—suffer from one or more types of **cardiovascular disease (CVD)**, diseases of the heart and blood vessels.[1] CVD has been the leading killer of U.S. adults every year since 1900, with the exception of the flu pandemic of 1918. Growing rates of obesity, hypertension, and diabetes contribute to CVD in the United States and worldwide.

An estimated 25.8 million Americans have diabetes,[2] which recently attained the dubious distinction of being the fastest growing chronic disease in American history. Though prevalence among Americans ages 20 to 44 is only 3.7 percent,[3] diabetes is increasing dramatically among younger adults,[4] children, and adolescents, largely due to obesity.[5] Approximately 231,000 people die each year of diabetes-related complications.[6]

As recently as 50 years ago, a cancer diagnosis was typically a death sentence. Today, early detection and better treatments have dramatically improved the prognosis for many people, particularly for those diagnosed early, although genetic factors continue to play an inescapable role.

Understanding the Cardiovascular System

■ **Identify the elements and functions of the cardiovascular system.**

The **cardiovascular system** is the network of organs and vessels through which blood flows as it carries oxygen and nutrients to all parts of the body. It includes the heart, arteries, arterioles (small arteries), veins, venules (small veins), and capillaries (minute blood vessels).

The Heart: A Mighty Machine

The heart is a muscular, four-chambered pump, roughly the size of your fist. It is a highly efficient, extremely flexible organ that contracts 100,000 times each day and pumps the equivalent of 2,000 gallons of blood to all areas of the body. In a 70-year lifetime, an average human heart beats 2.5 billion times.

The human body contains approximately 6 quarts of blood, which transports nutrients, oxygen, waste products, hormones, and enzymes throughout the body. Blood aids in regulating body temperature, cellular water levels, and acidity levels of body components and helps defend the body against toxins and harmful microorganisms. Adequate blood supply is essential to health.

The heart's four chambers work together to circulate blood constantly throughout the body. The two large upper chambers, **atria**, receive blood from the rest of the body; the two lower chambers, **ventricles**, pump the blood out again. Small valves regulate steady, rhythmic flow of blood and prevent leakage or backflow between chambers.

Flow of Blood through the Heart and Blood Vessels

Heart activity depends on a complex interaction of biochemical, physical, and neurological signals. To understand blood flow through the heart, follow the steps in **Figure 11.1**, from deoxygenated blood entering the heart to oxygenated blood being pumped into the blood vessels. Different types of blood vessels are required for different parts

of this process. **Arteries** carry blood away from the heart. All arteries carry oxygenated blood, *except* for the pulmonary arteries, which carry deoxygenated blood to the lungs, where the blood picks up oxygen and gives up carbon dioxide. The arteries branch off from the heart, then divide into smaller vessels called **arterioles**, then into even smaller **capillaries**. Capillaries have thin walls that permit the exchange of oxygen, carbon dioxide, nutrients, and waste products with body cells. Carbon dioxide and other waste products are transported to the lungs and kidneys through **veins** and **venules** (small veins).

Your heartbeat is governed by an electrical impulse that directs the heart muscle to move, resulting in sequential contraction of the chambers. This signal starts in a small bundle of highly specialized cells in the right atrium, called the **sinoatrial node (SA node)**, that serves as a natural pacemaker. The average adult heart at rest beats 70 to 80 times per minute.

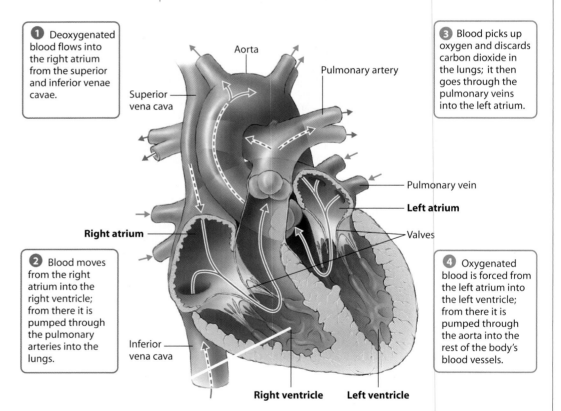

1 Deoxygenated blood flows into the right atrium from the superior and inferior venae cavae.

2 Blood moves from the right atrium into the right ventricle; from there it is pumped through the pulmonary arteries into the lungs.

3 Blood picks up oxygen and discards carbon dioxide in the lungs; it then goes through the pulmonary veins into the left atrium.

4 Oxygenated blood is forced from the left atrium into the left ventricle; from there it is pumped through the aorta into the rest of the body's blood vessels.

Aorta

Pulmonary artery

Superior vena cava

Pulmonary vein

Left atrium

Valves

Right atrium

Inferior vena cava

Right ventricle   **Left ventricle**

Figure 11.1 Blood Flow within the Heart

■ **Describe the pathway that blood follows as it circulates through the heart.**

Cardiovascular Disease: An Epidemiological Overview

learning outcomes

- **Describe patterns in the prevalence of cardiovascular disease relative to gender and ethnicity.**

Cardiovascular disease claims more lives each year than the next three leading causes of death combined (cancer, chronic lower respiratory diseases, and accidents), accounting for 33.6 percent of all deaths in the United States.[7] Consider the following:[8]

- More than 2,200 Americans die each day from CVD—an average of 1 death every 39 seconds. Many of these fatalities are **sudden cardiac deaths**, meaning an abrupt, profound loss of heart function (cardiac arrest) that causes death either instantly or shortly after symptoms occur.
- One in 2.9 women each year dies from CVD. In terms of total deaths, CVD has claimed the lives of more women than men every year since 1984. Only among people aged 20 to 39 is CVD significantly more prevalent among men than among women (**Figure 11.2**).
- African American adults have the highest rates of hypertension in the world, at 44 percent. Nearly 49 percent of African American adults have two or more CVD risks.
- Almost 10 percent of 12- to 19-year-olds already have metabolic syndrome (MetS), a major grouping of risk factors for CVD.
- Just under 26 percent of college graduates have multiple risk factors, compared to more than 52 percent among those having only a high school diploma.

Of the millions of Americans who currently live with one of the major categories of CVD, many lack health insurance and fail to receive appropriate screening and diagnostic tests. Others fail to recognize subtle symptoms until they result in a major cardiovascular event. Still others live in rural or remote areas where emergency transportation and care are not available. In spite of major improvements in medication, surgery, and other health care procedures, the prognosis for many of these individuals is not good.[9] Within 6 years of a recognized heart attack, 18 percent of men and 35 percent of women will have another, 7 percent of men and 6 percent of women will experience sudden death, and about 22 percent of men and 46 percent of women will be disabled with heart failure.

Although it is impossible to place a monetary value on human life, the economic burden of CVD on our society is huge—more than $503.2 billion estimated for 2010.[10] This figure includes the direct cost of medical services and medications, as well as indirect costs of lost productivity. Although economic concerns are huge, the effects of CVD on patients, their families, their communities, the health care system, and society may be even greater. And

CVD is not a uniquely American health problem; it accounts for 30 percent of all deaths globally.[11]

Several types of CVD are possible, including atherosclerosis, coronary heart disease (CHD), stroke, hypertension, angina pectoris, arrhythmia, congestive heart failure (CHF), and congenital cardiovascular defects. Many of these are potentially fatal; many can cause significant physical and psychological disability.

Although death rates are relatively easy to calculate, the short- and long-term psychological problems that occur after a person has a heart attack are harder to measure. Getting a grip on the fears that follow a cardiac event can be challenging. Knowing more about your specific CVD risks and what you can do about them is key to taking healthy action.

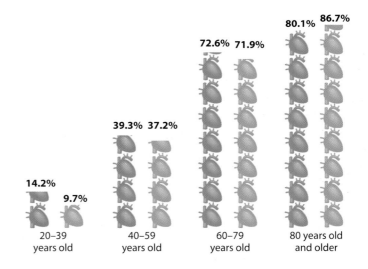

Figure 11.2 Prevalence of Cardiovascular Disease (CVD) in U.S. Adults Aged 20 and Older by Age and Sex

Source: Adapted from American Heart Association, *Heart Disease and Stroke Statistics—2011 Update* (Dallas: American Heart Association, 2011).

check yourself

- **What are some patterns in cardiovascular disease relative to gender and ethnicity?**

Key Cardiovascular Diseases: Atherosclerosis

learning outcomes

- **List the major factors contributing to atherosclerosis.**

The major cardiovascular diseases include atherosclerosis, coronary heart disease, stroke, and hypertension. Each of these cardiovascular diseases causes deaths and disabilities; their causes and treatments are discussed in the following modules.

Atherosclerosis comes from the Greek words *athero* (meaning gruel or paste) and *sclerosis* (hardness). In this condition, fatty substances, cholesterol, cellular waste products, calcium, and fibrin (a clotting material in the blood) build up in the inner lining of an artery. *Hyperlipidemia* (an abnormally high blood lipid level) is a key factor in this process, and the resulting buildup is called **plaque.**

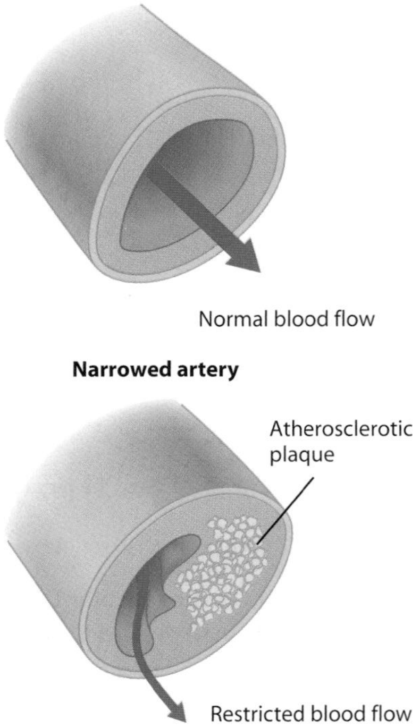

As plaque accumulates, vessel walls become narrow and may eventually block blood flow or cause vessels to rupture (**Figure 11.3**). The pressure buildup is similar to that achieved when putting your thumb over the end of a hose while water is on. Pressure builds within arteries just as pressure builds in the hose. If vessels are weakened and pressure persists, the vessels may burst or the plaque itself may break away from the walls of the vessels and obstruct blood flow. Even more importantly, fluctuation in the blood pressure levels within arteries can damage internal arterial walls, making it even more likely that plaque will stick to injured wall surfaces and accumulate.

Atherosclerosis is often called **coronary artery disease (CAD)** because of the damage to the body's main coronary arteries on the outer surface of the heart. These are the arteries that provide blood supply to the heart muscle itself. Most heart attacks result from blockage of these arteries. Atherosclerosis and other circulatory impairments also often reduce blood flow and limit the heart's blood and oxygen supply, a condition known as **ischemia**.

When atherosclerosis occurs in the lower extremities, such as in the feet, calves, or legs, or in the arms, it is called **peripheral artery disease (PAD)**. In recent years, increased attention has been drawn to PAD's role in subsequent blood clots and resultant heart attacks. In June 2008, when Tim Russert, a well-known NBC news correspondent, died suddenly of a heart attack after a long flight to Italy, there was speculation that he might have had a blood clot form in his legs from sitting for a prolonged period. This theory has not been confirmed; however, people are routinely advised to get up and walk around and flex or extend their legs to keep blood from pooling during long airplane flights or when sitting at a desk for long periods.

Whether from CAD or PAD, damage to vessels and the resulting threats to health can be severe. According to current thinking, five factors are responsible for this damage: inflammation, elevated levels of cholesterol and triglycerides in the blood, high blood pressure, heredity, and tobacco smoke. These factors are considered later in the chapter.

Normal artery

Normal blood flow

Narrowed artery

Atherosclerotic plaque

Restricted blood flow

Figure 11.3 Atherosclerosis and Coronary Artery Disease
In atherosclerosis, arteries become clogged by a buildup of plaque. When atherosclerosis occurs in coronary arteries, blood flow to the heart muscle is restricted and a heart attack may occur.

Sources: Adapted from Joan Salge Blake, *Nutrition and You*, 2nd ed. © 2012. Reprinted by permission of Pearson Education, Inc., Upper Saddle River, New Jersey.

check yourself

- **What is atherosclerosis, and what are its causes?**

Key Cardiovascular Diseases: Coronary Heart Disease

learning outcomes

- **List the major factors contributing to heart attack.**
- **Know the signs of a heart attack and how to respond to them.**

Of all the major cardiovascular diseases, **coronary heart disease (CHD)** is the greatest killer, accounting for about 1 in 6 deaths in the United States. Approximately 785,000 new heart attacks and 470,000 recurrent attacks occur each year. Another 195,000 people have silent heart attacks.[12]

A **myocardial infarction (MI),** or **heart attack**, involves an area of the heart that suffers permanent damage because its normal blood supply has been blocked. This condition is often brought on by a **coronary thrombosis** (clot) or an atherosclerotic narrowing that blocks a coronary artery (an artery supplying the heart muscle with blood). When a clot, or **thrombus,** becomes dislodged and moves through the circulatory system, it is called an **embolus.** Whenever blood does not flow readily, there is a corresponding decrease in oxygen flow to tissue below the blockage.

If the blockage is extremely minor, an otherwise healthy heart will adapt over time by enlarging existing blood vessels and growing new ones to reroute needed blood through other areas. This system, called **collateral circulation,** is a form of self-preservation that allows an affected heart muscle to cope with damage.

When a heart blockage is more severe, however, the body is unable to adapt on its own, and outside life-saving support is critical. The hour following a heart attack is the most crucial period—over 40 percent of heart attack victims die within this time.

It is important to know and recognize the symptoms of a heart attack so that help can be obtained immediately. Ignoring symptoms or delays in seeking treatment can have fatal consequences. Be sure to be familiar with heart attack symptoms and to know how to summon emergency help at home, work and school.

40%

of heart attack victims die within the first hour following a heart attack.

Skills for Behavior Change

WHAT TO DO IN THE EVENT OF A HEART ATTACK

People often miss the signs of a heart attack, or they wait too long to seek help. Knowing what to do in an emergency could save a life.

Know The Warning Signs

Symptoms of a heart attack can begin a few minutes or a few hours before the actual attack. All warning signs do not necessarily occur with every episode. The following are common heart attack symptoms:

- Discomfort (including uncomfortable pressure, squeezing, fullness, or pain) in the center of the chest lasting more than a few minutes or going away and coming back
- Pain or discomfort in one or both arms, back, neck, jaw, or stomach
- Shortness of breath, with or without chest discomfort
- Breaking out in a cold sweat
- Nausea or feelings of indigestion
- Lightheadedness or dizziness

For both men and women, the most common heart attack symptom is chest pain or discomfort. Women are more likely than men to experience some of the other common symptoms, particularly shortness of breath, nausea/vomiting, and back or jaw pain.

Be Prepared

- Keep a list of emergency rescue service numbers next to your telephone and in your pocket, wallet, or purse. Be aware of whether your local area has 9-1-1 emergency service.
- Expect the person to deny the possibility of anything as serious as a heart attack, particularly if that person is young and appears to be in good health. If you're with someone who appears to be having a heart attack, don't take no for an answer; insist on taking prompt action.
- If you are with someone who suddenly collapses, perform cardiopulmonary resuscitation (CPR). See www.heart.org for information on the new chest-compression-only techniques recommended by the American Heart Association. If you're trained and willing, use conventional CPR methods.

Sources: Adapted from American Heart Association, "Heart Attack, Stroke, and Cardiac Arrest Warning Signs," 2010, www.americanheart.org/presenter.jhtml?identifier=3053.

check yourself

- **What is a heart attack, and what are its causes?**
- **What should you do if someone shows signs of a heart attack?**

Key Cardiovascular Diseases: Stroke

- **List the major factors contributing to stroke.**
- **Know the signs of a stroke and how to respond to them.**

A **stroke** (or *cerebrovascular accident*) occurs when blood supply to the brain is interrupted, killing brain cells, which have little capacity to heal or regenerate.

Strokes may be *ischemic* (caused by plaque or a clot that reduces blood flow) or *hemorrhagic* (due to bulging or rupture of a weakened blood vessel). **Figure 11.4** illustrates blood vessel disorders that can lead to a stroke. An **aneurysm** is the most life threatening hemorrhagic stroke.

Mild strokes cause temporary dizziness, weakness, or numbness. More serious interruptions in blood flow may impair speech, memory, or motor control. Others affect heart and lung function regulation, killing within minutes. Every year an estimated 795,000 Americans suffer strokes; nearly 136,000 die as a result. Hypertension is a leading risk factor for stroke. Men have more strokes in their younger years; women more in their later years. Strokes account for 1 in 18 deaths each year.[13]

Many major strokes are preceded days, weeks, or months earlier by **transient ischemic attacks (TIAs)**, brief interruptions of the brain's blood supply that cause temporary impairment. Symptoms of TIAs include dizziness (particularly on rising), weakness, temporary paralysis or numbness in the face or other regions, temporary memory loss, blurred vision, nausea, headache, and difficulty speaking. Some people experience unexpected falls or have blackouts; others have no obvious symptoms.

The earlier a stroke is recognized and treatment started, the more effective the treatment. One of the great medical successes in recent years is the decline in the death rate from strokes, which in the United States has dropped by one-third since the 1980s.[14] Factors include improved diagnostics, better surgical options, clot-busting drugs injected soon after a stroke, acute care centers specializing in treatment and rehabilitation, and increased awareness of risk factors—especially high blood pressure, diabetes, and sodium consumption—and warning signals.

Despite improved treatments, stroke survivors do not always make a full recovery; often, problems with speech, memory, swallowing, and activities of daily living persist. Depression is also an issue for many survivors.

Skills for Behavior Change

WHAT TO DO IN THE EVENT OF A STROKE

People often misinterpret stroke warning signs, or wait too long to seek help. Warning signs include:

- Sudden numbness or weakness of the face, arm, or leg, especially on one side of the body
- Sudden loss of speech or trouble talking or understanding speech
- Sudden dimness or loss of vision in one or both eyes
- Sudden trouble walking, dizziness, or loss of balance or coordination
- Sudden, severe headache with no known cause

If you suspect someone is having a stroke, use the 60-second test. Ask the person to:

1. Smile.
2. Raise both arms.
3. Repeat a simple sentence, such as "It is sunny out today."

If the person has one or more signs above or has difficulty performing any of the three tasks, don't delay! Immediately call 9-1-1, and note the time the first symptoms appeared. If given within 3 hours of the start of symptoms, a clot-busting drug called *tissue plasminogen activator* (*tPA*) can reduce long-term disability from ischemic strokes.

Source: Adapted from American Heart Association, "Heart Attack, Stroke, and Cardiac Arrest Warning Signs," 2010, www.americanheart.org/presenter.jhtml?identifier=3053.

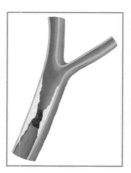

a A **thrombus** is a blood clot that forms inside a blood vessel and blocks the flow of blood at its origin.

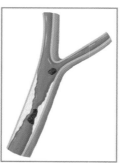

b An **embolus** is a blood clot that breaks off from its point of formation and travels in the bloodstream until it lodges in a narrowed vessel and blocks blood flow.

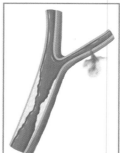

c A **hemorrhage** occurs when a blood vessel bursts allowing blood to flow into the surrounding tissue or between tissues.

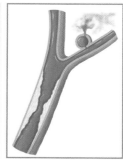

d An **aneurysm** is the bulging of a weakened blood vessel wall.

Figure 11.4 Blood Vessel Disorders That Can Lead to Stroke

- **What is stroke, and what are its causes?**
- **What should you do if someone shows signs of a stroke?**

Key Cardiovascular Diseases: Hypertension

learning outcomes

■ **Define hypertension and explain how it is measured.**

Hypertension refers to sustained high blood pressure. In general, the higher your blood pressure, the greater your risk for CVD. Hypertension is known as the silent killer—it often has few overt symptoms, and people often don't know they have it.

The prevalence of hypertension has increased by over 30 percent in the past 10 years; today 1 in 3 U.S. adults has blood pressure above recommended levels. The prevalence of high blood pressure (HBP) in African Americans in the United States, among the highest in the world, is increasing. More than 44 percent of African American women have HBP, compared to 28 percent of white women.[15]

Blood pressure is measured in two parts and expressed as a fraction—for example, 110/80, stated as "110 over 80." Both values are measured in *millimeters of mercury* (mm Hg). The first number refers to **systolic pressure**, the pressure applied to the walls of the arteries when the heart contracts, pumping blood to the rest of the body. The second value is **diastolic pressure**, the pressure applied to the walls of the arteries during the heart's relaxation phase, when blood reenters the chambers of the heart in preparation for the next heartbeat.

Normal blood pressure varies depending on weight, age, physical condition, and for different groups of people, such as women

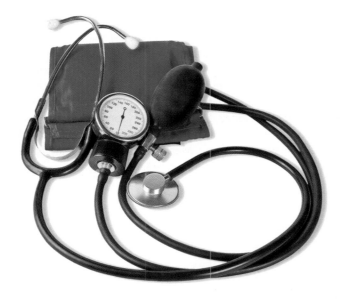

TABLE **11.1** Blood Pressure Classifications			
Classification	Systolic Reading (mm Hg)		Diastolic Reading (mm Hg)
Normal	Less than 120	and	Less than 80
Prehypertension	120–139	or	80–89
Hypertension			
Stage 1	140–159	or	90–99
Stage 2	Greater than or equal to 160	or	Greater than or equal to 100

Note: If systolic and diastolic readings fall into different categories, treatment is determined by the highest category. Readings are based on the average of two or more properly measured, seated readings on each of two or more health care provider visits.
Source: National Heart, Lung, and Blood Institute, *The Seventh Report of the Joint National Committee on Prevention, Detection, Evaluation, and Treatment of High Blood Pressure* (NIH Publication no. 03-5233), Bethesda, MD: National Institutes of Health, 2003.

and minorities. Systolic blood pressure tends to increase with age, whereas diastolic blood pressure increases until age 55 and then declines. As a rule, men have a greater risk for high blood pressure than do women until age 45, when the risks become about equal. After age 65, women are more likely than men to have high blood pressure.[16]

For the average person, 110/80 is a healthy blood pressure level. High blood pressure is usually diagnosed when systolic pressure is 140 or above. When only systolic pressure is high, the condition is known as *isolated systolic hypertension (ISH)*, the most common form of high blood pressure in older Americans. Diastolic pressure doesn't have to be high to indicate high blood pressure. See **Table 11.1** for a summary of blood pressure values and what they mean.

Treatment of hypertension can involve dietary changes (reducing sodium and calorie intake), weight loss (when appropriate), use of diuretics and other medications (when prescribed by a physician), regular exercise, treatment of sleep disorders such as sleep apnea, and the practice of relaxation techniques and effective coping and communication skills.

check yourself

■ **What is hypertension, and what are its causes and treatments?**

Other Cardiovascular Diseases

learning **outcomes**

- **Know the signs and symptoms of angina pectoris, arrhythmias, congestive heart failure, and childhood cardiovascular defects.**

Other cardiovascular diseases of concern include angina pectoris, arrhythmias, congestive heart failure, and childhood cardiovascular defects.

Angina Pectoris

People with ischemia often suffer from varying degrees of **angina** (pronounced "an-JY-nuh") **pectoris**, a condition caused by reduced oxygen flow to the heart; it often feels like pressure or squeezing in the chest or pain in the shoulders, arms, neck, jaw, or back. Over 7 million men and women suffer from this condition.[17] Although someone experiencing angina symptoms may think he or she is having a heart attack, it's not an actual attack. It can, however, provide an early warning of heart problems that should be checked out by trained medical personnel. It is important to remember that not all chest pain or discomfort is angina—an actual heart attack, lung problems (such as an infection or a clot), heartburn, or acute anxiety can trigger similar symptoms.

Mild angina cases are treated with rest. Treatments for more severe cases involve drugs that affect either supply of blood to the heart muscle or the heart's demand for oxygen. Pain and discomfort are often relieved with *nitroglycerin*, a drug used to relax (dilate) veins, reducing the amount of blood returning to the heart and so lessening its workload. Patients with angina caused by spasms of the coronary arteries are often given *calcium channel blockers*, which prevent calcium atoms from passing through the arteries and causing the contractions. *Beta blockers* control potential overactivity of the heart muscle.

Arrhythmias

Millions of Americans experience **arrhythmia**, an irregularity in heart rhythm that may result in dizziness; fainting; or heart fluttering, palpitations, or racing. Arrhythmia can be severe enough to result in death.[18] A person who complains of a racing heart in the absence of exercise or anxiety may be experiencing *tachycardia*, abnormally fast heartbeat. On the other end of the continuum is *bradycardia*, abnormally slow heartbeat. When a heart goes into **fibrillation**, it beats in a sporadic pattern that causes extreme inefficiency in moving blood through the cardiovascular system. If untreated, fibrillation may be fatal.

Not all arrhythmias are life threatening. Triggers can include excessive caffeine or nicotine consumption and panic attacks and other anxiety disorders. However, severe cases may require drug therapy or external electrical stimulus.

Congestive Heart Failure

When the heart muscle is damaged or overworked and lacks the strength to keep blood circulating normally through the body, **congestive heart failure (CHF)** can occur. CHF affects millions of Americans, particularly those over 65 with a history of heart disease or heart attack.[19] The heart may be injured by atherosclerosis, past heart attacks, high blood pressure, or congenital heart defects. The weakened heart muscle performs poorly, reducing blood flow out of the heart through the arteries. The return flow of blood through the veins begins to back up. The resulting pooling of blood enlarges the heart, makes it less efficient, and decreases the amount of blood that can be circulated. Fluid accumulates in areas such as the vessels in the legs, ankles, or lungs, causing swelling or difficulty in breathing.

CHF is a major cause of hospitalization in those with recurrent heart problems. If untreated, it can be fatal. However, most cases respond well to treatment, which includes *diuretics* (water pills) to relieve fluid accumulation; drugs such as *digitalis* that increase the heart's pumping action; and *vasodilators*, drugs that expand blood vessels and decrease resistance, making the heart's work easier.

Childhood Cardiovascular Defects

Approximately 36,000 children are born in the United States each year with some form of **congenital cardiovascular defect** (*congenital* means the problem is present at birth).[20] These may be relatively minor, such as slight *murmurs* (low-pitched sounds caused by turbulent blood flow through the heart) caused by valve irregularities, which many children outgrow. Other congenital problems are more serious and can be corrected only with surgery. Underlying causes are unknown but may be related to hereditary factors; maternal diseases, such as rubella, that occurred during fetal development; or a mother's chemical intake (particularly alcohol or methamphetamine) during pregnancy. With advances in pediatric cardiology, the prognosis for children with congenital heart defects is better than ever before.

Rheumatic heart disease can cause similar heart problems in children. It is attributed to rheumatic fever, an inflammatory disease caused by an unresolved *streptococcal infection* of the throat (strep throat). Over time, the strep infection can affect connective tissues of the heart, joints, brain, or skin. In some cases, the infection can lead to an immune response in which antibodies attack the heart as well as the bacteria. Many operations on heart valves are related to rheumatic heart disease.

check yourself

- **Name and describe several common cardiovascular diseases.**

Reducing CVD Risk: Metabolic Syndrome

learning outcomes

- **List the cluster of factors comprising metabolic syndrome.**

A large cluster of factors are related to increased risk for cardiovascular disease. Obesity, lack of physical activity, high cholesterol, and high blood pressure have all shown strong associations with subsequent CVD problems.[21]

Interestingly, though selected factors increase risks specific to CVD, the combination of these and other risk factors appears also to increase risks for insulin resistance and type 2 diabetes.[22] The term **cardiometabolic risks** refers to these combined risks, which indicate physical and biochemical changes that can lead to these major diseases. Some of these risks result from choices and behaviors, and so are modifiable, whereas others are inherited or intrinsic (such as age and gender) and cannot be modified.

Over the past decade, health professionals have attempted to establish diagnostic cutoff points for a cluster of combined cardiometabolic risks, variably labeled as *syndrome X, insulin resistance syndrome*, and, most recently, **metabolic syndrome (MetS)**. Historically, MetS is believed to increase risk for atherosclerotic heart disease by as much as three times normal rates. It has captured international attention, because an estimated 47 million people worldwide meet its criteria.[23] The more risk factors in the cluster, the greater the risk of CVD (**Figure 11.5**). Typically, for a diagnosis of MetS a person would have three or more of the following:

- Abdominal obesity (waist measurement of more than 40 inches in men or 35 inches in women)
- Elevated blood fat (triglycerides greater than 150 mg/dL)
- Low levels of high-density lipoprotein (HDL; "good" cholesterol) (less than 40 mg/dL in men and less than 50 mg/dL in women)
- Blood pressure greater than 130/85 mm Hg

- Fasting glucose greater than 100 mg/dL (a sign of insulin resistance or glucose intolerance)
- Levels of C-reactive proteins greater than 10 mg/L, indicating inflammation.

The use of MetS and similar terms has highlighted the relationship between the number of risks a person possesses and likelihood of developing CVD or diabetes. In this case, more appears to mean "worse." However, critics have questioned the usefulness of this risk profile, noting that data collection practices make it impossible to determine whether additional and compounded risk factors really contribute more to total risk. Research continues in this area; potential additional risks include constant low-grade inflammation in the body, a fatty liver, polycystic ovarian syndrome (a tendency to develop cysts on the ovaries), gallstones, and sleep apnea.[24] Having several characteristics of MetS can affect daily life even without CVD diagnosis.

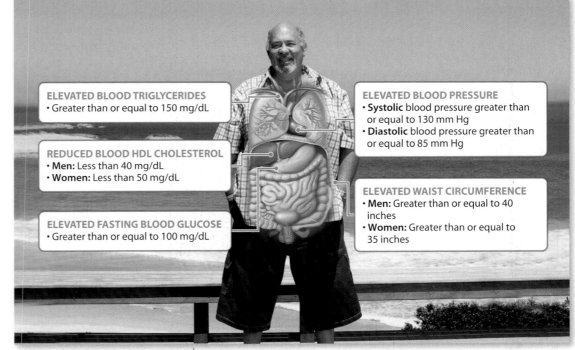

ELEVATED BLOOD TRIGLYCERIDES
• Greater than or equal to 150 mg/dL

REDUCED BLOOD HDL CHOLESTEROL
• **Men:** Less than 40 mg/dL
• **Women:** Less than 50 mg/dL

ELEVATED FASTING BLOOD GLUCOSE
• Greater than or equal to 100 mg/dL

ELEVATED BLOOD PRESSURE
• **Systolic** blood pressure greater than or equal to 130 mm Hg
• **Diastolic** blood pressure greater than or equal to 85 mm Hg

ELEVATED WAIST CIRCUMFERENCE
• **Men:** Greater than or equal to 40 inches
• **Women:** Greater than or equal to 35 inches

Figure 11.5 Risk Factors Associated with Metabolic Syndrome

check yourself

- **How does metabolic syndrome contribute to the risk of heart disease?**

Reducing CVD Risk: Modifiable Risks

■ **Describe modifiable factors affecting CVD risk.**

Although younger adults often see heart attacks and strokes as things that happen to "old" people, you may already be on course for significant risks. Hypertension, pre-diabetes, high cholesterol, and other risks have increased significantly among young people.

Hypertension affects 1 in 5 adults between the ages of 24 and 32. African Americans, Mexican American males, and white females are among the highest risk groups for obesity and hypertension, while male college students have higher rates of obesity, hypertension, and triglycerides than do female students.[25] Behaviors you choose today and in coming decades can actively affect your risk for CVD.

Avoid Tobacco Smoke

Risk of CVD is 70 percent greater for smokers than for nonsmokers. Smokers who have a heart attack are more likely to die within 1 hour. Chronic exposure to environmental tobacco smoke (ETS, or second-hand smoke) increases risk of heart disease by as much as 30 percent, with over 35,000 nonsmokers dying from ETS exposure each year.[26]

The good news is that if you stop smoking, your heart can mend itself. After 1 year, the former smoker's risk of heart disease drops by 50 percent. After 15 years, the risk drops to approximately equal that of nonsmokers. Between 5 and 15 years, the risk of stroke is similar to that of nonsmokers.[27]

Cut Back on Saturated Fat and Cholesterol

Cholesterol is a fat-like substance found in your bloodstream and cells. Your body produces about 2 grams per day, accounting for about 75 percent of blood cholesterol levels. The remaining 25 percent comes from diet. Cholesterol is carried in the blood by LDL and HDL lipoproteins (defined below); it plays a role in production of cell membranes and hormones, and helps process vitamin D. However, high levels increase CVD risk.

Diets high in saturated fat and *trans* fats are known to raise cholesterol levels and make the blood more viscous, increasing risk of heart attack, stroke, and atherosclerosis. Switching to a low-fat diet lowers the risk of clotting; even a 10 percent decrease in total cholesterol may result in a 30 percent reduction in incidence of heart disease.[28] If you have a hereditary predisposition to high cholesterol, it's even more important that you control it.

The type of cholesterol is just as important as total cholesterol. **Low-density lipoprotein (LDL)**, or "bad" cholesterol, is believed to build up on artery walls; **high-density lipoprotein (HDL)**, or "good" cholesterol, appears to remove such buildup. In theory, if LDL levels get too high or HDL levels too low, cholesterol will accumulate inside arteries and lead to cardiovascular problems.

Other blood lipid factors may also increase CVD risk. *Lipoprotein-associated phospholipase* A_2 *(Lp-PLA$_2$)* is an enzyme that circulates in the blood and attaches to LDL; it plays an important role in plaque accumulation and increased risk for stroke and coronary events, particularly in men.[29] Apolipoprotein B (apo B) is a primary component of LDL essential for cholesterol delivery to cells. Some researchers believe apo B levels may be more important to heart disease risk than total cholesterol or LDL levels.[30]

When you consume calories, the body converts any extra to **triglycerides**, which are stored in fat cells to provide energy. High counts of blood triglycerides are often found in people who are obese or overweight or who have high cholesterol levels, heart problems, or diabetes. A baseline cholesterol test (lipid panel or lipid profile) measures triglyceride, HDL, LDL, and total cholesterol; it should be taken at age 20, with follow-ups every 5 years, then annually for men over 35 and women over 45. (See **Table 11.2** for recommended levels of cholesterol and triglycerides.) The goal is to manage the ratio of HDL to total cholesterol by lowering LDL, raising HDL, or both.

Almost half of the more than 100 million Americans with high cholesterol should be able to reach their LDL and HDL goals through such diet and exercise changes. Others may also need cholesterol-lowering drugs.

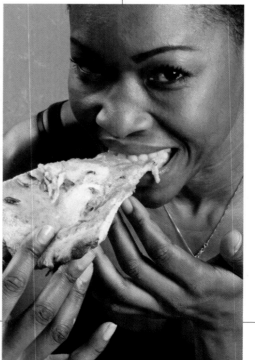

How can I improve my cholesterol level?

You get cholesterol from two primary sources: from your body (which involves genetic predisposition) and from food. The good news is that the 25% of the cholesterol you get from foods is the part where you can make real improvements in overall cholesterol profiles, even if you have a high genetic risk. Controlling your intake of saturated fats and *trans* fats will help you keep your cholesterol level in check.

Even low-intensity activity can reduce your risk of CVD. Exercise can increase HDL, lower triglycerides, and reduce coronary risks in several ways.

Modify Other Dietary Habits

Many Americans have added fish oil/omega 3, flaxseed, tea, soy, garlic, or coenzyme Q10 to their diets.[31] While dietary modifications such as these continue to be investigated, an overall approach, such as the DASH eating plan from the National Heart, Lung, and Blood Institute, has strong evidence to back up its claims of reducing CVD risk:

- Consume 5 to 10 milligrams per day of soluble fiber from sources such as oat bran, fruits, vegetables, legumes, and psyllium seeds.
- Consume about 2 grams per day of **plant sterols**,[32] which are present in many fruits, vegetables, nuts, seeds, cereals, legumes, vegetable oils, and other plant sources.
- Eat less sodium. Excess sodium has been linked to high blood pressure, which can affect CVD risk.

Maintain a Healthy Weight

Overweight people are more likely to develop heart disease and stroke even if they have no other risk factors. If you're heavy, losing even 5 to 10 pounds can make a significant difference. This is especially true if you're an "apple" (thicker around upper body and waist) rather than a "pear" (thicker around hips and thighs).

Exercise Regularly

Inactivity is a definite risk factor for CVD.[33] Even light activity—walking, gardening, housework, dancing—is beneficial if done regularly and over the long term.

Control Diabetes and Blood Pressure

People with diabetes have clear risks for a wide range of CVD problems.[34] In fact, CVD is the leading cause of death among diabetic patients. However, through diet, exercise, and medication, diabetics can control much of their increased risk for CVD.

Although blood pressure typically creeps up with age, lifestyle changes can dramatically lower CVD risk. Among the most benefi-

---

TABLE 11.2 — Recommended Cholesterol Levels for Adults

TOTAL CHOLESTEROL LEVEL (LOWER NUMBERS ARE BETTER)

Less than 200 mg/dL	Desirable level that puts you at lower risk for coronary heart disease.
200–239 mg/dL	Borderline high.
240 mg/dL and above	High blood cholesterol.

HDL CHOLESTEROL LEVEL (HIGHER NUMBERS ARE BETTER)

Less than 40 mg/dL (for men)	Low HDL cholesterol. A major risk factor for heart disease.
Less than 50 mg/dL (for women)	
60 mg/dL and above	High HDL cholesterol.

LDL CHOLESTEROL LEVEL (LOWER NUMBERS ARE BETTER)

Less than 100 mg/dL	Optimal.
100–129 mg/dL	Near or above optimal.
130–159 mg/dL	Borderline high.
160–189 mg/dL	High.
190 mg/dL and above	Very high.

TRIGLYCERIDE LEVEL (LOWER NUMBERS ARE BETTER)

Less than 150 mg/dL	Normal.
150–199 mg/dL	Borderline high.
200–499 mg/dL	High.
500 mg/dL and above	Very high.

Source: Adapted from American Heart Association, "Cholesterol Levels: AHA Recommendations," 2010, www.heart.org/HEARTORG/Conditions/Cholesterol/AboutCholesterol/What-Your-Cholesterol-Levels-Mean_UCM_305562_Article.jsp.

---

cial: losing extra pounds, cutting back on sodium, exercising more, reducing alcohol and caffeine intake, and quitting smoking.

Manage Psychological Factors and Stress Levels

High stress levels, chronic anxiety, depression, and high levels of anger or hostility can affect the cardiovascular system over time. While the exact mechanism is unknown, studies indicate that chronic stress may result in three times the risk of hypertension, CHD, and sudden cardiac death and that there is a link between anxiety, depression, and negative cardiovascular effects.[35]

check yourself

- **Of the risk factors described, which are of the most concern to you? What kind of changes could you make to improve in these areas?**

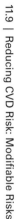

Reducing CVD Risk: Nonmodifiable Risks

■ **Identify nonmodifiable factors affecting CVD risk.**

Some risk factors for CVD cannot be prevented or controlled. Among these factors are:

■ **Ethnicity.** Though disparities in CVD death rates continue to decline, significant differences persist. In the United States, white Americans have the highest overall rate of heart disease, followed closely by African Americans. Asian American/Pacific Islanders have the highest rates of hypertension, followed by African Americans. **Figure 11.6** summarizes deaths from heart disease and stroke by ethnicity.

■ **Heredity.** Family history of heart disease appears to increase CVD risk significantly. Amount of cholesterol produced, tendencies to form plaque, and a host of other factors seem to have genetic links. Those with identified genetic risks can reduce future risks through diet, exercise, or medication.

■ **Age.** Although CVD can affect people of any age, 75 percent of heart attacks occur in people over 65. Increasing rates of obesity, diabetes, hypertension, and CVD risk factors among the young are reasons for concern.

■ **Gender.** Men are at greater risk for CVD until about 60, when women catch up and then surpass them. Women under 35 have a fairly low risk unless they have high blood pressure, kidney problems, or diabetes. Oral contraceptives and smoking also increase risk. Hormonal factors appear to reduce risk for women, though after menopause, women's LDL levels tend to rise.

Inflammation and C-Reactive Protein

Inflammation—which occurs when tissues are injured, for example by bacteria, trauma, toxins, or heat—may play a major role in atherosclerosis development,[36] because injured vessel walls are more prone to plaque formation. Cigarette smoke, high blood pressure, high LDL cholesterol, diabetes mellitus, certain forms of arthritis, and exposure to toxins have been linked to increased risk of inflammation. However, the greatest risk appears to be from infectious disease pathogens, most notably *Chlamydia pneumoniae* (a common cause of respiratory infections); *Helicobacter pylori* (a bacterium that causes ulcers); herpes simplex virus (which most of us have been exposed to); and *cytomegalovirus* (another herpes virus infecting most Americans before age 40).

During an inflammatory reaction, C-reactive proteins (CRPs) tend to be present in blood at high levels. This may signal elevated risk for angina and heart attack, though evidence that inflammatory processes prevent CHD is lacking.[37] Doctors can test patients using an assay called hs-CRP; if levels are high, action could be taken to prevent progression to a heart attack or other coronary event.[38]

Homocysteine

Homocysteine, an amino acid normally present in blood, at higher levels appears to increase risk for coronary heart disease, stroke, and peripheral vascular disease. Although research in this area is in its infancy, scientists hypothesize that homocysteine works much like CRP, inflaming the arterial lining and promoting fat deposits and development of blood clots.[39]

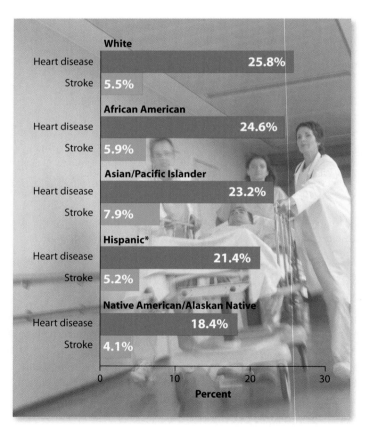

White
Heart disease — 25.8%
Stroke — 5.5%

African American
Heart disease — 24.6%
Stroke — 5.9%

Asian/Pacific Islander
Heart disease — 23.2%
Stroke — 7.9%

Hispanic*
Heart disease — 21.4%
Stroke — 5.2%

Native American/Alaskan Native
Heart disease — 18.4%
Stroke — 4.1%

Percent — 0   10   20   30

Figure 11.6 Deaths from Heart Disease and Stroke in the United States by Ethnicity

*Persons of Hispanic origin may be of any race.

Source: Data are from J. Xu, "Deaths: Leading Causes for 2007," *National Vital Statistics Reports* 58, no. 19 (2011): 1–100.

■ **Of the risk factors described, which is of the most concern to you and why?**

Diagnosing and Treating CVD

- **Describe techniques for diagnosing and treating CVD.**

CVD Diagnostic Techniques

An **electrocardiogram (ECG)** is a record of the heart's electrical activity. Patients may undergo a *stress test*—exercise on a stationary bike or treadmill with an electrocardiogram—or a *nuclear stress test*, which involves injecting a radioactive dye and taking images of the heart to reveal blood flow problems. In **angiography** (*cardiac catheterization*), a thin tube called a *catheter* is threaded through heart arteries, dye injected, and an X ray taken to identify blocked areas. A **positron emission tomography (PET) scan** produces three-dimensional images of the heart as blood flows through it. During a PET scan, a patient receives an intravenous injection of a radioactive tracer, which is tracked to produce images of the heart. Newer *single-photon emission computed tomography* (*SPECT*) scans provide an even better view. *Radionuclide imaging* involves injecting small nuclear isotopes or radionuclides into the bloodstream to aid in imaging. In *magnetic resonance imaging (MRI)*, powerful magnets look inside the body to help identify damage, congenital defects, and disease. *Ultrafast computed tomography (CT)*, an especially fast heart X ray, is used to evaluate bypass grafts, diagnose ventricular function, and identify irregularities. *Coronary calcium score* is derived from another type of ultrafast CT used to diagnose calcium levels in heart vessels; high levels increase risk. *Digital subtraction angiography (DSA)* is a modified form of computer-aided imaging that records pictures of the heart and blood vessels.

Surgical Options and Drug Therapies

Coronary bypass surgery has helped many patients survive coronary blockages or heart attacks. In a coronary artery bypass graft (CABG, referred to as a "cabbage"), a blood vessel is taken from another site in the patient's body (usually the saphenous vein in the leg or the internal thoracic artery [ITA] in the chest) and implanted to "bypass" blocked coronary arteries and transport blood to heart tissue.

With an **angioplasty** (sometimes called a *balloon angioplasty*), a catheter is threaded through blocked heart arteries. The catheter has a balloon at the tip, which is inflated to flatten fatty deposits against arterial walls, allowing blood to flow more freely. New forms of laser angioplasty and *atherectomy*, a procedure that removes plaque, are done in several clinics.

Many people with heart blockage undergo angioplasty and receive a **stent**, a steel mesh tube inserted to prop open the artery. Although stents are highly effective, in 30 to 60 percent of recipients gradual buildup around the stent can be great enough to cause the blockage to return.[40] Newer stents are usually medicated to reduce this risk.

Drugs that offer hope for prevention of, and reduction of harm from, heart attack include aspirin, which has been touted for its blood-thinning qualities.[41] Clot-busting therapy with **thrombolysis** can be performed within the first 1 to 3 hours after an attack. Thrombolysis involves injecting an agent such as *tissue plasminogen activator (tPA)* to dissolve the clot and restore some blood flow, thereby reducing the amount of tissue that dies from ischemia.[42]

Cardiac Rehabilitation and Recovery

Every year, more than 1 million Americans survive heart attacks. Over 7 million more have unstable angina, approximately 1.18 million have angioplasty, 640,000 have bypass procedures, 1.2 million have diagnostic angiograms, 111,000 receive implantable defibrillators, and nearly 358,000 have pacemakers implanted.[43] Strategies for rehabilitation may include exercise training and classes on nutrition and CVD risk management. Not all patients choose to participate, due to lack of insurance, fear of another attack due to exercise, or other barriers. However, the benefits of rehabilitation far outweigh the risks.

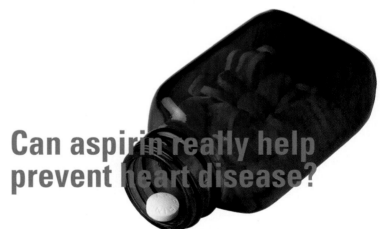

Can aspirin really help prevent heart disease?

In 2007, the American Heart Association recommended regular aspirin intake for its blood-thinning qualities, and in 2009, the Agency for Healthcare Research and Quality (AHRQ) recommended that men aged 45 to 79 take low-dose aspirin for heart attack prevention and women aged 55 to 79 take it to prevent stroke risks. Concerns over aspirin's side effects have surfaced, although others argue that people with multiple risk factors may benefit more from taking low-dose aspirin than not taking it.

check yourself

- **How is CVD commonly diagnosed and treated?**

What Is Cancer?

learning **outcomes**

- **Define the term** *cancer,* **and know the difference between benign and malignant tumors.**

Cancer is the name given to a large group of diseases characterized by the uncontrolled growth and spread of abnormal cells. When something interrupts normal cell programming, uncontrolled growth and abnormal cellular development result in a **neoplasm**, a new growth of tissue serving no physiological function. This neoplasmic mass often forms a clump of cells known as a **tumor**.

Not all tumors are **malignant** (cancerous); in fact, most are **benign** (noncancerous). Benign tumors are generally harmless unless they grow to obstruct or crowd out normal tissues. A benign tumor of the brain, for instance, may become life threatening if it grows enough to restrict blood flow and cause a stroke. The only way to determine whether a tumor is malignant is through **biopsy**, or microscopic examination of cell development.

Benign tumors generally consist of ordinary-looking cells enclosed in a fibrous shell or capsule that prevents their spreading to other body areas. In contrast, malignant tumors are usually not enclosed in a protective capsule and can therefore spread to other organs (**Figure 11.7**). This process, known as **metastasis**, makes some forms of cancer particularly aggressive in their ability to overwhelm bodily defenses. Malignant tumors frequently metastasize throughout the body, making treatment extremely difficult. Unlike benign tumors, which merely expand to take over a given space, malignant cells invade surrounding tissue, emitting clawlike protrusions that disturb the RNA and DNA within normal cells. Disrupting these substances, which control cellular metabolism and reproduction, produces **mutant cells** that differ in form, quality, and function from normal cells.

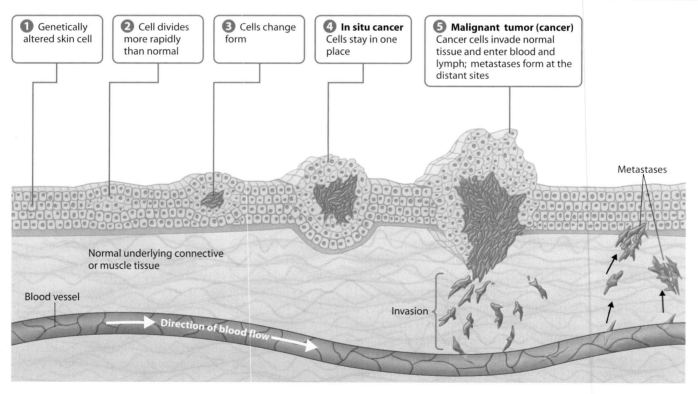

1 Genetically altered skin cell

2 Cell divides more rapidly than normal

3 Cells change form

4 In situ cancer Cells stay in one place

5 **Malignant tumor (cancer)** Cancer cells invade normal tissue and enter blood and lymph; metastases form at the distant sites

Metastases

Normal underlying connective or muscle tissue

Blood vessel

Direction of blood flow

Invasion

Figure 11.7 Metastasis
A mutation to the genetic material of a skin cell triggers abnormal cell division and changes cell formation, resulting in a cancerous tumor. If the tumor remains localized, it is considered in situ cancer. If the tumor spreads, it is considered a malignant cancer.

check yourself

- **What is cancer?**
- **What is the difference between benign and malignant tumors?**

Types and Sites of Cancer

learning outcomes

- **List the major types of cancer.**
- **List the most common sites of cancer.**

The word *cancer* refers not to a single disease, but to hundreds of different diseases. They are grouped into four broad categories based on the type of tissue from which the cancer arises:

- **Carcinomas.** Epithelial tissues (tissues covering body surfaces and lining most body cavities) are the most common sites for cancers; cancers occurring in epithelial tissue are called *carcinomas*. These cancers affect the outer layer of the skin and mouth as well as the mucous membranes. They metastasize initially through the circulatory or lymphatic system and form solid tumors.

- **Sarcomas.** Sarcomas occur in the mesodermal, or middle, layers of tissue—for example, in bones, muscles, and general connective tissue. In the early stages of disease, they metastasize primarily via the blood. These cancers are less common but generally more virulent than carcinomas. They also form solid tumors.

- **Lymphomas.** Lymphomas develop in the lymphatic system—the infection-fighting regions of the body—and metastasize through the lymphatic system. Hodgkin's disease is an example. Lymphomas also form solid tumors.

- **Leukemias.** Cancer of the blood-forming parts of the body, particularly the bone marrow and spleen, is called leukemia. A nonsolid tumor, leukemia is characterized by an abnormal increase in the number of white blood cells that the body produces.

Figure 11.8 shows the most common sites of cancer and the estimated number of new cases and deaths from each type in 2011.

265

Estimated New Cases of Cancer*		**Estimated Deaths from Cancer***	
Male	Female	Male	Female
Prostate 240,890 (29%)	**Breast** 230,480 (30%)	**Lung & bronchus** 85,600 (28%)	**Lung & bronchus** 71,340 (26%)
Lung & bronchus 115,060 (14%)	**Lung & bronchus** 106,070 (14%)	**Prostate** 33,720 (11%)	**Breast** 39,520 (15%)
Colon & rectum 71,850 (9%)	**Colon & rectum** 69,360 (9%)	**Colon & rectum** 25,250 (8%)	**Colon & rectum** 24,130 (9%)
Urinary bladder 52,020 (6%)	**Uterine corpus** 46,470 (6%)	**Pancreas** 19,360 (6%)	**Pancreas** 18,300 (7%)
Melanoma of the skin 40,010 (5%)	**Thyroid** 36,550 (5%)	**Liver & intrahepatic bile duct** 13,260 (4%)	**Ovary** 15,460 (6%)
Kidney & renal pelvis 37,120 (5%)	**Non-Hodgkin lymphoma** 30,300 (4%)	**Leukemia** 12,740 (4%)	**Non-Hodgkin lymphoma** 9,570 (4%)
Non-Hodgkin lymphoma 36,060 (4%)	**Melanoma of the skin** 30,220 (4%)	**Esophagus** 11,910 (4%)	**Leukemia** 9,040 (3%)
Oral cavity & pharynx 27,710 (3%)	**Kidney & renal pelvis** 23,800 (3%)	**Urinary bladder** 10,670 (4%)	**Uterine corpus** 8,120 (3%)
Leukemia 25,320 (3%)	**Ovary** 21,990 (3%)	**Non-Hodgkin lymphoma** 9,750 (3%)	**Liver & intrahepatic bile duct** 6,330 (2%)
Pancreas 22,050 (3%)	**Pancreas** 21,980 (3%)	**Kidney & renal pelvis** 8,270 (3%)	**Brain & other nervous system** 5,670 (2%)
All sites 822,300 (100%)	**All sites** 774,370 (100%)	**All sites** 300,430 (100%)	**All sites** 271,520 (100%)

*Excludes basal and squamous cell skin cancers and in situ carcinoma except urinary bladder. Percentages may not total 100% due to rounding.

Figure 11.8 Leading Sites of New Cancer Cases and Deaths, 2011 Estimates
Source: Adapted from American Cancer Society, *Cancer Facts & Figures 2011*. Atlanta: American Cancer Society, Inc. Used with permission.

check yourself

- **What are the major types of cancer?**
- **What sites are the most common sites of cancer?**

Risk Factors for Cancer

learning outcomes

- **List lifestyle, genetic, environmental, and medical risk factors for cancer.**

Specific risk factors for cancer fall into two major classes: hereditary risk and acquired (environmental) risk. Hereditary factors cannot be modified, whereas environmental factors are potentially modifiable.

Lifestyle Risks for Cancer

Anyone can develop cancer; however, about 78 percent of cancers are diagnosed at age 55 and above.[44] *Lifetime risk* refers to the probability that an individual, over the course of a lifetime, will develop cancer or die from it. In the United States, men have a lifetime risk of about 1 in 2 and women 1 in 3.[45]

Relative risk is a measure of the strength of the relationship between risk factors and a particular cancer. For example, a male smoker's relative risk of getting lung cancer is about 23 times that of a male nonsmoker.[46]

Tobacco Use Of all the risk factors for cancer, smoking is among the greatest. In the United States, tobacco is responsible for nearly 1 in 5 deaths annually, accounting for at least 30 percent of all cancer deaths and 87 percent of all lung cancer deaths.[47] Smoking is associated with increased risk of at least 15 different cancers, including nasopharynx, nasal cavity, paranasal sinuses, lip, oral cavity, pharynx, larynx, lung, esophagus, pancreas, uterine, cervix, kidney, bladder, stomach, and acute myeloid leukemia. Although smoking has never been shown to directly cause lung cancer, the evidence showing a direct association between heavy cigarette consumption and increased risk for lung cancer development is strong.

Of the several lifestyle risk factors for cancer, tobacco use is perhaps the most significant and the most preventable.

Alcohol and Cancer Risk One of the earliest comparisons of results from nearly 200 studies found strong and compelling associations between alcohol and cancers of the oral cavity, pharynx, esophagus, larynx, stomach, colon, rectum, liver, breast, and ovaries.[48] However, critics argued that the studies did not accurately measure dose and that threshold levels where alcohol significantly increased risk were not established. Today, evidence linking alcohol and cancer varies considerably by sex, consumption pattern, and other variables. Moderate alcohol intake (above one drink per day) in women appears to increase risk of cancers of the oral cavity and pharynx, esophagus, larynx, breast, and overall cancer risk. The more women drink, the greater their risk of cancer.[49] In men, heavy alcohol consumption (binge drinking) appears to significantly increase risk of pancreatic cancer[50] and of esophageal, liver, colon, stomach, prostate, and lung cancers.[51]

Poor Nutrition, Physical Inactivity, and Obesity About one-third of U.S. cancer deaths may be due to lifestyle factors such as overweight or obesity, physical inactivity, and nutrition.[52] Dietary choices and physical activity are the most important modifiable determinants of cancer risk (besides not smoking). Several studies indicate a relationship between high body mass index (BMI) and death rates for cancers, particularly cancers of the kidney, pancreas, colon, and endometrium.[53] The relative risk of breast cancer in postmenopausal women is 50 percent higher for obese women than for nonobese women, whereas the relative risk of colon cancer in men is 40 percent higher for obese men than for nonobese men. Numerous other studies support the link between cancer and obesity.[54]

Stress and Psychosocial Risks People who are under chronic, severe stress or who suffer from depression or other persistent emotional problems show higher rates of cancer than their healthy counterparts. Several newer studies support the premise that stress can play a role in cancer development.[55] Sleep disturbances or an unhealthy diet may weaken the body's immune system, increasing susceptibility to cancer. Another possible contributor to cancer development is poverty and the health disparities associated with low socioeconomic status.

Genetic and Physiological Risks

Scientists believe that about 5 percent of all cancers are strongly hereditary; some people may be more predisposed to the malfunctioning of genes that ultimately cause cancer.[56]

Suspected cancer-causing genes are called **oncogenes**. Though these genes are typically dormant, certain conditions such as age; stress; and exposure to carcinogens, viruses, and radiation may activate them, causing cells to grow and reproduce uncontrollably. Scientists are uncertain whether only people who develop cancer have oncogenes or whether we all have genes that can become oncogenes under certain conditions.

Certain cancers, particularly those of the breast, stomach, colon, prostate, uterus, ovaries, and lungs, appear to run in families. Hodgkin's disease and certain leukemias show similar familial patterns. Can we attribute these patterns to genetic susceptibility or to the fact that people in the same families experience similar environmental risks? The complex interaction of hereditary predisposition, lifestyle, and environment makes it a challenge to determine a single cause. Even among those predisposed to mutations, avoiding risks may decrease chances of cancer development.

Reproductive and Hormonal Factors Increased numbers of fertile years (early menarche, late menopause), not having children or having them later in life, recent use of birth control pills or hormone replacement therapy, and opting not to breastfeed all appear to increase risks of breast cancer.[57] However, although these factors appear to play a significant role in increased risk for non-Hispanic white women, they do not appear to have as strong of an influence on Hispanic women.[58] Breast cancer is also much more common in most Western countries than in developing countries. This is partly—and perhaps largely—accounted for by diets high in calories and fat, combined with later first childbirth, bearing fewer children, shorter periods of breast-feeding, higher obesity rates, and a longer life expectancy (people in less developed nations with shorter life expectancy may not live long enough to develop cancer).[59]

Occupational and Environmental Risks

Though workplace hazards account for only a small percentage of all cancers, several substances are known to cause cancer when exposure levels are high or prolonged. Asbestos, nickel, chromate, benzene, arsenic, and vinyl chloride are **carcinogens** (cancer-causing agents), as are certain dyes and radioactive substances, coal tars, inhalants, and possibly some herbicides and pesticides.

Radiation Ionizing radiation (IR)—radiation from X rays, radon, cosmic rays, and ultraviolet radiation (primarily UVB radiation)—is the only form of radiation proven to cause human cancer. Virtually any part of the body can be affected by IR, but bone marrow and the thyroid are particularly susceptible. Radon exposure in homes can increase lung cancer risk, especially in cigarette smokers. To reduce the risk of harmful effects, diagnostic medical and dental X rays are set at the lowest dose levels possible.

Nonionizing radiation produced by radio waves, cell phones, microwaves, computer screens, televisions, electric blankets, and other products has been a topic of great concern in recent years, though research has not proven excess risk to date.[60]

Some forms of cancer have strong genetic bases; daughters of women with breast cancer have an increased risk of developing the disease.

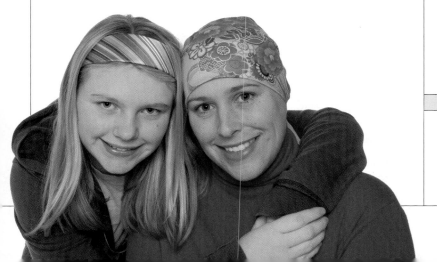

Chemicals in Foods Much of the concern about chemicals in food centers on possible harm from pesticide and herbicide residue. Continued research regarding pesticide and herbicide use is essential, and scientists and consumer groups stress the importance of a balance between chemical use and the production of high-quality food products.

Infectious Disease Risks

Infectious diseases can be triggers for cancer; over 25 percent of all malignancies in the United States are caused by viruses, bacteria, or parasites.[61] Although most of us are infected with potential cancer-causing pathogens during our lives, most never get cancer. Those who do appear to be particularly vulnerable to the genetic errors that oncogenes can trigger at the cellular level. Infections are thought to influence cancer development through chronic inflammation, suppression of the immune system, or chronic stimulation.

Chronic Hepatitis B, Hepatitis C, and Liver Cancer Viruses such as the ones that cause chronic forms of hepatitis B (HBV) and C (HCV) chronically inflame liver tissue, which may make it more hospitable for cancer development.

Human Papillomavirus and Cervical Cancer Nearly 100 percent of women with cervical cancer have evidence of human papillomavirus (HPV) infection. Fortunately, only a small percentage of HPV cases progresses to cervical cancer.[62] A vaccine is available to help protect young women from becoming infected with HPV.

Helicobacter Pylori and Stomach Cancer *Helicobacter pylori* is a bacterium found in the stomach lining of approximately 30 to 40 percent of Americans. It causes irritation, scarring, and ulcers for 20 percent of those infected; another 5 percent develop stomach cancer. *Helicobacter pylori* seems to trigger long-term inflammation, which speeds cell division, increasing chances of cancer. Antibiotic treatment often cures the ulcers, though it is not known whether it prevents cancer.[63]

Medical Factors

Some medical treatments can increase a person's risk for cancer. The use of estrogen and progesterone for relieving women's menopausal symptoms is now recognized to have contributed to multiple cancer risks. Prescriptions for estrogen therapy have declined dramatically; this is believed to have contributed to a recent large decline in breast cancer rates.[64] Some chemotherapy drugs have been shown to increase risks for other cancers; weighing the benefits versus harms of these treatments is always necessary.

check yourself

- **What are some major lifestyle, genetic, environmental, and medical risk factors for cancer?**

Lung Cancer

learning outcomes

- **Identify the major factors contributing to lung cancer.**

Over 221,000 new cases of lung cancer were expected to be diagnosed in 2011. Lung cancer, the leading cause of cancer deaths in the United States, killed an estimated 156,940 Americans in 2011.[65] Since 1987, more women have died each year from lung cancer than from breast cancer, which over the previous 40 years was the major cause of cancer deaths in women.[66]

Although lower smoking rates have boded well for cancer statistics, there is growing concern about the number of young people, particularly women and persons of low income and low educational levels, who continue to pick up the habit.

There is also concern about increase in lung cancers among *never smokers*—people who have never smoked, but nevertheless have as many as 15 percent of all lung cancers. Never smokers' lung cancer is believed to be related to exposure to secondhand smoke,

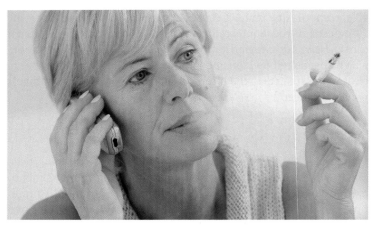

If my mom quits smoking now, will it reduce her risk of cancer, or is it too late?

It's never too late to quit. Stopping smoking at any time will reduce your risk of lung cancer, in addition to the numerous other health benefits that are gained. Studies of women have shown that within 5 years of quitting, their risk of death from lung cancer had decreased by 21 percent, when compared with people who had continued smoking.

radon gas, asbestos, indoor wood-burning stoves, and aerosolized oils caused by cooking with oil and deep fat frying.[67] This form of cancer seems resistant to traditional therapies; it may be a distinct type of lung cancer. Unfortunately, doctors often don't think

90% of all lung cancers could be avoided if people did not smoke.

of lung cancer when a never smoker presents with a cough. By the time they recognize that it's lung cancer, the prognosis is bleak.[68]

Detection, Symptoms, and Treatment

Symptoms of lung cancer include persistent cough, blood-streaked sputum, chest or back pain, and recurrent attacks of pneumonia or bronchitis. Many lung cancers are diagnosed in later stages because the imaging necessary to detect cancer is delayed due to cost. Treatment depends on type and stage of cancer. Surgery, radiation therapy, chemotherapy, and targeted biological therapies are all options.[69] If the cancer is localized, surgery is usually the treatment of choice. If it has spread, surgery is combined with radiation and chemotherapy. Unfortunately, despite advances in medical technology, survival rates 1 year after diagnosis are low, at 43 percent overall; and the 5-year survival rate for all stages combined is only 16 percent.[70] Newer tests, such as low-dose computerized tomography (CT) scans, molecular markers in sputum, and improved biopsy techniques, have helped improve diagnosis, but we still have a long way to go.

Risk Factors and Prevention

Risks for cancer increase dramatically based on the quantity of cigarettes and number of years of smoking, often referred to as *pack years*. Quitting smoking does reduce the risk of developing lung cancer.[71] People who have been exposed to industrial substances such as arsenic and asbestos or to radiation are at the highest risk for lung cancer. Exposure both to secondhand cigarette smoke and to radon gas (a gas that leaks into houses from naturally occurring uranium in the soil) is believed to play an important role in lung cancer development for smokers, past smokers, and never smokers.[72]

check yourself

- **What is lung cancer, and what are its causes?**
- **What can you do to protect yourself against lung cancer?**

Colon and Rectal Cancers

learning outcomes

- **Identify the major factors contributing to colorectal cancer.**

Colorectal cancers (cancers of the colon and rectum) continue to be the third most commonly diagnosed cancer in both men and women and the second leading cause of cancer deaths, even though death rates are declining.

If current rates of decline continue, experts predict a mortality rate reduction of 50 percent by 2020 due to earlier diagnosis and improved treatments. However, increasing incidence in those under the age of 50 has experts concerned, particularly because early diagnosis is critical and increasing numbers of people lack the health insurance that would cover necessary screening.[73] In 2010, there were over 141,210 cases of colorectal cancer diagnosed in the United States and 49,380 deaths.[74]

Detection, Symptoms, and Treatment

Because colorectal cancer tends to spread slowly, the prognosis is quite good if it is caught in the early stages. But in its early stages, colorectal cancer typically has no symptoms. As the disease progresses, bleeding from the rectum, blood in the stool, and changes in bowel habits are the major warning signals.

An excellent way to catch such cancers early is through testing. However, only 12.1 percent of all Americans over age 50 have had the most basic screening test—the at-home fecal occult blood test—in the past year, and only 43.1 percent have had an endoscopy test. Although these rates are low, it should be noted that rates are even lower among people aged 50 to 64 and especially lower among those who are non-white, have fewer years of education, lack health insurance, or are recent immigrants.[75]

Colonoscopies and other screening tests should begin at age 50 for most people. Virtual colonoscopies and fecal DNA testing are newer diagnostic techniques that have shown promise.

Treatment often consists of radiation or surgery. Chemotherapy, although not used extensively in the past, is today a possibility.

Risk Factors and Prevention

Anyone can get colorectal cancer, but people who are older than age of 50, who are obese, who have a family history of colon and rectal cancer, who have a personal or family history of polyps (benign growths) in the colon or rectum, or who have inflammatory bowel problems such as colitis run an increased risk. A history of diabetes also seems to increase risk. Other possible risk factors include diets high in fat or low in fiber, high consumption of red and processed meats, smoking, sedentary lifestyle, high alcohol consumption, and low intake of fruits and vegetables.

Regular exercise, a diet with lots of fruits and other plant foods, a healthy weight, and moderation in alcohol consumption appear to be among the most promising prevention strategies. Consumption of milk and calcium also appears to decrease risks. New research suggests that nonsteroidal anti-inflammatory drugs (NSAIDs) such as aspirin, postmenopausal hormones, folic acid, calcium supplements, selenium, and vitamin E may also help.[76]

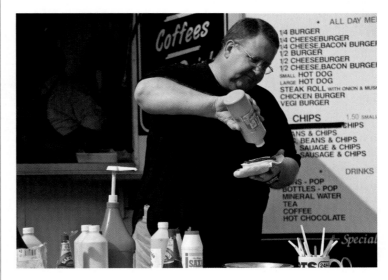

The consumption of red meat and processed meats is a risk factor for colorectal cancer, as is obesity. Food additives, particularly sodium nitrate, are used to preserve and give color to red meat and to protect against pathogens, particularly *Clostridium botulinum*, the bacterium that causes botulism. Concern about the carcinogenic properties of nitrates, which are often used in hot dogs, hams, and luncheon meats, has led to the introduction of meats that are nitrate-free or contain reduced levels of the substance.

check yourself

- **What is colorectal cancer, and what are its causes?**
- **What can you do to protect against colorectal cancer?**

Breast Cancer

- **Identify the major factors contributing to breast cancer.**

Breast cancer is a group of diseases that cause uncontrolled cell growth in breast tissue, particularly in the glands that produce milk and the ducts that connect those glands to the nipple. Cancers can also form in the connective and lymphatic tissues of the breast.

In 2010, approximately 230,480 women and 2,140 men in the United States were diagnosed with invasive breast cancer for the first time. In addition, 57,650 new cases of in situ breast cancer, a more localized cancer, were diagnosed. About 39,520 women and 450 men died, making breast cancer the second leading cause of cancer death for women.[77] The good news is that, as with many other cancers, numbers of new cases and numbers of deaths declined in 2010, each by as much as 2 percent.[78]

Detection

The earliest signs of breast cancer are usually observable on mammograms, often before lumps can be felt. However, mammograms are not foolproof, and there is debate regarding the optimal age at which women should start regularly receiving them. Hence, regular breast self-examination (BSE) is also important (see below for information on BSE). Mammograms detect between 80 and 90 percent of breast cancers in women without symptoms. A newer form of magnetic resonance imaging (MRI) appears to be even more accurate, particularly in women with genetic risks for tumors.[79]

Symptoms

Once breast cancer has grown enough that it can be felt by palpating the area, many women will seek medical care. Symptoms may include persistent breast changes, such as a lump in the breast or surrounding lymph nodes, thickening, dimpling, skin irritation, distortion, retraction or scaliness of the nipple, nipple discharge, or tenderness.

Treatment

Treatments range from lumpectomy to radical mastectomy to various combinations of radiation and chemotherapy. Among nonsurgical options, promising results have been noted among women using *selective estrogen-receptor modulators* (*SERMs*), such as tamoxifen and raloxifene, particularly among women whose cancers appear to grow in response to estrogen. These drugs, as well as new *aromatase inhibitors*, work by blocking estrogen.

The 5-year survival rate for people with localized breast cancer (which includes all people living 5 years after diagnosis, whether they are in remission, disease free, or under treatment) has risen from 63 percent in the early 1960s to 90 percent today.[80] However, these statistics vary dramatically by subgroup, based on the stage of a cancer when it is first detected and whether it has spread. If the cancer has spread to the lymph nodes or other organs, the 5-year survival rate drops as low as 23 percent.[81]

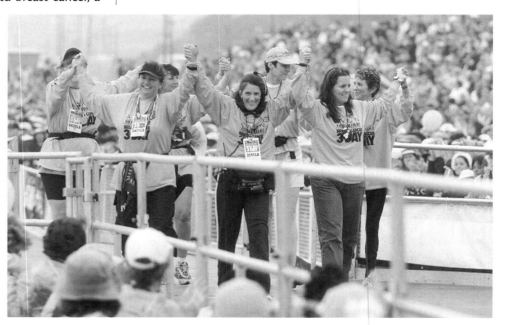

What are some of the challenges facing cancer survivors?

The journey through cancer survivorship is not always smooth. Even after the 5-year benchmark is reached, living a full, positive life in cancer's wake can be a major challenge. There may be physical, emotional, and financial issues to cope with for years after diagnosis and treatment. Survivors may find themselves struggling with access to health insurance and life insurance, financial strains, difficulties with employment, and the toll on personal relationships. Survivors also have to live with the possibility of a recurrence. However, cancer survivors can and do live active, productive lives despite these challenges.

Risk Factors and Prevention

The incidence of breast cancer increases with age. Although there are many possible risk factors, those well supported by research include family history of breast cancer, menstrual periods that started early and ended late in life, obesity after menopause, recent use of oral contraceptives or postmenopausal hormone therapy, never bearing children or bearing a first child after age 30, consuming two or more drinks of alcohol per day, and physical inactivity.[82] Note that it is only oral contraceptives that contain estrogen that are implicated in increased risk of breast cancer. The oral contraceptives that only contain progestin (the so-called minipills) have not been linked to any increase in breast cancer rates among the women who take them.

Having BRCA1 and BRCA2 gene mutations appears to account for approximately 5 to 10 percent of all cases of breast cancer; women who possess these genes have a 60 to 80 percent risk of developing breast cancer by age 70, as compared to a 7 percent risk in women without the mutations. Because these genes are rare, routine screening for them is not recommended unless there is a strong family history of breast cancer.[83]

International differences in breast cancer incidence correlate with variations in diet, especially fat intake, although a causal role for such dietary factors has not been firmly established. Sudden weight gain has also been implicated. Research also shows that regular exercise, even some forms of recreational exercise, can reduce risk.[84] In addition, preliminary studies in China indicate that higher dietary intake of soy may improve breast cancer outcomes. More research with different populations is necessary.[85]

Breast Awareness and Self-Exam

Combined with annual examinations, and with mammography as recommended, monthly breast self-exams can help women 20 and older who want to reduce their risk of a late breast cancer diagnosis (**Figure 11.9**). Women should know how their breasts normally look and feel and report any new breast changes to a health professional as soon as these changes are noted. Finding a breast change does not necessarily mean that there is a cancer.

The best time for a woman to examine her breasts is when the breasts are not tender or swollen. Women who do self-exams should have their technique reviewed during health check-ups by their health care professional. The American Cancer Society recommends the use of mammography and clinical breast exam in addition to self-examination.

To perform a breast self-exam:

- Lie down and place your right arm behind your head (1). When you are lying down, the breast tissue spreads evenly over the chest wall and is as thin as possible, making it much easier to feel all the breast tissue.
- Use the finger pads of the three middle fingers on your left hand to feel for lumps in the right breast (2). Use overlapping dime-sized circular motions of the finger pads to feel the tissue.
- Use three different levels of pressure to feel all the breast tissue. Light pressure is needed to feel the tissue closest to the skin; medium pressure to feel a little deeper; and firm pressure to feel the tissue closest to the chest and ribs. A firm ridge in the lower curve of each breast is normal. If you're not sure how hard to press, talk with your doctor or nurse. Use each pressure level to feel the breast tissue before moving on to the next spot.
- Move around the breast in an up-and-down pattern starting at an imaginary line drawn straight down your side from the underarm and moving across the breast to the middle of the chest bone (sternum or breastbone) (3). Be sure to check the entire breast area going down until you feel only ribs and up to the neck or collarbone (clavicle).
- Repeat the exam on your left breast, using the finger pads of the right hand.
- While standing in front of a mirror with your hands pressing firmly down on your hips, look at your breasts for any changes of size, shape, contour, or dimpling, or redness or scaliness of the nipple or breast skin. (The pressing down on the hips position contracts the chest wall muscles and enhances any breast changes.)
  - Examine each underarm while sitting up or standing and with your arm only slightly raised so you can easily feel in this area. Raising your arm straight up tightens the tissue in this area and makes it harder to examine.[86]

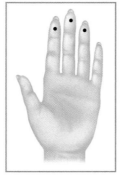 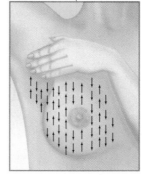

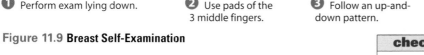

❶ Perform exam lying down.

❷ Use pads of the 3 middle fingers.

❸ Follow an up-and-down pattern.

Figure 11.9 Breast Self-Examination

check yourself

- **What is breast cancer, and what are its causes?**
- **What can you do to protect against breast cancer?**

Skin Cancer

- **Identify the major factors contributing to skin cancer.**

Skin cancer is the most common form of cancer in the United States today, affecting over 1 million people every year (1 in 5 of all adults). In 2010, an estimated 11,980 people died of skin cancer (8,790 from melanoma and 3,190 from other forms of skin cancer).[87]

The two most common types of skin cancer—basal cell and squamous cell carcinomas—are highly curable. **Malignant melanoma**, the third most common form of skin cancer, is the most dangerous, especially for women aged 25 to 29.[88] Between 65 and 90 percent of melanomas are caused by exposure to ultraviolet (UV) light or sunlight.

Detection, Symptoms, and Treatment

Potentially cancerous growths are often visible as abnormalities on the skin. Basal and squamous cell carcinomas show up most commonly on the face, ears, neck, arms, hands, and legs as warty bumps, colored spots, or scaly patches. Bleeding, itchiness, pain, or oozing are other symptoms that warrant attention. Although surgery may be necessary to remove these, they are seldom life threatening.

In striking contrast is melanoma, an invasive killer that may appear as a skin lesion. Typically, the lesion's size, shape, or color changes and it spreads to regional organs and throughout the body. Malignant melanomas account for over 75 percent of all skin cancer deaths. **Figure 11.10** shows melanoma compared to basal cell and squamous cell carcinomas. The *ABCD* rule can help you remember the warning signs of melanoma:

- **Asymmetry.** One half of the mole or lesion does not match the other half.
- **Border irregularity.** The edges are uneven, notched, or scalloped.
- **Color.** Pigmentation is not uniform. Melanomas may vary in color from tan to deeper brown, reddish black, black, or deep bluish black.
- **Diameter.** Diameter is greater than 6 millimeters (about the size of a pea).

Treatment of skin cancer depends on the type of cancer, its stage, and its location. Surgery, laser treatments, topical chemical agents, *electrodessication* (tissue destruction by heat), and *cryosurgery* (tissue destruction by freezing) are common treatments. For melanoma, treatment may involve surgical removal of the regional lymph nodes, radiation, or chemotherapy.

Risk Factors and Prevention

Anyone who overexposes himself or herself to ultraviolet (UV) radiation without adequate protection is at risk for skin cancer. The risk is greatest for people who:

- Have fair skin; blonde, red, or light brown hair; blue, green, or gray eyes
- Always burn before tanning, or burn easily and peel readily
- Don't tan easily but spend lots of time outdoors
- Use no or low-SPF (sun protection factor) sunscreens or expired suntan lotions
- Have had skin cancer or have a family history of skin cancer
- Experienced severe sunburns during childhood

Preventing skin cancer is a matter of limiting exposure to harmful UV rays. Upon exposure, the skin responds by increasing its thickness and the number of pigment cells (melanocytes), which produce the "tan" look. Ultraviolet light damages the skin's immune cells, lowering the normal immune protection of skin and priming it for cancer. Photodamage also causes wrinkling by impairing collagens that keep skin soft and pliable.

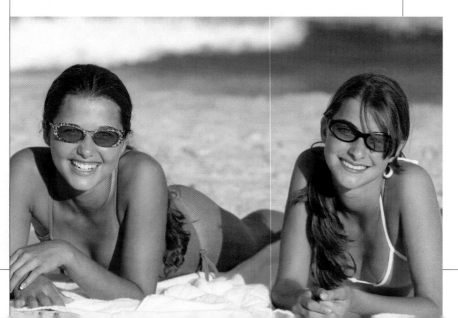

Is there any safe way to get a tan?

Unfortunately, no. There is no such thing as a "safe" tan, because a tan is visible evidence of UV-induced skin damage. The injury accumulated through years of tanning contributes to premature aging, as well as increasing your risk for disfiguring forms of skin cancer, eye problems, and possible death from melanoma. Whether the UV rays causing your tan came from the sun or from a tanning bed, the damage—and the cancer risk—is the same. Nor is an existing "base tan" protective against further damage. According to the American Cancer Society, tanned skin can provide only about the equivalent of sun protection factor (SPF) 4 sunscreen—much too weak to be considered protective.

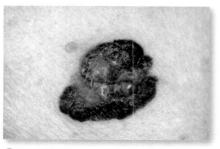 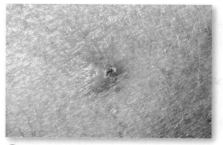 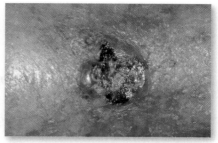

(a) Malignant melanoma (b) Basal cell carcinoma (c) Squamous cell carcinoma

Figure 11.10 Types of Skin Cancers
Preventing skin cancer includes keeping a careful watch for any new, pigmented growths and for changes to any moles. The ABCD warning signs of melanoma (a) include *asymmetrical* shapes, irregular *borders*, *color* variation, and an increase in *diameter*. Basal cell carcinoma (b) and squamous cell carcinoma (c) should be brought to your physician's attention but are not as deadly as melanoma.

Artificial Tans: Sacrificing Health for Beauty

In spite of the risks, many Americans, especially those under age 25, strive for a tan each year. Why? Recent research suggests a connection between high levels of UV light and endorphins. Those who tan in the sun or by artificial means may experience a short "high" for this reason.

Tanning is a multibillion-dollar industry that draws almost 30 million Americans into over 25,000 salons each year. The vast majority are teens or people in their twenties. In our culture, being tan is often equated with being healthy, chic, wealthy, and attractive, leading increasing numbers of men and women, but particularly adolescent girls, to seek quick tans in packaged visits to tanning beds.

Most tanning salon patrons incorrectly believe that tanning booths are safer than sitting in the sun. The truth is that there is no such thing as a safe tan from *any* source! Every time you tan, whether in the sun or in a salon, you expose your skin to harmful ultraviolet (UV) light rays. All tanning lamps emit UVA rays, and most emit UVB rays as well; both types can cause long-term skin damage and contribute to cancer. Consider the following:[89]

- Exposure to tanning beds at a young age increases melanoma risk by 75 percent.
- People who use tanning beds are 2.5 times more likely to develop squamous cell carcinoma and 1.5 times more likely to develop basal cell carcinoma.
- High-pressure sunlamps used in some salons emit doses of UV radiation that can be as much as 12 times that of the sun.
- Up to 90 percent of visible skin changes commonly blamed on aging are caused by the sun.
- Some tanning facilities don't calibrate the UV output of their tanning bulbs, which can lead to more or less exposure than is paid for.
- Patrons often try for a total-body tan. The buttocks and genitalia are particularly sensitive to UV radiation and prone to developing skin cancer.
- Tanning booths and beds pose significant hygiene risks. Don't assume that those little colored water sprayers used to "clean" the inside of the beds are sufficient to kill organisms. The busier the facility, the more likely you'll come into contact with germs that could make you ill.

Skills for Behavior Change

TIPS FOR PROTECTING YOUR SKIN IN THE SUN

- Avoid the sun or seek shade from 10 am to 4 pm, when the sun's rays are strongest. Even on a cloudy day, up to 80 percent of the sun's rays can get through.
- Apply an SPF 15 or higher sunscreen evenly to all uncovered skin before going outside. Look for a "broad-spectrum" sunscreen that protects against both UVA and UVB radiation. Check the label for the correct amount of time to allow between applying the product and going outdoors. If the label does not specify, apply the sunscreen 15 minutes before going outside.
- Check the expiration date on your sunscreen. Sunscreens lose effectiveness over time.
- Remember to apply sunscreen to your eyelids, lips, nose, ears, neck, hands, and feet. If you don't have much hair, apply sunscreen to the top of your head, too.
- Reapply sunscreen often. The label will tell you how often you need to do this. If it isn't waterproof, reapply it after swimming, or when sweating a lot.
- Wear loose-fitting, light-colored clothing. You can now purchase clothing that has SPF protection in most sporting goods stores. Wear a wide-brimmed, light-colored hat to protect your head and face.
- Use sunglasses with 99 to 100 percent UV protection to protect your eyes. Look for polarization in your shades.
- Check your skin for cancer, keeping an eye out for changes in birthmarks, moles, or sunspots.

Source: U.S. Food and Drug Administration, "Sun Safety: Save Your Skin!" Updated June 2010, www.fda.gov/ForConsumers/ConsumerUpdates/ucm049090.htm.

check yourself

- **What is skin cancer, and what are its causes?**
- **What can you do to protect against skin cancer?**

Prostate and Testicular Cancer

- **Identify the major factors contributing to prostate and testicular cancer.**

Prostate cancer and testicular cancer are two forms of the disease that all men need to be aware of.

Prostate Cancer

Cancer of the prostate is the second most frequently diagnosed cancer in American males today, after skin cancer, and is the second leading cause of cancer deaths in men after lung cancer. In 2010, about 240,890 new cases of prostate cancer were diagnosed in the United States. About 1 in 6 men will be diagnosed with prostate cancer during his lifetime, but only 1 in 36 will die of it, nearly 100 percent living with it for at least 5 years after diagnosis.[90] A man's probability of developing prostate cancer increases dramatically with age (**Table 11.3**).

Detection, Symptoms, and Treatment The prostate is a muscular, walnut-sized gland that surrounds part of a man's urethra, the tube that transports urine and sperm out of the body. A part of the reproductive system, its primary function is to produce seminal fluid. Symptoms of prostate cancer may include weak or interrupted urine flow; difficulty starting or stopping urination; feeling the urge to urinate frequently; pain on urination; blood in the urine; or pain in the low back, pelvis, or thighs. Many men have no symptoms in the early stages.

The American Cancer Society recommends that men aged 50 and over have an annual **prostate-specific antigen (PSA)** test and digital rectal prostate examination. Fortunately, prostate cancers tend to progress slowly, and 90 percent of all prostate cancers are detected while they are still in the local or regional stages. Over the past 20 years, the 5-year survival rate for all stages combined has increased from 69 percent to almost 100 percent, and the 15-year survival rate is 82 percent.[91]

Risk Factors and Prevention Chances of developing prostate cancer increase dramatically with age. Almost 2 out of every 3 prostate cancers are diagnosed in men over the age of 65.[92] Usually the disease has progressed to the point of displaying symptoms, or, more likely, men see a doctor for other problems and get a screening test or PSA test.

Race is also a risk factor in prostate cancer: African American men are 61 percent more likely to develop prostate cancer than white men and are much more likely to be diagnosed at an advanced stage. Prostate cancer is less common among Asian men and occurs at about the same rates among Hispanic men as it does among white men.[93]

Eating more fruits and vegetables, particularly those containing lycopene, a pigment found in tomatoes and other red fruits, may lower the risk of prostate cancer. Some studies have suggested that vitamin E or selenium may be beneficial, but in a major clinical trial of more than 35,000 men conducted over 5 years, neither supplement was found to lower prostate cancer risk.[94] The best advice is to follow recommendations for a balanced diet and to maintain a healthy weight.

Testicular Cancer

Testicular cancer is one of the most common types of solid tumors found in young adult men, affecting nearly 8,400 young men in 2010. Those between the ages of 15 and 35 are at greatest risk. Testicular cancer frequency over the past several years has steadily increased in this age group.[95] However, with a 96 percent 5-year survival rate, it is one of the most curable forms of cancer. Although the cause of testicular cancer is unknown, several risk factors have been identified. Men with undescended testicles appear to be at greatest risk, and some studies indicate a genetic influence.

In general, testicular tumors first appear as an enlargement of the testis or thickening in testicular tissue. Because this enlargement is often painless, it is important that young men practice regular testicular self-examination (**Figure 11.11**).

Testicular Self-Exam

Most testicular cancers can be found at an early stage. The American Cancer Society (ACS) advises men to be aware of testicular cancer and to see a doctor right away if they find a lump in a testicle. Because regular testicular self-exams have not been studied enough to show that they reduce the death rate from this cancer, the ACS does not have a recommendation on regular testicular self-exams for all men. If you have certain risk factors that increase your chance of developing testicular cancer (e.g., an undescended testicle, previous germ cell tumor in one testicle, or a family history), you should seriously consider monthly self-exam and talk about it with your doctor.

How To Examine Your Testicles

The best time to examine your testicles is during or after a shower, when the skin of the scrotum is relaxed.

- Hold the penis out of the way and examine each testicle separately.

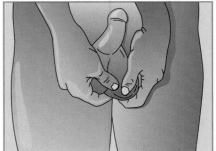

Figure 11.11 Testicular Self-Examination

TABLE 11.3 Probability of Developing Invasive Cancers during Selected Age Intervals by Sex, United States, 2005–2007*

Site	Sex	Birth to age 39	Ages 40 to 59	Lifetime
All sites[†]	Male	1 in 69	1 in 12	1 in 2
	Female	1 in 47	1 in 11	1 in 3
Breast	Female	1 in 207	1 in 27	1 in 8
Colon and rectum				
	Male	1 in 1,270	1 in 110	1 in 19
	Female	1 in 1,272	1 in 138	1 in 20
Lung and bronchus				
	Male	1 in 3,646	1 in 108	1 in 13
	Female	1 in 3,185	1 in 130	1 in 16
Melanoma of the skin[§]				
	Male	1 in 656	1 in 157	1 in 37
	Female	1 in 353	1 in 181	1 in 55
Prostate	Male	1 in 8,517	1 in 40	1 in 6
Uterine cervix	Female	1 in 656	1 in 377	1 in 147
Uterine corpus	Female	1 in 1,423	1 in 134	1 in 39

*For people free of cancer at beginning of age interval.
[†]Excludes basal and squamous cell skin cancers and in situ cancers except urinary bladder.
[§]Statistic is for whites only.
Source: DevCan Statistical Research, "Probability of Developing or Dying of Cancer," 6.5.0. Statistical Research and Applications Branch, National Cancer Institute, 2010, http://srab.cancer.gov/devcan; American Cancer Society, *Cancer Facts & Figures 2011*. Atlanta: American Cancer Society, Inc. Used with permission.

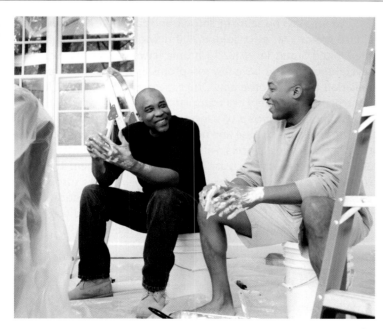

Having a father or brother with prostate cancer more than doubles a man's risk of getting prostate cancer himself. Men with a family history of prostate cancer need to be especially vigilant about their prostate health.

- Hold the testicle between your thumbs and fingers with both hands and roll it gently between the fingers.
- Look and feel for any hard lumps or nodules (smooth, rounded masses) or any change in the size, shape, or consistency of the testes.

You should be aware that each normal testis has an epididymis, which can feel like a small bump on the upper or middle outer side of the testis. Normal testicles also contain blood vessels, supporting tissues, and tubes that conduct sperm. Some men may confuse these with cancer at first. In addition, some noncancerous problems can sometimes cause swelling or lumps around a testicle. If you have any concerns, ask your doctor. Note that the ACS recommends a testicular exam as part of a routine cancer-related checkup.[96]

check yourself

- **What are prostate and testicular cancer, and what are their causes?**
- **What can you do to protect against prostate and testicular cancer?**

- **Understand screening recommendations for common cancers.**
- **Know the signs and symptoms of ovarian and uterine cancers, leukemia, and lymphoma.**

Table 11.4 shows screening recommendations for selected cancers. Other cancers are discussed below.

Ovarian Cancer

Ovarian cancer is the fifth leading cause of cancer deaths for women. In 2010, 21,990 women were diagnosed with ovarian cancer and 15,460 died from it.[97] It causes more deaths than any other cancer of the reproductive system; women tend not to discover it until the cancer is at an advanced stage. One-year survival rates are 75 percent, and 5-year survival rates are 46 percent.[98]

The most common symptom is enlargement of the abdomen. Abnormal vaginal bleeding or discharge is rarely a symptom until the disease is advanced. Other symptoms include vague digestive disturbances (stomach discomfort, gas, pressure, distention), fatigue, pain during intercourse, unexplained weight loss, unexplained changes in bowel or bladder habits, urinary frequency, and incontinence.[99]

Early-stage treatment typically includes surgery, chemotherapy, and occasionally radiation. Depending on the patient's age and desire to bear children, one or both ovaries, fallopian tubes, and the uterus may be removed. Chemotherapy and radiation are sometimes used.

Primary relatives (mother, daughter, sister) of a woman who has had ovarian cancer are at increased risk. A family or personal history of breast or colon cancer is also associated with increased risk. Women who have never been pregnant are more likely to develop ovarian cancer than those who have given birth to a child; the more children a woman has had, the less risk she faces. Use of fertility drugs may also increase a woman's risk.[100]

Using birth control pills, adhering to a low-fat diet, having multiple children, and breastfeeding can reduce risk of ovarian cancer.[101]

To protect yourself, get a complete pelvic examination annually. Women over 40 should have a cancer-related checkup every year. Uterine ultrasound or a blood test is recommended for those with risk factors or unexplained symptoms.

Cervical and Endometrial (Uterine) Cancer

Most uterine cancers develop in the body of the uterus, usually in the endometrium. The rest develop in the cervix, located at the base of the uterus. In 2010, an estimated 12,710 new cases of cervical cancer and 46,470 cases of endometrial cancer were diagnosed in the United States.[102] Overall incidence of cervical and uterine cancer has declined steadily over the past decade, perhaps due to more regular screenings of younger women using the **Pap test**, a procedure in which cells taken from the cervical region are examined for abnormal cellular activity. Pap tests are very effective for detecting early-stage cervical cancer, though less effective for detecting cancers of the uterine lining. Early warning signs of uterine cancer include bleeding outside the normal menstrual period or after menopause or persistent unusual vaginal discharge.

Risk factors for cervical cancer include early age at first intercourse, multiple sex partners, cigarette smoking, and certain sexually transmitted infections, including HPV (the cause of genital warts) and herpes. For endometrial cancer, age, estrogen, and obesity are strong risk factors. Risks are increased by treatment with tamoxifen for breast cancer, metabolic syndrome, late menopause, never bearing children, history of polyps in the uterus or ovaries, history of other cancers, and race (white women are at higher risk).[103]

Leukemia and Lymphoma

Leukemia is a cancer of the blood-forming tissues that leads to proliferation of millions of immature white blood cells. These abnormal cells crowd out normal white blood cells (which fight infection), platelets (which control hemorrhaging), and red blood cells (which carry oxygen to body cells). This results in symptoms such as fatigue, paleness, weight loss, easy bruising, repeated infections, nosebleeds, and other forms of hemorrhaging occur.

Leukemia can be acute or chronic and can strike both sexes and all age groups. An estimated 44,600 new cases were diagnosed in the United States in 2010.[104] Chronic leukemia can develop over several months and have few symptoms. It is usually treated with radiation and chemotherapy. Other methods of treatment include bone marrow and stem cell transplants.

Lymphomas, a group of cancers of the lymphatic system that include Hodgkin's disease and non-Hodgkin lymphoma, are among the fastest growing cancers, with an estimated 75,190 new cases in 2011.[105] Much of this increase has occurred in women. The cause is unknown; however, a weakened immune system is suspected—particularly one exposed to viruses such as HIV, hepatitis C, and Epstein-Barr virus (EBV). Treatment varies by type and stage; chemotherapy and radiotherapy are commonly used.

- **What are the screening recommendations for several common cancers?**
- **Have you been screened for any cancers for which you might be at risk? Why or why not?**
- **What are the signs and symptoms of ovarian and uterine cancers, leukemia, and lymphoma?**

TABLE 11.4 Screening Guidelines for the Early Detection of Cancer in Average-Risk Asymptomatic People

Cancer Site	Population	Test or Procedure	Frequency
BREAST	Women, aged 20+	Breast self-examination (BSE)	Beginning in their early 20s, women should be told about the benefits and limitations of BSE. The importance of prompt reporting of any new breast symptoms to a health professional should be emphasized. Women who choose to do BSE should receive instruction and have their technique reviewed during a periodic health examination. It is acceptable for women to choose not to do BSE or to do BSE irregularly.
		Clinical breast examination (CBE)	For women in their 20s and 30s, it is recommended that CBE be part of a periodic health examination, preferably at least every 3 years. Asymptomatic women aged 40 and over should continue to receive a CBE as part of a periodic health examination, preferably annually.
		Mammography	Begin annual mammography at age 40.*
COLON/RECTUM†	Men and women, aged 50+	*Tests that find polyps and cancer:*	
		Flexible sigmoidoscopy,‡ *or*	Every 5 years, starting at age 50
		Colonoscopy, *or*	Every 10 years, starting at age 50
		Double-contrast barium enema (DCBE),‡ *or*	Every 5 years, starting at age 50
		CT colonography (virtual colonoscopy)‡	Every 5 years, starting at age 50
		Tests that mainly find cancer:	
		Fecal occult blood test (FOBT) with at least 50% test sensitivity for cancer, or fecal immunochemical test (FIT), with at least 50% test sensitivity for cancer,‡§ *or*	Annual, starting at age 50
		Stool DNA test (sDNA)‡	Interval uncertain, starting at age 50
PROSTATE	Men, aged 50+	Prostate-specific antigen (PSA) with or without digital rectal examination (DRE)	Asymptomatic men who have at least a 10-year life expectancy should have an opportunity to make an informed decision with their health care provider about screening for prostate cancer after receiving information about the uncertainties, risks, and potential benefits associated with screening. Prostate cancer screening should not occur without an informed decision making process.
CERVIX	Women, aged 18+	Pap test	Cervical cancer screening should begin approximately 3 years after a woman begins having vaginal intercourse, but no later than 21 years of age. Screening should be done every year with conventional Pap tests or every 2 years using liquid-based Pap tests. At or after age 30, women who have had three normal test results in a row may get screened every 2 to 3 years with cervical cytology (either conventional or liquid-based Pap test) alone, or every 3 years with an HPV DNA test plus cervical cytology. Women aged 70 and older who have had three or more normal Pap tests and no abnormal Pap tests in the past 10 years and women who have had a total hysterectomy may choose to stop cervical cancer screening.
ENDOMETRIUM	Women, at menopause		At the time of menopause, women at average risk should be informed about risks and symptoms of endometrial cancer and strongly encouraged to report any unexpected bleeding or spotting to their physician.
CANCER-RELATED CHECKUP	Men and women, aged 20+		On the occasion of a periodic health examination, the cancer-related checkup should include examination for cancers of the thyroid; testicles; ovaries; lymph nodes; oral cavity; and skin; as well as health counseling about tobacco, sun exposure, diet and nutrition, risk factors, sexual practices, and environmental and occupational exposures.

*Beginning at age 40, annual CBE should be performed prior to mammography.

†Individuals with a personal or family history of colorectal cancer or adenomas, inflammatory bowel disease, or high-risk genetic syndromes should continue to follow the most recent recommendations for individuals at increased or high risk.

‡Colonoscopy should be done if test results are positive.

§For FOBT or FIT used as a screening test, the take-home multiple sample method should be used. An FOBT or FIT done during a DRE in the doctor's office is not adequate for screening.

Information should be provided to men about the benefits and limitations of testing so that an informed decision can be made with the clinician's assistance.

Source: American Cancer Society, *Cancer Facts & Figures 2011.* Atlanta: American Cancer Society, Inc. Used with permission.

Cancer Detection and Treatment

- **Describe several common cancer detection and treatment options.**

Detecting Cancer

Magnetic resonance imaging (MRI) uses a huge electromagnet to detect tumors by mapping the vibrations of atoms in the body on a computer screen. The **computerized axial tomography (CAT) scan** uses X rays to examine parts of the body. *Prostatic ultrasound* (a rectal probe using ultrasonic waves to produce an image of the prostate) is being investigated as a means to increase early detection of prostate cancer, combined with the PSA blood test.

Cancer Treatments

Treatments vary according to type and stage of cancer. Surgery to remove the tumor and surrounding tissue may be performed alone or with other treatments. The surgeon may operate using traditional surgical instruments or a laser, laparoscope, or other tools.

Radiotherapy (use of radiation) and **chemotherapy** (use of drugs) kill cancerous cells. Radiation is most effective in treating localized cancer because it can be targeted to a particular area. Side effects include fatigue, changes to skin in the affected area, and slightly greater chances of developing another type of cancer.

Chemotherapy may be used to shrink a tumor before or after surgery or radiation therapy or on its own. Powerful drugs are administered, usually in cycles so the body can recover from their effects. Side effects, which may include nausea, hair loss, fatigue, increased chance of bleeding, bruising, infection, and anemia, fade after treatment. Other effects, such as loss of fertility, may be permanent. Long-term damage to the cardiovascular and other body systems from radiotherapy and chemotherapy can be significant.

Participation in clinical trials (people-based studies of new drugs or procedures) has provided hope for many. Deciding whether to participate in a clinical trial can be difficult. Despite the risks, which should be carefully considered, thousands of clinical trial participants have benefited from treatments otherwise unavailable to them. Before beginning any form of cancer therapy, be a vigilant and vocal consumer. Read and seek information from cancer support groups. Check the skills of your surgeon, radiation therapist, and doctor in terms of clinical experience and interpersonal interactions. Look at Oncolink and other websites supported by the National Cancer Institute and the American Cancer Society (ACS) to check out clinical trials, reports on treatment effectiveness, experimental therapies, etc. And although you may like and trust your family doctor, it is always a good idea to seek consultation or advice from larger cancer facilities.

New Cancer Treatments

Surgery, chemotherapy, and radiation therapy remain the most common cancer treatments. However, newer techniques may be more effective for certain cancers or certain patients:

- **Immunotherapy.** Immunotherapy is designed to enhance the body's disease-fighting systems. Biological response modifiers such as interferon and interleukin-2 are under study.
- **Biological therapies.** *Cancer-fighting vaccines* alert the body's immune defenses to cells gone bad. Rather than preventing disease as other vaccines do, they help people who are already ill.
- **Gene therapies.** Viruses may carry genetic information that makes the cells they infect (such as cancer cells) susceptible to an antiviral drug. Scientists are also looking at ways to transfer genes that increase immune response to the cancerous tumor or that confer drug resistance to bone marrow so higher doses of chemotherapeutic drugs can be given.
- **Angiogenesis inhibitors.** Some compounds may stop tumors from forming new blood vessels, a process called *angiogenesis*. Without adequate blood supply, tumors either die or grow very slowly.
- **Disruption of cancer pathways.** Steps in the *cancer pathway* include oncogene actions, hormone receptors, growth factors, metastasis, and angiogenesis. Preliminary studies are under way to design compounds that inhibit actions at each of these steps.
- **Smart drugs.** *Targeted smart-drug therapies* attack only the cancer cells and not the entire body.
- **Enzyme inhibitors.** An enzyme inhibitor, *TIMP2*, shows promise for slowing metastasis of tumor cells. A metastasis suppressor gene, *NM23*, has also been identified.
- **Neoadjuvant chemotherapy.** This method uses chemotherapy to shrink the tumor before surgically removing it.
- **Stem cell research.** Transplants of stem cells from donor bone marrow are used when a patient's bone marrow has been destroyed by disease, chemotherapy, or radiation.

14%

of the estimated 10.8 million cancer survivors in the United States today were diagnosed more than 20 years ago.

- **What are some traditional and new treatments for cancer?**

What Is Diabetes?

- **Explain how glucose and insulin levels affect development of diabetes.**
- **Distinguish between type 1 and type 2 diabetes.**

Diabetes mellitus is a disease characterized by a persistently high level of sugar—glucose—in the blood. High blood glucose levels—or **hyperglycemia**—in diabetes can lead to serious health problems and premature death.

In a healthy person, carbohydrates from foods are broken down into a monosaccharide called *glucose*. Red blood cells use only glucose for fuel; brain and other nerve cells prefer glucose over other fuels. Excess glucose is stored as glycogen in the liver and muscles. The average adult has 5 to 6 grams of glucose in the blood at any given time, enough to provide energy for about 15 minutes of activity. Once circulating glucose is used, the body draws upon its glycogen reserves.

Whenever a surge of glucose enters the bloodstream, the **pancreas**, an organ just beneath the stomach, secretes a hormone called **insulin**, stimulating cells to take up glucose from the bloodstream and carry it into cells. Conversion of glucose to glycogen for storage in the liver and muscles is also assisted by insulin.

Type 1 diabetes (insulin-dependent diabetes) is an autoimmune disease in which the immune system attacks and destroys insulin-making cells in the pancreas, reducing or stopping insulin production. Without insulin, cells cannot take up glucose, and blood glucose levels become permanently elevated.

Type 1 diabetes used to be called *juvenile diabetes* because it most often appears during childhood or adolescence.[106] People with type 1 diabetes require daily insulin injections or infusions and must carefully monitor diet and exercise levels.

Type 2 diabetes (non-insulin-dependent diabetes) accounts for 90 percent of all diabetes cases.[107] In type 2, either the pancreas does not make sufficient insulin or the body cells become resistant to its effects and don't efficiently use available insulin (**Figure 11.12**), a condition referred to as **insulin resistance**. Unlike type 1 diabetes, which can appear suddenly, type 2 usually develops slowly.

In early stages of type 2 diabetes, cells begin to resist the effects of insulin. One contributor to insulin resistance is an overabundance of free fatty acids in fat cells (common in obese individuals). These free fatty acids inhibit cells' glucose uptake and diminish the liver's ability to self-regulate conversion of glucose into glycogen.

As blood levels of glucose gradually rise, the pancreas attempts to compensate by producing more insulin. Over time, more and more pancreatic insulin-producing cells sustain damage and become nonfunctional. As insulin output declines, blood glucose levels rise enough to warrant diagnosis of type 2 diabetes.

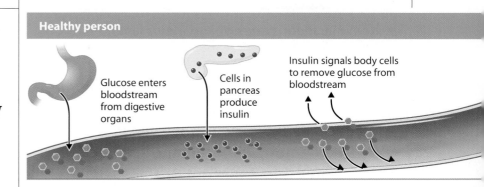

Healthy person

Glucose enters bloodstream from digestive organs

Cells in pancreas produce insulin

Insulin signals body cells to remove glucose from bloodstream

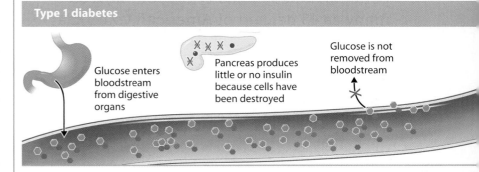

Type 1 diabetes

Glucose enters bloodstream from digestive organs

Pancreas produces little or no insulin because cells have been destroyed

Glucose is not removed from bloodstream

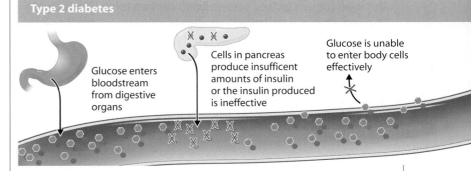

Type 2 diabetes

Glucose enters bloodstream from digestive organs

Cells in pancreas produce insufficent amounts of insulin or the insulin produced is ineffective

Glucose is unable to enter body cells effectively

Figure 11.12 Diabetes: What It Is and How It Develops
In a healthy person, a sufficient amount of insulin is produced and released by the pancreas and used efficiently by the cells. In type 1 diabetes, the pancreas makes little or no insulin. In type 2 diabetes, either the pancreas does not make sufficient insulin or cells are resistant to insulin and thus are not able to utilize it efficiently.

- **What is the role of glucose and insulin in diabetes?**
- **What is the difference between type 1 and type 2 diabetes?**

Diabetes: Risk Factors, Symptoms, and Treatment

- **Know incidence rates of and major factors affecting type 2 diabetes.**

One in five adults over age 65 has type 2 diabetes. The disease used to be referred to as *adult-onset diabetes*; now, however, it is often diagnosed among children and teens. Prior to 2000, only 1 to 2 percent of U.S. diabetes patients under 18 had type 2, but now as many as 45 percent of American youth diagnosed with diabetes have type 2.[108]

Risk Factors

Nonmodifiable risk factors include race and genetics. Among adults 20 and older, 12.6 percent of non-Hispanic blacks, 8.4 percent of Asian Americans, and 11.8 percent of those of Hispanic origin have type 2, in contrast to 7.1 percent of non-Hispanic whites.[109]

Having a close relative with type 2 diabetes is another significant risk factor. A group of "type 2 diabetes genes" has been identified.[110] But even though genetic susceptibility appears to play a role, given the fact that a population's gene pool shifts quite slowly—over centuries—the current epidemic of type 2 diabetes suggests that lifestyle factors are more to blame.

Modifiable risk factors are tied to lifestyle. In both children and adults, type 2 diabetes is linked to overweight and obesity. In adults, a body mass index (BMI) of 25 or greater increases the risk. In particular, a waistline measurement of 40 or more inches in males or 35 or more inches in females is highly correlated to development of type 2 diabetes.[111]

Sedentary lifestyle also increases risk, not only because inactivity fails to burn calories, but also because buildup of muscle tissue improves insulin uptake by cells.[112] People with type 2 diabetes who lose weight and increase physical activity can significantly improve their blood glucose levels. Inadequate sleep[113] and chronic psychological or physical stress[114] may also contribute to development of type 2 diabetes.

Pre-Diabetes

An estimated 57 million Americans 20 or older—25 percent of the adult population—have a set of symptoms known as **pre-diabetes**, a condition in which blood glucose levels are higher than normal, but not high enough to be classified as diabetes.[115] If this condition is not addressed, diabetes will eventually strike. Pre-diabetes is one of a cluster of six conditions linked to overweight and obesity that together constitute a dangerous health risk known as metabolic syndrome (MetS).[116] A person with MetS is five times more likely to develop type 2 diabetes than is a person without the syndrome.[117]

Gestational Diabetes

A third type of diabetes, **gestational diabetes**, is a state of high blood glucose during pregnancy, thought to be associated with metabolic stresses that occur in response to changing hormonal levels. Gestational diabetes occurs in 4 percent of pregnant women and often disappears after pregnancy.[118] However, between 50 and 70 percent of women with gestational diabetes may progress to type 2 diabetes if they fail to make significant lifestyle changes.[119]

Symptoms of Diabetes

Common symptoms of diabetes are similar for type 1 and type 2:

- **Thirst and excessive urination.** The kidneys filter excessive glucose from the blood, diluting it so it can be excreted in urine. This pulls too much water from the body, leading to dehydration, thirst, and excessive urination.

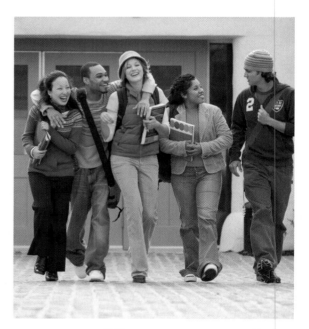

Do college students really need to be concerned about diabetes?

The rate of type 1 and type 2 diabetes among people aged 20 to 39 is 2.6%; however, more than 6% of college students in one study were found to have pre-diabetes.

- **Weight loss.** Because so many calories are lost in the glucose that passes into urine, a person with diabetes often loses weight.
- **Fatigue.** When glucose cannot enter cells, fatigue and weakness become inevitable.
- **Nerve damage.** High glucose levels damage the smallest blood vessels of the body, leading to numbness and tingling.
- **Blurred vision.** High blood glucose levels can dry out the cornea or damage microvessels in the eye.
- **Poor wound healing and increased infections.** High levels of glucose can affect ability to ward off infection and overall immune function.

Diabetes Complications

Poorly controlled diabetes can lead to a variety of complications:[120]

- **Diabetic coma.** In the absence of glucose, body cells break down stored fat for energy. This produces acidic molecules called *ketones*, excessive amounts of which dangerously elevate blood acid. The diabetic slips into a coma and, without prompt medical intervention, can die.
- **Cardiovascular disease.** More than 70 percent of diabetics have hypertension. Blood vessels become damaged as glucose-laden blood flows more sluggishly and nutrients and other substances are not transported as effectively.
- **Kidney disease.** Kidneys become scarred by their extraordinary workload and by high blood pressure in their vessels. Each year, almost 47,000 diabetics develop kidney failure.
- **Amputations.** More than 60 percent of nontraumatic amputations of legs, feet, and toes are due to diabetes. Impaired immune response combined with damaged blood vessels can enable minor infections to spread and resist treatment. Eventually, tissues die and the body part must be amputated.
- **Eye disease and blindness.** Each year, 12,000 to 24,000 people become blind because of diabetic eye disease.
- **Flu- and pneumonia-related deaths.** Each year, 10,000 to 30,000 people with diabetes die of complications from flu or pneumonia—a rate three times that of the general population.
- **Tooth and gum diseases.** Diabetics run an increased risk of periodontal disease.

Diagnosing, Monitoring, and Treating Diabetes

Generally, a physician orders one of two blood tests to diagnose pre-diabetes or diabetes:

- The *fasting plasma glucose (FPG) test* requires the patient to fast overnight; a small sample of blood is then tested for glucose concentration.
- The *oral glucose tolerance test (OGTT)* requires the patient to drink a fluid containing concentrated glucose. Blood is drawn for testing 2 hours later.

If you have any risk factors for type 2 diabetes, talk with your health care provider about having your blood glucose levels checked. If they're normal, testing should be repeated every 3 years.[121]

People with diagnosed diabetes should have blood glucose levels monitored with the *hemoglobin A1C test* at least twice a year.[122] Diabetics also must check their blood glucose levels several times a day, testing blood from a finger prick with a handheld glucose meter.

People with pre-diabetes can prevent or delay development of type 2 diabetes by up to 58 percent through modest weight loss and regular exercise.[123] For those with type 2 diabetes, such lifestyle changes can prevent or delay need for medication or insulin injections.

Weight loss significantly lowers risk of progressing from pre-diabetes to diabetes; the recommended goal is to lose 5 to 10 percent of current weight.[124] Weight loss is also important for people currently diagnosed with type 2 diabetes.

A low-fat, reduced-calorie diet aids weight loss. Researchers have also studied a variety of foods for their effect on blood glucose levels. A diet high in whole grains reduces risk of type 2 diabetes,[125] while foods high in fiber—fruits, vegetables, beans, nuts, and seeds—may improve blood sugar levels.[126] In one study, participants who ate foods high in fiber reduced their risk of diabetes by as much as 22 percent.[127] In addition, consumption of fish high in omega-3 fatty acids is linked with decreased progression of insulin resistance.[128]

People with diabetes should also pay attention to foods' glycemic index and glycemic load. A food's glycemic load is defined as its glycemic index (potential to raise blood glucose) multiplied by the grams of carbohydrates it provides, divided by 100. By combining high and low glycemic index foods, a diabetic can help control blood glucose levels throughout the day.

Thirty minutes of physical activity 5 days a week reduces risk of type 2 diabetes.[129] A recent study suggests that improved fitness is even more important than weight loss in improving quality of life for people with diabetes.[130]

When lifestyle changes fail to control type 2 diabetes, one of several oral medications may be prescribed,[131] each of which influences blood glucose in a different way—reducing the liver's glucose production, slowing absorption of carbohydrates from the small intestine, increasing pancreatic insulin production, or increasing cells' insulin sensitivity.

With type 1 diabetes, the pancreas cannot produce adequate insulin, making added insulin essential. People with type 2 diabetes whose blood glucose cannot be controlled with other treatments also require insulin. Insulin cannot be taken in pill form because it's a protein, and thus would be digested in the gastrointestinal tract. It must therefore be inserted into the fat layer under the skin, from which it is absorbed into the bloodstream.

Today, many diabetics use an insulin infusion pump rather than injections. The pump, small and easily hidden by clothes, delivers insulin in minute amounts throughout the day through a catheter inserted under the skin.[132]

check yourself

- **What factors put someone at greatest risk for type 2 diabetes?**

Your Health Inheritance: The Influence of Genetics on Disease

- **Explain how genes affect inheritance of disease-linked traits.**
- **Distinguish between single-gene, chromosome, and multifactorial disorders.**

Not only do we inherit our tendency to be short or tall or have blue or brown eyes, we also inherit a tendency for increased risk for certain conditions. However, inheritance is just one determinant of health—it doesn't dictate destiny. Health choices and behaviors can affect your quality of life and your risk of major disease and disability.

If that's the case, why find out your family health history? First, if you know that certain diseases run in your family, you can change your behaviors to reduce your risk. Second, you can share the information with health care providers so that they can provide better care, for instance, by looking for early warning signs of a condition. Third, a family health history is important if you are planning to have children. A handful of *genetic disorders* are controlled by inheritance; with a family history of any of these disorders, you could then talk to your health care provider about genetic testing and counseling.

Genes' Role in Inheritance

Inheritance is the process by which physical and biological characteristics—*traits*—are transmitted from parents to offspring. Within each of your cells is a sac called the *nucleus*, which is densely packed with **DNA (deoxyribonucleic acid)**, a molecule that stores the programming code your body uses for its assembly, growth, and functioning. DNA is a molecule shaped like a twisted ladder (a *double helix*), with two long side strands connected by "rungs." For much of the life of a cell, its DNA exists as tangled masses within the nucleus. But when a cell prepares to divide, its DNA becomes organized into 46 distinct bundles called **chromosomes** (**Figure 11.13**). These 46 chromosomes exist as two sets of 23; you get one set from each parent.

The ladder of DNA that makes up each chromosome contains hundreds of unique regions called **genes** that store the code for assembling particular

body proteins. Your full complement of DNA—including genes and noncoding regions—is your **genome**.

Genes can be likened to "pages" in the code book of DNA—they contain instructions for assembling—or *expressing*—specific body proteins. Essentially, all cells and tissues of the human body are composed of proteins. By controlling expression of proteins, genes control your body's appearance, structure, and function.

Proteins are made up of amino acids; the 20 amino acids in your body can be assembled into an estimated 10,000 to 50,000 unique body proteins.[133] For instructions indicating how to make each of these proteins, the cell turns to DNA: Each gene is a sequence of chemical instructions for combining amino acids into a specific protein. Minute differences in proteins result in differing physical and physiological characteristics, from height to color blindness.

Just as people inherit aspects of appearance, they can inherit genetic disorders or susceptibility to chronic diseases. But how are such traits passed down?

Cells have two sets of 23 chromosomes, one set from each parent. Your two gene copies may be similar, or they may be different. Different forms of the same gene are known as **alleles**.

For example, presence or absence of freckles is coded by just one gene, which has two alleles. Even if you inherited the freckle allele from just one parent, you'll still have freckles—the allele for freckles is **dominant**, whereas the allele for absence of freckles is **recessive**. A dominant allele always "dominates"—it always expresses the trait it codes for. In contrast, a recessive allele "recedes" in the presence of a dominant allele. When you inherit two recessive alleles, you express the recessive trait—in this case, no freckles. Or, if each parent has one dominant and one recessive allele, they will both have freckles. Yet they could both have transmitted their recessive allele to you, in which case you would not have freckles.

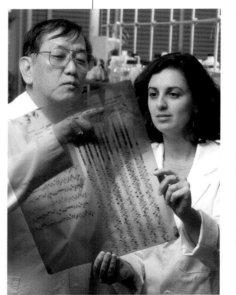

What makes genes so important to health?

Genes are important to health because they contain the code for assembling the proteins necessary for your body's structures and functions. The way that these proteins are put together can affect whether you are more at risk for certain conditions or have particular traits that can influence your health.

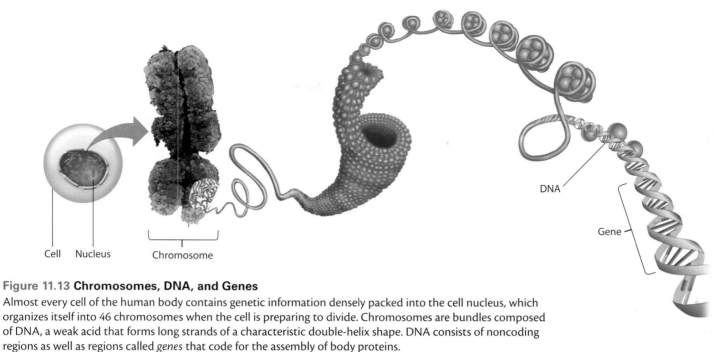

Figure 11.13 Chromosomes, DNA, and Genes
Almost every cell of the human body contains genetic information densely packed into the cell nucleus, which organizes itself into 46 chromosomes when the cell is preparing to divide. Chromosomes are bundles composed of DNA, a weak acid that forms long strands of a characteristic double-helix shape. DNA consists of noncoding regions as well as regions called *genes* that code for the assembly of body proteins.

Source: Adapted from Michael D. Johnson, *Human Biology: Concepts and Current Issues,* 5th ed. © 2010. Reprinted by permission of Pearson Education, Inc., Upper Saddle River, New Jersey.

Causes of Genetic Disorders

Just as humans can pass on physical traits, they can also pass on genetic disorders. **Single-gene disorders** occur as a result of a defect, or *mutation*, involving just one gene. **Chromosome disorders**, in contrast, are caused by errors in an entire chromosome or part of a chromosome.[134] A chromosome may be missing or broken or an extra chromosome may be present. These problems can be expressed as a wide range of abnormalities, including heart defects, kidney disorders, and mental retardation.

Multifactorial Disorders

Genes interact with one another and with many aspects of the environment, including diet, exposure to cigarette smoke and other toxins, viruses, and radiation. These factors can turn genes on or off so the proteins they code for are, or are not, assembled. Disorders in which genes play a role—but not the only role—are called **multifactorial disorders**. These include obesity, heart disease, type 2 diabetes, Alzheimer's disease, and certain types of cancer. Some researchers contend that nearly all conditions and diseases have a genetic component.[135] If a multifactorial disorder runs in your family, you should learn about other factors influencing the disorder and make healthy choices to reduce your risk.

The Role of Ethnicity

Some genetic disorders occur more frequently among people who trace their ancestry to a particular geographic area.[136] People in an ethnic group often share certain versions of their genes, passed down from common ancestors. If one of these genes contains a disease-causing mutation, a particular genetic disorder may be more frequent in this group.

Ethnicity is also believed to play some role in many multifactorial diseases. For example, hypertension, heart attack, and stroke are all more common among African Americans. Type 2 diabetes is more common among African Americans, Hispanic Americans, Native Americans, and Asian Americans than among Caucasian Americans. Also, although it's not clear why, African Americans are more likely, and Hispanic and Asian Americans less likely, to develop most cancers than are Caucasian Americans.[137] Still to be determined is how large a role genetics plays in these trends and how much is a result of environmental factors.

Genetic Counseling

Genetic counselors help couples identify their risk for giving birth to a baby with a genetic disorder, investigate disorders present within a family, and provide supportive counseling.[138] Gene tests can tell you whether you are a carrier of a genetic disorder. They can also be used for prenatal diagnosis, newborn screening, or to predict the presence of an adult-onset genetic disorder or confirm diagnosis of specific disorders in individuals with symptoms.[139]

check yourself

- **How do genes affect inheritance of disease-linked traits?**
- **What are the differences between single-gene, chromosome, and multifactorial disorders?**
- **What are the benefits of understanding your genetic inheritance?**

What's Your Personal CVD Risk?

An interactive version of this assessment is available online. Download it from the Live It section of www.pearsonhighered.com/donatelle.

Each of us has a unique level of risk for various diseases, including cardiovascular disease. Answer each of the following questions and total your points in each section.

1 Your Family Risk for CVD

	Yes (1 point)	No (0 points)	Don't Know
1. Do any of your primary relatives (parents, grandparents, siblings) have a history of heart disease or stroke?	○	○	○
2. Do any of your primary relatives have diabetes?	○	○	○
3. Do any of your primary relatives have high blood pressure?	○	○	○
4. Do any of your primary relatives have a history of high cholesterol?	○	○	○
5. Would you say that your family consumed a high-fat diet (lots of red meat, whole dairy, butter/margarine) during your time spent at home?	○	○	○

Total points:_____

2 Your Lifestyle Risk for CVD

	Yes (1 point)	No (0 points)	Don't Know
1. Is your total cholesterol level higher than it should be?	○	○	○
2. Do you have high blood pressure?	○	○	○
3. Have you been diagnosed as pre-diabetic or diabetic?	○	○	○
4. Do you smoke?	○	○	○
5. Would you describe your life as being highly stressful?	○	○	○

Total points:_____

3 Your Additional Risks for CVD

1. **How would you best describe your current weight?**
   a. Lower than what it should be for my height (0 points)
   b. About what it should be for my height (0 points)
   c. Higher than what it should be for my height (1 point)
2. **How would you describe the level of exercise that you get each day?**
   a. Less than how much I should be exercising each day (1 point)
   b. About how much I should be exercising each day (0 points)
   c. More than how much I should be exercising each day (0 points)
3. **How would you describe your dietary behaviors?**
   a. Eating only the recommended number of calories each day (0 points)
   b. Eating less than the recommended number of calories each day (0 points)
   c. Eating more than the recommended number of calories each day (1 point)
4. **Which of the following statements best describes your typical dietary behavior?**
   a. I eat from the major food groups, especially trying to get the recommended fruits and vegetables. (0 points)
   b. I eat too much red meat and consume too much saturated and *trans* fats from meat, dairy products, and processed foods each day. (1 point)
   c. Whenever possible, I try to substitute olive oil or canola oil for other forms of dietary fat. (0 points)

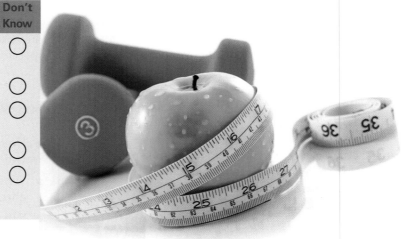

5. Which of the following (if any) describes you?
   a. I watch my sodium intake and try to reduce stress in my life. (0 points)
   b. I have a history of chlamydia infection. (1 point)
   c. I try to eat 5 to 10 milligrams of soluble fiber each day and to substitute a soy product for an animal product in my diet at least once each week. (0 points)

Total points: _____

Scoring

If you score between 1 and 5 in any section, consider your risk. The higher the number you've scored, the greater your risk. If you answered "don't know" for any question, talk to your parents or other family members as soon as possible to find out if you have any unknown risks.

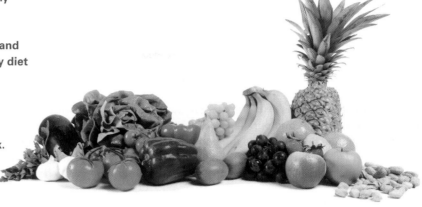

Your Plan for Change

The Assess Yourself activity evaluated your risk of heart disease. Based on your results and the advice of your physician, you may need to take steps to reduce your risk of CVD.

Today, you can:

◯ Get up and move! Take a walk in the evening, use the stairs instead of the escalator, or ride your bike to class. Start thinking of ways you can incorporate more physical activity into your daily routine.

◯ Begin improving your dietary habits by eating a healthier dinner. Replace the meat and processed foods you might normally eat with a serving of fresh fruit or soy-based protein and green leafy vegetables. Think about the amounts of saturated and *trans* fats you consume—which foods contain them, and how can you reduce consumption of these items?

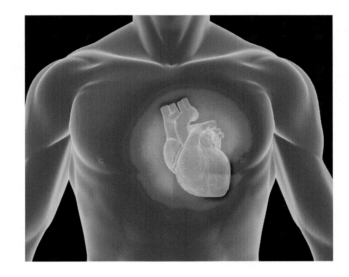

Within the next 2 weeks, you can:

◯ Begin a regular exercise program, even if you start slowly. Set small goals and try to meet them.

◯ Practice a new stress management technique. For example, learn how to meditate.

◯ Get enough rest. Make sure you get at least 8 hours of sleep per night.

By the end of the semester, you can:

◯ Find out your hereditary risk for CVD. Call your parents and find out if your grandparents or aunts or uncles developed CVD. Ask if they know their latest cholesterol LDL/HDL levels. Do you have a family history of diabetes?

◯ Have your own cholesterol and blood pressure levels checked. Once you know your levels, you'll have a better sense of what risk factors to address. If your levels are high, talk to your doctor about how to reduce them.

Assessyourself

What's Your Personal Risk for Cancer?

An interactive version of this assessment is available online. Download it from the Live It section of www.pearsonhighered.com/donatelle.

There are many cancer risk factors that you have the power to change. Once you carefully assess your risks, you can make lifestyle changes and pursue risk-reduction strategies that may lessen your susceptibility to various cancers.

Read each question and circle the number corresponding to each Yes or No. Be honest and accurate to get the most complete understanding of your cancer risks. Individual scores for specific questions should not be interpreted as a precise measure of relative risk, but the totals in each section give a general indication.

1 Breast Cancer

	Yes	No
1. Do you do a monthly breast self-exam?	1	2
2. Do you look at your breasts in the mirror regularly, checking for any irregular indentations/ lumps, discharge from the nipples, or other noticeable changes?	1	2
3. Has your mother, sister, or daughter been diagnosed with breast cancer?	2	1
4. Have you ever been pregnant?	1	2
5. Have you had lumps or cysts in your breasts or underarm?	2	1

Total points: _____

2 Skin Cancer

	Yes	No
1. Do you spend a lot of time outdoors, either at work or at play?	2	1
2. Do you use sunscreens with an SPF rating of 15 or more?	1	2
3. Do you use tanning beds or sun booths regularly to maintain a tan?	2	1
4. Do you examine your skin once a month, checking any moles or other irregularities, and using a hand mirror to check hard-to-see areas such as your back, buttocks, genitals, and neck, and under your hair?	1	2
5. Do you purchase and wear sunglasses that filter out harmful sunrays?	1	2

Total points: _____

3 Cancers of the Reproductive System

Men

	Yes	No
1. Do you examine your penis regularly for unusual bumps or growths?	1	2
2. Do you perform regular testicular self-exams?	1	2
3. Do you have a family history of prostate or testicular cancer?	2	1
4. Do you practice safe sex and wear condoms with every sexual encounter?	1	2
5. Do you avoid exposure to harmful environmental hazards such as mercury, coal tars, benzene, chromate, and vinyl chloride?	1	2

Total points: _____

Women

	Yes	No
1. Do you have regularly scheduled Pap tests?	1	2
2. Have you been infected with the human papillomavirus, Epstein-Barr virus, or other viruses believed to increase cancer risk?	2	1
3. Has your mother, sister, or daughter been diagnosed with breast, cervical, endometrial, or ovarian cancer (particularly at a young age)?	2	1
4. Do you practice safe sex and use condoms with every sexual encounter?	1	2
5. Are you obese, taking estrogen, or consuming a diet that is very high in saturated fats?	2	1

Total points: _____

4 Cancers in General

	Yes	No		Yes	No
1. Do you smoke cigarettes on most days of the week?	2	1	6. Do you limit your overall consumption of alcohol?	1	2
2. Do you consume a diet that is rich in fruits and vegetables?	1	2	7. Do you eat foods rich in lycopenes (such as tomatoes) and antioxidants?	1	2
3. Are you obese, or do you lead a primarily sedentary lifestyle?	2	1	8. Are you "body aware" and alert for changes in your body?	1	2
4. Do you live in an area with high air pollution levels or work in a job where you are exposed to several chemicals on a regular basis?	2	1	9. Do you have a family history of ulcers or of colorectal, stomach, or other digestive-system cancers?	2	1
5. Are you careful about the amount of animal fat in your diet, substituting olive oil or canola oil for animal fat whenever possible?	1	2	10. Do you avoid unnecessary exposure to radiation, cell phone emissions, and microwave emissions?	1	2

Total points: _____

Analyzing Your Scores

Look carefully at each question for which you circled a 2. Are there any areas in which you received mostly 2s? Did you receive total points of 6 or higher in parts 1 through 3? Did you receive total points of 11 or higher in part 4? If so, you have at least one identifiable risk. The higher your score, the more risks you may have.

Your Plan for Change

The Assess Yourself activity identifies certain behaviors that can contribute to increased cancer risks. If you have identified particular risky behaviors, consider steps you can take to change these behaviors and improve your future health.

Today, you can:

○ Perform a breast or testicular self-exam and commit to doing one every month.

○ Take advantage of the salad bar in your dining hall for lunch or dinner, and load up on greens, or request veggies such as steamed broccoli or sautéed spinach.

Within the next 2 weeks, you can:

○ Buy a bottle of sunscreen (with SPF 15 or higher) and begin applying it as part of your daily routine. (Be sure to check the expiration date, particularly on sale items!) Also, stay in the shade from 10 AM to 2 PM, as this is when the sun is strongest.

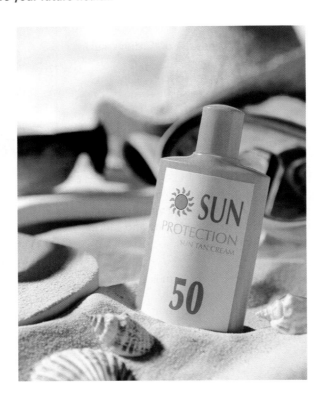

○ Find out your family health history. Talk to your parents, grandparents, or an aunt or uncle to find out if family members have developed cancer. This will help you assess your own genetic risk.

By the end of the semester, you can:

○ Work toward achieving a healthy weight. If you aren't already engaged in a regular exercise program, begin one now. Maintaining a healthy body weight and exercising regularly will lower your risk for cancer.

○ Stop smoking, avoid secondhand smoke, and limit your alcohol intake.

11.26 | Assess Yourself: What's Your Personal Risk for Cancer?

287

CVD, Cancer, and Diabetes

Summary

- The cardiovascular system consists of the heart and circulatory system, a network of vessels that supplies the body with nutrients and oxygen.
- Cardiovascular diseases include atherosclerosis, coronary artery disease, peripheral artery disease, coronary heart disease, stroke, hypertension, angina pectoris, arrhythmias, congestive heart failure, and congenital and rheumatic heart disease.
- Many risk factors for cardiovascular disease can be modified, such as cigarette smoking, high blood cholesterol and triglyceride levels, hypertension, lack of exercise, a diet high in saturated fat, obesity, diabetes, and emotional stress. Some risk factors, such as age, gender, and heredity, cannot be modified.
- Cancer is a group of diseases characterized by uncontrolled growth and spread of abnormal cells. These cells may create tumors.
- Lifestyle factors for cancer include smoking, obesity, poor diet, lack of exercise, and stress. Biological factors include inherited genes, age, and gender. Infectious agents that may cause cancer are chronic hepatitis B and C, human papillomavirus, and genital herpes.
- There are many different types of cancer. Common cancers include those of the lung, breast, colon and rectum, skin, prostate, testis, ovary, and uterus; leukemia; and lymphomas.
- Early diagnosis improves survival rate. Self-exams for breast, testicular, and skin cancer aid early diagnosis.
- Diabetes mellitus is characterized by a persistently high level of glucose in the blood. In type 1 diabetes, the immune system attacks insulin-making cells in the pancreas, dangerously elevating insulin levels. In type 2 diabetes, the pancreas doesn't make sufficient insulin, or the cells don't use it efficiently.
- Genetics has an enormous influence on disease. Single-gene disorders occur as a result of a defect involving just one gene. Chromosome disorders are caused by errors in an entire chromosome or part of a chromosome.

Pop Quiz

1. What does a person's cholesterol level indicate?
   a. The formation of fatty substances, called *plaque*, which can clog the arteries
   b. The level of triglycerides in the blood, which can increase risk of coronary disease
   c. Hypertension, which leads to thickening and hardening of the arteries
   d. None of the above.

2. A stroke results
   a. when a heart stops beating.
   b. when cardiopulmonary resuscitation has failed to revive a stopped heart.
   c. when blood flow in the brain has been compromised, either due to blockage or hemorrhage.
   d. when blood pressure rises above 120/80 mm Hg.

3. The "bad" type of cholesterol found in the bloodstream is known as
   a. high-density lipoprotein (HDL).
   b. low-density lipoprotein (LDL).
   c. total cholesterol.
   d. triglycerides.

4. Which of the following is true of metabolic syndrome?
   a. It is decreasing among the general population.
   b. It lowers your risk of cardiovascular disease.
   c. Obesity, high triglyceride levels, and hypertension are some of its symptoms.
   d. All of the above.

5. When cancer cells have *metastasized*,
   a. they have grown into a malignant tumor.
   b. they have spread to other parts of the body, including vital organs.
   c. the cancer is retreating and cancer cells are dying off.
   d. None of the above.

6. A cancerous *neoplasm* is a
   a. type of biopsy.
   b. form of benign tumor.
   c. type of treatment for a tumor.
   d. malignant group of cells or tumor.

7. "If you are male and smoke, your chances of getting lung cancer are 23 times greater than those of a nonsmoker." This statement refers to a type of risk assessed statistically, known as
   a. relative risk.
   b. comparable risk.
   c. cancer risk.
   d. genetic predisposition.

8. The more serious and life-threatening type of skin cancer is
   a. basal cell carcinoma.
   b. squamous cell carcinoma.
   c. melanoma.
   d. lymphoma.

9. Which of the following is *not* true of type 2 diabetes?
   a. It is the most common type of diabetes.
   b. It is an autoimmune disorder.
   c. Its primary symptom is elevated blood glucose levels.
   d. It is highly correlated with obesity and sedentary lifestyle.

10. What is a multifactorial disorder?
    a. A disorder resulting from a mutation involving just one gene
    b. A disorder resulting from an error in a chromosome containing many genes
    c. A disorder having both a genetic component and an environmental or behavioral component
    d. A disorder involving one dominant and one recessive gene

Answers to these questions can be found on page A-1.

Web Links

1. **American Heart Association.** Information, statistics, and resources regarding cardiovascular care, including an opportunity to test your risk for CVD. www.heart.org
2. **American Cancer Society.** Information, statistics, and resources regarding cancer. www.cancer.org
3. **American Diabetes Association.** Information and resources for those with diabetes. www.diabetes.org

Infectious Conditions

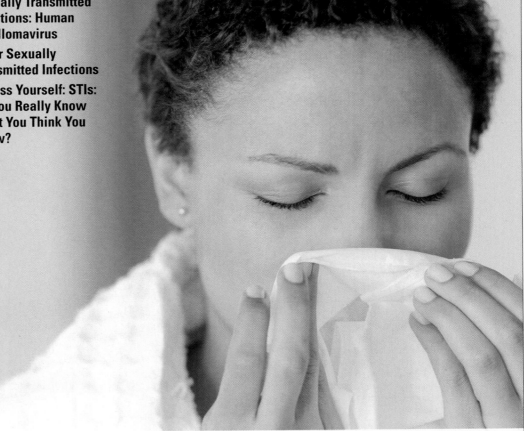

Disease-causing agents, or **pathogens**, are found throughout our world. New varieties arise constantly; others have existed for as long as there has been life on this planet. At times, infectious diseases wiped out whole groups of people through **epidemics**; bubonic plague, for example, killed up to one-third of the population of Europe in the 1300s. A **pandemic**, or global epidemic, of influenza killed more than 20 million people in 1918. Today, new, resistant forms of older organisms—such as H1N1 flu and the methicillin-resistant *Staphylococcus aureus*, or MRSA, staph infection—defy current pharmacological weapons.

Despite constant bombardment by pathogens, however, our immune systems are remarkably adept at protecting us. Exposure to invading microorganisms actually helps build resistance to pathogens. Millions of *endogenous microorganisms* live in and on our bodies, usually in peaceful coexistence. *Exogenous microorganisms*, in contrast, are those that don't normally inhabit the body. When they do, they are apt to produce infection or illness. The more easily these pathogens can gain a foothold and sustain themselves, the more **virulent**, or aggressive, they may be in causing disease.

The Process of Infection

- **Explain the process of infection and defenses against pathogens.**
- **List common risk factors for infection.**

Most diseases are **multifactorial**, caused by the interaction of several factors inside and outside a person. For a disease to occur, the person, or *host*, must be *susceptible*, which means that the immune system must be in a weakened condition (**immunocompromised**); an *agent* capable of *transmitting* a disease must be present; and the *environment* must be *hospitable* to the pathogen. Although all pathogens pose a threat if they gain entry and begin to grow in the body, the chances that they will do so are actually quite small.

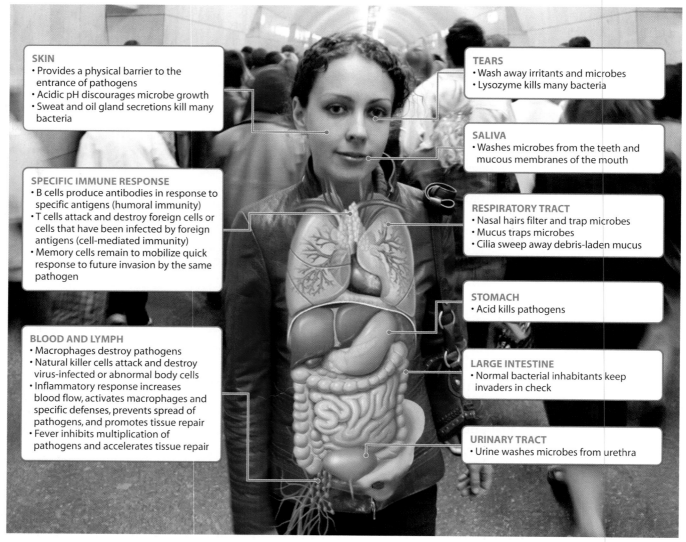

SKIN
- Provides a physical barrier to the entrance of pathogens
- Acidic pH discourages microbe growth
- Sweat and oil gland secretions kill many bacteria

SPECIFIC IMMUNE RESPONSE
- B cells produce antibodies in response to specific antigens (humoral immunity)
- T cells attack and destroy foreign cells or cells that have been infected by foreign antigens (cell-mediated immunity)
- Memory cells remain to mobilize quick response to future invasion by the same pathogen

BLOOD AND LYMPH
- Macrophages destroy pathogens
- Natural killer cells attack and destroy virus-infected or abnormal body cells
- Inflammatory response increases blood flow, activates macrophages and specific defenses, prevents spread of pathogens, and promotes tissue repair
- Fever inhibits multiplication of pathogens and accelerates tissue repair

TEARS
- Wash away irritants and microbes
- Lysozyme kills many bacteria

SALIVA
- Washes microbes from the teeth and mucous membranes of the mouth

RESPIRATORY TRACT
- Nasal hairs filter and trap microbes
- Mucus traps microbes
- Cilia sweep away debris-laden mucus

STOMACH
- Acid kills pathogens

LARGE INTESTINE
- Normal bacterial inhabitants keep invaders in check

URINARY TRACT
- Urine washes microbes from urethra

Figure 12.1 The Body's Defenses against Disease-Causing Pathogens
In addition to the defenses listed, many of the body's defensive secretions and fluids, such as earwax, tears, mucus, and blood, contain enzymes and other proteins that can kill some invading pathogens or prevent or slow their reproduction.

Preventing Pathogens from Entering the Body

Pathogens can enter the body through several routes of transmission. They may be transmitted by *direct contact* between infected persons, such as during sexual relations, kissing, or touching, or by *indirect contact*, such as by touching an object the infected person has had contact with. You may also **autoinoculate** yourself, or transmit a pathogen from one part of your body to another. For example, you may touch a herpes sore on your lip, then transmit the virus to your eye by touch.

Dogs, cats, livestock, and wild animals can spread *animal-borne pathogens* through bites or feces or by carrying infected insects into living areas. Although *interspecies transmission* of diseases (diseases passed from humans to animals and vice versa) is rare, it does occur.

Your body constantly protects against and defends you from pathogens that could make you ill. For pathogens to gain entry into your body, they must overcome barriers that prevent pathogens from entering your body, mechanisms that weaken organisms that breach these barriers, and substances that counteract the threat that these organisms pose. **Figure 12.1** summarizes some of the body's defenses against invasion.

Risk Factors You Can Control

With all these pathogens floating around, how can you avoid getting sick? Fortunately, there are ways to take care of yourself. Too much stress, inadequate nutrition, a low fitness level, lack of sleep, misuse or abuse of legal and illegal drugs, poor personal hygiene, and high-risk behavior significantly increase the risk for many diseases. College students, in particular, often are at higher risk because of many of the above factors, in addition to the fact that alcohol and other drugs, increasing numbers of sexual experiences, and close living conditions all create higher risk for exposure to pathogens. You can make changes in your community to clean up toxins, set policies on contaminant levels, and reduce the likelihood of exposure to pathogens or toxins. The chain of infection between pathogen, environment, and host presents multiple opportunities for individuals and communities to intercede and "break the chain," preventing and controlling disease transmission.

Risk Factors You Typically Cannot Control

Unfortunately, some factors that make you susceptible to a certain disease are either hard to control or completely beyond your control:

- **Heredity.** Perhaps the single greatest factor influencing disease risk is genetics. It is often unclear whether hereditary diseases are due to inherited genetic traits or to inherited insufficiencies in the immune system. Some believe that we may inherit the quality of our immune system, so some people are naturally more resistant to disease and infection.
- **Aging.** People over age 65 are often more vulnerable to infectious diseases because body defenses are reduced. Thinning of the skin, reduced sweating, and other physical changes can make the elderly more vulnerable to disease. In addition, as people age certain **comorbidities** (diseases that occur at the same time) overwhelm the body's ability to ward off enemies and increase the risk of infection. In these situations, **opportunistic infections** can cause illness.
- **Environmental conditions.** Unsanitary conditions and the presence of drugs, chemicals, and hazardous pollutants and wastes in food and water probably have a great effect on our immune systems. A growing body of research points to changes in the climate, where, for example, increases in mosquito populations increase the spread of diseases such as malaria.[1] In addition, natural disasters and long-term exposure to toxic chemicals are believed to be significant contributors to increasing numbers of infectious diseases.[2] Environmental crises such as earthquakes and floods that contaminate food and water and leave victims without medical care also create perfect conditions for the spread of infectious disease.
- **Organism virulence and resistance.** Some organisms, such as the foodborne organism that causes *botulism*, are particularly virulent, and even tiny amounts may make the hardiest of us ill. Other organisms have mutated and become resistant to the body's defenses and to medical treatments. Multidrug-resistant strains of tuberculosis, *Staphylococcus*, and other organisms are emerging in many parts of the world.
- **College environment.** Living and studying in close quarters, lack of sleep, and poor cleaning habits all can contribute to increased susceptibility to disease.

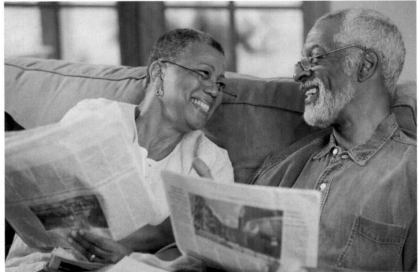

As we age, our risk from infectious disease increases. It is important to maintain a healthy diet, get plenty of exercise, and avoid exposure to pathogens.

check yourself

- **What are three common routes of infection?**
- **What are some ways your body fights off infection?**

Your Immune System

- ■ **Explain how the immune system defends against invasion by pathogens**.

Immunity is a condition of being able to resist a particular disease by counteracting the substance that produces the disease. Any substance capable of triggering an immune response is called an **antigen**. An antigen can be a virus, a bacterium, a fungus, a parasite, a toxin, or a tissue or cell from another organism.

How the Immune System Works

As soon as an antigen breaches the body's initial defenses, the body responds by forming substances called **antibodies** that are matched to that specific antigen, much as a key is matched to a lock. The body analyzes the antigen, considers its size and shape, verifies that the antigen is not part of the body itself, and then produces a specific antibody to destroy or weaken it. This process, which is much more complex than described here, is part of a system called *humoral immune responses*. **Humoral immunity** is the body's major defense against many bacteria and the poisonous substances, called **toxins**, that they produce.

In **cell-mediated immunity**, specialized white blood cells called **lymphocytes** attack and destroy the foreign invader. Lymphocytes constitute the body's main defense against viruses, fungi, parasites, and some bacteria, and they are found in the blood, lymph nodes, bone marrow, and certain glands. Other key players in this immune response are **macrophages** (a type of phagocytic, or cell-eating, white blood cell).

Two forms of lymphocytes in particular, the *B lymphocytes* (B cells) and *T lymphocytes* (T cells), are involved in the immune response. *Helper T cells* are essential for activating B cells to produce antibodies. They also activate other T cells and macrophages. Another form of T cell, known as the *killer T cell*, directly attacks infected or malignant cells. *Suppressor T cells* turn off or suppress the activity of B cells, killer T cells, and macrophages. After a successful attack on a pathogen, some of the attacker T and B cells are preserved as *memory T and B cells*, enabling the body to recognize and respond quickly to subsequent attacks by the same kind of organism.

Once people have survived certain infectious diseases, they become immune to those diseases, meaning that in all probability they will not develop them again. Upon subsequent attack by the same disease-causing microorganisms, their memory T and B cells are quickly activated to come to their defense. **Figure 12.2** provides a summary of the cell-mediated immune response.

When the Immune System Misfires: Autoimmune Diseases Although the immune response generally works in our favor, the body sometimes makes a mistake and targets its own tissue as the enemy, builds up antibodies against that tissue, and attempts to destroy it. This is known as **autoimmune disease** (*auto* means "self"). The National Institutes of Health estimates that over 24 million Americans suffer from some form of autoimmune disease and that the numbers are increasing. Researchers estimate that there are between 80 and 140 different types of autoimmune disease, many of which are chronic, debilitating, and life threatening. Common autoimmune disorders include *rheumatoid arthritis, systemic lupus erythematosus (SLE), type 1 diabetes*, and *multiple sclerosis*. Many people do not realize that autoimmune diseases are among the leading causes of death in girls and women younger than age 65.[3]

Inflammatory Response, Pain, and Fever If an infection is localized, pus formation, redness, swelling, and irritation often occur. These symptoms are components of the body's inflammatory response, and they indicate that the invading organisms are being fought systemically. The four cardinal signs of inflammation are redness, swelling, pain, and heat.

Pain is often one of the earliest signs that an injury or infection has occurred. Pathogens can kill or injure tissue at the site of infection, causing swelling that puts pressure on nerve endings in the area, causing pain. Although pain does not feel good, it plays a valuable role in the body's response to injury or invasion. For example, it can cause a person to avoid activity that may aggravate the injury or site of infection, thereby protecting against further damage.

Another frequent indicator of infection is *fever*, or a body temperature above the average norm of 98.6 °F. Fever is frequently caused by toxins secreted by pathogens that interfere with the control of body temperature. Although extremely elevated temperatures are harmful to the body, a mild fever is protective: Raising body temperature by one or two degrees destroys some disease-causing organisms. A fever also stimulates the body to produce more white blood cells, which destroy more invaders. Of course, with fevers beyond 101 or 102 °F risks to the patient outweigh any benefits. In these cases, medical treatment should be obtained.

Vaccines: Bolstering Your Immunity

Recall that once people have been exposed to a specific pathogen, subsequent attacks activate their memory T and B cells, thus giving them immunity. This is the principle on which **vaccination** is based.

A vaccine consists of killed or weakened versions of a disease-causing microorganism or an antigen similar to but less dangerous than the disease antigen. It is administered to stimulate the immune system to produce antibodies against future attacks without actually causing the disease (or by causing a very minor case of it). Vaccines typically are given orally or by injection; this form of immunity

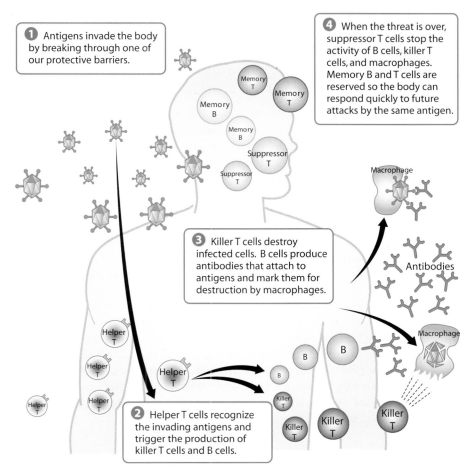

① Antigens invade the body by breaking through one of our protective barriers.

④ When the threat is over, suppressor T cells stop the activity of B cells, killer T cells, and macrophages. Memory B and T cells are reserved so the body can respond quickly to future attacks by the same antigen.

③ Killer T cells destroy infected cells. B cells produce antibodies that attach to antigens and mark them for destruction by macrophages.

② Helper T cells recognize the invading antigens and trigger the production of killer T cells and B cells.

Figure 12.2 The Cell-Mediated Immune Response

is termed *artificially acquired active immunity*, in contrast to *naturally acquired active immunity* (which is obtained by exposure to antigens in the normal course of daily life) or *naturally acquired passive immunity* (as occurs when a mother passes immunity to her fetus via their shared blood supply or to an infant via breast milk). Because of their close living quarters and frequent interactions with other people, college students face a higher than average risk

TABLE 12.1 Recommended Vaccinations for Teens and College Students

- Tetanus-diphtheria-pertussis vaccine (Td/Tdap)
- Meningococcal vaccine*
- HPV vaccine series
- Hepatitis B vaccine series
- Polio vaccine series
- Measles-mumps-rubella (MMR) vaccine series
- Varicella (chickenpox) vaccine series
- Influenza vaccine
- Pneumococcal polysaccharide (PPV) vaccine
- Hepatitis A vaccine series

*Recommended for previously unvaccinated college first-year students living in dormitories.
Source: Centers for Disease Control and Prevention, "2011 Child and Adolescent Immunization Schedules," 2011, www.cdc.gov/vaccines/recs/schedules/child-schedule.htm.

of infection from diseases that are largely preventable. Vaccines that should be a high priority among 20-somethings include the tetanus-diphtheria-pertussis vaccine (Tdap), the meningococcal conjugate vaccine (MCV4), and the human papillomavirus (HPV) vaccine. **Table 12.1** shows recommended vaccines for teens and college students.

While some advise against vaccinations, avoiding a potentially deadly or disabling disease outweighs any risks. If you develop minor rashes or other symptoms after being immunized, let your doctor know.

Skills for Behavior Change

Reduce Your Risk of Infectious Disease

■ **Limit your exposure to pathogens.** Stay home if you are not feeling well; encourage others to do the same. Don't drag yourself to classes or work and infect others. Don't share utensils or drinking glasses, keep your toothbrush away from those of other people, and wash your hands often. Sneeze or cough into your arm or sleeve rather than your hands. Keep hands away from your mouth, nose, eyes, and other body orifices. Use disposable tissues rather than reusable handkerchiefs.

■ **Exercise regularly.** Regular exercise raises core body temperature and kills pathogens. Sweat and oil make the skin a hostile environment for many bacteria. Avoid excessive exercise that could overtax the immune system.

■ **Get enough sleep.** Sleep allows the body time to refresh itself, produce necessary cells, and reduce inflammation. Even a single night without sleep can increase inflammatory processes and delay wound healing.

■ **Stress less.** Rest and relaxation, stress management practices, laughter, and calming music have all been shown to promote healthy cellular activity and bolster immune functioning.

■ **Optimize eating.** Enjoy a healthy diet, including adequate amounts of water, protein, and complex carbohydrates. Eat more omega-3 fatty acids to reduce inflammation, and restrict saturated fats, replacing them with good fats such as olive oil. Antioxidants are believed to be important in immune functioning, so get your daily fruits and vegetables.

check yourself

■ **How do vaccines help your body resist viruses?**

■ **What are four steps you can take to reduce your overall chances of infection?**

Disease-Causing Pathogens: Bacteria

learning outcomes

- **List several common bacterial infections.**

We can categorize pathogens into six major types: bacteria, viruses, fungi, protozoans, parasitic worms, and prions (see **Figure 12.3**). Each has a particular route of transmission and characteristic elements that make it unique. In the following pages, we discuss each of these categories and give an overview of some of the diseases that they cause.

Bacteria (singular: *bacterium*) are simple, single-celled microscopic organisms. Although there are several thousand known species of bacteria (and many thousands more that are unknown), just over 100 lead to disease in humans. In many cases, it is not the bacteria themselves that cause disease, but rather the toxins that they produce.

Diseases caused by bacteria can be treated with **antibiotics**. However, today's arsenal of antibiotics is becoming less effective, as strains of bacteria with **antibiotic resistance** become more common. Such "superbugs" can result when successive generations of bacteria mutate to develop an ability to withstand the effects of specific drugs.

Staphylococcal Infections

Staphylococci are present on the skin or in the nostrils of 20 to 30 percent of us at any given time, without problems or symptoms. However, with a cut or break in the *epidermis*, or outer layer of skin, staphylococci may enter the system and cause an **infection**. If you have suffered from acne, boils, styes (infections of the eyelids), or infected wounds, you've probably had a "staph" infection.

Although most of these infections are readily defeated by the immune system, resistant forms of staph are on the rise. One, **methicillin-resistant *Staphylococcus aureus*** (**MRSA**), has come under intense scrutiny.[4] Symptoms of MRSA infection often start with a rash or pimplelike skin irritation. Within hours, symptoms may progress to redness, inflammation, pain, and deeper wounds. If untreated, MRSA may invade blood, bones, joints, surgical wounds, heart valves, and lungs; it can be fatal.[5]

Health care-associated or *health care-acquired MRSA (HA-MRSA)* cases arise in settings, such as hospitals or nursing homes, where invasive treatments, infectious pathogens, and weakened immune systems converge. In *community-acquired MRSA (CA-MRSA)*, people are infected during normal daily activities. *Linezolid-resistant* Staphylococcus aureus, or LRSA, is a particularly potent and resistant bacterium that has evolved among patients using the antibiotic linezolid to

treat MRSA. Because linezolid was one of the few remaining effective treatments for the most severe forms of MRSA, many wonder whether the antibiotic "well" may finally be running dry.

Streptococcal Infections

At least five types of the **Streptococcus** microorganism are known to cause bacterial infections. Group A streptococci (GAS) cause the most common diseases, such as streptococcal pharyngitis ("strep throat") and scarlet fever, which is often preceded by a sore throat.[6] One particularly virulent group of GAS can lead to a rare but serious disease called *necrotizing fasciitis* (often referred to as "flesh-eating strep").[7] Group B streptococci can cause illness in newborns, pregnant women, older adults, and adults with illnesses such as diabetes or liver disease.[8]

Streptococcus pneumoniae causes thousands of cases of meningitis and pneumonia and 7 million cases of ear infections in the United States each year. About 30 percent of these cases are resistant to penicillin, the primary treatment; many penicillin-resistant strains are also resistant to other antibiotics.

Meningitis

Meningitis is an infection and inflammation of the *meninges*, the membranes that surround the brain and spinal cord. Some forms of bacterial meningitis are contagious and can be spread through contact; *pneumococcal meningitis* is the most common and the most dangerous. Several thousand cases of meningitis are reported in the United States each year. *Meningococcal meningitis*, a virulent form of meningitis, has risen dramatically on college campuses in recent years.[9]

The signs of meningitis are sudden fever, severe headache, and a stiff neck, particularly causing difficulty touching chin to chest. Persons suspected of having meningitis should receive immediate, aggressive medical treatment. Vaccines are available for some types of meningitis.

Pneumonia

Pneumonia is a general term for a range of conditions that result in inflammation of the lungs and difficulty breathing. It is characterized by chronic cough, chest pain, chills, high fever, fluid accumulation, and eventual respiratory failure.

Bacterial pneumonia responds readily to antibiotic treatment in the early stages, but can be deadly in more advanced stages. Pneumonias caused by viruses, fungi, chemicals, or other substances in the lungs are more difficult to treat. Vulnerable populations include children; the poor; those displaced by war, famine, and natural disasters; older adults; those occupation-

Ticks are a vector for several devastating bacterial diseases.

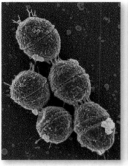 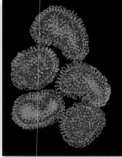 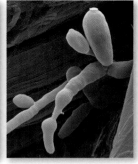 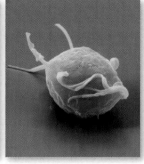 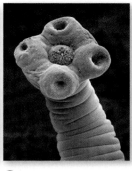

ⓐ Bacteria ⓑ Viruses ⓒ Fungi ⓓ Protozoan ⓔ Parasitic worm

Figure 12.3 Examples of Five Major Types of Pathogens
(a) Color-enhanced scanning electron micrograph (SEM) of *Streptococcus* bacteria, magnified 40,000×.
(b) Colored transmission electron micrograph (TEM) of influenza (flu) viruses, magnified 32,000×.
(c) Color SEM of *Candida albicans*, a yeast fungus, magnified 50,000×. (d) Color TEM of *Trichomonas vaginalis*, a protozoan, magnified 9,000×. (e) Color-enhanced SEM of a tapeworm, magnified 50×.

ally exposed to chemicals and particulates that damage the lungs; and those suffering from other illnesses.

Tuberculosis (TB)

Once a major killer in the United States, **tuberculosis (TB)** was largely controlled by 1950 as a result of improved sanitation, isolation of infected persons, and treatment with drugs such as *rifampin* or *isoniazid*. However, during the past 20 years, several factors have led to its resurgence: deteriorating social conditions, including overcrowding and poor sanitation; failure to isolate active cases; a weakening of public health infrastructure, leading to less funding for screening; and migration of TB to the United States through immigration and international travel. In 2009, the most recent year for which data are available, there were 11,545 active cases of TB in the United States, compared to 85,000 in 1950.[10]

Almost 2 billion people—a third of the world's population—have been exposed to TB. Some 81 percent of tuberculosis-related deaths occur in developing countries, where it accounts for 26 percent of preventable deaths.[11] TB is the number-one infectious killer of women of reproductive age worldwide, as well as the leading cause of death among HIV-positive patients.

Symptoms include persistent coughing, weight loss, fever, and spitting up blood. Airborne transmission via the respiratory tract is the primary mode of transmission, and infected people can be contagious without actually showing any symptoms themselves. Those at highest risk include the poor, especially children, and the chronically ill; people in crowded prisons and homeless shelters who continuously inhale the same contaminated air are also at higher risk, as are persons with compromised immune systems.

Multidrug-resistant TB (MDR-TB) is a form of TB that is resistant to at least two of the best anti-TB drugs. An even more dangerous form, **extensively drug-resistant TB (XDR-TB)**, is extremely difficult to treat. These newer strains of tuberculosis are reaching epidemic proportions in many regions of the world.

Tickborne Bacterial Diseases

Certain tickborne diseases have become major health threats in the United States. The most noteworthy include two bacterially caused diseases, *Lyme disease* and *ehrlichiosis*, both of which spike in the summer and can cause significant disability to humans and animals.

Once believed to be closely related to viruses, **rickettsia** are now considered a form of bacteria. They multiply within small blood vessels, causing vascular blockage and tissue death. Rickettsia require an insect vector (carrier) for transmission to humans. Two common forms of human rickettsial disease are *Rocky Mountain spotted fever* (*RMSF*), carried by a tick, and *typhus*, carried by a louse, flea, or tick. These produce similar symptoms, including high fever, weakness, rash, and coma; both can be life threatening.

For all insect-borne diseases, the best protection is to stay indoors at dusk and early morning to avoid high insect activity. If you must go out, wear protective clothing or use bug sprays containing natural oils, pyrethrins, or DEET (diethyl toluamide). If you are traveling where insect-borne diseases are prevalent, bed nets and other protective measures may be necessary.

Peptic Ulcers

A **peptic ulcer** is a chronic ulcer or lesion that occurs in the lining of the stomach (gastric ulcer) or in the *duodenum* (duodenal ulcer), a section of the small intestine. For decades, nobody thought ulcers had anything to do with infectious diseases. We now know that more than 60 percent of peptic ulcers result from infection by a common bacterium, *Helicobacter pylori*.[12] Factors that increase risk include smoking, caffeine consumption, stress, excess levels of digestive enzymes and stomach acids, and regular use of nonsteroidal anti-inflammatory drugs (NSAIDs) such as aspirin, ibuprofen, and naproxen sodium. The disorder, which affects more than 4.5 million Americans every year, generally responds to antibiotics, avoidance of NSAIDs, or antisecretory therapy.[13]

check yourself

- **List three illnesses or conditions that can result from bacterial infection.**

Disease-Causing Pathogens: Viruses

- **Identify the causes and symptoms of common viral infections.**

Viruses are the smallest known pathogens, approximately 1/500th the size of bacteria.

Essentially, a virus consists of a protein structure that contains either *ribonucleic acid* (*RNA*) or *deoxyribonucleic acid* (*DNA*). Viruses are incapable of carrying out any life processes on their own. To reproduce, viruses must invade and inject their own DNA and RNA into a host cell, take it over, and force it to make copies of themselves. The new viruses then erupt out of the host cell and seek other cells to invade.

Because viruses cannot reproduce outside living cells, they are especially difficult to culture in a laboratory, making detection and study extremely time consuming. Viral diseases can be difficult to treat, because many viruses can withstand heat, formaldehyde, and large doses of radiation with little effect on their structure. Some viruses have **incubation periods** (the length of time required to develop fully and cause symptoms in their hosts) that last for years, which delays diagnosis. Drug treatment is also limited; drugs powerful enough to kill viruses generally kill the host cells, too, though some medications block stages in viral reproduction without damaging host cells.

The Common Cold

Colds can be caused by any number of viruses (there may be over 200), though the rhinovirus is responsible for up to 40 percent of all colds, followed by the coronavirus, at 20 percent.[14] Colds are **endemic** (always present to some degree) throughout the world. Otherwise healthy people carry cold viruses in their noses and throats most of the time; these are held in check until the host's resistance is lowered. It is possible to "catch" a cold—from airborne droplets of a sneeze or from skin-to-skin or mucous membrane contact—though the hands are the greatest avenue for virus transmission. Cover your nose and mouth with a tissue or elbow when sneezing. You cannot catch a cold from getting a chill, though chills may lower your resistance to a pathogenic virus.

Although numerous theories exist concerning how to "cure" the common cold, including taking vitamin C, zinc, or echinacea, there's little proof of their efficacy.[15] The best rule of thumb is to keep your resistance high via diet, rest, reduced stress, and exercise. Avoid people with newly developed colds (during the first 24 hours of onset). Wash your hands often, and keep them away from your nose, mouth, and eyes.

If you contract a cold, rest, fluids, and a healthy diet can help you recover quickly. Children should not be given aspirin for colds or flu; this could lead to development of *Reye's syndrome*, a potentially fatal disease. Nonaspirin over-the-counter preparations are effective for alleviating symptoms.

36,000

Americans die of the flu each year.

Influenza

In otherwise healthy people, **influenza**, or flu, is usually not life threatening (see **Figure 12.4**). However, for individuals over 65, under 5, or with respiratory problems or heart disease, it can be very serious. Five to 20 percent of Americans get the flu each year; of these, 200,000 need hospitalization.[16] Treatment is *palliative*—focused on symptom relief rather than cure.

Three varieties of flu virus have been discovered, with many strains within each. The A form of the virus is generally the most virulent, followed by B and C. Immunity to one form doesn't necessarily convey immunity to others. New strains appear all the time; in 2009, H1N1 (swine flu) rose to pandemic levels.

Some vaccines have proven effective against certain strains of flu virus, but ineffective against others. In spite of minor risks, people over age 65, pregnant women, people with heart or lung disease, and people with certain other illnesses should be vaccinated. Flu shots take 2 to 3 weeks to become effective, so people at risk should get these shots in the fall before the flu season begins.

Infectious Mononucleosis

Initial symptoms of **mononucleosis**, or "mono," include sore throat, fever, headache, nausea, chills, and pervasive weakness or fatigue. Later, lymph nodes and the spleen may enlarge, and body rashes, aching joints, and jaundice (yellowing of the whites of the eyes and the skin) may occur.

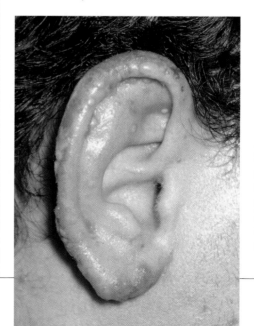

A series of fluid-filled blisters on the face, neck, or torso can be a sign of herpes gladiatorum. This form of herpes is easily spread, especially among athletes.

SYMPTOMS	COLD	FLU
Fever	Rare	Usual; high (100–102°F, occasionally higher, especially in children); lasts 3–4 days
Headache	Rare	Common
General aches and pains	Slight	Usual; often severe
Fatigue, weakness	Sometimes	Usual; can last up to 2–3 weeks
Extreme exhaustion	Never	Usual; at the beginning of the illness
Stuffy nose	Common	Sometimes
Sneezing	Usual	Sometimes
Sore throat	Common	Sometimes
Chest discomfort, cough	Common; mild to moderate, hacking cough	Common; can become severe
TREATMENT	Antihistamines, decongestants, nonsteroidal anti-inflammatory medicines	Antiviral medicines—see your doctor
PREVENTION	Wash your hands often with soap and water; avoid close contact with anyone with a cold	Annual vaccination; antiviral medicines—see your doctor
COMPLICATIONS	Sinus congestion, middle ear infection, asthma	Bronchitis, pneumonia; can worsen chronic conditions; can be life threatening

Figure 12.4 Is It a Cold or the Flu?
Source: Adapted from the National Institute of Allergy and Infectious Diseases, "Is It a Cold or the Flu?", 2008, www.niaid.nih.gov/topics/flu/documents/sick.pdf.

major health problem, with over 400 million chronic carriers and an estimated 620,000 deaths each year.[19]

Hepatitis C (HCV) infections are on an epidemic rise, because resistant forms of the virus are emerging. Some cases can be traced to blood transfusions or organ transplants. An estimated 17,000 new cases occur in the United States each year, with approximately 3.2 million people chronically infected.[20] Between 75 and 85 percent develop chronic infections; without treatment, infected people may develop cirrhosis of the liver, liver cancer, or liver failure.[21] Currently, no vaccine is available for HCV.

To prevent spread of HBV and HCV, use latex condoms every time you have sex; don't share personal-care items that might have blood on them, such as razors or toothbrushes; get a blood test for HBV; never share needles; if you are having body art done, go only to reputable artists or piercers who follow established sterilization and infection-control protocols.

Herpes Viruses

Herpes viruses are among the more common viruses infecting humans; painful, blistering rashes are hallmarks of these infections. These diseases are easily transmitted via physical contact and can become chronic problems.

Caused by the *herpes varicella zoster virus (HVZV)*, **chickenpox** produces symptoms of fever and fatigue 13 to 17 days after exposure, followed by skin eruptions that itch, blister, and produce a clear fluid. The virus is present in these blisters for approximately 1 week. A vaccine for chickenpox is available.

Without vaccination, the chickenpox virus can become reactivated under high stress or when the immune system is taxed by other diseases. This painful, blistering rash with other possible complications is called **shingles**; it affects over 1 million people in the United States, most over age 60. A vaccine for those over age 60 is now recommended.[22]

Herpes gladiatorum is caused by the herpes simplex type 1 virus. It is prevalent among those engaging in contact sports such as wrestling. Highly contagious via mats used by many people, for example, in a yoga studio or gym, or body-to-body contact, herpes gladiatorum is also referred to as "mat pox" or "wrestler's herpes." Symptoms of blistering rash and pain are common, particularly on the face, neck, and torso.

Herpes infections that are sexually transmitted are discussed later in this chapter.

Caused by the Epstein-Barr virus, mononucleosis is readily detected through a blood test. Despite its nickname "the kissing disease," mono does not appear to be easily contracted through normal, everyday personal contact. Treatment is often a lengthy process that involves bed rest, balanced nutrition, and medications.

Hepatitis

Hepatitis is a virally caused inflammation of the liver. Symptoms include fever, headache, nausea, loss of appetite, skin rashes, pain in the upper right abdomen, dark yellow-brown urine, and jaundice. Hepatitis has several known forms (A, B, C, D, and E), with A, B, and C the most common.

Hepatitis A (HAV) is contracted by eating food or drinking water contaminated with human feces. Since vaccinations became available, U.S. HAV rates have declined by nearly 90 percent. However, over 25,000 people per year are still infected.[17] Handlers of infected food, children at day care centers, those having sexual contact with HAV-positive individuals, or those traveling to regions where HAV is endemic are at higher risk, as are those who ingest seafood from contaminated water or use contaminated needles. Fortunately, individuals infected with hepatitis A don't become chronic carriers. Many are asymptomatic (symptom-free).

Hepatitis B (HBV) is spread through unprotected sex; sharing needles when injecting drugs; needlesticks on the job; or, for newborns, an infected mother. It can lead to chronic liver disease or liver cancer. In spite of vaccine availability, over 1.2 million people in the United States are chronically infected, with over 43,000 new cases each year.[18] Although global HBV infections have declined, they continue to be a

check yourself

- List three illnesses or conditions that can result from viral infection.

Other Pathogens and Emerging Diseases

■ **Describe how fungi, protozoans, parasitic worms, and prions cause infection.**

■ **Explain the problem of emerging and resurgent diseases.**

Bacteria and viruses account for many, but not all, common diseases. Other organisms can also infect a host.

Our environment is inhabited by hundreds of species of **fungi**, multi- or unicellular organisms that obtain food by infiltrating the bodies of other organisms, both living and dead. Many fungi, such as edible mushrooms, penicillin, and the yeast used to make bread, are useful to humans, but some species can produce infections. *Candidiasis* (vaginal yeast infection), ringworm, jock itch, and toenail fungus are common fungal diseases.

Protozoans are microscopic single-celled organisms associated with tropical diseases such as African sleeping sickness and malaria. The most common protozoan disease in the United States is the often sexually transmitted *trichomoniasis*. A common waterborne protozoan disease, *giardiasis*, can cause intestinal pain and discomfort.

Parasitic worms are the largest of the pathogens. Ranging in size from small pinworms to large tapeworms, most are more a nuisance than a threat.

A **prion** is a self-replicating, protein-based agent that can infect humans and other animals. One is believed to cause *bovine spongiform encephalopathy* (BSE, or "mad cow disease"). A similar prion causes *variant Creutzfeldt-Jakob disease* (vCJD) in humans.[23] Both are fatal brain diseases with multiyear incubation periods.

Emerging and Resurgent Diseases

Although our immune systems are adept at responding to challenges, microbes and other pathogens appear to be gaining ground. Rates of infectious diseases have rapidly increased over the past decade, due to a combination of overpopulation, inadequate health care, increasing poverty, environmental degradation, and drug resistance.[24]

Dengue *Dengue* viruses are the most widespread mosquito-borne viruses. Fifty to 100 million infections occur yearly with over 22,000 deaths, mostly among children.[25] Several thousand U.S. citizens get dengue each year, mostly in Puerto Rico, the U.S. Virgin Islands, Samoa, and Guam.[26] Symptoms include nausea, aches, and chronic fatigue and weakness. *Dengue hemor-*

Mosquitoes spread many diseases, including dengue and malaria.

rhagic fever, a more serious form of the disease, causes capillaries to spill fluid and blood into surrounding tissue.

West Nile Virus *West Nile virus* (WNV) is spread by infected mosquitoes. Several thousand cases surface in the United States every year; though most people have mild or no symptoms, WNV can result in chronic disability or death, most often for the elderly and those with impaired immune systems.[27] Symptoms include fever, headache, and body aches (often with skin rash and swollen lymph glands) and encephalitis (inflammation of the brain). No vaccine or specific treatment is available; avoiding mosquito bites is the best prevention.[28]

Avian (Bird) Flu *Avian influenza* is an infectious disease of birds. A recent strain, H5N1, is capable of crossing the species barrier and causing severe illness in humans.[29] Although the virus has yet to mutate into a form highly infectious to humans, outbreaks in which people contract the disease from birds have occurred. As of August 2010, the WHO had recorded 503 cases in humans, with 299 deaths.[30]

***Escherichia coli* O157:H7** *Escherichia coli* O157:H7 is one of over 170 types of *E. coli* bacteria that can infect humans. Most *E. coli* organisms are harmless and live in the intestines of healthy animals and humans. *E. coli* O157:H7, however, produces a lethal toxin and can cause severe illness or death. Eating ground beef that is rare or undercooked, drinking unpasteurized milk or juice, or swimming in sewage-contaminated water or public pools can also cause infection via ingestion of infected fecal matter.

Listeriosis Foods that are improperly cooked or that don't require cooking (such as luncheon meats) are susceptible to transmitting the bacterium responsible for listeriosis. Symptoms begin with mild fever and progress to headache and inflammation of the brain. The immunocompromised and pregnant women are at greatest risk. Listeria-tainted cantaloupes recently caused 16 deaths in Colorado.

Malaria *Malaria*, a disease caused by a parasite and transmitted by the *Anopheles* mosquito, causes more than 500 million cases of illness and 1 million deaths each year, mostly in sub-Saharan Africa, Latin America, the Middle East, and parts of Europe.[31] Travelers from malaria-free regions are highly vulnerable.[32]

■ **What are three emerging or resurgent diseases that threaten global health?**

Antibiotic Resistance

■ **Explain the phenomenon of antibiotic resistance.**

Antibiotics are supposed to wipe out bacteria that are susceptible to them. However, many common antibiotics are becoming ineffective against resistant strains of bacteria. How this happens: Bacteria and other microorganisms that cause infections and diseases can evolve rapidly, developing ways to survive drugs that had once been able to kill or weaken them. Through this process, some of the bacteria and microorganisms are becoming "superbugs" that cannot be stopped with existing medications.

Antibiotic Resistance on the Rise

Antibiotic resistance is a problem today for several reasons:[33]

■ **Improper use of antibiotics and resulting growth of superbugs.** When used improperly, antibiotics kill only the weak bacteria, leaving the strongest to thrive and replicate. Bacteria can swap genes with one another under the right conditions, so hardy drug-resistant germs can share their resistance mechanisms with other germs. These germs adapt and mutate, and eventually an entire colony of resistant bugs grows and passes on its resistance traits to new generations of bacteria.

Over time, most pathogens evolve, but human negligence can speed the resistant ones on their journey. If a patient begins an antibiotic regimen, but stops taking the drug as soon as symptoms abate rather than finishing the course of antibiotics, then the surviving bacteria build immunity to the drugs used to treat them. Doctors also overprescribe antibiotics: The Centers for Disease Control and Prevention (CDC) estimates that one-third of the 150 million antibiotic prescriptions written each year are unnecessary, resulting in bacterial strains that are tougher than the drugs used to fight them.

■ **Overuse of antibiotics in food production.** About 70 percent of antibiotic production today is used to treat sick animals living in crowded feedlots and to encourage growth in livestock and poultry. Farmed fish may also be given antibiotics to fight off disease in controlled water areas. Although research in this area is in its infancy, many believe that ingesting meats, animal products, and fish full of antibiotics may contribute to antibiotic resistance in humans. In addition, water runoff and sewage from feedlots can contaminate the water in rivers and streams with antibiotics.

■ **Misuse and overuse of antibacterial soaps and other cleaning products.** Preying on the public's fear of germs and disease, the cleaning industry adds antibacterial ingredients to many of its dish soaps, hand cleaners, shower scrubs, surface scrubs, and other household products. Just how much these products contribute to overall resistance is difficult to assess; as with antibiotics, the germs these products do not kill may become stronger than before.

What Can You Do?

You can take the following steps to prevent antibiotic resistance:

■ **Be responsible with medications.** To help prevent antibiotic resistance, use antimicrobial drugs only for bacterial, not viral, infections. Take medications as prescribed and finish the full course. Consult with your health care provider if you feel it is necessary to stop your medication.

■ **Use regular soap, not antibacterial soap, when washing your hands.** Some experts say that antibacterial cleaning products do more harm than good. Research suggests that antibacterial agents contained in soaps actually may kill normal bacteria, thus creating an environment for resistant, mutated bacteria that are impervious to antibacterial cleaners and antibiotics.

■ **Avoid food treated with antibiotics.** Buy meat from animals that were not unnecessarily dosed with antibiotics. (Look for that information on the label of meat products.)

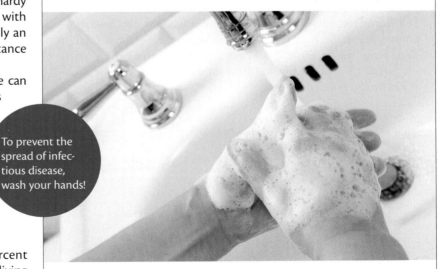

To prevent the spread of infectious disease, wash your hands!

check yourself

■ **How do bacteria become resistant to antibiotics?**
■ **What can you do to prevent antibiotic resistance?**

Sexually Transmitted Infections

- **Identify how sexually transmitted infections are transmitted.**

- **List steps to take to protect yourself against sexually transmitted infections.**

There are more than 20 known types of **sexually transmitted infections (STIs)**. Once referred to as *venereal diseases* and then *sexually transmitted diseases*, the current terminology is more reflective of the number and types of these communicable diseases and also of the fact that they are caused by infecting pathogens. More virulent strains and antibiotic-resistant forms spell trouble in the days ahead.

If you live in the United States, you have a 1 in 2 chance of getting an STI by age 25. Every year, there are at least 19 million new cases of STIs, only some of which are curable.[34] STIs affect men and women of all backgrounds and socioeconomic levels. However, they disproportionately affect women, minorities, and infants. In addition, STIs are most prevalent in teens and young adults.[35]

Early symptoms of STIs are often mild and unrecognizable. Left untreated, however, some of these infections can have grave consequences, such as sterility, blindness, central nervous system destruction, disfigurement, and even death. Infants born to mothers carrying the organisms for these infections are at risk for a variety of health problems.

As with many communicable diseases, much of the pain and suffering associated with STIs can be eliminated through education, responsible action, simple preventive strategies, and prompt treatment. Anyone can contract an STI, but you can avoid them if you take appropriate precautions when you decide to engage in a sexual relationship.

What's Your Risk?

Several reasons have been proposed to explain the present high rates of STIs. The first relates to the moral and social stigmas associated with these infections. Shame and embarrassment often keep infected people from seeking treatment. Unfortunately, the infected usually continue to be sexually active, thereby infecting unsuspecting partners. People who are uncomfortable discussing sexual issues may also be less likely to use, and ask their partners to use, condoms to protect against STIs and pregnancy.

Another reason proposed for the STI epidemic is our casual attitude about sex. Bombarded by a media that glamorizes sex, many people take sexual partners without considering the consequences. Others are pressured into sexual relationships they don't really want. Generally, the more sexual partners a person has, the greater the risk for contracting an STI.

Ignorance—about the infections, their symptoms, and the fact that someone can be asymptomatic but still infected—is also a factor. A person who is infected but asymptomatic can unknowingly spread an STI to an unsuspecting partner, who may, in turn, ignore or misinterpret any symptoms. By the time either partner seeks medical help, he or she may have infected several others. In addition, many people mistakenly believe that certain sexual practices—oral sex, for example—carry no risk for STIs. In fact, oral sex practices among young adults may be responsible for increases

High-risk behaviors	Moderate-risk behaviors	Low-risk behaviors	No-risk behaviors
Unprotected vaginal, anal, and oral sex—any activity that involves direct contact with bodily fluids, such as ejaculate, vaginal secretions, or blood—are high-risk behaviors.	Vaginal, anal, or oral sex with a latex or polyurethane condom and a water-based lubricant used properly and consistently can greatly reduce the risk of STI transmission. Dental dams used during oral sex can also greatly reduce the risk of STI transmission.	Mutual masturbation, if there are no cuts on the hand, penis, or vagina, is very low risk. Rubbing, kissing, and massaging carry low risk, but herpes can be spread by skin-to-skin contact from an infected partner.	Abstinence, phone sex, talking, and fantasy are all no-risk behaviors.

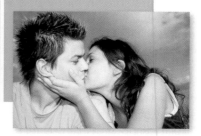

Figure 12.5 Continuum of Risk for Various Sexual Behaviors
Different behaviors have different levels of risk for various sexually transmitted infections (STIs); however, no matter what, any sexual activity involving direct contact with blood, semen, or vaginal secretions is high risk.

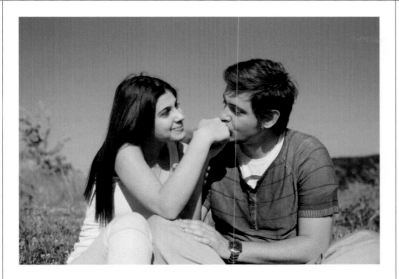

How can I tell if someone I'm dating has an STI?

You can't tell if someone has an STI just by looking at them; it isn't something broadcast on a person's face, and many people with STIs are themselves unaware of the infection because it could be asymptomatic. The only way to know for sure is to go to a clinic and get tested. In addition, partners need to be open and honest with each other about their sexual histories, and practice safer sex.

in herpes and other STIs. **Figure 12.5** shows the continuum of risk for various sexual behaviors. The Skills for Behavior Change offers tips for ways to practice safer sex.

Routes of Transmission

STIs are generally spread through some form of intimate sexual contact. Sexual intercourse, oral–genital contact, hand–genital contact, and anal intercourse are the most common modes of transmission. Less likely, but still possible, modes of transmission include mouth-to-mouth contact and contact with fluids from body sores that may be spread by the hands. Although each STI is a different infection caused by a different pathogen, all STI pathogens prefer dark, moist places, especially the mucous membranes lining the reproductive organs. Most of them are susceptible to light and excess heat, cold, and dryness, and many die quickly on exposure to air. Like other communicable infections, STIs have both pathogen-specific incubation periods and periods of time during which transmission is most likely, called *periods of communicability*.

Where to Go for Help

If you are concerned about your own risk or that of a friend, arrange a confidential meeting with a health professional at your college health service or community STI clinic. He or she will provide you with the information that you need to decide whether you should be tested for an STI.

Skills for Behavior Change

SAFE IS SEXY

Practicing the following behaviors will help you reduce your risk of contracting a sexually transmitted infection (STI):

- Avoid casual sexual partners. All sexually active adults who are not in a lifelong monogamous relationship should practice safer sex.
- Use latex condoms consistently and correctly. Remember that condoms do not provide 100 percent protection against all STIs.
- Postpone sexual involvement until you are assured that your partner is not infected; discuss past sexual history and, if necessary, get tested for any potential STIs.
- Avoid injury to body tissue during sexual activity. Some pathogens can enter the bloodstream through microscopic tears in anal or vaginal tissues.
- Avoid unprotected oral, anal, or vaginal sexual activity in which semen, blood, or vaginal secretions could penetrate mucous membranes or enter through breaks in the skin.
- Always use a condom or a dental dam (a sensitive latex sheet about the size of a tissue that can be placed over the female genitals to form a protective layer) during vaginal, oral, or anal sex.
- Avoid using drugs and alcohol, which can dull your senses and affect your ability to take responsible precautions with potential sex partners.
- Wash your hands before and after sexual encounters. Urinate after sexual relations and, if possible, wash your genitals.
- Total abstinence is the only absolute way to prevent the transmission of STIs, but abstinence can be a difficult choice to make. If you have any doubt about the potential risks of having sex, consider other means of intimacy (at least until you can assure your safety)—massage, dry kissing, hugging, holding and touching, and masturbation (alone or with a partner).
- Think about situations ahead of time to avoid risky behaviors, including settings with alcohol and drug use.
- If you are worried about your own HIV or STI status, have yourself tested. Don't risk infecting others.

Sources: American College of Obstetricians and Gynecologists (ACOG), *How to Prevent Sexually Transmitted Diseases*, ACOG Education Pamphlet AP009 (Washington, DC: American College of Obstetricians and Gynecologists, 2011), www.acog.org/publications/patient_education/bp009.cfm; American Social Health Association, "Sexual Health: Prevention Tips," 2010, www.ashastd.org/sexualhealth/reduce_risk_prevention_tips.cfm.

check yourself

- **How are STIs transmitted?**
- **What can you do to protect yourself against STIs?**

Sexually Transmitted Infections: HIV/AIDS

learning **outcomes**

- **Define HIV/AIDS and explain its transmittal and treatment.**

Acquired immunodeficiency syndrome (AIDS) is a significant global health threat. Since 1981, when AIDS was first recognized, approximately 65 million people worldwide have become infected with **human immunodeficiency virus (HIV)**, the virus that causes AIDS.

At the end of 2009, approximately 33.3 million people worldwide were living with HIV.[36] In the United States, approximately 1.1 million people have been infected with HIV and at least 576,384 have died.[37] In 2009, approximately 20,185 new HIV/AIDS cases were diagnosed in the United States.[38]

Initially, people were diagnosed as having AIDS only when they developed blood infections, the cancer known as Kaposi's sarcoma, or other indicator diseases common in male AIDS patients. The CDC has expanded the indicator list to include pulmonary tuberculosis, recurrent pneumonia, and invasive cervical cancer. Perhaps the most significant indicator today is a drop in the level of the body's master immune cells, CD4 cells (also called helper T cells), to one-fifth the level in a healthy person.

How HIV Is Transmitted

HIV typically enters one person's body via another person's infected body fluids (e.g., semen, vaginal secretions, blood), often through a break in the mucous membranes of the genital organs or the anus. After initial infection, HIV multiplies rapidly, progressively destroying helper T cells (which call the rest of the immune response to action), weakening the body's resistance to disease.

HIV cannot reproduce outside its living host, except in a controlled laboratory environment, and does not survive well in open air. It cannot be transmitted through casual contact.[39] Insect bites do not transmit HIV.[40]

High-Risk Behaviors AIDS is not a disease of gay people or minority groups; rather, it is related to high-risk behaviors such as having unprotected sexual intercourse and sharing needles. People who engage in high-risk behaviors increase their risk for the disease; people who do not have minimal risk. **Figure 12.6** shows the breakdown of sources of HIV infection among U.S. men and women.

The majority of HIV infections arise from the following high-risk behaviors:

- **Exchange of body fluids.** The greatest risk factor is the exchange of HIV-infected body fluids during vaginal or anal intercourse. Blood, semen, and vaginal secretions are the major fluids of concern.

- **Injecting drugs.** A significant percentage of AIDS cases in the United States result from sharing or using HIV-contaminated needles and syringes. Although users of illegal drugs are commonly considered the only members of this category, others may also share needles—for example, people with diabetes who inject insulin or athletes who inject steroids.

Mother-to-Child (Perinatal) Transmission This can occur during pregnancy, during labor and delivery, or through breastfeeding. Without antiretroviral treatment, approximately 25 percent of HIV-positive pregnant women will transmit the virus to their infants.[41]

Body Piercing and Tattooing Body piercing and tattooing can be done safely, but dangerous pathogens can be transmitted with any puncture of the skin. Unsterile needles can transmit staph, HIV, hepatitis B and C, tetanus, and other diseases. If you opt for tattooing or body piercing, take the following safety precautions:[42]

- Look for clean, well-lighted work areas and inquire about sterilization procedures.
- Packaged, sterilized needles should be used once, then discarded. A piercing gun cannot be sterilized properly. Watch that the artist uses new needles and tubes from a sterile package.
- Immediately before piercing or tattooing, the body area should be carefully sterilized. The artist should wash his or her hands and put on new latex gloves for each procedure.

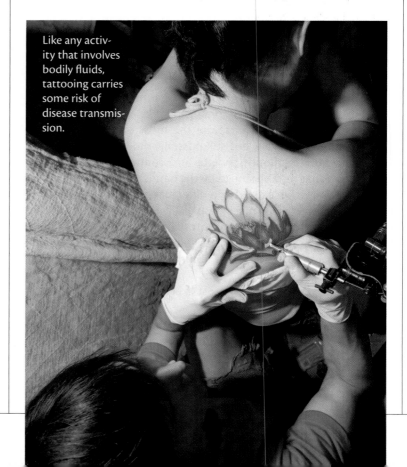

Like any activity that involves bodily fluids, tattooing carries some risk of disease transmission.

95%

of people with HIV worldwide live in developing nations

■Leftover tattoo ink should be discarded after each procedure. Do not allow the artist to reuse ink that has been used for other customers. Used needles should be disposed of in a "sharps" container.

Symptoms of HIV/AIDS

A person may go for months or years after infection by HIV before any significant symptoms appear; incubation time varies greatly from person to person. For adults who receive no medical treatment, it takes an average of 8 to 10 years for the virus to cause the slow, degenerative changes in the immune system that are characteristic of AIDS. During this time, the person may experience *opportunistic infections* (infections that gain a foothold when the immune system is not functioning effectively). Colds, sore throats, fever, tiredness, nausea, and night sweats commonly appear. Later symptoms include wasting syndrome, swollen lymph nodes, and neurological problems. As the immune system continues to decline, the body becomes more vulnerable to infection. A diagnosis of AIDS, the final stage of HIV infection, is made when the infected person has either a dangerously low CD4 (helper T) cell count (below 200 cells per cubic milliliter of blood) or has contracted one or more opportunistic infections characteristic of the disease (such as Kaposi's sarcoma or *Pneumocystis carinii* pneumonia).

Testing for HIV Antibodies

Once antibodies have formed in reaction to HIV, a blood test known as the *ELISA* (enzyme-linked immunosorbent assay) may detect their presence. It can take 3 to 6 months after initial infection for sufficient antibodies to develop in the body to show a positive test result. Therefore, individuals with negative test results should be retested within 6 months. When a person who previously tested *negative* (no HIV antibodies present) has a subsequent test that is *positive,* seroconversion is said to have occurred. In such a situation, the person would typically take another ELISA test, followed by a more precise test known as the *Western blot.* These are not AIDS tests per se. Rather, they detect antibodies for HIV, indicating the presence of the virus in the person's system.

Health officials distinguish between *reported* and *actual* cases of HIV infection because it is believed that many HIV-positive people avoid being tested. One reason is fear of knowing the truth. Another is the fear of recrimination from employers, insurance companies, and medical staff. However, early detection and reporting are important, because immediate treatment for someone in the early stages of HIV disease is critical.

Treatments and Prevention

New drugs have slowed the progression from HIV to AIDS and prolonged life expectancies for most AIDS patients. *Protease*

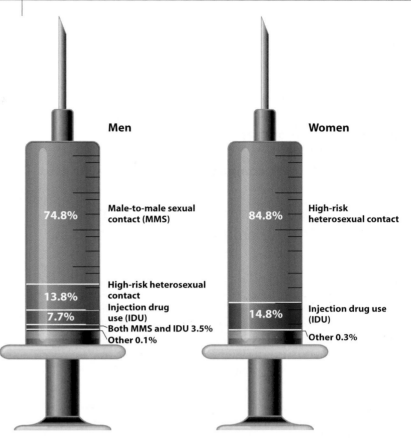

Men

74.8% — **Male-to-male sexual contact (MMS)**

13.8% — **High-risk heterosexual contact**

7.7% — **Injection drug use (IDU)**

Both MMS and IDU 3.5%

Other 0.1%

Women

84.8% — **High-risk heterosexual contact**

14.8% — **Injection drug use (IDU)**

Other 0.3%

Figure 12.6 Sources of HIV Infection in Men and Women in the United States, 2009

Source: Data from Centers for Disease Control and Prevention, *HIV Surveillance Report, 2009*, vol. 21, June 2011, www.cdc.gov/hiv/surveillance/resources/reports/2009report.

inhibitors (e.g., amprenavir, ritonavir, and saquinavir) act to prevent production of the virus in cells HIV has already invaded. Other drugs, such as AZT, ddI, ddC, d4T, and 3TC, inhibit the HIV enzyme *reverse transcriptase* before the virus has invaded the cell, thereby preventing infection of new cells.

Although these drugs provide longer survival rates for people with HIV, we are still a long way from a cure. Newer drugs that held promise are becoming less effective as HIV develops resistance to them. Costs of taking multiple drugs are prohibitive, and side effects are common.

Although scientists have been working on a variety of HIV vaccine trials, no vaccine is currently available. The only way to prevent HIV infection is through the choices you make in sexual behaviors and drug use and by taking responsibility for your own health and the health of your loved ones. So what should you do?

Of course, the simplest answer is abstinence. If you don't exchange body fluids, you won't get the disease. If you do decide to be intimate, the next best option is to use a condom.

check yourself

- **What are three common routes of transmission for HIV?**
- **What can you do to prevent the spread of HIV and to protect yourself against it?**

Sexually Transmitted Infections: Chlamydia and Gonorrhea

- **List the symptoms and treatment of chlamydia and gonorrhea.**
- **Identify common complications of STIs in women.**

Two of the most common sexually transmitted infections are chlamydia and gonorrhea.

Chlamydia

Chlamydia, an infection caused by the bacterium *Chlamydia trachomatis* that often presents no symptoms, is the most commonly reported STI in the United States. Chlamydia infects an estimated 2.8 million Americans annually, the majority of them women.[43] This estimate could be higher, because many cases go unreported.

Signs and Symptoms In men, early symptoms may include painful and difficult urination; frequent urination; and a watery, puslike discharge from the penis. Symptoms in women may include a yellowish discharge, spotting between periods, and occasional spotting after intercourse. However, many chlamydia victims display no symptoms and therefore do not seek help until the disease has done secondary damage. Women are especially likely to be asymptomatic; over 70 percent do not realize they have the disease, which can put them at risk for secondary damage.[44]

Complications The secondary damage resulting from chlamydia is serious in both men and women. Men can suffer injury to the prostate gland, seminal vesicles, and bulbourethral glands, and they can suffer from arthritis-like symptoms and inflammatory damage to the blood vessels and heart. Men can also experience epididymitis, inflammation of the area near the testicles. In women, chlamydia-related inflammation can injure the cervix or fallopian tubes, causing sterility, and it can damage the inner pelvic structure, leading to **pelvic inflammatory disease (PID)**. If an infected woman becomes pregnant, she has a high risk for miscarriage and stillbirth. Chlamydia may also be responsible for one type of *conjunctivitis*, an eye infection that affects not only adults but also infants, who can contract the disease from an infected mother during delivery (**Figure 12.7**). Untreated conjunctivitis can cause blindness.[45]

Diagnosis and Treatment Diagnosis of chlamydia is determined through a laboratory test. A sample of urine or fluid from the vagina or penis is collected to identify the presence of the bacteria. Unfortunately, chlamydia tests are not a routine part of many health clinics' testing procedures. Usually a person must specifically request one. If detected early, chlamydia is easily treatable with antibiotics such as tetracycline, doxycycline, or erythromycin.

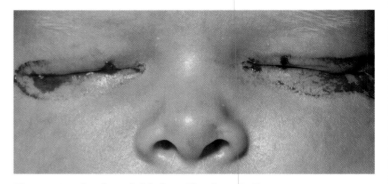

Figure 12.7 Conjunctivitis in a Newborn's Eyes
Untreated chlamydia and gonorrhea in a pregnant woman can be passed to her child during delivery, causing the eye infection conjunctivitis.

Gonorrhea

Gonorrhea is one of the most common STIs in the United States, surpassed only by chlamydia in number of cases. The CDC estimates that there are over 700,000 cases per year, plus numbers that go unreported.[46] Caused by the bacterial pathogen *Neisseria gonorrhoeae*, gonorrhea primarily infects the linings of the urethra, genital tract, pharynx, and rectum. It may spread to the eyes or other body regions by the hands or through body fluids, typically during vaginal, oral, or anal sex. Most cases occur in individuals between the ages of 20 and 24.[47]

Signs and Symptoms In men, a typical symptom is a white, milky discharge from the penis accompanied by painful, burning urination 2 to 9 days after contact (**Figure 12.8**). Epididymitis can also occur as a symptom of infection. However, some men with gonorrhea are asymptomatic.

In women, the situation is just the opposite: Most women do not experience any symptoms, but if a woman does experience symptoms, they can include vaginal discharge or a burning sensation on urinating.[48] The organism can remain in the woman's vagina, cervix, uterus, or fallopian tubes for long periods with no apparent symptoms other than an occasional slight fever. Thus a woman can be unaware that she has been infected and that she is infecting her sexual partners.

Complications In a man, untreated gonorrhea may spread to the prostate, testicles, urinary tract, kidney, and bladder. Blockage of the vasa deferentia due to scar tissue may cause sterility. In some cases, the penis develops a painful curvature during erection. If the infection goes undetected in a woman, it can spread to the fallopian tubes and ovaries, causing sterility or, at the very least, severe inflammation and PID. The bacteria can also spread up the reproductive tract or, more rarely, through the blood and infect the joints, heart valves, or brain. If an infected woman becomes pregnant, the infection can be transmitted to her baby during delivery, potentially causing blindness, joint infection, or a life-threatening blood infection.

Diagnosis and Treatment Diagnosis of gonorrhea is similar to that of chlamydia, requiring a sample of either urine or fluid from the vagina or penis to detect the presence of the bacteria. If detected early, gonorrhea is treatable with antibiotics, but the *Neisseria gonorrhoeae* bacterium has begun to develop resistance to some antibiotics. Chlamydia and gonorrhea often occur at the same time, though different antibiotics are needed to treat each infection separately.[49]

Complications of STIs in Women: PID and UTIs

Women disproportionately experience the long-term consequences of STIs. If not treated, up to 40 percent of women infected with *Neisseria gonorrhoeae* or *Chlamydia trachomatis* may develop pelvic inflammatory disease (PID). PID is a catchall term for infections of the uterus, fallopian tubes, and ovaries resulting from untreated STIs.[50]

Symptoms of PID vary but generally include lower abdominal pain, fever, unusual vaginal discharge, painful intercourse, painful urination, and irregular menstrual bleeding. The vague symptoms associated with chlamydial and gonococcal PID cause 85 percent of infected women to delay seeking medical care, thereby increasing the risk of permanent damage and scarring that can lead to infertility and ectopic pregnancy. Among women with PID, ectopic pregnancy (in which an embryo begins to develop outside of the uterus, usually in a fallopian tube) occurs in 9 percent and chronic pelvic pain in 18 percent.[51]

Women are also at greater risk than men for developing general urinary tract infection (UTIs).[52] UTIs can be caused by various factors, including untreated STIs. Women are disproportionately affected by UTIs because a woman's urethra is much shorter than a man's, making it easier for bacteria to enter the bladder. In addition, a woman's urethra is closer to her anus than is a man's, allowing bacteria to spread into her urethra and cause an infection. Symptoms of a UTI in women include a burning

sensation during urination and lower abdominal pain. A UTI can be diagnosed through a urine test and treated by antibiotics. If left untreated, UTIs can cause kidney damage.

Note that men can also get UTIs, although they are rarer than UTIs in women. One form is nongonoccocol urethritis, which is most commonly caused by *Chlamydia trachomatis*. Infections should be taken seriously—if you have a milky penile discharge and/or burning during urination, contact your health care provider.

The serious complications that can result from untreated STIs in women further illustrate the need for early diagnosis and treatment. Regular screening is particularly important, because women are often asymptomatic, increasing their risk of complications such as PID and UTIs. Data from a randomized trial of chlamydia screening in a managed care setting suggested that screening programs can reduce the incidence of PID by as much as 60 percent.

Skills for Behavior Change

COMMUNICATING ABOUT SAFER SEX

At no time in your life is it more important to communicate openly than when you are starting an intimate relationship. The following will help you communicate with your partner about potential risks:

- Plan to talk before you find yourself in an awkward situation.
- Select the right moment and place for both of you to discuss safer sex; choose a relaxing environment in a neutral location, free of distractions.
- Remember that you have a responsibility to your partner to disclose your own health status. You also have a responsibility to yourself to stay healthy.
- Be direct, honest, and determined in talking about sex before you become involved.
- Discuss the issues without sounding defensive or accusatory. Reassure your partner that your reasons for desiring abstinence or safer sex arise from respect and not distrust.
- Analyze your own beliefs and values ahead of time. Know where you will draw the line on certain actions, and be very clear with your partner about what you expect.
- Decide what you will do if your partner does not agree with you. Anticipate potential objections or excuses, and prepare your responses accordingly.

Source: Adapted from Queensland Health, "Talking to Your Partner about Sex," 2010, www.health.qld.gov.au/istaysafe/lets-talk-about-sex/talking-to-partner .aspx.

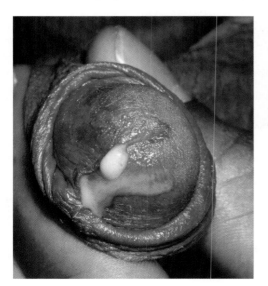

Figure 12.8
Gonorrhea
One common symptom of gonorrhea in men is a milky discharge from the penis, accompanied by burning sensations during urination. Whereas these symptoms will cause most men to seek diagnosis and treatment, women with gonorrhea are often asymptomatic, so they may not be aware they are infected.

check yourself

- **What are the primary signs of chlamydia? Of gonorrhea?**
- **How does PID affect fertility in women?**

Sexually Transmitted Infections: Syphilis

- **List the symptoms and treatment of syphilis in men and women.**

Syphilis is caused by a bacterium, the spirochete *Treponema pallidum*. The incidence of syphilis is highest in both men and women aged 20 to 24. The incidence of syphilis in newborns has continued to increase in the United States.[53] Because it is extremely delicate and dies readily on exposure to air, dryness, or cold, the organism is generally transferred only through direct sexual contact or from mother to fetus.

Signs and Symptoms

Syphilis is known as the "great imitator," because its symptoms resemble those of several other infections. It should be noted, however, that some people experience no symptoms at all. Syphilis can occur in four distinct stages:[54]

- **Primary syphilis.** The first stage of syphilis, particularly for men, is often characterized by the development of a **chancre** (pronounced "shank-er"), a sore located most frequently at the site of initial infection that usually appears 3 to 4 weeks after initial infection (see **Figure 12.9**). In men, the site of the chancre tends to be the penis or scrotum; in women, the site of infection is often internal, on the vaginal wall or high on the cervix, where the chancre is not readily apparent and the likelihood of detection is not great. Whether or not it is detected, the chancre is oozing with bacteria, ready to infect an unsuspecting partner. In both men and women, the chancre will disappear in 3 to 6 weeks.
- **Secondary syphilis.** If the infection is left untreated, a month to a year after the chancre disappears, secondary symptoms may appear, including a rash or white patches on the skin or on the mucous membranes of the mouth, throat, or genitals. Hair loss may occur, lymph nodes may enlarge, and the victim may develop a slight fever or headache. In rare cases, sores develop around the mouth or genitals. As during the active chancre phase, these sores contain infectious bacteria, and contact with them can spread the infection.
- **Latent syphilis.** After the secondary stage, if the infection is left untreated, the syphilis spirochetes begin to invade body organs, causing lesions called *gummas*. The infection now is rarely transmitted to others, except during pregnancy, when it can be passed to the fetus.

- **Tertiary/late syphilis.** Years after syphilis has entered the body, its effects become all too evident if still untreated. Late-stage syphilis indications include heart and central nervous system damage, blindness, deafness, paralysis, premature senility, and, ultimately, dementia.

Complications

Pregnant women with syphilis can experience complications such as premature births, miscarriages, and stillbirths. An infected pregnant woman may transmit the syphilis to her unborn child. The infant will then be born with *congenital syphilis*, which can cause death; severe birth defects such as blindness, deafness, or disfigurement; developmental delays; seizures; and other health problems. Because in most cases the fetus does not become infected until after the first trimester, treatment of the mother during this time will usually prevent infection of the fetus.

Diagnosis and Treatment

Two methods can be used to diagnose syphilis. In the primary stage, a sample from the chancre is collected to identify the bacteria. Another method of diagnosing syphilis is through a blood test. Syphilis can easily be treated with antibiotics, usually penicillin, for all stages except the late stage.

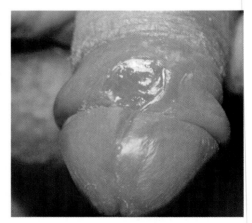

Figure 12.9 Syphilis A chancre on the site of the initial infection is a symptom of primary syphilis.

- **What are the four stages of untreated syphilis?**

Sexually Transmitted Infections: Herpes

learning outcomes

- **List the symptoms and treatment of both types of herpes simplex virus.**

Herpes is a general term for a family of infections characterized by sores or eruptions on the skin that are caused by the herpes simplex virus. The herpes family of diseases is not transmitted exclusively by sexual contact; kissing or sharing eating utensils can also transmit the infection.

Herpes infections range from mildly uncomfortable to extremely serious. **Genital herpes** affects approximately 16.2 percent of the population aged 14 to 49 in the United States.[55]

The two types of herpes simplex virus are HSV-1 and HSV-2. Only about 1 in 6 Americans currently has HSV-2; however, 50 to 80 percent of adults have HSV-1, usually appearing as cold sores on the mouth.[56] Both herpes simplex types 1 and 2 can infect any area of the body, producing lesions (sores) in and around the vaginal area; on the penis; and around the anal opening, buttocks, thighs, or mouth (see **Figure 12.10**). Herpes simplex virus remains in nerve cells for life and can flare up when the body's ability to maintain itself is weakened.

Signs and Symptoms

The precursor phase of a herpes infection is characterized by a burning sensation and redness at the site of infection. During this time, prescription or over-the-counter medications can keep the disease from spreading. However, this phase is quickly followed by the second phase, in which a blister filled with a clear fluid containing the virus forms. If you pick at this blister or otherwise spread this fluid with fingers, lipstick, etc., you can autoinoculate other body parts. Particularly dangerous is the possibility of spreading the infection to your eyes, which can cause blindness.

Over a period of days, the blister will crust over, dry up, and disappear, and the virus will travel to the base of an affected nerve supplying the area and become dormant. Only when the victim becomes overly stressed, when diet and sleep are inadequate, when the immune system is overworked, or when excessive exposure to sunlight or other stressors occur will the virus become reactivated (at the same site) and begin the blistering cycle again. Each time a sore develops, it casts off (sheds) viruses that can be highly infectious. However, a herpes site also can shed the virus when no overt sore is present, particularly during the interval between the earliest symptoms and blistering. People may get genital herpes by having sexual contact with others who don't know they are infected or who are having outbreaks of herpes without any sores. A person with genital herpes can also infect a sexual partner during oral sex. The virus is spread rarely, if at all, by touching objects such as a toilet seat.

Complications

Genital herpes is especially serious in pregnant women because the baby can be infected as it passes through the vagina during birth. Many physicians recommend cesarean deliveries for infected women. Additionally, women with a history of genital herpes appear to have a greater risk of developing cervical cancer.

Diagnosis and Treatment

Diagnosis involves a blood test or analyzing a sample from the suspected sore. Although there is no cure for herpes at present, certain drugs can be used to treat symptoms. Unfortunately, they seem to work only if the infection is confirmed during the first few hours after contact. The effectiveness of other treatments, such as L-lysine, is largely unsubstantiated. Over-the-counter medications may reduce the length of time of sores/symptoms. Other drugs, such as famciclovir (FAMVIR), may reduce viral shedding between outbreaks, possibly reducing risks to sexual partners.[57]

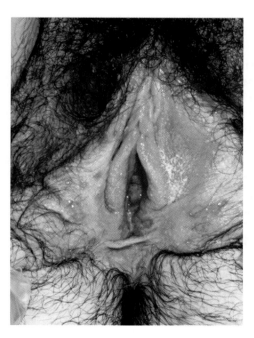

Figure 12.10 Herpes
Both genital and oral herpes can be caused by either herpes simplex virus type 1 or 2.

check yourself

- **What are the primary signs of and treatments for herpes?**

Sexually Transmitted Infections: Human Papillomavirus

- **List the various problems caused by human papillomavirus.**

Genital warts (*venereal warts or condylomas*) are caused by a group of viruses known as **human papillomavirus (HPV)**. There are over 100 different types of HPV; more than 30 types are sexually transmitted and classified as either low risk or high risk.

A person becomes infected when certain types of HPV penetrate the skin and mucous membranes of the genitals or anus. This is among the most common STIs, with 20 million Americans infected with genital HPV and approximately 6 million new cases each year.[58]

Signs and Symptoms

Genital HPV appears relatively easy to catch. The typical incubation period is 6 to 8 weeks after contact. People infected with low-risk HPV may develop genital warts, a series of bumps or growths on the genitals (see **Figure 12.11**).

Complications

Infection with high-risk types of HPV may lead to cervical *dysplasia*, or changes in cells that may lead to a precancerous condition. Exactly how high-risk HPV infection leads to cervical cancer is uncertain. Six out of 10 cervical cancers occur in women who have never received a Pap test or have not been tested for HPV in the past 5 years.[59]

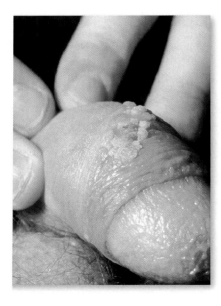

Figure 12.11
Genital Warts
Genital warts are caused by certain types of the human papillomavirus.

Of those cases that become precancerous and are left untreated, 70 percent result in cancer. In addition, HPV may pose a threat to a fetus exposed to the virus during birth.

Diagnosis and Treatment

Diagnosis of genital warts from low-risk types of HPV is determined through visual examination by a health care provider. High-risk types can be diagnosed in women through microscopic analysis of cells from a Pap smear or by collecting a sample from the cervix to test for HPV DNA. There is currently no HPV DNA test for men.

Treatment is available only for the low-risk forms of HPV that cause genital warts. The warts can be treated with topical medication or frozen with liquid nitrogen and then removed. Large warts may require surgical removal.

HPV Vaccines

Most sexually active people will contract some form of human papillomavirus (HPV) at some time in their lives, though they may never know it. Of the approximately 40 types of sexually transmitted HPV, most cause no symptoms and go away on their own. Low-risk types can cause genital warts, but some high-risk types can cause cervical cancer in women and other less common genital cancers. Currently, two HPV vaccines, Cervarix and Gardasil, can help prevent women from becoming infected with HPV and subsequently developing cervical cancer.

HPV vaccines are recommended for 11- and 12-year-old girls and can also be given to girls 9 or older. It is also recommended for girls and women aged 13 through 26 who have not yet been vaccinated or completed the vaccine series. One of the HPV vaccines, Gardasil, is also licensed for males aged 9 through 26; they may choose to get this vaccine to prevent genital warts. (Only Gardasil protects against low-risk HPV types 6 and 11; because these HPV types cause 90 percent of cases of genital warts in females and males, Gardasil is approved for use with males as well as females.[60]) New research is being done on the vaccines' safety and efficacy in those over 26.

Note that neither vaccine protects against all types of HPV or prevents all cases of cervical cancer. Women should continue getting screened for cervical cancer (through regular Pap tests). Also, the vaccines do not prevent other STIs, so it is still important for sexually active persons to lower their risk for other STIs.

- **How can women guard themselves against HPV-linked cervical cancer?**

Other Sexually Transmitted Infections

■ **List the symptoms and treatment of other common STIs.**

Several other sexually transmitted infections have less serious effects than infections such as HIV and syphilis, but nevertheless should be avoided.

Candidiasis (Moniliasis)

Most STIs are caused by pathogens that come from outside the body; however, the yeastlike fungus *Candida albicans* is a normal inhabitant of the vaginal tract in most women. (See **Figure 12.3** for a micrograph of this fungus.) Only when the normal chemical balance of the vagina is disturbed will these organisms multiply and cause the fungal disease **candidiasis**, also sometimes called *moniliasis* or a *yeast infection*.

Signs and Symptoms Symptoms of candidiasis include severe itching and burning of the vagina and vulva and a white, cheesy vaginal discharge.[61] When this microbe infects the mouth, whitish patches form, and the condition is referred to as *thrush*. Thrush infection can also occur in men and is easily transmitted between sexual partners. Symptoms of candidiasis can be aggravated by contact with soaps, douches, perfumed toilet paper, chlorinated water, and spermicides.

Diagnosis and Treatment Diagnosis of candidiasis is usually made by collecting a vaginal sample and analyzing it to identify the pathogen. Antifungal drugs applied on the surface or by suppository usually cure candidiasis in just a few days.

Trichomoniasis

Unlike many STIs, **trichomoniasis** is caused by a protozoan, *Trichomonas vaginalis*. (See **Figure 12.3** for a micrograph of this organism.) An estimated 7.4 million new cases occur in the United States each year, although most people who contract it remain free of symptoms.[62]

Signs and Symptoms Symptoms among women include a foamy, yellowish, unpleasant-smelling discharge accompanied by a burning sensation, itching, and painful urination. Most men with trichomoniasis do not have any symptoms, though some men experience irritation inside the penis, mild discharge, and a slight burning after urinating.[63] Although usually transmitted by sexual contact, the "trich" organism can also be spread by toilet seats, wet towels, or other items that have discharged fluids on them.

Diagnosis and Treatment Diagnosis of trichomoniasis is determined by collecting fluid samples from the penis or vagina to test for the presence of the protozoan. Treatment includes oral metronidazole, usually given to both sexual partners to avoid the possible "ping-pong" effect of repeated cross-infection typical of STIs.

Pubic Lice

Pubic lice, often called "crabs," are small parasitic insects that are usually transmitted during sexual contact (see **Figure 12.12**). More annoying than dangerous, they move easily from partner to partner during sex. They have an affinity for pubic hair and attach themselves to the base of these hairs, where they deposit their eggs (nits). One to 2 weeks later, the nits develop into adults that lay eggs and migrate to other body parts, thus perpetuating the cycle.

Signs and Symptoms Symptoms of pubic lice infestation include itchiness in the area covered by pubic hair, bluish-gray skin color in the pubic region, and sores in the genital area.

Diagnosis and Treatment Diagnosis of pubic lice involves an examination by a health care provider to identify the eggs in the genital area. Treatment includes washing clothing, furniture, and linens that may harbor the eggs. It usually takes 2 to 3 weeks to kill all larval forms. Although sexual contact is the most common mode of transmission, you can "catch" pubic lice from lying on sheets or sitting on a toilet seat that an infected person has used.

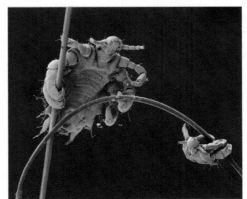

Figure 12.12
Pubic Lice
Pubic lice, also known as "crabs," are small, parasitic insects that attach themselves to pubic hair.

■ **Describe symptoms and treatment of candidiasis and trichomoniasis.**

■ **How are pubic lice transmitted and treated?**

Assessyourself

STIs: Do You Really Know What You Think You Know?

The following quiz will help you evaluate whether your beliefs and attitudes about sexually transmitted infections (STIs) lead you to behaviors that increase your risk of infection. Indicate whether you believe the following items are true or false, then consult the answer key that follows.

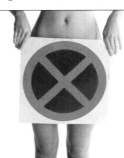

An interactive version of this assessment is available online. Download it from the Live It! section of www.pearsonhighered.com/donatelle.

TRUE **FALSE**

1. You can always tell when you've got an STI because the symptoms are so obvious. ○ ○

2. Some STIs can be passed on by skin-to-skin contact in the genital area. ○ ○

3. Herpes can be transmitted only when a person has visible sores on his or her genitals. ○ ○

4. Oral sex is safe sex. ○ ○

5. Condoms reduce your risk of both pregnancy and STIs. ○ ○

6. As long as you don't have anal intercourse, you can't get HIV. ○ ○

7. All sexually active females should have a regular Pap smear. ○ ○

8. Once genital warts have been removed, there is no risk of passing on the virus. ○ ○

9. You can get several STIs at one time. ○ ○

10. If the signs of an STI go away, you are cured. ○ ○

11. People who get STIs have a lot of sex partners. ○ ○

12. All STIs can be cured. ○ ○

13. You can get an STI more than once. ○ ○

Answer Key

1. **False.** The unfortunate fact is that many STIs show no symptoms. This has serious implications: (a) you can be passing on the infection without knowing it and (b) the pathogen may be damaging your reproductive organs without you knowing it.

2. **True.** Some viruses can be present on the skin around the genital area. Herpes and genital warts are the main culprits.

3. **False.** Herpes is most easily passed on when the sores and blisters are present, because the fluid in the lesions carries the virus. But the virus is also found on the skin around the genital area. Most people contract herpes this way, unaware that the virus is present.

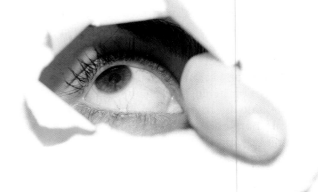

4. False. Oral sex is not safe sex. Herpes, genital warts, and chlamydia can all be passed on through oral sex. Condoms should be used on the penis. Dental dams should be placed over the female genitals during oral sex.

5. True. Condoms significantly reduce the risk of pregnancy when used correctly. They also reduce the risk of STIs. It is important to point out that abstinence is the only behavior that provides complete protection against pregnancy and STIs.

6. False. HIV is present in blood, semen, and vaginal fluid. Any activity that allows for the transfer of these fluids is risky. Anal intercourse is a high-risk activity, especially for the receptive (passive) partner, but other sexual activity is also a risk. When you don't know your partner's sexual history and you're not in a long-term monogamous relationship, condoms are a must.

7. True. A Pap smear is a simple procedure involving the scraping of a small amount of tissue from the surface of the cervix (at the upper end of the vagina). The sample is tested for abnormal cells that may indicate cancer. All sexually active women should have regular Pap smears.

8. False. Genital warts, which may be present on the penis, the anus, and inside and outside the

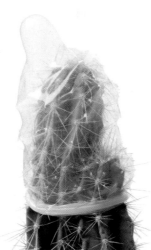

vagina, can be removed. However, the virus that caused the warts will always be present in the body and can be passed on to a sexual partner.

9. True. It is possible to have many STIs at one time. In fact, having one STI may make it more likely that a person will acquire more STIs. For example, the open sore from herpes creates a place where HIV can easily be transmitted.

10. False. The symptoms may go away, but your body is still infected. For example, syphilis is characterized by various stages. In the first stage, a painless sore called a chancre appears for about a week and then goes away.

11. False. If you have sex once with an infected partner, you are at risk for an STI.

12. False. Some STIs are viruses and therefore cannot be cured. There is no cure at present for herpes, HIV/AIDS, or genital warts. These STIs are treatable (to lessen the pain and irritation of symptoms), but not curable.

13. True. Experiencing one infection with an STI does not mean that you can never be infected again. A person can be reinfected many times with the same STI. This is especially true if a person does not get treated for the STI and thus keeps reinfecting his or her partner with the same STI.

Sources: Adapted from Jefferson County Public Health, "STD Quiz," Modified March 2009, www.co.jefferson.co.us/health/health_T111_R69.htm. Used with permission; Adapted from Family Planning Victoria, "Play Safe," Updated July 2005, www.fpv.org.au/1_2_2.html. © Family Planning Victoria. Used by permission.

12.14 | Assess Yourself: STIs: Do You Really Know What You Think You Know?

311

Your Plan for Change

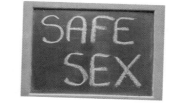

The Assess Yourself activity lets you consider your beliefs and attitudes about STIs and identify possible risks you may be facing. Now that you have considered these results, you can begin to change behaviors that may be putting you at risk for STIs and for infection in general.

Today, You Can:

○ Put together an "emergency" supply of condoms. Outside of abstinence, condoms are your best protection against an STI. If you don't have a supply on hand, visit your local drugstore or health clinic. Remember that both men and women are responsible for preventing the transmission of STIs.

○ To prevent infections in general, get in the habit of washing your hands regularly. After you cough, sneeze, blow your nose, use the bathroom, or prepare food, find a sink, wet your hands with warm water, and lather up with soap. Scrub your hands for about 20 seconds (count to 20 or recite the alphabet), rinse well, and dry your hands.

Within the Next 2 Weeks, You Can:

○ Talk with your significant other honestly about your sexual history. Make appointments to get tested if either of you think you may have been exposed to an STI.

○ Adjust your sleep schedule so that you're getting an adequate amount of rest every night. Being well rested is one key aspect of maintaining a healthy immune system.

By the End of the Semester, You Can:

○ Check your immunization schedule and make sure you're current with all recommended vaccinations. Make an appointment with your health care provider if you need a booster or vaccine.

○ If you are due for an annual pelvic exam, make an appointment. Ask your partner if he or she has had an annual exam and encourage him or her to make an appointment if not.

Summary

- Your body has several defense systems to keep pathogens from invading. The skin is the body's major protection. The immune system creates antibodies to destroy antigens. Fever and pain play a role in defending the body. Vaccines bolster the body's immune system against specific diseases.

- The major classes of pathogens are bacteria, viruses, fungi, protozoans, parasitic worms, and prions. Bacterial infections include staphylococcal infections, streptococcal infections, meningitis, pneumonia, tuberculosis, tickborne diseases, and peptic ulcers. Major viral infections include the common cold; influenza; hepatitis; and the herpes viruses, including chickenpox, shingles, and herpes gladiatorum.

- Emerging and resurgent diseases such as avian flu, West Nile virus, and dengue pose significant threats for future generations. Many factors contribute to these risks. Possible solutions focus on a public health approach to prevention.

- Sexually transmitted infections (STIs) are spread through sexual intercourse, oral–genital contact, anal sex, hand–genital contact, and sometimes mouth-to-mouth contact. STIs include chlamydia, gonorrhea, syphilis, herpes, human papillomavirus (HPV) and genital warts, candidiasis, trichomoniasis, and pubic lice. Sexual transmission may also be involved in some urinary tract infections (UTIs).

- Acquired immunodeficiency syndrome (AIDS) is caused by the human immunodeficiency virus (HIV). Globally, HIV/AIDS has become a major threat to the world's population. Anyone can get HIV by engaging in high-risk sexual activities that include exchange of body fluids, by having received a blood transfusion before 1985, and by injecting drugs (or having sex with someone who does). You can reduce your risk for contracting HIV significantly by not engaging in risky sexual activities or IV drug use.

Pop Quiz

1. Which of the following do *not* assist the body in fighting disease?
   a. Antigens
   b. Antibodies
   c. Lymphocytes
   d. Macrophages

2. Which of the following diseases is caused by a prion?
   a. Shingles
   b. Listeria
   c. Mad cow disease
   d. Trichomoniasis

3. An example of passive immunity is
   a. inoculation with a vaccine containing weakened antigens.
   b. when the body makes its own antibodies to a pathogen.
   c. the antibody-containing part of the vaccine that came from someone else.
   d. None of the above.

4. One of the best ways to prevent contagious viruses from spreading is to
   a. wash your hands frequently.
   b. cover your mouth when sneezing.
   c. keep your hands away from your mouth and eyes.
   d. All of the above.

5. Which of the following is a *viral* disease?
   a. Hepatitis
   b. Pneumonia
   c. Malaria
   d. Streptococcal infection

6. Which of the following STIs cannot be treated with antibiotics?
   a. Chlamydia
   b. Gonorrhea
   c. Syphilis
   d. Herpes

7. Pelvic inflammatory disease (PID) is a(n)
   a. sexually transmitted infection.
   b. type of urinary tract infection.
   c. infection of a woman's fallopian tubes or uterus.
   d. disease that both men and women can get.

8. The most widespread sexually transmitted bacterium is
   a. gonorrhea.
   b. chlamydia.
   c. syphilis.
   d. chancroid.

9. Jennifer touched her viral herpes sore on her lip and then touched her eye. She ended up with the herpes virus in her eye as well. This is an example of
   a. acquired immunity.
   b. passive spread.
   c. autoinoculation.
   d. self-vaccination.

10. Which of the following is *not* true about HIV?
    a. Potential sex partners will show signs of HIV if they are infected.
    b. The virus can be spread through semen or vaginal fluids.
    c. You cannot get HIV from an insect bite.
    d. Unprotected anal sex increases risk of exposure to HIV.

Answers to these questions can be found on page A-1.

Web Links

1. **American Social Health Association.** This site provides facts, support, resources, and referrals about sexually transmitted infections and diseases. www.ashastd.org

2. **San Francisco AIDS Foundation.** This community-based AIDS service organization focuses on ending the HIV/AIDS pandemic through education, patient services, advocacy, and global programs. www.sfaf.org

3. **Specialized CDC sites.** These sites focus on infectious diseases:
   - National Center for Immunization and Respiratory Diseases. www.cdc.gov/ncird/index.html
   - National Center for Preparedness, Detection and Control of Infectious Diseases. www.cdc.gov/ncpdcid
   - National Center for HIV/AIDS, Viral Hepatitis, STD and TB Prevention. www.cdc.gov/nchhstp

4. **AVERT.** An international site with information on HIV/AIDS, global STI statistics, interactive quizzes, and graphics displaying current statistics for vulnerable populations. www.avert.org

Violence and Unintentional Injuries

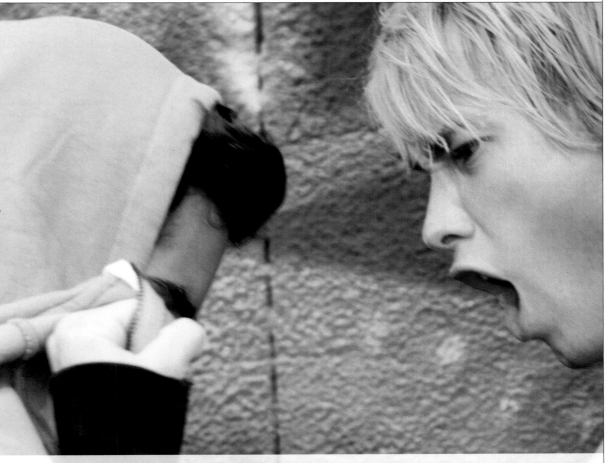

The World Health Organization (WHO) defines **violence** as "the intentional use of physical force or power, threatened or actual, against oneself, another person, or against a group or community, that either results in or has a high likelihood of resulting in injury, death, psychological harm, maldevelopment or deprivation."[1] Today, most experts realize that emotional and psychological forms of violence can be as devastating as physical blows.

The U.S. Public Health Service categorizes violence resulting in injuries into either intentional injuries or unintentional injuries. **Intentional injuries**—those committed with intent to harm— typically include assaults, homicides, and self-directed injuries. **Unintentional injuries** are those committed without intent to harm.[2]

Why do we focus attention on violence and injury in an introductory health text for college and university students? The answer is simple: Violent and abusive interactions are common problems for young adults, as are unintentional—and often preventable—injuries. This chapter discusses common instances of both violence and unintentional injuries, identifying steps you can take to reduce your risk as well as strategies for managing a violent or injurious situation should one occur.

Crime Rates and Causes of Violence

learning outcomes

■ **List individual and social factors contributing to violence.**

Violence has been a part of the American landscape since colonial times; however, it wasn't until the 1980s that the U.S. Public Health Service identified violence as a leading cause of death and disability and gave it chronic disease status, indicating that it was a pervasive threat to society.

Statistics from the Federal Bureau of Investigation (FBI) have shown that, after steadily increasing from 1973 to 2006, rates of overall crime and certain types of violent crime have been decreasing over the past few years (**Figure 13.1**).[3]

Why be so concerned about violence if the major forms of violent crime are on a downward trend? The answer is that *any* violence affects us all. Even if we have never been victimized personally, we all are victimized by violent acts that cause us to be fearful; impinge on our liberty; and damage the reputation of our campus, city, or nation.

Violence on Campus

In 2007 and 2008, deadly mass shootings took place at Virginia Tech and Northern Illinois University, sending shock waves across college campuses. Today, it would be hard to find a campus without a safety plan in place to prevent and respond to this type of violent crime.

93% of crimes against college students occur at off-campus locations.

Relationship violence is one of the most prevalent problems on college campuses. In the most recent American College Health Association's survey, 11.6 percent of women and 6.6 percent of men reported being emotionally abused in the past 12 months by a significant other. Two percent of men and 2 percent of women reported being involved in a physically abusive relationship. Another 1 percent of men and 2 percent of women reported being in a sexually abusive relationship.[4]

The statistics on reported violence on campus represent only a glimpse of the big picture. It is believed that fewer than 25 percent of campus crimes in general are reported to *any* authority. And reports suggest that up to 95 percent of women raped or sexually assaulted on campus never report these crimes.[5]

Factors Contributing to Violence

Several factors increase the likelihood of violent acts:[6]

■ **Poverty.** Low socioeconomic status can create an environment of hopelessness in which some people view violence as the only way of obtaining what they want.
■ **Unemployment.** Financial strain, losing or fear of losing a job, economic downturns, and living in economically depressed areas can increase rates and severity of violence.[7]
■ **Parental influence.** Children raised in environments in which shouting, hitting, emotional abuse, antisocial behavior, and other forms of violence are commonplace are more apt to act out these behaviors as adults.[8]
■ **Cultural beliefs.** Cultures that objectify women and empower men to be tough and aggressive show higher rates of violence in the home.[9]

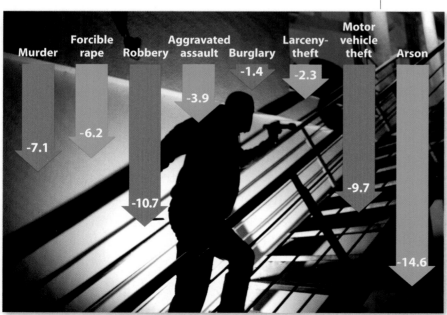

Figure 13.1 Declining Crime Rates
According to the FBI's Preliminary Semiannual Uniform Crime Report, in the United States violent crime dropped 6.2% and property crime declined 2.8% during the first 6 months of 2010, compared to the same period in 2009.
Source: Adapted from Federal Bureau of Investigation, *Crime in the United States, Preliminary Semiannual Uniform Crime Report 2010,* Table 3, www.fbi.gov/about-us/cjis/ucr/crime-in-the-u.s/2010/preliminary-crime-in-the-us-2009/prelimiucrjan-jun_10_excels/table-3.

Murder -7.1, Forcible rape -6.2, Robbery -10.7, Aggravated assault -3.9, Burglary -1.4, Larceny-theft -2.3, Motor vehicle theft -9.7, Arson -14.6

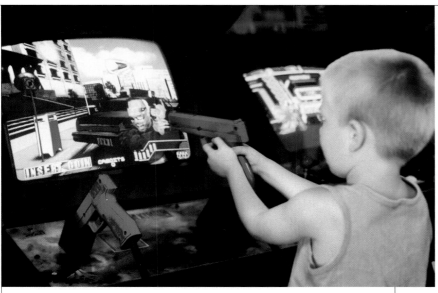

Does violence in the media cause violence in real life?

Evidence of the real-world effects of violence in the media is inconclusive. Arguably, Americans today—especially children—are exposed to more depictions of violence in the news, movies, music, and games than ever before, but research has not shown a clear link between a person's exposure to violent media and his or her propensity to engage in violent acts. Regardless, many people are concerned that children today are being exposed to more violence than they have the emotional or cognitive maturity to handle.

- **Discrimination or oppression.** Whenever one group is oppressed or perceives that its members are oppressed by those of another group, violence against others is more likely.
- **Religious beliefs and differences.** Strong religious beliefs can lead people to think that violence against others is justified.
- **Political differences.** Civil unrest and differences in political beliefs have historically been triggers for violent acts.
- **Breakdowns in the criminal justice system.** Overcrowded prisons, lenient sentences, early releases from prison, and trial errors subtly encourage violence in many ways.
- **Stress.** People who are in crisis or under stress are more apt to be highly reactive, striking out at others or acting irrationally.[10]
- **Heavy use of alcohol and other substances.** Alcohol and drug abuse are often catalysts or risk factors for violence.[11]

What Makes People Prone to Violence?

Personal factors also can increase risks for violence. Problems with anger and substance abuse are both predictors of future aggressive behavior.[12] *Anger* is a spontaneous, usually temporary, biological feeling or emotional state of displeasure that occurs most frequently during times of personal frustration. Anger can range from slight irritation to *rage*, a violent and extreme form of anger.

People who anger quickly often have low tolerance for frustration. The cause may be genetic or physiological; typically, however, anger-prone people come from families that are disruptive, chaotic, and unskilled in emotional expression.[13] And people taught not to express anger in public often don't know how to handle it when it reaches a level they can no longer hide.

Aggressive behavior is often a key aspect of violent interactions. **Primary aggression** is goal-directed, hostile self-assertion that is destructive in nature. **Reactive aggression** is more often part of an emotional reaction brought about by frustration.

For some, sudden episodes of rage are related to **intermittent explosive disorder (IED)**, a psychological disorder characterized by repeated episodes of aggressive, violent behavior grossly out of proportion to the situation.

Substance abuse is also linked to violence.[14] Consumption of alcohol—by perpetrators of the crime, the victim, or both—immediately precedes over half of all violent crimes. Criminals using illegal drugs commit robberies and assaults more frequently than criminals who do not use them, and do so especially during periods of heavy drug use. In domestic assault cases, more than 86 percent of the assailants and 42 percent of victims reported using alcohol at the time of the attack. Nearly 15 percent of victims and assailants reported using cocaine at the time of the attack. Alcohol abuse, particularly binge drinking, is associated with physical victimization among males and sexual victimization (particularly rape) among females on college and university campuses.

315

How Much Impact Does the Media Have?

Several early studies seemed to support a link between excessive exposure to violent media and subsequent violent behavior.[15] Yet, just as media violence has exploded, rates of violent crime and victimization among teens 10 to 17 have fallen to the lowest rates ever recorded.[16] According to the National Crime Victimization Survey, the violent crime rate declined by 39 percent and the property crime rate by 29 percent from 2000 to 2009.[17] A meta-analysis of 26 studies examining the relationship between exposure to media violence and violent aggression did not support the association.[18] And some critics argue that playing violent video games or watching violent movies is cathartic for some who report relieved stress and feelings of exhaustion afterward.[19] Concern has also been raised that people who spend too much time in front of screens may miss the important communication lessons that come from talking in person and learning to get along with others. Debate also continues over whether viewers of media violence become desensitized to violence.

check yourself

- **What are three factors that might make a person prone to violence?**

Interpersonal Violence

- **Identify and define the various types of interpersonal violence.**

Intentional injury can be categorized into three major types: *interpersonal violence, collective violence*, and *self-directed violence*—although there is some degree of overlap among these groups.[20] **Interpersonal violence** includes violence inflicted against one individual by another, or a small group of others; homicide, hate crimes, domestic violence, child abuse, elder abuse, and sexual victimization all fit into this category.

Homicide

Homicide, defined as murder or non-negligent manslaughter, is the 15th leading cause of death in the United States but the second leading cause of death for persons aged 15 to 24. It accounts for

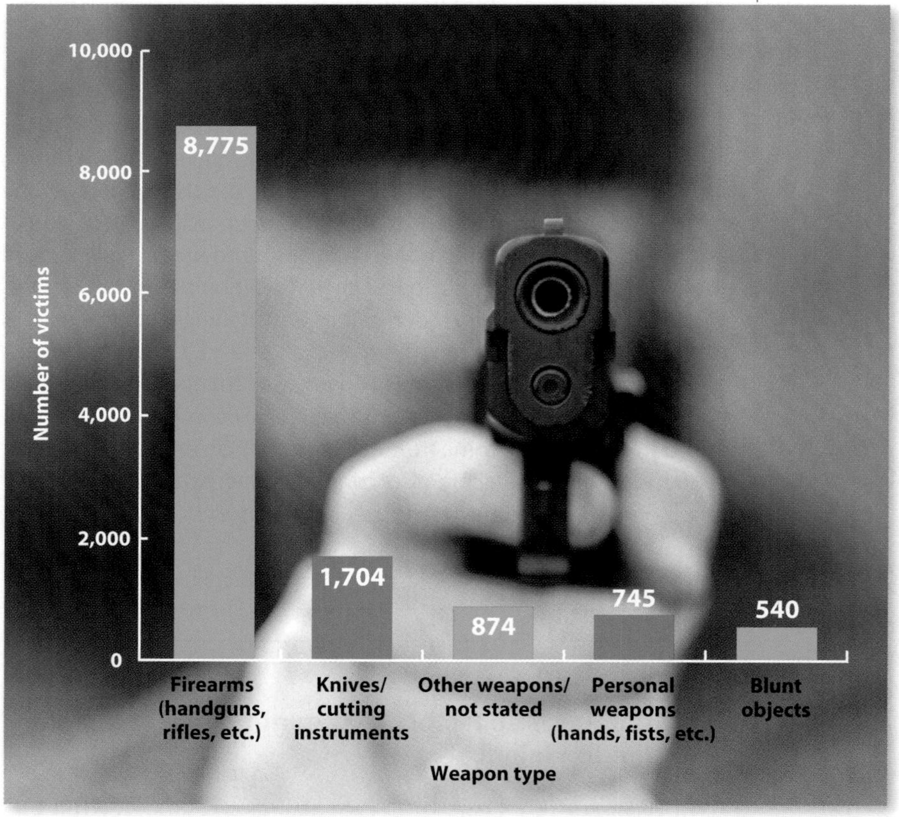

Figure 13.2 Homicide in the United States by Weapon Type, 2010

Sixty-seven percent of murders in the United States are committed using firearms, far outweighing all other weapons combined.

Source: Data from U.S. Department of Justice, Federal Bureau of Investigation, Crime in the United States, 2010, Expanded Homicide Data, Table 8, http://www.fbi.gov/about-us/cjis/ucr/crime-in-the-u.s/2010/crime-in-the-u.s.-2010/tables/10shrtbl08.xls.

more than 18,000 premature deaths in the United States annually, the majority of which are caused by firearms.[21] Most homicides are not random acts of violence: Over half of all homicides occur among people who know one another. In two-thirds of these cases, the perpetrator and the victim are friends or acquaintances; in one-third, they belong to the same family.[22]

Homicide rates reveal clear differences across races and ages. Whereas overall homicide rates in the United States have fluctuated minimally, and have even decreased in some populations, those involving young victims and perpetrators, particularly young black males, have surged. From 2002 to 2007, the number of homicides involving black male victims aged 15 to 24 rose by 31 percent, and those involving them as perpetrators increased by 41 percent.[23] How do homicide rates compare by race in general? Overall, in 2008 in the United States population-based rates of homicide were 3.3 per 100,000 for whites, 20.6 per 100,000 for blacks, and 2.5 per 100,000 for all other races combined.[24]

The rates of homicide in the United States are higher than in many other developed nations (**Table 13.1**). As **Figure 13.2** shows, the number of gun-related homicides in the United States is particularly high; handguns are consistently responsible for more murders than any other single type of weapon.[25] Today, 35 percent of American homes have a gun on the premises, with more than 283 million privately owned guns registered—40 percent of which are handguns.[26] However, the number of guns available doesn't entirely account for the high rates of gun-related homicide in the United States. Countries such as Canada with similar household possessions of guns have much different gun-related crime rates than does the United States: In 2006, there were 12,791 murders by firearms in the United States, compared to only 190 in Canada.[27]

Hate Crimes

A **hate crime** is a crime committed against a person, property, or group of people that is motivated by the offender's bias against a race, religion, disability, sexual orientation, or ethnicity. In spite of national efforts to promote understanding and appreciation of diversity in workplaces, schools, and communities, intolerance of differences continues to smolder in many parts of

U.S. society. According to the FBI's most recent *Hate Crime Statistics* report, there were 8,336 reported victims of hate crimes in 2009 (**Figure 13.3**).[28] More than 62 percent of the persons who committed these crimes were white, 18.5 percent were black, and the remaining offenders' race was unknown.[29]

Bias-related crime, both on campus and in the community, is sometimes referred to as **ethnoviolence**, a word that describes violence among ethnic groups in the larger society that is based on prejudice and discrimination. **Prejudice** is an irrational attitude of hostility directed against an individual; a group; a race; or the supposed characteristics of an individual, group, or race. **Discrimination** constitutes actions that deny equal treatment or opportunities to a group of people, often based on prejudice. Often prejudice and discrimination stem from a fear of change and a desire to blame others when forces such as the economy and crime seem to be out of control.

Common reasons given to explain bias-related and hate crimes include (1) *thrill seeking* by multiple offenders through a group attack, (2) *feeling threatened* that others will take their jobs or property or best them in some way, (3) *retaliating* for some real or perceived insult or slight, and (4) *fearing the unknown or differences*. For other people, hate crimes are a part of their mission in life, either due to religious zeal or distorted moral beliefs.

Nearly 12 percent of all bias-related and hate crimes occur on campuses, and schools and colleges have the fastest growing risks for such crimes.[30] Campuses have responded to reports of hate crimes by offering courses that emphasize diversity, training faculty appropriately, and developing policies that strictly enforce punishment for hate crimes.[31] Sadly, many minor assaults do go unreported because the victims fear retaliation or continued stigmatization.

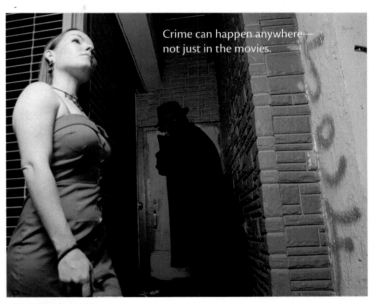
Crime can happen anywhere—not just in the movies.

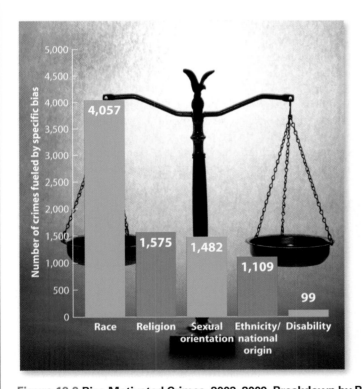

Figure 13.3 Bias-Motivated Crimes, 2003–2009, Breakdown by Bias
When hate crime victims were asked the type of bias they suspect motivated the crime, about 58% believed that the crime was motivated by racial bias. About a third of victims suspected that they were targeted due to their ethnicity, and a quarter said it was because of their associations with persons having particular characteristics.

Note: Data do not sum to 100% because victims may have reported more than one type of bias motivating the hate crime.

Source: Data from Federal Bureau of Investigation, "Hate Crime Statistics, 2009," www.fbi.gov/ucr/hc2009, 2010.

TABLE 13.1	Homicide Rates in Selected Nations

Country	Homicide Rate per 100,000 People
Uganda	36.3
South Africa	33.8
Mexico	18.1
Russia	11.2
Philippines	5.4
United States	5.0
India	3.4
Canada	1.8
France	1.4
Australia	1.2
Saudi Arabia	1.0
Japan	0.5

Source: Data from United Nations Office on Drugs and Crime, "UNODC Homicide Statistics," 2011, www.unodic.org/unodc/en/data-and-analysis/homicide.html.

check yourself

- **What factors are correlated with increased homicide rates in the United States?**
- **List three reasons given to explain hate crimes.**

Violence in the Family

- **Explain how personal and social factors can lead to domestic violence and child and elder abuse.**

Sadly, victims of violence and abuse may find that the perpetrators of these crimes are their own spouse, partner, parent, or child. Why do people commit acts of violence against their own loved ones?

Domestic Violence

Domestic violence refers to the use of force to control and maintain power over another person in the home environment. It can occur between parent and child, between spouses or intimate partners, or between siblings or other family members. The violence may involve emotional abuse; verbal abuse; threats of physical harm; and physical violence ranging from slapping and shoving to beatings, rape, and homicide.

Women are more likely than men to become victims of violent acts perpetrated by spouses, lovers, ex-spouses, and ex-lovers. This form of domestic violence is known as **intimate partner violence (IPV)**. The aggression often includes pushing, slapping, and shoving, but it can take more severe forms.

In 2009, women experienced about 4.8 million IPV-related physical assaults and rapes. Men were the victims of about 2.9 million IPV-related assaults. Of these assaults, there were 2,340 deaths, 70 percent of which occurred in women.[32] Homicide committed by a current or former intimate partner is the leading cause of death of pregnant women in the United States.[33] In addition, 74 percent of all murder-suicides in the United States involve an intimate partner.[34]

Have you ever heard of a woman who is repeatedly beaten by her partner and wondered, "Why doesn't she just leave him?" There are many reasons some women find it difficult to break their ties with their abusers. Some, particularly those with small children, are financially dependent on their

partners. Others fear retaliation against themselves or their children. Some hope the situation will change with time, and others stay because cultural or religious beliefs forbid divorce. Finally, some women still love the abusive partner and are concerned about what will happen to him if they leave.

In the 1970s, psychologist Lenore Walker developed a theory called the *cycle of violence* that explained predictable, repetitive patterns of psychological and/or physical abuse in abusive relationships.[35] Over the years, Walker's initial work has been criticized for its lack of scientific rigor, anecdotal approach, and seeming overstatement of selected patterns as universal truths. In her most recent book, *The Battered Woman Syndrome*, Walker responds to many of her early critics with improved quantitative analysis, reviews of recent research, and an extensive list of experts in the field of violence.[36]

Today, the cycle of violence continues to be important to understanding why people stay in otherwise unhealthy relationships. The cycle consists of three major phases:

1. **Tension building.** This phase typically occurs prior to the overtly abusive act and includes breakdowns in communication, anger, psychological aggression and violent language, growing tension, and fear.
2. **Incident of acute battering.** At this stage, the batterer usually is trying to "teach her a lesson"; when he feels he has inflicted enough pain, he stops. When the acute attack is over, he may respond with shock and denial about his own behavior or blame her for making him do it.
3. **Remorse/reconciliation.** During this "honeymoon" period, the batterer may be kind, loving, and apologetic, swearing that he

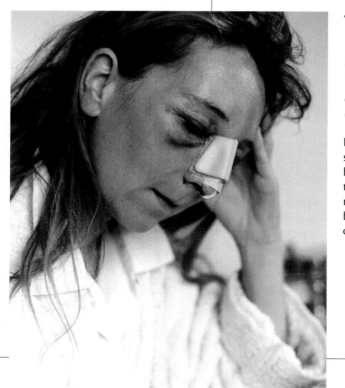

Why do people stay in abusive relationships?

People who stay with their abusers may do so because they are dependent on the abuser, because they fear the abuser, or even because they love the abuser. In some cultures, women may not be free to leave an abusive relationship because of restrictive laws, religious beliefs, or social mores.

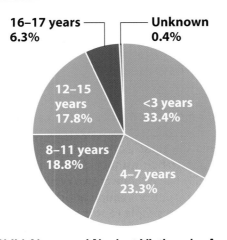

Figure 13.4 Child Abuse and Neglect Victims, by Age, 2009

Source: U.S. Department of Health and Human Services, Administration on Children, Youth and Families, *Child Maltreatment 2009* (Washington, DC: U.S. Government Printing Office, 2010), www.acf.hhs.gov/programs/cb/pubs/cm09.

will never act violently again and will work to change his behavior. However, when things that triggered past abuse resurface, the cycle starts over.

For a woman caught in this cycle, it is often very hard to summon the resolution to extricate herself. Most need effective outside intervention.

No single reason explains why people tend to be abusive in relationships. Alcohol abuse is often associated with such violence, and marital dissatisfaction is also a predictor. Numerous studies also point to differences in communication patterns between abusive and nonabusive relationships. Many experts believe that men who engage in severe violence are more likely than other men to suffer from personality disorders.[37]

Child Abuse and Neglect

Children living in families in which domestic violence or sexual abuse occurs are at great risk for damage to personal health and well-being. **Child abuse** refers to the harm of a child by a caregiver, generally a parent. The abuse may be sexual, psychological, physical, or any combination of these. **Neglect** includes failure to provide for a child's basic needs for food, shelter, clothing, medical care, education, or proper supervision.

How serious are the problems of child abuse and neglect? Although exact figures are difficult to obtain, a new report to Congress includes results of several studies based largely on information obtained from nearly 11,000 sentinels—people who deal with probable cases on a daily basis and report their findings. These studies indicate that an estimated 1.25 million children (1 out of every 58) experienced maltreatment in one form or another between 2005 and 2006. Of those children, an estimated 553,000 (44%) were abused. Most of the abused children (58%) experienced physical abuse, slightly more than 27 percent were emotionally abused, and slightly more than 24 percent experienced sexual abuse.[38] **Figure 13.4** shows the rates of abuse among children of different ages.

Sexual abuse of children by adults or older children includes sexually suggestive conversations; inappropriate kissing; touching;

petting; oral, anal, or vaginal intercourse; and other sexual interactions. Recent studies indicate that the rates of sexual abuse in children range from 3 to 32.2 percent of all children, with girls being at greater risk than young boys, even though young boys are abused in significant numbers.[39]

Most experts believe that as high as these numbers are, the shroud of secrecy surrounding this problem makes it very likely that they grossly underestimate the number of actual cases. Unfortunately, the programs taught in schools today may give children the false impression that they are more likely to be assaulted by a stranger, when in reality 90 percent of child sexual abuse victims know their perpetrator in some ways, with nearly 70 percent of children abused by family members, usually an adult male.[40]

People who were abused as children bear spiritual, psychological, or physical scars. Studies have shown that child sexual abuse has an impact on later life; children who experience sexual abuse are at increased risk for anxiety disorders, depression, eating disorders, post-traumatic stress disorder (PTSD), and suicide attempts.[41] Youth who have been sexually abused are 25 percent more likely to experience teen pregnancy, 30 percent more likely to abuse their own children, and are much more likely to have problems with alcohol abuse or drug addiction.[42]

There is no single profile of a child abuser. The most common perpetrators in child maltreatment cases are biological parents. Frequently, the perpetrator is a young adult in his or her mid-twenties without a high school diploma, living at or below the poverty level, depressed, socially isolated, with a poor self-image, and having difficulty coping with stressful situations. In many instances, the perpetrator has experienced violence and is frustrated by life.

Not all violence against children is physical. Health can be severely affected by psychological violence—assaults on personality, character, competence, independence, or general dignity as a human being. The negative consequences of this kind of victimization can include depression, low self-esteem, and a pervasive fear of offending the abuser.[43]

Elder Abuse

Elder abuse is a problem for many of today's seniors; best estimates indicate that between 700,000 and 3.5 million older Americans are abused, neglected, or exploited each year, with fewer than 1 in 6 cases ever identified.[44] Many victims fail to report because they are embarrassed that a family member is an abuser, they don't want the abuser to get in trouble or retaliate by putting them in a nursing home, they feel guilty because someone has to take care of them, or they fear that after a report things will get worse. Others suffer from dementia and therefore aren't aware that the abuse is happening. Today, a variety of social service and public health groups are exploring options for protecting our elderly citizens in much the same way that we endeavor to protect children in our society.

check yourself

- **How does the cycle of violence explain why people stay in dangerous or unhealthy relationships?**

- **What steps can be taken to reduce child and elder abuse?**

Sexual Victimization

learning outcomes

- **Identify the types and prevalence of rape and sexual abuse.**

The term *sexual victimization* refers to any situation in which an individual is coerced or forced to comply with or endure another's sexual acts or overtures. It can run the gamut from harassment to stalking to assault and rape. As with all forms of violence, both men and women are susceptible to sexual victimization. Young people are especially vulnerable; 60 percent of female victims of rape and 69 percent of male victims were first raped before the age of 18.[45]

Sexual victimization and violence can have devastating and far-reaching effects on people of any age. Depression, suicide risks, drug and alcohol abuse, traumatic stress disorders, self-harm, and a host of interpersonal problems often increase among women and men who have been victimized sexually.[46]

Sexual Assault and Rape

Sexual assault is any act in which one person is sexually intimate with another person without that person's consent. This may range from touching to forceful penetration and may include, for example,

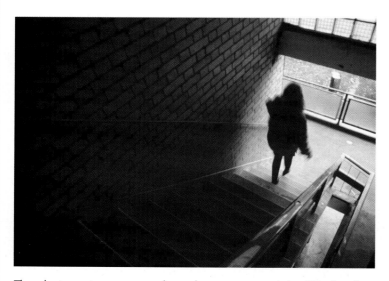

The reluctance to report sexual assault on campus and the difficulty of pursuing criminal proceedings in the campus environment can create turmoil in victims' lives, while too rarely leading to punishment of offenders.

ignoring indications that intimacy is not wanted, threatening force or other negative consequences, and actually using force.

Considered the most extreme form of sexual assault, **rape** is defined as "penetration without the victim's consent."[47] Incidents of rape generally fall into one of two types. An **aggravated rape** is any rape involving one or multiple attackers, strangers, weapons, or physical beatings. A **simple rape** is a rape perpetrated by one person, whom the victim knows, and does not involve a physical beating or use of a weapon. Most rapes are classified as simple rape, but that terminology should not be taken to mean that a simple rape is any less violent or criminal. The FBI ranks rape as the second most violent crime, trailing only murder.[48]

According to the National Center for Injury Prevention and Control, 1 in 6 women and 1 in 33 men reported experiencing an attempted or completed rape at some time in their lives.[49] An estimated 79 percent of all sexual assaults reported by women victims in 2009 were committed by someone the victim knew: 41 percent of perpetrators were the victim's friend or acquaintance and 39 percent were intimates.[50] Men can also be victims of rape and sexual assault, and a growing number have come forward to report their abusers. Over 41 percent of male victims were first raped before the age of 12, and 28 percent were first raped between the ages of 12 and 17. These first rapes were committed by acquaintances (32.3%), family members (17.7%), friends (17.6%), or intimate partners (15.9%).[51]

By most indicators, reported cases of rape appear to have declined in the United States since the early 1990s, even as reports of other forms of sexual assault have increased. This decline is thought to be due to shifts in public awareness and attitudes about rape, combined with tougher crime policies, major educational campaigns, and media attention. These changes enforce the idea that rape is a violent crime and should be treated as such.

Although these declines in reported cases may be encouraging, studies indicate that only 16 percent of all rapes are actually reported to law enforcement.[52] Why do so many victims never report the crimes committed against them? Typically major barriers include not wanting others to know, fear of retaliation, perception of insufficient evidence, uncertainty about how to report, and uncertainty whether a crime was committed or harm intended.

The terms *date rape* and *acquaintance rape* have been used interchangeably in the past. However, most experts now believe that the term *date rape* is inappropriate because it minimizes the criminal nature of the rape. **Acquaintance rape** refers to any rape in which

84%

of sexual assaults that occur on college campuses are acquaintance rapes.

What does *date rape* mean?

The term *date rape* was formerly applied to a sexual assault occurring in the context of a dating relationship. The term has fallen out of favor because the word *date* implies something reciprocal or arranged, thus minimizing the crime. The term *acquaintance rape* is now more commonly used, referring to any rape in which the rapist is known to the victim, even if only minimally. Acquaintance rape is particularly common on college campuses, where alcohol and drug use can impair young people's judgment and self-control.

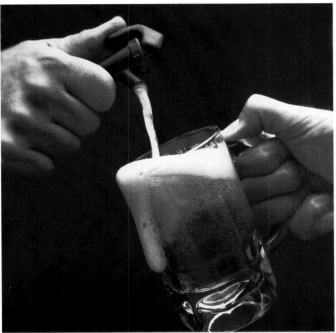

A lot of campus rapes start here.

Whenever there's drinking or drugs, things can get out of hand. So it's no surprise that many campus rapes involve alcohol.

But you should know that under any circumstances, sex without the other person's consent is considered rape. A felony, punishable by prison. And drinking is no excuse.

That's why, when you party, it's good to know what your limits are. You see, a little sobering thought now can save you from a big problem later.

the rapist is known to the victim. It may be a dating situation or a situation in which two strangers meet in a social setting. Acquaintance rape is more common in venues in which alcohol, drugs, and partying are the norm. Most acquaintance rapes happen to women aged 15 to 24; the most likely victim is the new college student.[53]

An estimated 673,000 of the nearly 6 million women (about 12%) currently attending college in the United States have been raped.[54] By some estimates, as many as 25 percent of college women have experienced an attempted or completed rape in college.[55] Over 80 percent of these rapes were committed by an attacker the victim knew, most occurred on campus, and alcohol was commonly involved, as were the two most commonly used rape-facilitating drugs, Rohypnol and gamma-hydroxybutyrate (GHB).[56]

Although its legal definition varies within the United States, **marital rape** can be any unwanted intercourse or penetration (vaginal, anal, or oral) obtained by force, threat of force, or when the spouse is unable to consent.[57] Marital rape may account for 25 percent of all rapes. This problem has undoubtedly existed since the origin of marriage as a social institution, though it is noteworthy that marital rape did not become a crime in all 50 states until 1993. Even more noteworthy is the fact that 33 states still allow exemptions from marital rape prosecution, meaning that the judicial system may treat it as a lesser crime.

In general, women under 25 and those from lower socioeconomic groups are at highest risk of marital rape. Women from homes where other forms of domestic violence are common and where there is a high rate of alcoholism or substance abuse also tend to be victimized at greater rates. Women subjected to marital rape often report multiple offenses over time; these events are likely to be forced anal and oral experiences.[58]

Social Contributors to Sexual Violence

Sexual violence and intimate partner violence share factors that increase their likelihood:[59]

- **Minimization.** Many people assume that sexual assault is rare. However, rape is the most underreported of all serious crimes.
- **Trivialization.** Because rape is underreported, many are not aware they know rape victims. Many consider rape by an intimate partner not serious.
- **Blaming the victim.** In spite of efforts to combat such thinking, there is still the belief that an attractive or scantily clad woman "asks" for sexual advances.
- **Male socialization.** Many still believe "boys will be boys." Women are often *objectified*, or treated as sexual objects, which contributes to the idea that it's natural for men to be predatory and women to be passive targets.
- **Male misperceptions.** With media implying that sex is the focus of life, it's not surprising that some men believe that when a woman says no, she is really asking to be seduced.
- **Situational factors.** Dates in which the male makes all the decisions are more likely to end in an aggressive sexual scenario. Alcohol and other drugs increase the risk and severity of assaults.

Organizational, institutional, and patriarchal structures in society that lead to unequal power and control in the workplace, home, and in relationships can also contribute to sexual violence. Also, societies that condone dominant male stereotypes in media, athletics, and other settings may lead to increased risks. Clearly, there is no single cause or contributor to sexual violence, and several factors are likely to converge to increase chances of a sexually violent action.

check yourself

- **What are three types of rape and sexual abuse?**
- **What are two social contributors to sexual violence?**

Other Forms of Sexual Violence

- **Explain the definitions of, and ways to address, sexual harassment and stalking.**

Sexual harassment and stalking are two common forms of sexual violence, even when they do not involve physical harm.

Sexual Harassment

Sexual harassment is defined as unwelcome sexual conduct related to any condition of employment or evaluation of student performance. Commonly, people think of harassment as involving persons in power; however, peers can also harass one another.

Sexual harassment may include unwanted touching; unwarranted sex-related comments or pressure for sexual favors; deliberate or repeated humiliation or intimidation based on sex; and gratuitous comments, jokes, questions, or remarks.

If you feel you are being harassed:

- **Tell the harasser to stop.** Be clear about what is bothering you. Tell the person if it continues that you will report it to authorities. If harassing is via phone or Internet, block the person from your listings.
- **Document the harassment.** Save copies of all communication that the harasser sends you.
- **Avoid being alone with the harasser.** Witnesses can ensure appropriate validation of the event.
- **Complain to authority.** Talk to your instructor, adviser, or counseling center psychologist. If he or she doesn't take you seriously, investigate your school's internal grievance procedures.
- **Remember that you have not done anything wrong.**

Stalking

Stalking can be defined as conduct directed at a person that would cause a reasonable person to feel fear. This may include repeated visual or physical proximity, nonconsensual written or verbal communication, and implied or explicit threats.[60] More than 1 in 4 victims report being stalked via some form of technology.[61]

Millions of women and men are stalked annually in the United States; the vast majority of stalkers are persons involved in relationship breakups or other dating acquaintances. Adults 18 to 24 experience the highest rates of stalking.

Stalkers may have deficient social skills or may not have learned how to deal with complex social relationships and situations; they may have free time and little accountability for daily activities.[62] Stalkers may be surprised to learn that their actions trigger fear and anxiety.

Emotional and Psychological Abuse

Emotional abuse can occur in any intimate relationship, but it is particularly prevalent in romantic and sexual relationships. It can take the form of constant criticisms, verbal attacks, displays of anger, or controlling behavior. Psychological abusers seek to intimidate and debase, gaining control. Often this can lead to or accompany physical abuse and sexual coercion.

Victims of psychological or emotional abuse often experience a form of overt or subtle brainwashing in which their self-confidence and self-respect are slowly whittled away. Tactics the abuser uses may include:

- **Domination:** The victim is controlled in nearly every aspect of life. If the abuser doesn't get his or her way, there is some form of penalty.
- **Verbal assaults:** Constant put downs, name calling, fault-finding, and blaming serve to humiliate the victim and damage his or her self-esteem.
- **Control of social interactions:** The victim's world revolves around the other person's needs. Time and social contacts are monitored and controlled, and social isolation increases.
- **Emotional blackmail:** The abuser plays on the victim's fears and insecurities, striking at vulnerabilities and weaknesses to influence actions. There may be threats to leave, to damage personal property, or to harm pets or children.
- **Volatility:** The abuser's sudden and unpredictable bursts of anger, kindness, violent demonstrations of force, and other conflicting responses to situations can cause anxiety, fear, and emotional upheaval in the victim.

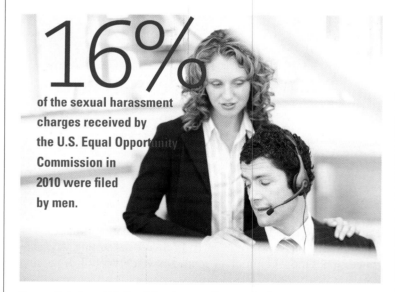

16% of the sexual harassment charges received by the U.S. Equal Opportunity Commission in 2010 were filed by men.

Source: Data from U.S. Equal Employment Opportunity Commission, "Sexual Harassment Charges," 2011, www.eeoc.gov/eeoc/statistics/enforcement/sexual_harassment.cfm.

- **How can sexual harassment be prevented and controlled?**

Collective Violence

learning **outcomes**

■ **List the factors associated with terrorism and gang violence.**

Collective violence is violence perpetrated by groups. It includes political party, militia, and governmental violence; religious or cultural clashes; national or international violence; mobs; riots after sporting events; and other group-against-group forms of violence. Gang violence and terrorist threats are two forms of collective violence that have surfaced as major threats in recent years.

Terrorism

On September 11, 2001, terrorist attacks on the World Trade Center and the Pentagon revealed the vulnerability of our nation to domestic and international threats. Today, threats against our airlines, mass transportation systems, cities, national monuments, and our population fuel fears of looming terrorist attacks. Effects on our economy, travel restrictions, additional security measures, and military buildups are but a few of the examples of how terrorist threats have affected our lives. As defined in the Code of Federal Regulations, **terrorism** is the "unlawful use of force or violence against persons or property to intimidate or coerce a government, the civilian population, or any segment thereof in furtherance of political or social objectives."[63]

Over the past decade, the Centers for Disease Control and Prevention (CDC) consolidated many resources into its Emergency Preparedness and Response division. The division is set up to monitor potential problems, develop a plan for mobilizing communities in the case of attack, and provide resources and information to help Americans respond to terrorist threats and prepare for possible attacks. The Department of Homeland Security was established to prevent future attacks, and the FBI and other government agencies have also prepared a set of procedures and guidelines to ensure citizens' health and safety.

Gang Violence

The growing influence of street gangs has had a harmful impact on our country. Gang violence, including drug trafficking, sex trafficking, shootings, beatings, thefts, carjackings, and bystanders literally being caught in the crossfire of gang shootouts, have caused entire neighborhoods to live in fear. Once thought to occur only in urban areas, gang violence now is a growing threat in rural and suburban communities as well, particularly in the West, Pacific Northwest, Southwest, and Midwest regions of the country.[64]

Why do young people join gangs? Although the reasons are complex, gangs seem to meet many of the personal needs of young people. Often, gangs give members a sense of self-worth, companionship, security, and excitement. In other cases, gangs provide economic security through criminal activity, drug sales, or prostitution. Once young people become involved in gang subculture, it is difficult for them to leave. Threats of violence or fear of not making it on their own discourage even those who are seriously trying to get out.

Who is at risk for joining a gang? The age range of gang members is typically 12 to 22. Risk factors include low self-esteem, academic problems, low socioeconomic status, alienation from family and society, a history of family violence, and living in gang-controlled neighborhoods.[65]

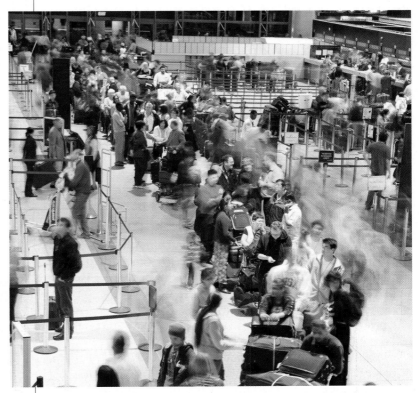

The threat of terrorism has affected many aspects of our daily lives. From increased security at airports to restrictions on public transit, steps taken to protect against terrorism have changed day-to-day activities.

check yourself

■ **What is collective violence?**
■ **What factors contribute to collective violence?**

How to Avoid Becoming a Victim of Violence

learning **outcomes**

- **List strategies to prevent violence against yourself and others.**

After a violent act is committed against someone we know, we may acknowledge the horror of the event, express sympathy, and go on with our lives, but it may take the brutalized person months or years to recover both physically and emotionally. For this reason, preventing a violent act is far better than recovering from it. Both individuals and communities can play important roles in the prevention of violence and intentional injuries. Assaults and threats can arise from in-person encounters or they may develop from online encounters.

Social Networking Safety

At any given time, millions of people are chatting away on social networking sites with friends, family, and strangers and posting photos and personal information that may be available to people they barely know, sometimes placing them at considerable risk. These sites raise some concerns about potential risks—from stalking and identity theft to embarrassment and defamation. For example:

- A first-year student at Virginia Commonwealth University was murdered by someone she met on MySpace.
- A student at the University of Kansas learned the consequences of revealing too much information on Facebook when she was stalked by a man who encountered her class schedule online.
- In Britain, 4.5 million Web users between ages 14

and 21 were vulnerable to identity fraud because of information provided on their social networking sites when security measures were hacked.

- Hiring and firing decisions have been influenced by information employees and job applicants made publicly available on Facebook and Twitter.
- Underage users may pose as adults, leading to claims of inappropriate sexual contact with minors and other criminal offenses on the part of people interacting with them online.

Although very real threats to health, reputation, financial security, and future employment lie in wait for those who post indiscriminately and unwisely to the Web, social networking sites are far from wholly dangerous. To safely enjoy the benefits and to avoid the risks of social networking sites, you'll need to practice a little caution and use some common sense. The following tips will help you to remain safe, protect your identity, and feel free to express yourself without fear of repercussions:

- Don't post anything on the Web that you wouldn't want someone to pick out of your trashcan and read. Your address, phone numbers, banking information, calendar, family secrets, and other information should be kept off the sites.
- Don't post compromising pictures, videos, or other things that you wouldn't want your mother or coworkers to see.
- Never meet a stranger in person whom you've met only online without bringing a trusted friend along or, at the very least, notifying a close friend of where you will be and when you will return. Arrange a ride home with a friend in advance and choose a well-established, public place to meet during daylight hours. Don't give your address or traceable phone numbers to the person you are meeting.

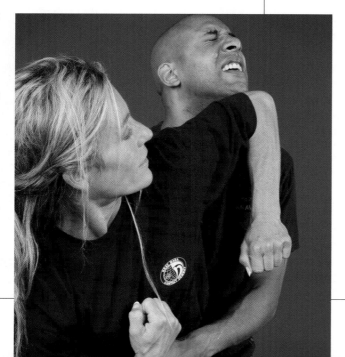

How can I protect myself from becoming a victim of violence?

One of the best ways to protect yourself from violence is to avoid situations or circumstances that could lead to it. Another way to protect yourself is to learn self-defense techniques, such as shown here. College campuses often offer safety workshops and self-defense classes to arm students with the physical and mental skills that may help them to repel or deter an assailant.

Self-Defense against Rape and Personal Assault

Assault can occur no matter what preventive actions you take, but commonsense self-defense tactics can lower the risk. Self-defense is a process that includes increasing your awareness, developing self-protective skills, taking reasonable precautions, and having the judgment necessary to respond quickly to changing situations. Because rape on campus often occurs in social or dating settings, it is important to know ways to avoid and extract yourself from potentially dangerous situations. **Skills for Behavior Change**, below, identifies practical tips for preventing dating violence.

Most attacks by unknown assailants are planned in advance. Many rapists use certain ploys to initiate their attacks. Examples include asking for help; offering help; staging a deliberate "accident," such as bumping into you; or posing as a police officer or other authority figure. Sexual assault frequently begins with a casual, friendly conversation.

Listen to your feelings and trust your intuition. Be assertive and direct to someone who is getting out of line or becoming threatening. Stifle your tendency to be nice, and don't fear making a scene. Use the following tips to let a potential assailant know that you mean what you say and are prepared to defend yourself:

- **Speak in a strong voice.** Use commands such as, "Leave me alone!" rather than questions such as, "Will you please leave me alone?" Avoid apologies and excuses. Sound like you mean it.
- **Maintain eye contact with a would-be attacker.** Eye contact keeps you aware of the person's movements and conveys an aura of strength and confidence.
- **Stand up straight, act confident, and remain alert.** Walk as if you own the sidewalk.

If you are attacked, act immediately. Draw attention to yourself and your assailant. Scream, "Fire!" Research has shown that passersby are much more likely to help if they hear the word *fire* rather than just a scream.

What to Do if a Rape Occurs

If you are a rape victim, report the attack. This gives you a sense of control. Follow these steps:

- Call 9-1-1 (if a phone is available).
- Do not bathe, shower, douche, clean up, or touch anything that the attacker may have touched.
- Save the clothes you were wearing, and do not launder them. They will be needed as evidence. Bring a clean change of clothes to the clinic or hospital.
- Contact the rape assistance hotline in your area, and ask for advice on therapists or counseling if you need additional help or advice.

If a friend is raped, here's how you can help:

- Believe her. Don't ask questions that may appear to implicate her in the assault.
- Recognize that rape is a violent act and that the victim was not looking for this to happen.

- Encourage your friend to see a doctor immediately, because she may have medical needs but feel too embarrassed to seek help on her own. Offer to go with her.
- Encourage her to report the crime.
- Be understanding, and let her know you will be there for her.
- Recognize that this is an emotional recovery, and it may take months or years for her to bounce back.
- Encourage your friend to seek counseling.

One of the most important things you can do is to be supportive. Don't put your friend on the defensive with questions such as "Why didn't you leave?" or "What were you thinking by taking that drink?" Better options for questions might be "What happened? What do you feel that you want to do now? Is there anyone in particular you want to call or talk to? Is there anything I can do for you?"

Skills for Behavior Change
REDUCING YOUR RISK OF DATING VIOLENCE

- **Prior to your date, think about your values; set personal boundaries before you walk out the door.**
- **If a situation feels like it is getting out of control, stop and talk, speak directly, and don't worry about hurting feelings. Be firm.**
- **Watch your alcohol consumption. Drinking might get you into situations you'd otherwise avoid.**
- **Do not accept beverages or open-container drinks from anyone you do not know well and trust. At a bar or a club, accept drinks only from the bartender or wait staff.**
- **Never leave a drink or food unattended. If you get up to dance, have someone you trust watch your drink or take it with you.**
- **Go out with several couples or in groups when dating someone new.**
- **Stick with your friends. Agree to keep an eye out for one another at parties, and have a plan for leaving together and checking in with one another. Never leave a bar or party alone with a stranger.**
- **Pay attention to your date's actions. If there is too much teasing and all the decisions are made for you, it could mean trouble. Trust your intuition.**
- **Practice what you will say to your date if things go in an uncomfortable direction. You have the right to express your feelings, and it is OK to be assertive. Do not be swayed by arguments such as "What about my feelings?" "You were leading me on," and "If you really cared about me, you would."**

check yourself

- **What are three things you can do to reduce your risk of personal assault?**
- **How can you support a friend who has been raped or assaulted?**

Campus and Community Responses to Violence

- **Describe how college campuses are responding to the threat of violence.**

Increasingly, campuses have become microcosms of the greater society, complete with the risks, hazards, and dangers that people face in the world. They also are uniquely different in that they are open to the public and offer an opportunity for predators of all types to exploit young men and women in environments in which they feel safe. Many college administrators have been proactive in establishing violence-prevention policies, programs, and services. They have also begun to examine the aspects of campus culture that promote and tolerate violent acts.[66]

Prevention and Early Response Efforts

The Virginia Tech and Northern Illinois tragedies of 2007 and 2008 prompted vast restructuring of existing policies and strategies for prevention, as well as implementation of methods for notifying students and faculty of immediate risk. Historically, prevention efforts have focused on rape-awareness programs, safety workshops, anti-theft programs, and grounds safety measures such as good lighting, escort services, and well-placed emergency call boxes. Newer programs being developed include emergency response drills that enable campus police, campus administration, community law enforcement, and emergency medical teams to practice how they would respond in the event of a major threat, such as a shooter on campus.

Campuses are reviewing the effectiveness of emergency messaging systems. E-mail alerts can reach only those campus community members who are either at their computers or who receive e-mail updates on mobile devices; campuses are also working to implement cell phone alert systems. The REVERSE 9-1-1 system uses database and geographic information system (GIS) mapping technologies to notify campus police and community members in the event of problems, whereas systems developed by companies such as Rave Wireless allow campus administrators to send out alerts in text, voice, e-mail, or instant message format. Some schools program the phone numbers, photographs, and basic student information for all incoming first-year students into a university security system so that in the event of a threat students need only hit a button on their phones, whereupon campus police will be notified and tracking devices will pinpoint their location.

Changes in the Campus Environment

Recognizing that they may be liable for not protecting their students, and out of a genuine concern for faculty, staff, and student health, administrators are asking key questions about the safety of the campus environment. Campus lighting, parking lot security, call boxes for emergencies, removal of overgrown shrubbery along bike paths and walking trails, and stepped-up security are increasingly on the radar of campus safety personnel. Buildings themselves are designed with better lighting and more security provisions, and in some cases security cameras have been installed in hallways, classrooms, and public places throughout campus. Safe rides are provided for students who have consumed too much alcohol; campus leaders have become more involved in campus safety issues; and health promotion programs have stepped up their violence prevention efforts through seminars on acquaintance rape, sexual assault, harassment, and other topics.

Hazing, which can be defined as "any activity expected of someone joining or participating in a group that humiliates, degrades, abuses, or endangers them regardless of a person's willingness to participate" can contribute to an atmosphere of violence and intimidation on campus.[67]

Each year, deaths and injuries are caused by the stunts and tasks involved in hazing. Students participating in the hazing seldom report problems to authorities, and the prevalence of hazing may come to light on campus only after a serious injury or death occurs.

According to a recent study, 55 percent of college students involved in clubs, teams, and organizations experience hazing. In 95 percent of the cases in which students identified their experience as hazing, they did not report the events to campus officials.[68] There may be several reasons for this, but one seems to be that more students perceive positive rather than negative outcomes of hazing, for example, a sense of accomplishment or belonging.

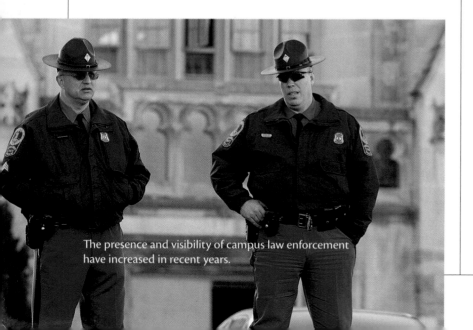

The presence and visibility of campus law enforcement have increased in recent years.

Campus Law Enforcement

Campus law enforcement has changed over the years by increasing both numbers of its members and its authority to prosecute student offenders. Campus police are responsible for emergency responses to situations that threaten safety, human resources, the general campus environment, traffic and bicycle riders, and other dangers. They have the power to enforce laws with students in the same way those laws are handled in the general community. In fact, many campuses now hire state troopers or local law enforcement officers to deal with campus issues rather than maintain a separate police staff.

Many of these law enforcement groups follow a community policing model in which officers have specific responsibilities for certain areas of campus, departments, or events. Narrowing the scope of each officer's territory in this way helps officers get to know people in the area and makes them better able to anticipate risky situations and prevent problems. Schools around the country are also enhancing the ability of campus law enforcement to respond to emergencies. Many officers receive special training in handling crisis and hostage situations, as well as being issued stun guns and other equipment meant to disable potential offenders.

Community Strategies for Preventing Violence

You can take a number of steps to ensure your personal safety (see **Skills for Behavior Change** below). However, it is also necessary to address issues of violence and safety at a community level. Because the factors that contribute to violence are complex and interrelated, community strategies for prevention must also be multidimensional, focusing on individuals, schools, families, communities, policies, programs, and services designed to reduce risk. The CDC's Injury Response initiatives include interventions designed to prevent violence before it begins:

- Develop policies, intervention programs, and laws that prevent violence, such as counseling services, education programs focused on parenting skills or dating behavior, and assistance in giving individuals the confidence to protect themselves against physical and emotional assaults.
- Work with individuals in skills-based educational programs that teach the basics of interpersonal communication, anger management, conflict resolution, appropriate assertiveness, stress management, and other health-based behaviors.
- Beginning at an early age, involve families, schools, community programs, athletics, music, faith-based groups, and so on, providing experiences that help young people develop self-esteem and self-efficacy.
- Promote tolerance and acceptance, and establish and enforce policies that forbid discrimination on the basis of religion, gender, race, sexual orientation, age, marital status, income, or other differences.
- Improve community services focused on family planning, mental health services, day care and respite care, and alcohol and substance abuse prevention.
- Improve the built environment in communities by making sure walking trails, parking lots, and other public areas are well lit, unobstructed, and patrolled regularly.
- Improve community-based support and treatment for victims, and ensure that individuals have choices available when trying to stop the violence in their lives.

Skills for **Behavior Change**

STAY SAFE ON ALL FRONTS

You can take a number of steps to protect yourself from assault. Follow these tips to increase your awareness and reduce your risk of a violent attack.

Outside Alone
- Carry a cell phone; keep it turned on, but don't use it. Be aware of what is happening around you.
- If you are being followed, don't go home. Head for a location where there are other people. If you decide to run, run fast and scream loudly to attract attention.
- Vary your routes; walk or jog with others. Stay close to others.
- Park near lights; avoid dark areas where people could hide.
- Carry pepper spray or other deterrents. Consider using your campus escort service.
- Tell others where you are going and when you expect to be back.

In Your Car
- Lock your doors. Do not open your doors or windows to strangers.
- If someone hits your car while you are driving, drive to the nearest gas station or other public place. Call the police or road service for help, and stay in your car until help arrives.
- If a car appears to be following you, do not drive home. Drive to the nearest police station.

In Your Home
- Install deadbolts on all doors and locks on all windows. Don't leave a spare key outside. Consider installing a home alarm system.
- Lock doors when at home, even during the day. Close blinds and drapes whenever you are away and in the evening when you are home.
- Rent apartments that require a security code or clearance to gain entry; avoid easily accessible apartments such as first-floor units. When you move into a new residence, pay a locksmith to change the keys and locks.
- Don't let repair people in without asking for identification; have someone with you when repairs are made.
- Keep a phone near your bed and program it to dial 9-1-1.
- If you return to find your residence has been broken into, don't enter. Call the police. If you encounter an intruder, it is better to give up your money than to fight back.

327

check yourself

- **What can schools and communities do to prevent or reduce violence?**

Reducing Your Risk on the Road

■ **List the major causes of motor vehicle accidents, and how to stay safe on the road.**

Almost 34,000 people died in motor vehicle accidents (MVAs) in 2009—nearly 100 Americans every day.[69]

Factors Contributing to MVAs

Five factors—distracted driving, impaired driving, speeding, vehicle safety issues, and driver age—contribute to the majority of MVAs.[70] Most of these are within your personal control.

Distracted Driving Driving while being distracted by a cell phone is deadly. In 2009, 5,474 people were killed and an estimated 448,000 were injured in crashes that were reported to involve distracted driving. Studies show that 31 percent of drivers aged 16 to 24 text while driving, and 70 percent of all drivers report talking on their cell phones regularly while driving.

Recognizing that increased reliance on cell phones could be contributing to motor vehicle accidents, officials are enacting laws that restrict their use. Thirty states ban all phone use for novice drivers, 31 states ban texting while driving, and 8 states ban the use of handheld phones completely but allow hands-free phone calls.[71]

Other common distractions include manipulating handheld devices, adjusting CD players or the radio, looking in the mirror, calling out the window, and eating. Nearly 8 out of 10 MVAs happen within just 3 seconds of a driver becoming distracted.[72] The next time you're tempted to text, make a call, or even swat an insect while driving, pull over. Handle the distraction. Then rejoin traffic when you're ready.

Impaired Driving Every day, 32 people in the United States die in MVAs that involve an alcohol-impaired driver. This amounts to nearly 12,000 deaths. Sixty-five percent of alcohol-impaired drivers involved in fatal crashes are young, aged 21 to 34.[73] Use of drugs other than alcohol is also a significant cause of MVA injury and death.[74] And many researchers contend that driving while sleep deprived is as dangerous as driving drunk.

Public health and law enforcement agencies are cooperating on measures to keep impaired drivers off the road:

■ Designated driver programs, including public funding of "safe rides" and free nonalcoholic beverages for designated drivers

■ Strict enforcement of laws defining impaired driving and the legal drinking age

■ Measures to prevent repeat offenses, including mandatory alcohol or drug abuse treatment, ignition interlock systems that prevent vehicle operation by anyone with a blood alcohol concentration above a specified level, stricter testing for and punishment of those who abuse prescription medicines and/or drive when sleep impaired, and license revocation

Speeding Speeding is a factor in 1 of 3 fatal crashes. Many people speed because they don't perceive it as dangerous. Unfortunately, such attitudes lead to more than 13,000 deaths each year.[75]

Vehicle Safety Issues Wearing a safety belt cuts your risk of death or serious injury in a crash by about half.[76] If you're transporting an infant or child, follow state laws governing use and location of age-appropriate safety seats.

Vehicles can include many safety features, from airbags to stability control. Unfortunately, people who don't have the financial resources to drive vehicles with state-of-the-art features—and that often includes college students—are at increased risk during MVAs. Still, the next time you're planning to purchase a car, new or used, look for features recommended by the Insurance Institute for Highway Safety:

1. Does the car have front airbags? Side airbags? (Airbags don't eliminate the need for safety belts.)
2. Does the car have antilock brakes? Traction and stability control?
3. Does the car have impact-absorbing crumple zones?
4. Are there strengthened passenger compartment side walls?
5. Is there a strong roof support? (The center doorpost on four-door models gives you an extra roof pillar.)

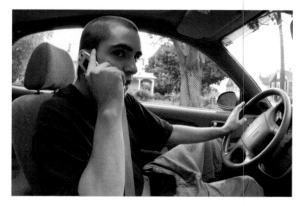

What's wrong with talking on a cell phone while driving?

Talking on a cell phone while driving puts you at a four times greater risk of being in a motor vehicle accident. It also increases the risk of injury and death to other drivers, passengers, and pedestrians and is illegal in many states.

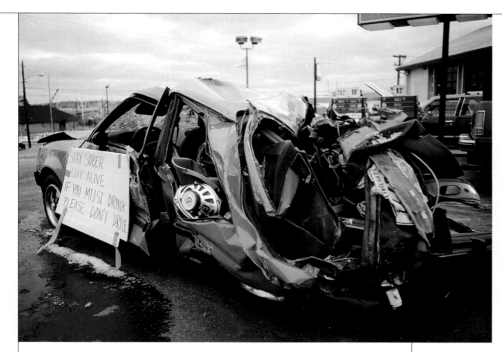

Another factor is the size of the vehicles involved. All cars sold in the United States must meet U.S. Department of Transportation standards for crash worthiness. However, in crashes involving multiple vehicles, the death rate in 2007 for people in subcompacts was almost twice the rate for people in very large cars.[77] Many college students drive small cars because they are more affordable and use less gas, but the laws small cars of physics make such cars more dangerous, especially in frontal collisions with larger cars.

What about motorcycles? Per vehicle mile traveled, motorcyclists are about 37 times more likely than passenger car occupants to die in an MVA, and 9 times more likely to be injured. In 2008, this translated into more than 5,000 motorcyclist deaths and 96,000 injuries.

Many motorcyclists involved in MVAs have avoided severe injuries because they were wearing a helmet. Although the benefits of helmets and protective clothing are well established, only 20 states have full helmet requirements for anyone riding a motorcycle. To find out your state requirements, go to www.iihs.org/laws/helmetusecurrent.aspx.[78]

Driver Age While sensory impairments and slowed reflexes can increase accident rates among people 65 and older, rates are at their peak among teen drivers, especially in the first year a teen has a license.[79] Graduated driver licensing (GDL) programs have been shown to reduce MVA fatalities in crashes involving teens by nearly 20 percent,[80] and to reduce the risk of all MVAs involving teen drivers by 20 to 40 percent.[81]

Risk-Management Driving Techniques

Although you can't control what other drivers are doing, you can reduce your risk of injury in an MVA:

- Don't manipulate electronic devices or talk on a cell phone while driving, even if the phone is hands-free.

Driving under the influence of alcohol greatly increases the risk of being involved in a motor vehicle crash. Of all drivers between the ages of 15 and 20 involved in fatal crashes, nearly 1 out of 3 had been drinking.

- Don't drink and drive. If you plan to party, designate a sober driver, arrange for a taxi or "safe ride," or spend the night where you are.
- Don't drive when tired or when in a highly emotional or stressed state.
- Surround your car with a safety "bubble." The rear bumper of the car ahead of you should be at least 3 seconds away.
- Scan the road ahead of you and to both sides.
- Drive with your low-beam headlights on, *day and night*, to make your car more visible to other drivers.
- Anticipate the actions of others as much as you can; be on the alert for unsignaled lane changes, sudden braking, or other unexpected maneuvers.
- Obey all traffic laws.
- Whether you're the driver or a passenger, always wear a seat belt.

Road Rage

The National Highway Traffic Safety Administration defines aggressive driving as "the operation of a motor vehicle in a manner that endangers or is likely to endanger persons or property."[82] An extreme version of such behavior is *road rage*, which is believed to be a leading cause of highway deaths. Although you cannot control or predict the behavior of others, there are steps you can take to avoid becoming a victim of road rage:

- **Avoid eye contact and engagement.** If you're driving or in public and someone tries to get a reaction from you, avoid confrontation and remove yourself from the situation.
- **Don't antagonize.** Slowing down in traffic to bug someone in an obvious hurry, honking your horn, flashing your high beams, or other passive-aggressive gestures can upset even the most mild-mannered people.
- **If someone follows you after a nasty interaction, either in a car or on foot, do not immediately go home or to your workplace.** Head for the nearest police station or busy area. Never isolate yourself.
- **Take names.** If you don't know the person, try keeping a mental description or get a license plate number. Report offenders, even if you're afraid of getting involved.
- **Stay calm.** Think before opening your mouth, and practice stress management whenever possible.

check yourself

- **What are three factors linked to increased risk of motor vehicle accidents?**
- **What can you do to stay safe on the road?**

Safe Recreation

learning **outcomes**

- **Explain how to stay safe while biking, skateboarding, skiing, snowboarding, swimming, and boating.**

Recreational activities among young people that commonly involve injury include biking, skateboarding, snow sports, and swimming and boating. By following some basic guidelines while doing these activities, you can have fun and be safe.

Bike Safety

Over 63 million Americans of all ages ride bicycles for transportation, recreation, and fitness. The National Highway Traffic Safety Administration (NHTSA) reports about 630 deaths per year from cycling accidents. The majority of cycling deaths (64%) involve cyclists aged 16 and older.[83] Most fatal collisions are due to cyclists' errors, usually failure to yield at intersections. However, alcohol also plays a significant role in bicycle deaths and injuries: In 2009, nearly one-fourth (24%) of cyclists killed were legally drunk.[84]

All cyclists should wear a properly fitted bicycle helmet every time they ride (**Figure 13.5**). The NHTSA reports that a helmet is the single most effective way to prevent head injury resulting from a bicycle crash. Moreover, bear in mind that cyclists are considered vehicle operators; they are required to obey the same rules of the road as do drivers.

Cyclists should consider the following suggestions:

- Wear a helmet approved by the American National Standards Institute (ANSI) or the Snell Memorial Foundation.
- Watch the road and listen for traffic sounds! Never listen to an MP3 player or talk on a cell phone, even hands free, while cycling.

- Don't drink and ride.
- Follow all traffic laws, signs, and signals.
- Ride with the flow of traffic.
- Wear light or brightly colored, reflective clothing that is easily seen at dawn, dusk, and during full daylight.
- Avoid riding after dark. If you must ride at night, use a front light and a red reflector or flashing rear light, as well as reflective tape or other markings on your bike and clothing.
- Know and use proper hand signals.
- Keep your bicycle in good condition.
- Use bike paths whenever possible.
- Stop at stop signs and traffic lights.

Safe Skateboarding

According to the U.S. Consumer Product Safety Commission (CPSC), approximately 26,000 people are treated in hospital emergency rooms each year with skateboard-related injuries. These injuries are most commonly due to falls or collisions, and some are fatal. Three factors commonly contribute to skateboard injury: lack of protective equipment, poor board maintenance, and irregular riding surfaces. Both inexperience and overconfidence also play a role: One-third of all injuries happen to people who have been skateboarding for less than a week, but the majority occur among people who have been skating for more than a year, typically when they are attempting difficult stunts.[85]

Skateboard safety tips from the CPSC:

- Wear an approved helmet, padded clothes, special skateboarding gloves, and padding for your knees and other joints. Padding should be snug but loose enough to allow movement.
- Between uses, check your board for loose, broken, sharp, or cracked parts, and have it repaired if necessary.
- Examine the surface where you'll be riding for holes, bumps, and debris.
- Never skateboard in the street.
- Never hitch a ride from a car, bicycle, or other vehicle.
- Practice complicated stunts in specially designed areas, wearing protective padding.
- Practice safe falling: If you start to lose your balance, crouch down; if you fall, "relax and roll."
- Don't drink and ride.

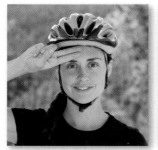 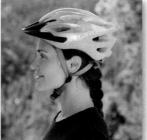 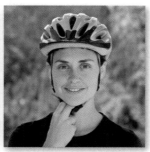

1 The helmet should sit level on your head and low on your forehead—one or two finger-widths above your eyebrows.

2 The sliders on the side straps should be adjusted to form a "V" shape under, and slightly in front of, your ears. Lock the sliders if possible.

3 The chin strap buckle should be centered under your chin. Tighten the strap until it is snug, so that no more than two fingers fit under the strap.

Figure 13.5 Fitting a Bicycle Helmet
When your helmet is fitted correctly, opening your mouth wide in a yawn should cause the helmet to pull down on your head. Also, you should not be able to rock the helmet back more than the width of two fingers above the eyebrows or forward into your eyes.

Safety in the Snow

The National Ski Areas Association (NSAA) reports that a skiing or snowboarding fatality occurs at the rate of 3.8 per 1 million participants per year.[86] Severe nonfatal injuries, such as head trauma and spinal cord injury, also occur, but at a similarly low rate. This makes snow sports much safer, overall, than bicycling, swimming, and many others. The rate of injury has also been declining for decades, largely because of shorter skis, improved safety features on equipment, and increased safety efforts at resorts, such as having more monitors on the slopes, setting aside special family skiing areas, and encouraging helmet use.

One of the most important ways to protect yourself while skiing or snowboarding is to wear an approved helmet; helmet use reduces the risk of any head injury by 30 to 50 percent. It's also important to keep skis and snowboards in good condition and to choose trails according to your ability. Pay attention to the locations of others; if you stop, move to the side of the trail. Observe all posted signs and warnings.

Water Safety

Drowning is the sixth most common cause of accidental death among Americans of all ages, with 1 in 5 of those deaths occurring in children 14 and younger. Males are nearly four times more likely than females to die from unintentional drowning.[87] About half of all fatal drownings involve alcohol.[88]

Swimming Almost half of adults surveyed say they've had an experience in which they nearly drowned.[89] Most drownings occur during water recreation—swimming, diving, or just simply having fun—in unorganized or unsupervised areas, such as ponds or pools without lifeguards present. Many drowning victims were strong swimmers.

All swimmers should take the following precautions:

- Don't drink alcohol before or while swimming.
- Don't enter the water without a life jacket unless you can swim at least 50 feet unassisted.
- Know your limitations; get out of the water when you start to feel even slightly fatigued.
- Never swim alone, even if you are a skilled swimmer. You never know what might happen.
- Never leave a child unattended, even in extremely shallow water.
- Before entering water, check the depth. Most neck and back injuries result from diving into water that is too shallow.
- Never swim in a river with currents too swift for easy, relaxed swimming.
- Never swim in muddy or dirty water that obstructs your view of the bottom. Water that is discolored and choppy or foamy may indicate a rip current.
- If you're caught in a rip current, swim parallel to the shore. Once you are free of the current, swim toward the shore.
- Learn cardiopulmonary resuscitation (CPR). CPR performed by bystanders has been shown to improve outcomes in drowning victims.[90]

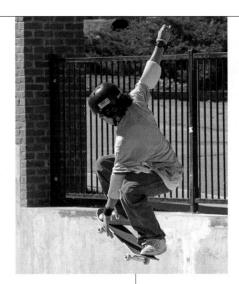

Do I really have to wear a helmet while I'm skateboarding?

The majority of skateboarding injuries occur among people who have been practicing the sport for more than a year, often when they attempt a stunt beyond their level of skill. Wearing a helmet, no matter how experienced a skateboarder you are, will help protect you in case of a fall.

Boating In 2009, the U.S. Coast Guard received reports of 3,358 injured boaters and 736 deaths. About 70 percent of boating fatalities are drownings; of those who drowned, 9 out of 10 were not wearing a **personal flotation device**—a life jacket. Other boating fatalities are due to trauma, hypothermia, carbon monoxide poisoning, and other causes.[91]

About one-third of all boating fatalities involve alcohol. When boat operators are drinking, both collisions with other boats and falls overboard are much more likely. If someone who has been drinking does fall overboard, he or she is more likely to drown or to die of hypothermia. Unfortunately, the "designated driver" concept does not apply to boating—intoxicated passengers often cause or contribute to boating accidents. The U.S. Coast Guard and every state have "Boating Under the Influence" (BUI) laws that carry stringent penalties, including fines, license revocation, and even jail time.[92]

Consider the following safety tips from the American Boating Association:[93]

- Before leaving home, let others know where you are going, who will be with you, and when you expect to return.
- Check the weather. Listen to advisories regarding high winds, storms, and other environmental factors.
- Even for short trips, make sure the vessel doesn't leak, has enough fuel (if powered), and has proper safety equipment.
- Make sure you have enough life jackets for all on board; make life jackets easily accessible.
- Carry an emergency radio and cell phone.
- Don't drink alcohol before you leave, and don't bring any aboard.

The U.S. Coast Guard recommends that before setting out, you put on your life jacket. Most modern life jackets are thin and flexible and can be worn comfortably all day. Children must wear a life jacket once the vessel is under way, unless they are below deck. Wear a life jacket not only when sailing or motor boating, but also when canoeing, kayaking, and rafting.

check yourself

- **What are three strategies that can help keep you safe when biking or skateboarding? In the snow? On the water?**

Avoiding Injury from Excessive Noise

- **List factors contributing to noise-induced hearing loss.**
- **Explain how to protect your hearing.**

Take a look at **Figure 13.6**, which shows the decibel (dB) levels of common sounds. In general, noise levels above 85 dB (about as loud as a diesel truck) increase risks for hearing loss. When you consider the many such noises people are exposed to every day, it should be no surprise that more than 36 million U.S. adults have hearing loss. Although you might think it's only a problem for the old, 26 million Americans between 20 and 69 have hearing loss due to exposure to loud sounds at work or in leisure activities.[94]

Noise-induced hearing loss results when exposure to high-decibel (dB) noise, usually over time, damages sensory receptors in the cochlea, or inner ear. One of the highest rates of sudden noise-induced hearing loss is among adults 20 to 29. Ironically, more than 75 percent of students in a recent study reported awareness of the danger, yet more than half continued to expose themselves to such noise.[95] More than 66 percent of these reported tinnitus (ringing in the ears), which can be a precursor to hearing loss. Most rock musicians use earplugs when performing or rehearsing, and their audiences would be wise to do the same. If you can't hear the person standing next to you at a concert, put in earplugs or look for a quieter spot.

Increasingly, children and young adults are experiencing hearing loss due to use of portable music devices. Three factors make these devices more likely to damage hearing than listening to music from an external speaker: frequency of use, duration of use, and volume. The high level of sound quality and portability of MP3 players mean people are listening to music more often and for longer periods. And because playing a tune at high volume on modern MP3 players doesn't distort its sound, people may be less likely to turn down the volume than they would have been with older devices.[96]

What can you do to avoid hearing loss while still enjoying your music? Keep the volume at or below 80 dB—a level at which you can carry on a conversation—and you won't need to limit time spent listening to music. If a friend nearby can hear your music, it's definitely too loud. And though debate continues over the relative safety of over-the-ear earphones versus ear buds, earphones seem to be safer.[97]

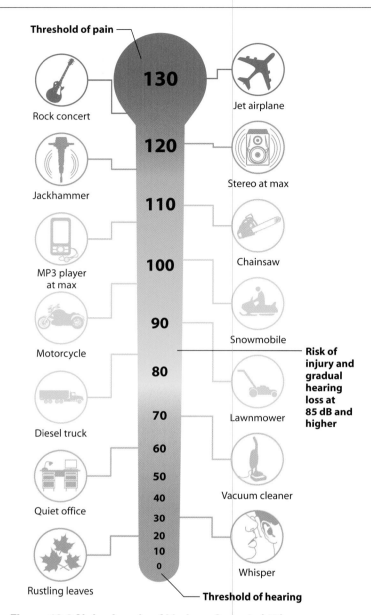

Figure 13.6 Noise Levels of Various Sounds (dB)
Decibels increase logarithmically, so each increase of 10 dB represents a 10-fold increase in loudness.
Source: Adapted from National Institute on Deafness and Other Communication Disorders, "How Loud Is Too Loud? Bookmark," Updated July 2011, www.nidcd.nih.gov/health/hearing/ruler.asp.

- **What are three things you can do to avoid hearing loss?**

Safety at Home

learning outcomes

- **List steps to take to prevent and address common household safety hazards.**

Poisoning

A **poison** is any substance that is harmful when ingested, inhaled, injected, or absorbed through the skin. Every day in the United States, about 75 people die as a result of unintentional poisoning, and another 2,000 are treated in emergency departments.[98] To prevent poisoning:

- Read and follow all usage and warning labels before taking medications or working with chemicals, including household products.
- Never share or sell prescription drugs.
- Never mix household products together; combinations can give off toxic fumes.
- When working with chemicals, wear a protective mask and make sure the area in which you work is well ventilated. Wear gloves and other protective clothing, and eyeglasses or an eye guard if splashing could occur.
- Keep medications, dietary supplements, and alcohol out of sight of children, preferably in a locked cabinet.
- Program the 24-hour national poison control number, 1-800-222-1222, into your phone.

If you suspect you have ingested or inhaled a poison or you are with someone who has collapsed, dial 9-1-1. If the victim is not breathing and you are trained in CPR, provide CPR until paramedics arrive. If the victim is awake and alert, dial the poison control hotline (1-800-222-1222). Follow the instructions given. If you go to a hospital emergency room, bring the suspected poison, if possible.

Falls

Falls are the third most common cause of death from unintentional injury and the most common cause of traumatic brain injury.[99] Although falls are most common among older adults, people of all ages experience them. To reduce your risk of falls:

- Leave nothing lying around on the floor or stairs.
- Avoid using small scatter rugs and mats. Use rubberized liners to secure large rugs to the floor.
- Train pets to stay away from your feet.
- Install slip-proof mats, treads, or decals in showers and tubs and on the stairs.
- If you need to reach something or to change a ceiling light, use an appropriate stool or ladder.
- Wear supportive shoes. Flip-flops and loose shoes can trip you.

Fire

In the United States, a residential fire claims a life every 3 hours.[100] The three main causes of fires in campus housing are cooking, careless

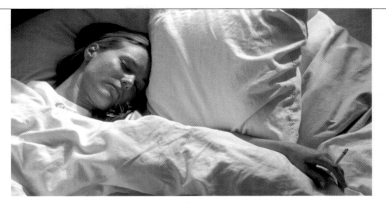

What's the top cause of fire-related deaths?

Smoking is the number one cause of fire-related deaths. If you fall asleep with a lit cigarette, bedding and clothing can quickly ignite. If you can't quit, take it outside.

smoking, and arson. However, a variety of other factors typically contribute to injuries from dormitory fires: alcohol use, ignoring of fire drills and actual alarms, poorly maintained or vandalized alarm systems, and failure to call 9-1-1.[101] To prevent fires:

- Extinguish cigarettes in ashtrays. Never smoke in bed!
- Set lamps away from drapes, linens, and paper.
- Keep kitchen cloths and sleeves away from stove burners. Use caution when lighting barbecue grills.
- Keep candles away from combustibles. Never leave candles unattended.
- Avoid overloading electrical circuits with appliances and cords.
- Have the proper fire extinguishers ready; replace batteries in smoke alarms and test them periodically.

If a fire breaks out, your priority is to get out *as soon as possible*. First, feel the door handle: If it's hot, don't open the door! Go to a window, open it wide, and call for help. Hang a sheet from the window to alert rescuers. Call 9-1-1. If smoke is entering your room, seal cracks in the door with blankets or towels. Stay low—there's less smoke close to the floor.

If the handle is not hot, open the door cautiously. If the hallway is clear, get out, yelling, "Fire!" and knocking on doors as you leave. If you encounter smoke, stay low—crawl if necessary. If you pass a fire alarm, pull it. Always use stairs, never an elevator. Once you're outside, dial 9-1-1.

check yourself

- **What are two things each that you can do to prevent household poisoning, falls, and fire?**

Avoiding Workplace Injury

■ **Identify common workplace injuries and how to avoid them.**

American adults spend most of their waking hours on the job. Although most job situations are pleasant and productive, others pose hazards. Transportation incidents make up the largest number of fatal work injuries (41%). An additional 23 percent of fatal work injuries occur on highways, mostly involving truck drivers. Overall, workers in the transportation and material moving, construction and extraction, and service industries are at the highest risk of fatal injuries; fishing workers, farmers, and loggers are also at high risk.[102]

Although on-the-job deaths capture media attention, workers may also be seriously injured or disabled at their jobs. Common work injuries include cuts and lacerations, chemical burns, fractures, sprains, and strains (often of the back), and repetitive motion disorders. Because so many work injuries are due to overexertion, poor body mechanics, or repetitive motion, they are largely preventable. We discuss these problems and share some prevention strategies here.

Protect Your Back

Low back pain (LBP), usually as a result of injury, is the major cause of disability for people ages 20 to 45 in the United States, who suffer more frequently and severely from this problem than older people do.[103] It is one of the most commonly experienced chronic ailments among college students.

Most injuries to the back are in the lumbar spine area (lower back); strengthening core muscle groups and stretching muscles to avoid cramping and spasms reduce risks. Frequently, sports injuries, stress on spinal bones and tissues, the sudden jolt of a car accident, or other obvious causes are the culprits. Other times, sitting too long in the same position or hunching over your computer while pulling an all-nighter can leave you with pain so severe you can't stand up or walk comfortably. Carrying heavy backpacks is another frequent source of LBP.

Avoid typical risks by using common sense when engaging in activities that could injure your back. Get up and stretch intermittently while working in a static position. Good posture can also reduce back problems.

Other measures you can take to reduce the risk of back pain:

■ Invest in a high-quality, supportive mattress.
■ Avoid long hours in high-heeled shoes, which tilt the pelvis forward.
■ Control your weight. Extra weight puts increased strain on your knees, hips, and back.
■ Warm up and stretch before exercising or lifting heavy objects.
■ When lifting something heavy, use proper form (**Figure 13.7**). Do not bend from the waist or take the weight load on your back.
■ Buy a desk chair with good lumbar support.

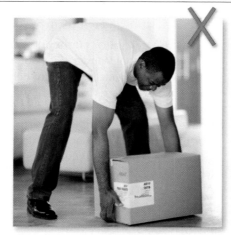

ⓐ Attempting to lift a heavy object by bending at your waist is a common cause of back injury.

Figure 13.7 Lifting a Heavy Object

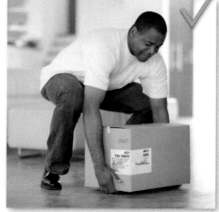

ⓑ Start as close to the object as possible, with it positioned between your knees as you squat down. Keep your feet parallel, or stagger one foot in front of the other. Keep the object close to your body as you stand, using your legs, not your back, to lift.

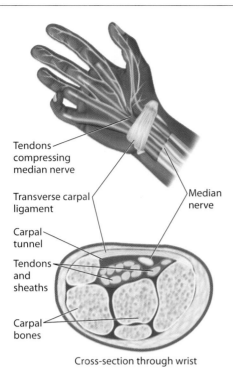

Figure 13.8 Carpal Tunnel Syndrome
The carpal tunnel is a space beneath the transverse carpal ligament and above the carpal bones of the wrist. The median nerve and the tendons that allow you to flex your fingers run through this tunnel. Carpal tunnel syndrome occurs when repetitive use prompts inflammation of the tissues and fluids of the tunnel. This, in turn, compresses the median nerve.

■ Move your car seat forward so your knees are elevated slightly.
■ Engage in regular exercise, particularly core exercises that strengthen and stretch abdominal muscles and back muscles.
■ Downsize your backpack.

Maintain Alignment while Sitting

Think back over your day: How many hours have you sat glued to a computer or book? Were you slouching, hunched over, or sitting up straight? Your answers are probably reflected in the degree of aching and stiffness you may be feeling right now. So how can you maintain healthy alignment while you work? Try these strategies:

1. Sit comfortably with your feet flat on the floor or on a footrest, and your knees level with your hips. Raise or lower your chair, or move to a different chair, to achieve this position.
2. Your middle back should be firmly against the back of the chair. The small of your back should be supported, too. If you can't feel the chair back supporting your lumbar region, try placing a small cushion or rolled towel behind the curve of your lower back.
3. Keep your shoulders relaxed and straight, not rolled or hunched forward.
4. The angle of your elbows should be 90 degrees to your upper arms. Adjust your position or the position of your device to achieve this angle.
5. Ideally, you should be looking straight ahead, not peering down at the device's screen.

Avoid Repetitive Motion Disorders

It's the end of the term, and you've finished the last of several papers. After hours of nonstop typing, your hands are numb and you feel intense pain that makes the thought of typing one more word unbearable. You may be suffering from one of several **repetitive motion disorders (RMDs)**, sometimes called *overuse syndrome*, *cumulative trauma disorders*, or *repetitive stress injuries*. These refer to a family of soft tissue injuries that begin with inflammation and gradually become disabling.

Repetitive motion disorders include carpal tunnel syndrome, bursitis, tendonitis, and ganglion cysts, among others.[104] Twisting of the arm or wrist, overexertion, and incorrect posture or position are usually contributors. The areas most likely to be affected are the hands, wrists, elbows, and shoulders, but the neck, back, hips, knees, feet, ankles, and legs can be affected, too. Over time, RMDs can cause permanent damage to nerves, soft tissue, and joints. Usually, RMDs are associated with repeating the same task and gradually irritating the area in question. Certain sports (tennis, golf, and others), gripping the wheel while driving, keyboarding or texting, and a number of technology-driven activities can also result in RMDs.

Because many of these injuries occur in everyday work, play, and athletics, they are often not reported to national agencies that keep track of injury statistics. Nevertheless, cases of "BlackBerry thumb," carpal tunnel syndrome, and other maladies are widespread.

One of the most common RMDs is **carpal tunnel syndrome (CTS)**, an inflammation of the soft tissues and fluids within the "tunnel" through the carpal bones of the wrist (**Figure 13.8**). This puts pressure on the median nerve, which runs down the forearm through the tunnel. Symptoms include numbness, tingling, and pain in the fingers and hands. Carpal tunnel syndrome typically results from spending hours typing at the computer keyboard, flipping groceries through computerized scanners, or manipulating other objects in jobs "made simpler" by technology. The risk for CTS can be reduced by proper design of workstations, protective wrist pads, and worker training. Physical and occupational therapy is an important part of treatment and recovery.

Strategies for avoiding repetitive motion disorders include:[105]

■ If you are doing repetitive motion activities such as taking notes in class by hand, reduce your force and relax your grip. There are pens available that offer oversized grips and free-flowing ink, which lessen the strain on your hand.
■ Take frequent breaks to stretch your hands and wrists.
■ Keep your hands and fingers warm. A cold environment can lead to stiffness and hand pain. You may need to wear fingerless gloves if you can't control your environment.

check yourself

■ **What are two strategies to protect your back?**
■ **What workplace factors contribute to repetitive motion disorders?**

Are You at Risk for Violence or Injury?

How often are you at risk for sustaining an intentional or unintentional injury? Answer the questions below to find out.

An interactive version of this assessment is available online. Download it from the Live It! section of www.pearsonhighered.com/donatelle.

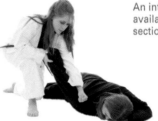

1 Relationship Risk

How often does your partner:

	Never	Sometimes	Often
1. Criticize you for your appearance (weight, dress, hair, etc.)?	○	○	○
2. Embarrass you in front of others by putting you down?	○	○	○
3. Blame you or others for his or her mistakes?	○	○	○
4. Curse at you, shout at you, say mean things, insult, or mock you?	○	○	○
5. Demonstrate uncontrollable anger?	○	○	○
6. Criticize your friends, family, or others who are close to you?	○	○	○
7. Threaten to leave you if you don't behave in a certain way?	○	○	○
8. Manipulate you to prevent you from spending time with friends or family?	○	○	○
9. Express jealousy, distrust, and anger when you spend time with other people?	○	○	○
10. Make all the significant decisions in your relationship?	○	○	○
11. Intimidate or threaten you, making you fearful or anxious?	○	○	○
12. Make threats to harm others you care about, including pets?	○	○	○
13. Control your telephone calls, monitor your messages, or read your e-mail without permission.	○	○	○
14. Punch, hit, slap, or kick you?	○	○	○
15. Make you feel guilty about something?	○	○	○
16. Use money or possessions to control you?	○	○	○
17. Force you to perform sexual acts that make you uncomfortable or embarrassed?	○	○	○
18. Threaten to kill himself or herself if you leave?	○	○	○
19. Follow you, call to check on you, or demonstrate a constant obsession with what you are doing?	○	○	○

2 Risk for Vehicular Injuries

How often do you:

	Never	Sometimes	Often
1. Drive after you have had one or two drinks?	○	○	○
2. Drive after you have had three or more drinks?	○	○	○
3. Drive when you are tired?	○	○	○
4. Drive while you are extremely upset?	○	○	○
5. Drive while using your cell phone?	○	○	○
6. Drive or ride in a car while not wearing a seat belt?	○	○	○
7. Drive faster than the speed limit?	○	○	○
8. Accept rides from friends who have been drinking?	○	○	○

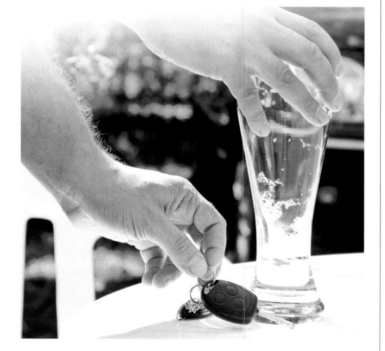

3 Online Safety

How often do you:

	Never	Sometimes	Often
1. Give out your name/address on the Internet?	○	○	○
2. Put personal identifying information on your blog, Facebook, or other websites?	○	○	○
3. Post personal pictures, travel/vacation plans and other private material on social networking sites?	○	○	○
4. Date people you meet online?	○	○	○
5. Use a shared or public computer to check e-mail without clearing the browser cache?	○	○	○
6. Make financial transactions online without confirming security measures?	○	○	○

4 Risk for Assault or Rape

How often do you:

	Never	Sometimes	Often
1. Drink more than 1 or 2 drinks while out with friends or at a party?	○	○	○
2. Leave your drinks unattended while you get up to dance or go to the bathroom?	○	○	○
3. Accept drinks from strangers while out at a bar or party?	○	○	○
4. Leave parties with people you barely know or just met	○	○	○
5. Walk alone in poorly lit or unfamiliar places?	○	○	○
6. Open the door to strangers?	○	○	○
7. Leave your car or home door unlocked?	○	○	○
8. Talk on your cell phone, oblivious to your surroundings?	○	○	○

Analyzing Your Responses

Look at your responses to the list of questions in each of these sections. Part 1 focused on relationships—if you answered "sometimes" or "often" to several of these questions, you may need to evaluate your situation. In Parts 2 through 4, if you answered "often" to any question, you may need to adjust your behavior and educate yourself about steps you can take to remain safe.

13.14 | Assess Yourself:
Are You at Risk for Violence or Injury?

337

VIOLENCE AND UNINTENTIONAL INJURIES

Your Plan for Change

The Assess Yourself activity gave you a chance to consider symptoms of abuse in your relationships and signs of unsafe behavior in other realms of your life. Now that you are aware of these signs and symptoms, you can work on changing behaviors to reduce your risk.

Today, you can:

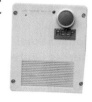

○ Pay attention as you walk your normal route around campus and think about whether you are taking the safest route. Is it well lit? Do you walk in areas that receive little foot traffic? Are there any emergency phone boxes along your route? Does campus security patrol the area? If part of your route seems unsafe, look around for alternate routes. Vary your route when possible.

○ Look at your residence's safety features. Is there a secure lock, dead bolt, or keycard entry system on all outer doors? Can windows be shut and locked? Is there a working smoke alarm in every room and hallway? Are the outside areas well lit? If you live in a dorm or apartment building, is there a security guard at the main entrance? If you notice any potential safety hazards, report them to your landlord or campus residential life administrator right away.

Within the next 2 weeks, you can:

○ If you are worried about potentially abusive behavior in a partner or in a friend's partner, visit the campus counseling center and ask about resources on campus or in your community to help you deal with potential relationship abuse. Consider talking to a counselor about your concerns or sitting in on a support group.

○ Next time you attend a party, set limits for yourself in order to remain in control of your behavior and to avoid putting yourself in a dangerous or compromising position. Decide ahead of time on the number of drinks you will have, arrange with a friend to monitor each other's behavior during the party, and be sure you have a reliable, safe way of getting home.

By the end of the semester, you can:

○ Learn ways to protect yourself by signing up for a self- defense workshop or violence prevention class on campus or in the community.

○ Get involved in an on-campus or community group dedicated to promoting safety. You might want to attend a meeting of an antiviolence group, join in a Take Back the Night rally, or volunteer at a local rape crisis center or battered women's shelter.

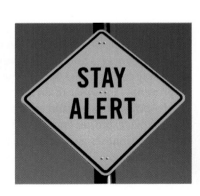

Summary

- Factors that lead people to be violent include economic difficulties, parental influence, cultural beliefs, discrimination, political differences, stress, substance abuse, stress, excessive fear, anger, and a history of violence.

- Interpersonal violence includes homicide, domestic violence, child abuse, elder abuse, and sexual victimization.

- Forms of collective violence, including gang violence and terrorism, continue to result in fear, anxiety, and issues of discrimination.

- Recognizing how to protect yourself, knowing where to get help, and having honest, straightforward dialogue in dating situations can help reduce risk of becoming a victim of violence.

- Shootings and extreme acts of violence on campuses have resulted in a groundswell of activities designed to protect students. Preventing violence means community activism; prioritizing mental and emotional health; and skills training in anger management, coping, parenting, and other key areas.

- Distracted driving, impaired driving, and road rage are factors in an overwhelming number of motor vehicle accidents. A well-designed and well-maintained vehicle can reduce the likelihood and severity of accidents, as can simple risk-management techniques.

- Basic safety guidelines—including wearing appropriate safety gear and staying sober—can help people stay safe during sports and recreation.

- High-decibel noise can lead to hearing loss; music listeners should keep earphone volume to a reasonable level and use earplugs or distance themselves from speakers to protect hearing at concerts and similar events.

- To stay safe at home, know how to prevent—and what to do in the event of—poisoning, fire, and injury. In the workplace, proper ergonomics can help prevent injuries and repetitive motion disorders.

Pop Quiz

1. An example of an *intentional injury* is:
   a. a car crash.
   b. murder.
   c. drowning.
   d. road rage.

2. Jack beats his wife Melissa "to teach her a lesson." Afterward, he denies attacking her. The phase of the cycle of violence that this illustrates is
   a. acute battering.
   b. chronic battering.
   c. remorse/reconciliation.
   d. tension building.

3. When Jane began her new job with all male coworkers, her supervisor told her that he enjoyed having an attractive woman in the workplace, and he winked at her. His comment constitutes
   a. acquaintance rape.
   b. sexual assault.
   c. sexual harassment.
   d. sexual battering.

4. In a sociology class, students were discussing sexual assault. One student commented that some women dress too provocatively. The social assumption this student made is
   a. minimization.
   b. trivialization.
   c. blaming the victim.
   d. "boys will be boys."

5. Rape by a person the victim knows and that does not involve a physical beating or use of a weapon is called
   a. simple rape.
   b. sexual assault.
   c. simple assault.
   d. aggravated rape.

6. Which of the following is an example of stalking?
   a. Making intimate and sexually implied comments to another person
   b. Repeated visual, physical, or virtual seeking out of another person
   c. Unwelcome sexual conduct by the perpetrator
   d. Sexual abuse of a child

7. Which of the following is *not* a good response to another driver's road rage?
   a. Avoid eye contact.
   b. Remember the person's license plate number.
   c. Drive home immediately.
   d. Drive to the nearest police station.

8. The majority of skateboarding accidents happen to riders who
   a. are new to the sport.
   b. have been riding for more than a year.
   c. are trying out new equipment.
   d. are skating on public property.

9. Above what decibel level do risks for hearing loss increase?
   a. 70 dB (vacuum cleaner)
   b. 85 dB (diesel truck engine)
   c. 108 dB (MP3 player at maximum volume)
   d. 130 dB (jet airplane engine)

10. Which of the following is *not* a common factor in repetitive motion disorders?
   a. Lifting from the back rather than the knees
   b. Prolonged typing
   c. Poor sitting posture
   d. Incorrectly aligned computer workstation setup

Answers to these questions can be found on page A-1.

Web Links

1. **Communities against Violence Network.** Information about violence against women, from domestic violence to legal information and statistics. www.cavnet2.org

2. **National Center for Injury Prevention and Control.** Statistics and information on fatal and nonfatal injuries, both intentional and unintentional. www.cdc.gov/injury

3. **National Center for Victims of Crime.** Resources for victims of crimes ranging from hate crimes to sexual assault. www.ncvc.org

4. **National Sexual Violence Resources Center.** An excellent resource for victims of sexual violence. www.nsvrc.org

5. **Workplace Safety and Health.** Data and resources on a range of workplace safety issues. www.cdc.gov/workplace

Environmental Health

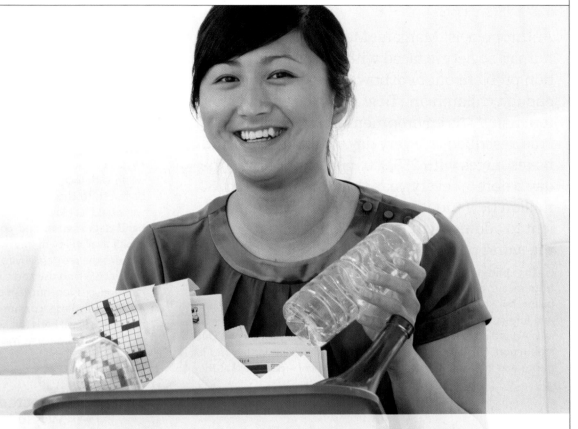

339

The threat from climate change is serious, it is urgent, and it is growing. Our generation's response to this challenge will be judged by history, for if we fail to meet it—boldly, swiftly, and together—we risk consigning future generations to an irreversible catastrophe.

> —President Barack Obama, United Nations Summit on Climate Change, 2009

The global population has grown more in the past 50 years than at any other time in history. Polar ice caps are melting at rates that defy even the direst predictions, and threats of rising sea levels loom. One in 4 existing mammals is threatened with extinction as humans destroy habitat, exacerbate drought and flooding through climate change, and pollute the environment. Clean water is becoming increasingly scarce, fossil fuels are dwindling quickly, and solid and hazardous wastes are growing in proportion to population.

Have we crossed the point at which we will be unable to restore the balance between humans and nature, or are there actions we can take to bring the environmental health of Earth back into balance? Individuals, communities, and political powers must take action now to make positive change. This chapter gives an overview of factors contributing to our global environmental crisis.

Overpopulation

- **List factors affecting population growth and overpopulation.**

Anthropologist Margaret Mead wrote, "Every human society is faced with not one population problem but two: how to beget and rear enough children and how not to beget and rear too many."[1] As environmental scientist Robert H. Friis described it, "Every day we share Earth and its resources with 250,000 more people than the day before ... every year, there are more than 80 million new mouths to feed. This is the equivalent to adding a city the size of Philadelphia to the world population every week."[2]

The United Nations projects that the world population will grow from its current level of 7 billion to 9.3 billion by 2050 and to 10.1 billion by 2100 (**Figure 14.1**).[3] Meanwhile, fertile land, clean water, rain forests, and natural resources are disappearing at a phenomenal rate. According to a recent United Nations Global Environmental Outlook report (GEO-4), the human population is living far beyond its means and inflicting damage on the environment—damage that may

already be irreparable.[4] Population experts believe that the most critical environmental challenge today is slowing population growth. Evidence of the effects of unchecked population growth, excessive consumption, and toxic byproducts of human use and waste is everywhere:

- **Impact on other species.** Changes in the **ecosystem** are resulting in destruction of whole species. Twelve percent of birds are threatened with extinction, with 23 percent of mammals and more than 30 percent of amphibians already gone or nearly gone. Many that survive have chemically induced ailments or genetic disfigurement.[5]
- **Impact on our food supply.** We are currently fishing our oceans at rates 250 percent greater than those they need to regenerate. At current rates, scientists project a global collapse of all fish species by 2050. Food shortages and famine occur in many regions of the world with increasing frequency. Faced with these issues, we may be forced to change how we think about food. Many experts say we should "eat lower on the food chain" by eating more plants.
- **Land degradation and contamination of drinking water.** Per capita availability of freshwater is declining; contaminated water remains the greatest environmental cause of human disease. Unsustainable land use and climate change are increasing land degradation, erosion, nutrient depletion, and deforestation.
- **Impact on energy consumption.** Despite a shift away from nonrenewable **fossil fuels** (oil, coal, natural gas) and toward renewable energy sources, such as hydropower and solar, wind, and biomass

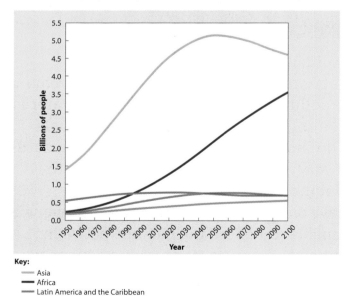

Key:
— Asia
— Africa
— Latin America and the Caribbean
— Europe
— Northern America
— Oceania

Figure 14.1 Estimated and Projected World Population Growth, 1950–2100

Source: United Nations, Department of Economic and Social Affairs, Population Division, *World Population Prospects: The 2010 Revision*, 2011, http://esa.un.org/unpd/wpp/Analytical-Figures/htm/fig_2.htm.

TABLE 14.1 Selected Total Fertility Rates Worldwide, 2011

Country	Number of Children Born per Woman*	Rank
Niger	7.60	1
Uganda	6.69	2
Afghanistan	5.59	13
Iraq	3.67	42
India	2.62	79
Mexico	2.29	101
United States	2.06	123
Australia	1.78	157
Canada	1.58	178
China	1.54	182
Russia	1.42	197
Japan	1.21	219

*Indicates the average number of children that would be born per woman if all women lived to the end of their childbearing years and bore children according to a given fertility rate at each age.

Source: Data from Central Intelligence Agency, "The World Factbook: Country Comparison: Total Fertility Rate," 2011, https://www.cia.gov/library/publications/the-world-factbook/rankorder/2127rank.html.

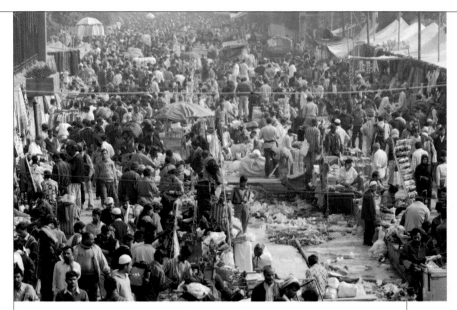

Why is population growth an environmental issue?

Every year the global population grows by 90 million, but Earth's resources are not expanding. Population increases are believed responsible for most current environmental stress.

power, most of us still use fossil fuels. In many developing regions, demand for fossil fuels is growing at unprecedented rates.

Factors Affecting Population Growth

The **total fertility rate** is a measure of the hypothetical average number of children born to women during their lifetime (typically assessed as ages 15 to 44), given prevailing fertility and mortality rates. In the United States today, the fertility rate is just over 2.0.[6] In many developing countries, rates range from over 5.0 to nearly 8.0 (see **Table 14.1**).[7]

High fertility rates lead to rapid increases in overall population in poorer countries and create a significant impact on environmental resources. Even in wealthy countries, slight changes in fertility rates affect energy use.

Mortality rates from both chronic and infectious diseases have declined in both developed and developing regions as a result of improved public health infrastructure, availability of drugs and vaccines, disaster preparedness, and other factors. Longer life spans put pressure on the environment.

Different Nations, Different Growth Rates

India is expected to add another 600 million people by the year 2050, surpassing China as the world's most populous country.[8] The preference for large families in many developing nations has historically been related to several factors: high infant mortality rates; the traditional view of children as "social security" (working from a young age to assist families in daily survival and supporting aging parents); the low educational and economic status of women, which often leaves women with few reproductive choices; and the traditional desire for sons, which keeps parents of daughters reproducing until they have male offspring.

In contrast, population sizes in wealthier nations are static or declining, with one notable exception—the United States, which had a growth rate of nearly 1 percent in 2010.[9] Each year, the United States adds nearly 3 million more people, or 8,000 per day.[10]

Although the United States makes up only 5 percent of the world's population, it is responsible for nearly 25 percent of total global resource consumption.[11] According to the World-watch Institute, "between 1950 and 2000, the United States was responsible for 212 gigatons of carbon dioxide, whereas India was responsible for less than 10 percent as much. . . .

The richest people on the planet are appropriating more than their fair share of 'environmental space.'"[12] Industrial countries, with less than 20 percent of the world's population, have contributed roughly 40 percent of global carbon emissions and are responsible for more than 60 percent of the total carbon dioxide that fossil fuels have added to the atmosphere.[13]

Meanwhile, China and other industrializing countries are becoming major consumers of fossil fuels as they emulate Western lifestyles. Emissions in China are now rising at a rate of approximately 10 percent a year—10 times the rate of increase in industrialized nations.[14]

Zero Population Growth

Many countries have enacted population control measures or encouraged citizens to limit family size. Proponents of *total zero population growth* think each couple should produce two or fewer offspring, allowing the population to stabilize or decrease. Currently, more than 20 countries have zero or negative population growth, meaning that deaths equal or surpass births (this doesn't include the effects of immigration or emigration). Based on current rates, Ukraine is expected to lose 28 percent of its population between the present and 2050, with Russia losing 22 percent and Japan losing 21 percent.[15] Although some praise these declines, others worry about their social and cultural implications.

As education levels of women increase and women achieve equality in pay, job status, and social status, fertility rates decline. Also, as women gain choices in birth control, access to health care, and information about family planning, they tend to marry later and have fewer children. Policies that encourage low birth rates in society and that educate citizens about the consequences of unchecked population growth may be effective.

check yourself

- **What are some effects of overpopulation worldwide?**
- **What is zero population growth?**

- ■ **Identify the major factors contributing to air pollution.**

The term *air pollution* refers to the presence of substances (suspended particles and vapors) not found in perfectly clean air.[16] Natural events, living creatures, and toxic byproducts have always polluted the environment. What is new is the vast array of **pollutants**, their concentrations, and their potential interactive effects.

Generally, air pollutants are either *naturally occurring* or *anthropogenic* (human caused). Naturally occurring air pollutants include particulate matter, such as ash from volcanic eruptions. Anthropogenic sources include those caused by *stationary sources* (e.g., the 2010 BP oil spill in the Gulf of Mexico) and *mobile sources* such as vehicles.[17] According to Environmental Protection Agency (EPA) estimates, mobile sources are the major contributors of key air pollutants such as carbon monoxide (CO), sulfur oxides (SO$_x$), and nitrogen oxides (NO$_x$). In fact, motor vehicles alone contribute about 60 percent of all CO emissions nationwide, with nonroad sources contributing another 22 percent. Some say that "clean coal" offers a good alternative to oil, but critics argue that coal-burning plants contribute the major portion of sulfur oxide pollution and that petroleum refineries and some older diesel engines continue to be large sources of pollution. Primary sources of NO$_x$ pollution include motor vehicles, electric utilities, and other fuel-burning sources.[18]

Components of Air Pollution

Concern about air quality prompted Congress to pass the Clean Air Act in 1970 and to amend it in 1977 and again in 1990. The goal was to develop standards for six of the most widespread air pollutants that seriously affect health: sulfur dioxide, particulates, carbon monoxide, nitrogen dioxide, ground-level

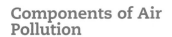

Acid deposition has many harmful effects on the environment. Because its toxins seep into groundwater and enter the food chain, it also poses health hazards to humans.

When the AQI is in this range:	... air quality conditions are	... as symbolized by this color:
0 to 50	Good	Green
51 to 100	Moderate	Yellow
101 to 150	Unhealthy for sensitive groups	Orange
151 to 200	Unhealthy	Red
201 to 300	Very unhealthy	Purple
301 to 500	Hazardous	Maroon

Figure 14.2 Air Quality Index (AQI)
The EPA provides individual AQIs for ground-level ozone, particle pollution, carbon monoxide, sulfur dioxide, and nitrogen dioxide. All AQIs are presented using the general values, categories, and colors of this figure.
Source: U.S. Environmental Protection Agency, "Air Quality Index: A Guide to Air Quality and Your Health," Updated July 2010, www.airnow.gov/index.cfm?action=aqibasics.aqi.

ozone, and lead. Other common air pollutants include carbon dioxide and hydrocarbons. Today, ozone and particle air pollution are the most widespread and dangerous of the air pollutants.[19] Some of the components of air pollution, most notably carbon dioxide, are also greenhouse gases that play a role in global warming and climate change.

Photochemical Smog

Photochemical smog is a mix of particulates and gases that forms when oxygen-containing compounds of nitrogen and hydrocarbons react in the presence of sunlight. It is sometimes called *ozone pollution*, because ozone is one of the products of this reaction. In most cases, smog forms via a **temperature inversion**, a weather condition in which a cool layer of air is trapped under a layer of warmer air, which prevents air circulation. When gases such as hydrocarbons and nitrogen oxides are released into the cool air, they remain suspended until winds remove the warmer air layer. Smog is more likely to occur in valley regions blocked by hills or mountains—for example, Los Angeles.

The most noticeable adverse effects of smog are difficulty breathing, burning eyes, headaches, and nausea. Long-term exposure poses serious health risks, particularly for children, older adults, pregnant women, and people with chronic respiratory disorders such as asthma and emphysema.

Air Quality Index

Air quality can change from day to day or even hour to hour. The EPA's Air Quality Index (AQI) (**Figure 14.2**) measures how clean or polluted air is and notes health effects that can happen within a few hours or

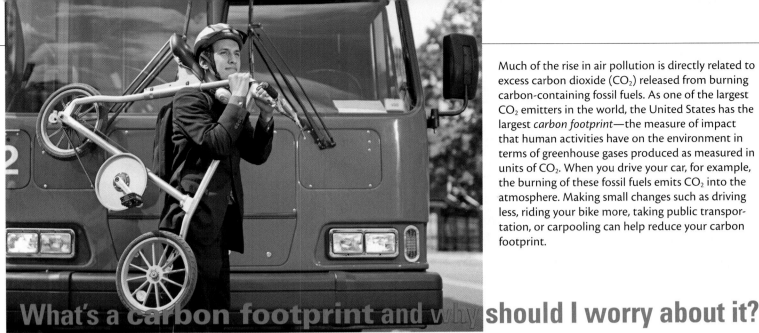

Much of the rise in air pollution is directly related to excess carbon dioxide (CO_2) released from burning carbon-containing fossil fuels. As one of the largest CO_2 emitters in the world, the United States has the largest *carbon footprint*—the measure of impact that human activities have on the environment in terms of greenhouse gases produced as measured in units of CO_2. When you drive your car, for example, the burning of these fossil fuels emits CO_2 into the atmosphere. Making small changes such as driving less, riding your bike more, taking public transportation, or carpooling can help reduce your carbon footprint.

What's a carbon footprint and why should I worry about it?

days after breathing polluted air. It reflects national air quality standards for five major air pollutants regulated by the Clean Air Act.

The higher the AQI number (0 to 500), the greater the air pollution and associated health risks. At levels above 100, air quality is considered unhealthy—at first for certain groups of people, then at higher levels for everyone. The EPA has divided the AQI scale into six color-coded categories that help the public assess daily air quality.

Acid Deposition and Acid Rain

Acid deposition (replacing the term *acid rain*) refers to precipitation that has fallen through air that contains molecules that turn to acid when mixed with water (sulfur dioxides and nitrogen oxides).

In the United States, roughly two-thirds of all sulfur dioxide and one-fourth of all nitrogen oxides come from electric power generation that relies on burning fossil fuels.[20] When coal-powered plants, ore smelters, oil refineries, and steel mills burn fuels, the sulfur and nitrogen in the emissions combine with oxygen and sunlight to become sulfur dioxide and nitrogen oxides (precursors of sulfuric acid and nitric acids, respectively). Small acid particles are then carried by the wind and combine with moisture to produce acidic rain or snow. Acidic pollutants can be deposited in two ways. *Wet deposition* refers to acidic rain, fog, and snow. In *dry deposition*, chemicals may become incorporated into dust or smoke before falling to the ground.[21]

When it falls into lakes and ponds, acid deposition gradually acidifies the water. Once the acidity reaches a certain level, plant and animal life cannot survive.[22] Ironically, acidified lakes and ponds become a clear deep blue, giving the illusion of beauty and health. Every year, acid deposition destroys millions of trees; much of the world's forestlands are now experiencing damaging levels of acid deposition.[23]

Acid deposition aggravates and may even cause bronchitis, asthma, and other respiratory problems, and people with emphysema or heart disease may suffer from exposure, as may developing fetuses.[24] Acid deposition can cause metals such as aluminum, cadmium, lead, and mercury to **leach** out of the soil. If these metals make their way into water or food supplies, they can cause cancer in humans.

Ozone Layer Depletion

The ozone layer forms a protective stratum in Earth's stratosphere—the highest level of our atmosphere, 12 to 30 miles above Earth's surface. It protects our planet and its inhabitants from ultraviolet B (UVB) radiation, a primary cause of skin cancer. Such radiation damages DNA and weakens immune systems in both humans and animals.

In the 1970s, instruments developed to test atmospheric contents indicated that chemicals used on Earth, especially **chlorofluorocarbons (CFCs**, used in products such as refrigerants and hair sprays), were contributing to the ozone layer's rapid depletion. When released into the air through spraying or offgassing, CFCs migrate into the ozone layer, where they decompose and release chlorine atoms. These atoms cause ozone molecules to break apart and ozone levels to be depleted.

The U.S. government banned the use of aerosol sprays containing CFCs in the 1970s. The discovery of an ozone "hole" over Antarctica led to the 1987 Montreal Protocol treaty, whereby the United States and other nations agreed to further reduce the use of CFCs and other ozone-depleting chemicals. The treaty was amended in 1995 to ban CFC production in developed countries. Today, over 190 countries have signed the treaty as the international community strives to preserve the ozone layer.[25]

What can you do to combat the process of ozone layer depletion? Two important steps are to purchase products labeled "ozone friendly" or "CFC-free" and to be sure that old refrigerators, freezers, and air conditioners are recycled and that the CFCs from them are recovered rather than being released into the atmosphere.

check yourself

■ **What are four factors contributing to air pollution?**

learning outcomes

- **Identify pollutants that affect indoor air quality.**

A growing body of evidence indicates that the air *inside* buildings can be much more hazardous than outdoor air even in the most industrialized cities. The higher the dose of pollutants, and the more airtight the house, the greater the health risk.

Age, preexisting medical conditions, and respiratory function can affect your risk of being affected by indoor air pollution.[26] Those with allergies may be particularly vulnerable. Health effects may develop over years of exposure or may occur in response to toxic levels of pollutants.

Prevention of indoor air pollution should focus on three main areas: *source control* (eliminating or reducing individual contaminants), *ventilation improvements* (increasing the amount of outdoor air coming indoors), and *air cleaners* (removing particulates from the air).[27] In an attempt to reduce pollutants, many manufacturers are offering green building products and furnishings, such as natural-fiber fabrics, untreated wood, and low- or no-volatile organic compound paints.

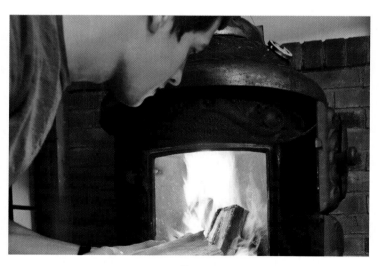

How can air pollution be a problem indoors?

The air within homes can be 10 to 40 times more hazardous than outside air. Indoor air pollution comes from wood stoves, furnaces, cigarette smoke, asbestos, formaldehyde, radon, lead, mold, and household chemicals.

20 to 100

potentially dangerous chemical compounds can be found in the air of the average American home.

Sources of Indoor Air Pollution

The main sources of indoor air pollution are as follows.

Environmental Tobacco Smoke Perhaps the greatest source of indoor air pollution is *environmental tobacco smoke* (*ETS*)—smoke from cigarette, cigar, and pipe smoking. The only effective way to eliminate ETS is to enact strict no-smoking policies. Many U.S. cities ban smoking in public places, at worksites, and in automobiles where children are present.

Home Heating If you rely on wood or on oil- or gas-fired furnaces for home heating, make sure your heating appliance is properly installed, vented, and maintained. In wood stoves, burning properly seasoned wood reduces particulates. Thorough cleaning and maintenance can prevent carbon monoxide buildup in the home. Inexpensive home monitors are available to detect high carbon monoxide levels.

Asbestos **Asbestos** is a mineral compound used to insulate vinyl flooring, roofing materials, heating pipe coverings, and many other products in buildings constructed before 1970. When bonded to other materials, asbestos is relatively harmless, but if its tiny fibers become loosened and airborne, they can embed themselves in the lungs. If asbestos is detected in the home, it must be removed or sealed off by a professional.

Formaldehyde **Formaldehyde** is a colorless, strong-smelling gas released from building materials or new carpet in a process called *offgassing*. Offgassing is highest in new products, but the process can continue for many years.

To limit your formaldehyde exposure, ask about the formaldehyde content of products you purchase, and avoid those that contain it, or buy used furniture. Some houseplants, such as philodendrons and spider plants, help clean formaldehyde from the air.

Radon **Radon is** an odorless, colorless gas found in soil that can penetrate homes through cracks or other openings in the basement or foundation. Radon is the second leading cause of lung cancer, after smoking.[28]

The EPA estimates that as many as 8.1 million U.S. homes (1 out of every 15) have elevated radon levels.[29] Homes below the third floor should be tested for radon, ideally every 2 years or when moving into a new home. Inexpensive test kits are available in hardware stores.

Lead **Lead** is a metal pollutant sometimes found in paint, batteries, drinking water, pipes, dishes with lead-based glazes, dirt, soldered cans, and some candies made in Mexico. Recently, several toys produced in China have been recalled due to unsafe levels of lead in their paint.

Up to 25 percent of U.S. homes still have lead-based paint hazards, and an estimated 250,000 American children under 5 have unsafe blood lead levels.[30] To reduce lead exposure, keep areas where children play as dust-free as possible, and do not remove lead paint yourself. Many cities have free lead-testing programs.

Mold Molds are fungi that live both indoors and outdoors. They produce tiny reproductive spores that continually waft through air. These spores can irritate lungs and cause other health problems. For ways to reduce mold exposure, see **Skills for Behavior Change**.

Sick Building Syndrome **Sick building syndrome (SBS)** is said to exist when 80 percent of a building's occupants report air pollution-related problems (many complain of maladies that lessen or vanish when they leave the building.). Poor ventilation is a primary cause of SBS. Other causes include faulty furnaces that emit carbon monoxide, nitrogen dioxide, and sulfur dioxide; biological air pollutants such as dander (dried skin and hair from pets), molds, and dust; volatile organic compounds from products such as hairspray, cleaners, and adhesives; and heavy metals such as lead. Symptoms include eye irritation, sore throat, queasiness, and worsened asthma.

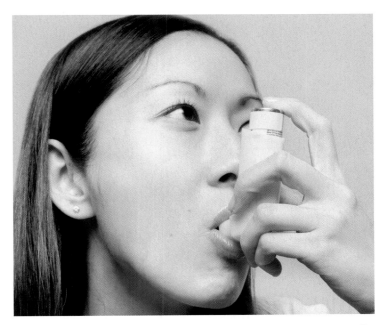

What causes asthma?

Asthma is caused by inflammation of the airways in the lungs, restricting airflow and leading to wheezing, chest tightness, shortness of breath, and coughing. In most people, asthma is brought on by contact with allergens or irritants in the air; some people also have exercise-induced asthma. People with asthma can generally control their symptoms through the use of inhaled medications, and most asthmatics keep a "rescue" inhaler of bronchodilating medication on hand to use in case of a flare-up.

Indoor air pollution and SBS are increasing concerns in the classroom and workplace. Many U.S. schools have unsatisfactory indoor air quality, often due to poor ventilation, construction techniques that block outside air, and the use of synthetic construction materials.[31] Poor air quality can trigger allergies, asthma, and other health problems.[32]

Air Pollution and Asthma

Asthma is a long-term, chronic inflammatory disorder that causes tiny airways in the lung to spasm in response to triggers. Symptoms include wheezing, difficulty breathing, shortness of breath, and coughing. Although most asthma attacks are mild, severe attacks can trigger potentially fatal contractions of the bronchial tubes.[33]

Asthma falls into two types: extrinsic and intrinsic. The more common form, *extrinsic* or *allergic asthma*, is associated with allergic triggers; it tends to run in families and develop in childhood. *Intrinsic* or *nonallergic asthma* may be triggered by anything except an allergy. Several factors can increase your risk of developing asthma—one of the most significant is environmental allergens and irritants.[34]

Asthma rates have increased by more than 65 percent since the 1980s;[35] many blame increasing pollution rates, especially in poor and nonwhite communities, as well as triggers such as dust mites in mattresses, chemicals in carpets and furniture, and airtight modern buildings.

Skills for Behavior Change

BE MOLD FREE

- Keep the humidity level in your home between 40 and 60 percent.
- Use an air conditioner or a dehumidifier during humid months.
- Be sure your home has adequate ventilation, including exhaust fans in the kitchen and bathrooms. If there are no fans, open windows.
- Buy paints with mold-resistant properties or add mold inhibitors.
- In the bathroom, wipe down shower doors, keep surfaces dry, and, if necessary, use environmentally safe mold-killing products. Do not carpet bathrooms and basements or other rooms that are routinely damp.
- Many antimold products commonly used in outdoor areas are extremely toxic; pets and wildlife may wander through these after they've been applied. Use them sparingly or not at all.
- Wash rugs used in entryways and other areas where moisture can accumulate.
- Throw away mattresses and furniture exposed to excessive moisture.
- Dry clothing thoroughly before putting it away.
- When buying a house, don't skimp on mold inspections. Check for mold growth regularly, especially in rental units where landlords may not pay attention to these risks.

check yourself

- **What are four common indoor air pollutants and their sources?**

Global Warming and Climate Change

- **Describe how greenhouse gas buildup contributes to climate change.**

More than 100 years ago, scientists theorized that carbon dioxide emissions from the burning of fossil fuels would create a buildup of greenhouse gases in Earth's atmosphere that could have a warming effect on Earth's surface.[36] In recent years, these predictions have been supported by reports from leading international scientists in the field and accounts in the popular media, such as the 2006 documentary film *An Inconvenient Truth*, all detailing startling indicators of a planet in trouble.

Consequences of the Greenhouse Effect

The *greenhouse effect* is a natural phenomenon in which **greenhouse gases**, such as **carbon dioxide (CO_2)**, warm the planet (see **Figure 14.3**). Human activities such as burning fossil fuels and land clearing have increased greenhouse gases in the atmosphere, resulting in the **enhanced greenhouse effect**, in which excess solar heat is trapped, raising the planet's overall temperature and leading to an increase in extreme weather and climate change in areas around the globe. According to data from the National Oceanic and Atmospheric Administration (NOAA) and the National Aeronautics and Space Administration (NASA), Earth's surface temperature has risen about 1.2 to 1.4 °F since 1900, with accelerated warming occurring in the past two decades.[37] Furthermore, the consensus is that temperatures will continue to rise, perhaps by as much as 5 to 10 degrees in the next 100 years, unless immediate steps are taken to reverse the trend. Projected results of such a temperature increase—which might include rising sea levels (potentially flooding entire countries), glacier retreat, arctic shrinkage at the poles, altered patterns of agriculture (including changes in growing seasons and alterations of climatic zones), deforestation, drought, extreme weather events, increases in tropical diseases, changes in disease trends and patterns, loss of biological species, and economic devastation—would be catastrophic.

The greenhouse gases include carbon dioxide, nitrous oxide, methane, CFCs, and hydrocarbons. The most predominant is carbon dioxide, which accounts for 49 percent of all greenhouse gases. The United States is the planet's greatest producer of greenhouse gases, responsible for over 22 percent of all output—a number expected to increase by 43 percent by 2025.[38] Rapid deforestation of the tropical rain forests of Central and South America, Africa, and southeast Asia also contributes to the rapid rise in greenhouse gases. Trees take in carbon dioxide, transform it, store the carbon for food, and release oxygen into the air. As our planet loses forests, at the rate of hundreds of acres per hour, it loses the capacity to dissipate carbon dioxide.

A United Nations treaty signed in Kyoto in 1997 outlined an international plan to reduce the manmade emissions responsible for climate change. The Kyoto Protocol, which went into effect in 2005, required participating countries to reduce their emissions between 2008 and 2012 by at least 5 percent below 1990 levels.[39] More than 160 countries signed on to the Kyoto Protocol, including more than 30 industrialized countries.[40] The treaty would require the United States to reduce emissions by 33 percent, but, despite support for the treaty from many Americans, then-president George W. Bush chose not to sign because of concerns that major developing nations, including India and China, are not required to reduce emissions under the treaty. A follow-up summit in Copenhagen in 2009 sought to restrict global temperatures to a rise of 2 °C by 2050 but was marked by

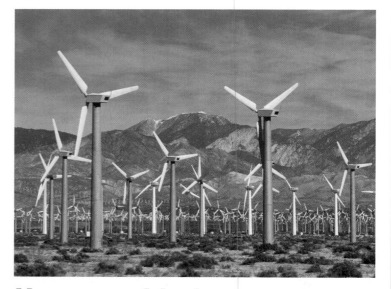

How can I help prevent global warming?

Global warming, sometimes referred to as *climate change*, is a global problem. We need to work with other nations to ensure that everyone does their part. By reducing use of fossil fuels, using high-efficiency vehicles, and supporting increased use of renewable resources such as solar, wind, and water power, you can help combat global warming. For example, the National Renewable Energy Laboratory predicts that, with proper development, wind power could provide 20% of U.S. energy needs.

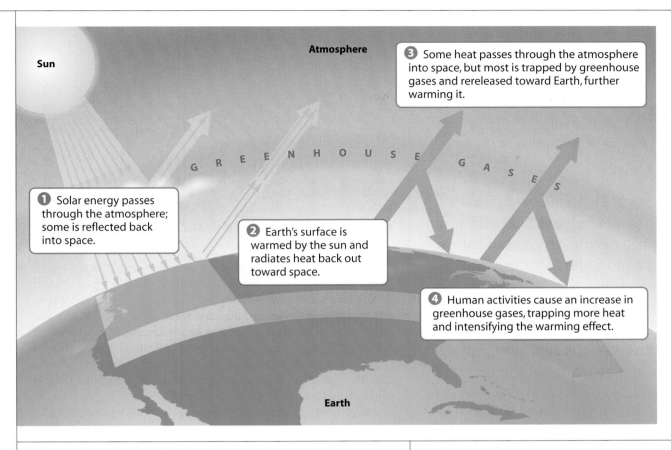

Figure 14.3

The Enhanced Greenhouse Effect

The natural greenhouse effect is responsible for making Earth habitable; it keeps the planet 33 °C (60 °F) warmer than it would otherwise be. An increase in greenhouse gases resulting from human activities is creating the enhanced greenhouse effect, trapping more heat and causing dangerous global climate change.

Sun

Atmosphere

③ Some heat passes through the atmosphere into space, but most is trapped by greenhouse gases and rereleased toward Earth, further warming it.

GREENHOUSE GASES

① Solar energy passes through the atmosphere; some is reflected back into space.

② Earth's surface is warmed by the sun and radiates heat back out toward space.

④ Human activities cause an increase in greenhouse gases, trapping more heat and intensifying the warming effect.

Earth

disagreement among the major participants. A more successful summit, held in December 2010 in Cancun, Mexico, produced commitments from more than 80 countries to cut emissions. To make the agreement binding, a formal treaty will need to be signed, which is still in progress.[41]

Reducing Air Pollution and the Threat of Global Warming

Air pollution and climate change problems are rooted in our energy, transportation, and industrial practices. Clearly, we must develop comprehensive national strategies that encourage the use of renewable resources such as solar, wind, and water power. Because industrial production is a key contributor to fossil fuel emission, clean energy, green factories, improved technology, and governmental regulation are necessary for slowing climate change.

Most experts agree that reducing consumption of fossil fuels in cars and shifting to alternative fuels, improving gas mileage, and using mass transportation are crucial to air pollution reduction. Many cities have taken steps in this direction by setting high parking fees and road-usage tolls in congested areas and by imposing bans on city driving. Local governments should be encouraged to provide convenient and inexpensive public transportation and to motivate people to use it regularly.

Meanwhile, many U.S. communities are creating bicycle lanes and holding "bike to work" days. Scooters and other low-energy modes of transportation are becoming increasingly popular. Some college campuses have enacted new policies allowing increased skateboard and in-line skate use on campus. Other campuses provide scooter and bike garages to protect students from theft and vandalism and to encourage students to bring energy-efficient vehicles to campus.

You can participate in this effort by finding ways to reduce your own **carbon footprint**, or the amount of CO_2 emissions you contribute to the atmosphere in your daily life. Go to www.nature.org/greenliving/carboncalculator to assess your carbon footprint and learn how to reduce it. To see how your college or university handles sustainability, check out the College Sustainability Report Card at www.greenreportcard.org.

You can reduce your carbon footprint by making thoughtful choices about everyday consumption:

- **Refuse the "buy new" impulse.** Cars, cell phones, MP3 players—they all take new energy to produce. Keep such products until they no longer work, rather than succumbing to the urge to get the latest and greatest.
- **Reduce power consumption by unplugging.** Chargers, laptops, clocks, stereos, and TVs all consume power when plugged in, even if they are turned off. Unplug your appliances or buy a power strip that shuts them all off at once.
- **Buy less food and use what you buy.** We waste far too much food. If you find yourself buying food and then throwing half of it away before you get around to eating it, take a closer look at your shopping habits.

check yourself

- **What are some possible effects of uncontained global warming?**
- **What is a carbon footprint, and what behaviors can help reduce yours?**

Pollution in the Water

- **Identify the major factors contributing to water pollution.**

Seventy-five percent of Earth is covered with water in the form of oceans, seas, lakes, rivers, streams, and wetlands. Beneath the landmass are reservoirs of groundwater. We draw our drinking water from either these underground sources or from surface freshwater. However, just 1 percent of the entire water supply is available for human use—the rest is too salty, too polluted, or locked away in polar ice caps.[42]

Over half the global population faces a shortage of clean water. More than 2.6 billion people, about 40 percent of the planet's population, have no access to basic sanitation or adequate toilet facilities. More than 1.5 million deaths each year, mostly among children under 5 years of age, are attributed to illnesses caused by lack of safe water and sanitation.[43]

By 2025, approximately 2.8 billion people will live in countries with severe shortages of clean water. By 2050, these numbers will increase to 4 billion people in 54 countries.[44]

Considering how little water is available to meet the world's agricultural, manufacturing, community, personal, and sanitation needs, it is no wonder that clean water is a precious commodity. In the United States, water consumption—for domestic consumption, recreational use, energy (primarily cooling at power plants), food production, and industry—totals 1,500 gallons per person per day. That's about three times the world average.[45]

Water Contamination

Any substance that gets into the soil can enter the water supply. Industrial pollutants and pesticides work their way into soil, then into groundwater. Underground storage tanks containing gasoline may leak. Drugs, from pain killers to deodorants, wind up in sewers, making their way into waste treatment plants. A comprehensive U.S. Geological Survey investigation discovered many chemical compounds in 139 streams across the United States; both surface water and some of our deepest underground aquifers appear to be affected.[46] Although some studies indicate that concentrations of these contaminants are not yet high enough to result in high risks of reproductive disruptions, developmental toxicity, or cancer development, others question the risk of long-term, continued low-dose and/or cumulative exposure.[47]

2,000,000
kilograms of water pollutants are released daily in the United States.

Tap water in the United States is among the safest in the world. Under the Safe Drinking Water Act (SDWA), the EPA sets standards for drinking water quality. Cities and municipalities have strict policies and procedures governing water treatment, filtration, and disinfection to screen out pathogens and microorganisms. However, according to a recent Associated Press (AP) inquiry, a "vast array of pharmaceuticals—including antibiotics, anticonvulsants, mood stabilizers and hormones—have been found in the drinking water supplies of at least 41 million Americans."[48]

Many other toxic substances also flow into our waterways. **Point source pollutants** enter a waterway at a specific location such as a ditch or pipe; the two major entry points are sewage treatment plants and industrial facilities. **Nonpoint source pollutants**—*runoff* and *sedimentation*—drain or seep into waterways from soil erosion and sedimentation, construction wastes, pesticide and fertilizer runoff, street runoff, acid mine drainage, wastes from engineering projects, leakage from septic tanks, and sewage sludge (see **Figure 14.4**).

Six categories of pollutants cause the most concern and the greatest potential harm:

- **Gasoline and petroleum products.** In the mid-1980s, Congress authorized funds to plug leaking, underground storage tanks as

Air pollution spreads across the landscape and is often overlooked as a major nonpoint source of pollution. Airborne nutrients and pesticides can be transported far from their area of origin.

Point-source contamination can be traced to specific points of discharge from wastewater treatment plants and factories or from combined sewers.

Eroded soil and sediment can transport considerable amounts of some nutrients, such as organic nitrogen and phosphorus, and some pesticides, such as DDT, to rivers and streams.

Wastewater

Runoff

Runoff

Seepage   Groundwater discharge to streams   Seepage

Figure 14.4 Potential Sources of Groundwater Contamination
Source: Adapted from U.S. Geological Survey, Wisconsin Water Science Center, "Learn More about Groundwater," 2008, http://wi.water.usgs.gov/gwcomp/learn.

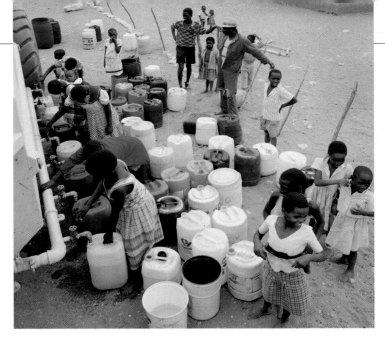

Is there such a thing as water scarcity?

Lack of clean water and sanitation is a major global problem. Another issue is the lack of water available relative to demand. *Closed basins* are defined as regions where existing water cannot meet the agricultural, industrial, municipal, and environmental needs of all; the Stockholm International Water Institute estimates that 1.4 billion people live in closed basins. The problem is expected to worsen rapidly: the Food and Agriculture Organization estimates that the number of people worldwide suffering from water scarcity will increase to 1.8 billion by 2025.

part of the Solid Waste Disposal Act. By 2009, cleanup or containment had occurred at over 80 percent of nearly 500,000 release sites. Funding challenges remain for the remaining sites, which continue to pose threats to nearby underground water sources. Programs to replace tanks, secure tanks, and remove threats are ongoing.[49]

■ **Chemical contaminants.** *Organic solvents* are chemicals designed to dissolve grease and oil. Many household products (stain and spot removers, drain cleaners, septic system cleaners, and paint removers) also contain these toxic chemicals. Organic solvents work their way into the water supply when consumers dump leftover products into the toilet or street drains and when industries bury leftovers in barrels from which solvents may leach into groundwater.

■ **Polychlorinated biphenyls. Polychlorinated biphenyls (PCBs)** were once used as insulation in high-voltage electrical equipment. The human body does not excrete ingested PCBs, but rather stores them in fatty tissues and the liver—they *bioaccumulate*. Exposure to PCBs is associated with birth defects, cancer, and various skin problems. The manufacture of PCBs was discontinued in the United States in 1977, but approximately 500 million pounds have been dumped into landfills and waterways, where they continue to pose an environmental threat.[50]

■ **Dioxins.** Dioxins are chlorinated hydrocarbons found in herbicides (chemicals used to kill vegetation). Dioxins also bioaccumulate; they're much more toxic than PCBs. Long-term effects include possible immune system damage and increased risk of infections

and cancer. Short-term exposure to high concentrations of PCBs or dioxins can have severe consequences, including nausea; vomiting; diarrhea; painful rashes and sores; and chloracne, in which the skin develops painful pimples that may never go away.

■ **Pesticides. Pesticides** are chemicals designed to kill insects, rodents, plants, and fungi. Over 1,055 active ingredients are sold as pesticides throughout the world.[51] Americans use millions of pounds each year, though only small amounts reach targeted organisms. The rest settles on land, floats in air, or runs off into waterways. Pesticides evaporate readily and are often dispersed by wind. Residues cling to fresh fruits and vegetables and can accumulate in the body when people eat these items. Several groups have published consumer guides to the fruits and vegetables likely to be the best and worst when it comes to pesticide contaminants; see www.foodnews.org for one example. Potential hazards associated with exposure to pesticides include birth defects, liver and kidney damage, and nervous system disorders.

■ **Lead.** Lead can leach into water from pipes or water lines, usually in older homes. The EPA has issued new standards to reduce levels of lead in drinking water: no more than 15 parts per billion (ppb). (Previous standard allowed an average of 50 ppb.) If lead is present in your home's water, reduce your risk by running tap water for several minutes before drinking or cooking with it. This flushes out water that has been standing overnight in lead-contaminated lines.

Skills for **Behavior Change**

WASTE LESS WATER!

In The Kitchen
■ Turn off the tap while washing dishes.
■ Check faucets and pipes for leaks. Leaky faucets can waste more than 3,000 gallons of water each year.
■ Equip faucets with aerators to reduce water use by 4 percent.
■ Wash only full dishwasher loads; use the energy-saving mode.

In The Laundry Room
■ Wash only full laundry loads.
■ Upgrade to a high-efficiency washing machine.

In The Bathroom
■ Detect and fix leaks. A leaky toilet can waste 200 gallons of water every day.
■ Install a high-efficiency toilet that uses 60 percent less water.
■ Take showers instead of baths; limit showers to the time it takes to lather and rinse.
■ Replace old showerheads with efficient models that use 60 percent less water.
■ Turn off the tap while brushing your teeth to save up to 8 gallons of water per day.

check yourself

■ **What are three major sources of water pollution?**

■ **What are four steps that you can take to reduce water waste?**

learning outcomes

- **List the major factors contributing to pollution on land.**

Much of the waste that ends up polluting the water starts out polluting the land. For generations, humans have gathered their garbage together in designated areas, creating uninhabitable dumps and landfills. The more people on the planet, the more waste they create, and the more pressure is put on the land to accommodate increasing amounts of refuse—much of which is nonbiodegradable, and some of which is directly harmful to living organisms, including ourselves.

Solid Waste

One of the most common ways that people try to preserve the environment is by participating in recycling programs (**Figure 14.5**). However, each day, every person in the United States generates an average of more than 4.3 pounds of **municipal solid waste (MSW)**, more commonly known as trash or garbage—containers and packaging; discarded food; yard debris; and refuse from residential, commercial, institutional, and industrial sources (see **Figure 14.6**).[52] The total comes to about 243 million tons of MSW each year.[53] Although experts believe that up to 90 percent of our trash is recyclable, we still fall far short of this goal with respect to most types of trash. In the United States, 33.8 percent of all MSW is recovered and recycled or composted, almost 12 percent is burned at combustion facilities, and the remaining 54.3 percent is disposed of in landfills.[54]

Approximately 2 percent, or 3,190 tons, of the MSW is made up of electronic waste.[55] Several options are available for reducing electronic waste in MSW, including recycling, participating in electronic reuse programs, and donating your consumer electronics. Visit www.digitaltips.org/green/default.asp and www.ecyclingcentral.com to find information about locations for electronic waste recycling in your state and to learn how to reduce electronic waste in your MSW.

The number of landfills in the United States has actually decreased in the past decade, but their sheer mass has increased. Many people worry that we are rapidly losing our ability to dispose of all of the waste we create. As communities run out of landfill space, it is becoming more common to haul garbage out to sea to dump, where it contaminates ocean ecosystems, or to ship it to landfills in other states or to developing countries, where it becomes someone else's problem. In today's throwaway society, we need to become aware of the amount of waste we generate every day and to look for ways to recycle, reuse, and—most desirable of all—reduce what we consume.

Communities, businesses, and individuals can adopt several strategies to control waste:

- *Source reduction* (*waste prevention*) involves altering the design, manufacture, or use of products and materials to reduce the amount and toxicity of what gets thrown away. The most effective MSW-reducing strategy is to prevent waste from ever being generated in the first place.
- *Recycling* involves sorting, collecting, and processing materials to be reused in the manufacture of new products. This process diverts items such as paper, glass, plastics, and metals from the waste stream.
- *Composting* involves collecting organic waste, such as food scraps and yard trimmings, and allowing it to decompose with the help of microorganisms (mainly bacteria and fungi). Individuals and communities have increased composting processes in recent years and composted waste is increasingly used for a variety of products. Most commonly, organic waste is combined

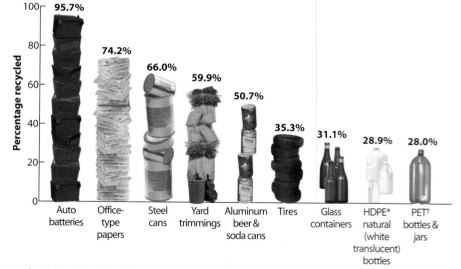

†High-density polyethylene
*Polyethylene terephthalate

Figure 14.5 How Much Do We Recycle?

Source: Data from U.S. Environmental Protection Agency, *Municipal Solid Waste Generation, Recycling, and Disposal in the United States: Facts and Figures for 2009* (Washington, DC: U.S. Environmental Protection Agency, 2010), Available at www.epa.gov/epawaste/nonhaz/municipal/pubs/msw2009-fs.pdf.

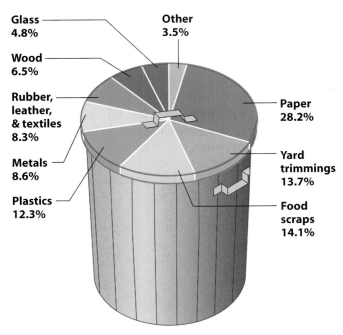

Glass 4.8%
Other 3.5%
Wood 6.5%
Rubber, leather, & textiles 8.3%
Metals 8.6%
Plastics 12.3%
Paper 28.2%
Yard trimmings 13.7%
Food scraps 14.1%

Figure 14.6 What's in Our Trash?

Source: Data from U.S. Environmental Protection Agency, *Municipal Solid Waste Generation, Recycling, and Disposal in the United States: Facts and Figures for 2009* (Washington, DC: U.S. Environmental Protection Agency, 2010), Available at www.epa.gov/epawaste/nonhaz/municipal/pubs/msw2009-fs.pdf.

to produce a humus-like substance that is suitable for use in gardens and for soil enhancement.

■ *Combustion with energy recovery* typically involves the use of boilers and industrial furnaces to generate energy and material recovery or incinerators, which primarily destroy waste but can also recover waste for material use. Energy recovery has become an increasing source of energy for many communities.

Do you know anyone who throws recyclable items away rather than recycling them? What do you think motivates their behavior? What might encourage them to recycle more than they do now?

Hazardous Waste

Hazardous waste is defined as waste with properties that make it capable of harming human health or the environment. In 1980, the Comprehensive Environmental Response, Compensation, and Liability Act, or **Superfund**, was enacted to provide funds for cleaning up hazardous waste dump sites that endanger public health and land. This fund is financed through taxes on the chemical and petroleum industries (87%) and through general federal tax revenues (13%). To date, 32,500 potentially hazardous waste sites have been identified across the nation, and 90 percent of these have been cleared or "recovered."[56] Currently, 50 priority sites are being actively cleared, with thousands more sites waiting for future cleanup that will cost billions of dollars. Newer cleanup technologies are being investigated, including nanotechnologies, that could reduce these cleanup costs by as much as 75 percent.

The large number of hazardous waste dump sites in the United States indicates the severity of our toxic chemical problem. American manufacturers generate more than 1 ton of chemical waste per

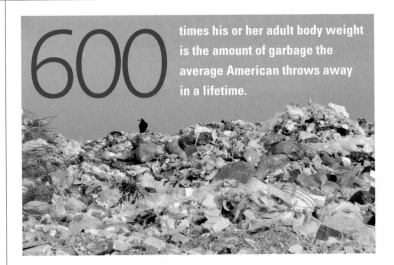

600 times his or her adult body weight is the amount of garbage the average American throws away in a lifetime.

person per year (275 million tons annually). Many wastes are now banned from land disposal or are treated to reduce their toxicity before they become part of land disposal sites. The EPA has developed protective requirements for land disposal facilities, such as double liners, detection systems for substances that may leach into groundwater, and groundwater monitoring systems.

It's likely that you have hazardous waste sitting on a garage shelf or under a kitchen or bathroom sink. Pesticides, paints and paint thinners, solvents, moss killers, batteries, old gasoline cans, many cleaning products, glues, and adhesives as well as paint and stain removers and hot tub or pool chemicals are all examples of potential hazardous wastes.

To be a thoughtful consumer, read the labels on products before buying them. Whenever possible, substitute less toxic, natural products for hazardous ones. Remember to never pour old pesticides, cleaning agents, gasoline, or solvents down the drain or dump them on the ground.

There are many effective substitutes for harsh cleaning products:

■ To get out laundry or carpet stains, use club soda.
■ To get rid of moths in your pantry or clothes, use cedar shavings or lavender.
■ To clean dirty windows and surfaces, mix water with vinegar or ammonia.
■ To clean your showers, sinks, and tubs, skip the toxic chemical sprays. Use a vinegar/water solution or baking soda. Wipe surfaces dry after showering to avoid build-up.

351

check yourself

■ **How can we reduce the amount of municipal solid waste generated?**

■ **What is hazardous waste, and what are its dangers?**

Radiation

- **Explain the environmental and personal risks associated with radiation.**

Radiation is energy that travels in waves or particles. Many different types of radiation make up the electromagnetic spectrum. Exposure to radiation is an inescapable part of life on this planet, and only some of it poses a threat to human health.

Nonionizing Radiation

Nonionizing radiation is radiation at the lower end of the electromagnetic spectrum. This radiation moves in relatively long wavelengths and has enough energy to move atoms but not enough to remove electrons or alter molecular structure. Examples of nonionizing radiation are radio waves, TV signals, microwaves, infrared waves, and visible light.

Although many believe that *electromagnetic fields* (*EMFs*) generated by electric power delivery systems increase one's risk for cancer, reproductive dysfunction, and other ailments, others point to major inconsistencies in the research and little resulting hazard to health. However, one particular form of EMF—radio-frequency (RF) energy emitted by cell phones—is currently the subject of much debate and research. Depending on how close a phone's antenna is to the head, as much as 60 percent of the microwave radiation it emits may actually penetrate the head, reaching an inch to an inch-and-a-half into the brain. In infants and children, whose skulls are thinner, potential penetration may be even greater.

Many countries, including the United States, use standards set by the Federal Communications Commission (FCC) for radio-frequency energy based on research by several scientific groups. These groups identified a whole-body *specific absorption rate* (*SAR*) value for exposure to RF energy. Four watts per kilogram was identified as a level above which harmful biological effects may occur. The FCC requires wireless phones to comply with a limit of 1.6 watts per kg. (To find the SAR level for your phone, go to www.fcc.gov/cgb/sar.)

Three large studies have found no correlation between cell phone use and brain tumors.[57] However, a recent large-scale study by the International Agency for Research on Cancer suggests that the risk of developing gliomas (a type of tumor) may be higher among those who use cell phones the most.[58]

To lower any potential risk:

- If your "talk time" is long, switch to a landline phone, on which RF levels are lower. If you talk a lot, buy a hands-free device.

- Children under 14 should be limited in their talk time. Text messages (within limits), headsets, and hands-free devices or speaker phones are the best option.
- When your signal level is low, stay off the phone. Phones that have to work to pull in a signal may increase RF levels.
- Use a wireless earpiece only when on the phone; the earpiece is always emitting RFs.
- Men shouldn't keep a cell phone in their pocket or on their belt; cell phone radiation can reduce sperm counts.

Ionizing Radiation

Ionizing radiation is caused by the release of particles and electromagnetic rays from atomic nuclei during the normal process of disintegration. Some naturally occurring elements, such as uranium, emit radiation. The sun is another source of ionizing radiation, in the form of high-frequency ultraviolet rays—those against which the ozone layer protects us.

Exposure is measured in **radiation absorbed doses (rads)**, also called *roentgens*. Harm can occur with dosages as low as 100 to 200 rads, including nausea, diarrhea, fatigue, anemia, sore throat, and hair loss. At 350 to 500 rads, symptoms become more severe, and death may result because the radiation hinders bone marrow production of white blood cells that protect us from disease. Dosages above 600 to 700 rads are invariably fatal.

Recommended maximum "safe" dosages range from 0.5 to 5 rads per year.[59] Approximately 50 percent of the radiation to which we are exposed comes from natural sources, including radon and cosmic radiation. Another 48 percent comes from medical exposure (e.g., CAT scans and X rays). The remaining 2 percent is nonionizing

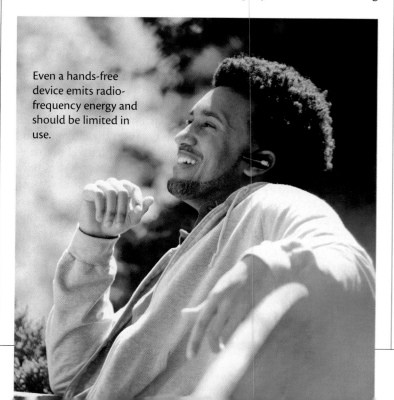

Even a hands-free device emits radio-frequency energy and should be limited in use.

radiation from such sources as computer monitors, microwave ovens, televisions, and radar screens.[60] Most of us are exposed to far less radiation than the safe maximum dosage per year. The effects of long-term exposure to relatively low levels of radiation are unknown.

Nuclear Power Plants

Nuclear power plants account for less than 1 percent of the total radiation to which we are exposed in the United States, but they are symbols of many of the dangers of radiation and controversial sources of energy. The debate over nuclear energy has gone on for many years and has been affected by several disasters and near-disasters surrounding nuclear power plants.

Based on the most recent statistics, there are 433 active nuclear power plants in 30 countries and another 65 under construction. Of the active plants, 103 are in the United States. The United States has the most reactors and generates the most electricity from nuclear energy of any nation; however nuclear power only makes up about 20 percent of our total energy production. In contrast, over 75 percent of the electricity generated in France is from nuclear power.[61]

For some, the lure of nuclear energy is that it's cheap to make. Initial costs of building nuclear power plants are high, but actual power generation is relatively inexpensive. A 1,000-megawatt reactor produces enough energy for 650,000 homes and saves 420 million gallons of fossil fuels each year. Nuclear reactors discharge fewer carbon oxides into the air than fossil fuel–powered generators.[62]

However, nuclear power does have its downside. Disposal of nuclear wastes is extremely problematic. Another major concern is the possibility of a **nuclear meltdown**, which occurs when the temperature in a nuclear reactor's core increases enough to melt both the nuclear fuel and the containment vessel that holds it. Most modern facilities seal their reactors and containment vessels in concrete buildings with pools of cold water on the bottom. If a meltdown occurs, the building and the pool are supposed to prevent the escape of radioactivity.

In March 2011, a massive earthquake and tsunami hit northern Japan, endangering several nuclear power plants in the region, most notably the Fukushima Daiichi plant on the island of Honshu. The 9.0-magnitude quake triggered automatic shutdown of the nation's nuclear reactors—a major source of Japan's power—at the same time the quake and tsunami affected operation of backup generators designed to cool the reactors' cores in an emergency, leading to the collapse of an outer building (though not the reactor it contained). To release the resulting dangerous pressure buildup inside the reactors, plant workers released radioactive steam into the air.

The Fukushima accident was the most serious since a 1986 reactor core fire and explosion at the Chernobyl nuclear power plant in Ukraine. Unlike Fukushima, the Chernobyl plant had no containment structure. Radioactive fallout from the Chernobyl disaster spread over most of the Northern Hemisphere and led to extremely elevated cancer rates in the immediate area. While both disasters were rated 7 out of 7 for severity, immediate damage from Chernobyl was higher, although Fukushima's radiation leaks continue and could eventually exceed those at Chernobyl.[63]

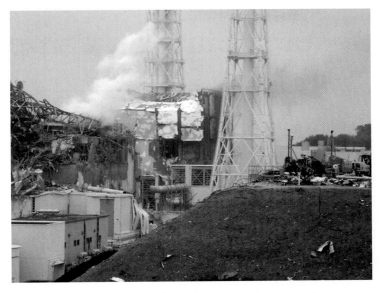

The 2011 accident at the Fukushima Daiichi plant in Japan, following an earthquake and tsunami, raised new questions about the safety of nuclear power.

In recent years, our dependence on declining oil reserves had sparked public interest in the potential benefits of nuclear power. However, the Fukushima disaster illustrated starkly how even an extremely well-run and safety-focused nuclear power program like Japan's could be devastated—with terrible global effects—by an act of nature beyond anyone's control. Nations around the world, including the United States, continue to watch Japan for outcomes while slowing or stopping nuclear power development on their own soil.

Despite recent occurrences, some proponents argue that nuclear power is more efficient and cheaper than fossil fuels. Nuclear power generation emits relatively low amounts of CO_2. Greenhouse gas emissions and the contribution of nuclear power plants to global warming are relatively minor. Unlike solar power, the technology is readily available; it does not have to be developed. In addition, the construction and staffing of new nuclear power plants create jobs.[64]

Opponents of nuclear power argue that nuclear power may appear cheap, but the building of reactors is heavily dependent on taxpayer subsidies. We still have no foolproof way of disposing of nuclear waste. Uranium is a scarce resource—as with fossil fuels, it will run out one day. And, as Fukushima and Chernobyl illustrate, they contend that the risks of major nuclear accidents are not worth any savings in cost of generating electricity.[65]

check yourself

- **What is the difference between ionizing and nonionizing radiation?**

- **What are some benefits and drawbacks to the use of nuclear power?**

Sustainability on Campus

learning outcomes

- **Identify what you can do to live sustainably on campus.**

You are moving into a new dorm room, along with hundreds of other students, and are excited to decorate, meet your new roommate, and make your room the place to be. As a student, this is also your chance to make a positive difference and minimize your ecological footprint. Your actions, and those of your friends, roommates, and school, can have a lasting impact on your life and the future of the environment.

More and more universities and colleges are recognizing that students want to attend schools that reflect their values and beliefs with regards to sustainability. The annual College Sustainability Report Card (www.greenreportcard.org) grades colleges and universities on their responses to a survey assessing commitment to sustainability in the areas of administration, climate change and energy, food and recycling, green building, student involvement, transportation, endowment transparency, investment priorities, and shareholder engagement. The Sierra Club annually rates colleges and universities on their efforts to be green, with special emphasis on where each school obtains its energy (**Table 14.2**). Initiatives recognized by the program include striving to become carbon neutral, integrating sustainability studies across the curriculum, and providing incentives for alternative modes of transportation.

Another issue to take into consideration may be the physical environment in which the school exists. A recent report from the American Lung Association rated the cleanest and dirtiest U.S. cities in terms of air pollution.[66] Among the top 10 in ozone pollution were Los Angeles, Houston, and Charlotte (North Carolina); Los Angeles, Phoenix, and Pittsburgh were all high in particle pollution. The lowest in ozone pollution included Honolulu, Fargo (North Dakota), and Rochester (Minnesota); the lowest in particle pollution included Cheyenne (Wyoming), Santa Fe (New Mexico), and Tucson. In the future, will students consider air pollution and other environmental factors when making their choices about schooling? Would you consider moving to or from a given urban environment based on air quality and other "green" issues?

The green sustainability movement is picking up steam and turning ideas into realities. You do not need to be an environmental science major or a self-proclaimed "hippie" to make a difference. Going green on campus can be a goal for your apartment, your sorority or fraternity, or your residence hall.

Start making a positive impact by turning off lights when you leave a room or restroom. See if your residence has a way of minimizing the amount of lights used on a floor. Sometimes lights are connected through several outlets; turning off a strand might still provide enough light but minimize the amount of energy consumed. Find out whether your administration supports the use of CFLs—compact fluorescent lights—longer-lasting, energy-conserving bulbs that give off the same amount of light as an incandescent bulb at a fraction of the energy used. Next time you go to the store, buy a couple for your new lighting fixtures and start making a positive impact.

TABLE 14.2 The 10 Most Eco-Enlightened U.S. Colleges and Universities

1. University of Washington (WA)
2. Green Mountain College (VT)
3. University of California, San Diego
4. Warren Wilson College (NC)
5. Stanford University (CA)
6. University of California, Irvine
7. University of California, Santa Cruz
8. University of California, Davis
9. Evergreen State College (WA)
10. Middlebury College (MA)

Source: Sierra Club, "America's Coolest Schools: Fifth Annual List," *Sierra Magazine,* August 2011. Copyright © 2011 by Sierra Club. Reprinted with permission. This text originally appeared in *Sierra,* the national magazine of the Sierra Club.

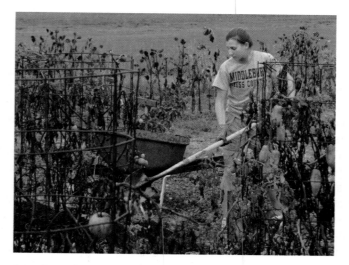

Schools can "go green" by supporting organic gardens and other sustainable activities.

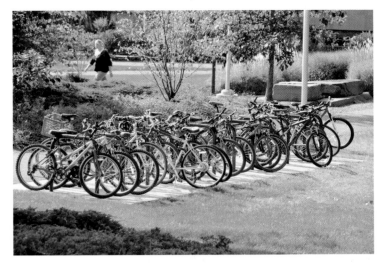

Does receiving support, such as plentiful bicycle racks, for alternative forms of transportation around campus make it more likely that you can contribute to a greener environment?

Making Green Consumer Choices

When buying a new appliance, look for the Energy Star logo, indicating that the appliance meets energy-efficiency standards set by the EPA and U.S. Department of Energy. Adjust the con-

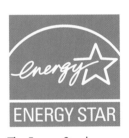

The Energy Star logo signals that an appliance meets energy conservation standards.

trols on your new appliances so that they do not run at full power all the time. This will help curb unnecessary energy usage and lower the cost of your monthly energy bills. Better yet, consider unplugging items such as iPods, TVs, computers, hair dryers, coffee pots, and cell phones, all of which still consume energy when not in use.

What about your computer? While in school, you will probably use it for everything from social networking to writing papers. Fortunately, you have many options to help you make better energy-

conserving choices when it comes to computer use. When buying a computer, always look for the Energy Star logo. (Go to www .energystar.gov/index.cfm?c=higher_ed.bus_dormroom for more information about creating an Energy Star dorm room.)

Consider buying a laptop rather than a desktop computer, because laptops use less energy. You can also set your computer to sleep or hibernate mode when not in use. When you look for a printer, choose one that prints double-sided, which will help reduce the amount of paper you use. Do not print unnecessary documents, and make sure you recycle used paper—don't just throw it away.

Something else to consider when you are looking at your energy consumption is your television. In general, the bigger the screen, the greater the power consumption; moving from a 36-inch to a 60-inch set can make for a major hit on your electric bill. In addition, LCD and plasma sets often use more electricity than comparable sized LED sets. There are several online resources for comparing energy consumption levels. Sets purchased after 2010 have to meet

even more stringent qualifications for an Energy Star rating due to changes in regulations.

If you must have a 40-inch or higher set, there are things you can do to reduce your energy use:

- Adjust your brightness and contrast controls downward. Most people don't need the standard brightness settings that make sets "pop" in the showroom.
- Buy one size down from what you think you need.
- Pay careful attention to Energy Star ratings. Newer sets have better ratings overall, with old tube sets being the worst culprits of all.

Skills for Behavior Change

SHOPPING TO SAVE THE PLANET

- Look for products with less packaging or with refillable, reusable, or recyclable containers.
- Bring your own reusable, washable grocery bags to the store. (Be sure to wash bags after carrying meat in them.)
- Buy foods that are produced sustainably.
- Purchase organic or locally produced foods or foods produced with fewer chemicals and pesticides.
- Do not buy plastic bottles of water. Purchase a hard plastic or stainless steel, wide-mouth water bottle and fill it from a filtered source. Wash it regularly.
- Do not use caustic cleansers. Simple vinegar or a dilute mixture of water and bleach is usually just as effective and less harsh on your home and the environment.
- Buy laundry products that are free of dyes, fragrances, and sulfates.
- Use soap and water to clean surfaces, not disposable cleaning cloths and spray-on shower cleaners. Avoid antibacterial soaps and cleaners, because they contribute to microbial resistance.
- Purchase appliances with the Energy Star logo. Remember that your big-screen TV may be a huge energy drain, along with your old refrigerator. Replace outdated appliances when you can, and watch those energy levels.
- Buy CFLs instead of less energy-efficient incandescent bulbs. Use caution when installing and removing CFLs and avoid breakage—CFLs contain mercury. Clear the room for at least 30 minutes after any accidental breakage.
- Use reusable mugs, plates, napkins, and silverware rather than disposable products. Wash and reuse plastic silverware.
- Buy recycled paper products when you can.
- Purchase bed linens and bath towels that are made from bamboo, hemp, or organic cotton.

check yourself

- **What are three changes you can make now to help the environment?**
- **What, if any, are reasons that prevent you from making choices that are environmentally aware?**

What Are You Doing to Preserve the Environment?

Environmental problems often seem too big for one person to make a difference. Each day, though, there are things you can do that contribute to the planet's health. For each statement below, indicate how often you follow the described behavior.

An interactive version of this assessment is available online. Download it from the Live It! section of www.pearsonhighered.com/donatelle.

	Always	Usually	Sometimes	Never
1. Whenever possible, I walk or ride my bicycle rather than drive a car.	1	2	3	4
2. I carpool with others to school or work.	1	2	3	4
3. I have my car tuned up and inspected every year.	1	2	3	4
4. When I change the oil in my car, I make sure the oil is properly recycled, rather than dumped on the ground or into a floor drain.	1	2	3	4
5. I avoid using the air conditioner except during extreme conditions.	1	2	3	4
6. I turn off the lights when a room is not being used.	1	2	3	4
7. I take a shower rather than a bath most of the time.	1	2	3	4
8. I have water-saving devices installed on my shower, toilet, and sinks.	1	2	3	4
9. I make sure faucets and toilets in my home do not leak.	1	2	3	4
10. I use my bath towels more than once before putting them in the wash.	1	2	3	4
11. I wear my clothes more than once between washings when possible.	1	2	3	4
12. I make sure that the washing machine is full before I wash a load of clothes.	1	2	3	4
13. I purchase biodegradable soaps and detergents.	1	2	3	4
14. I use biodegradable trash bags.	1	2	3	4
15. At home, I use dishes and silverware rather than disposable products.	1	2	3	4
16. When I buy prepackaged foods, I choose the ones with the least packaging.	1	2	3	4
17. I do not subscribe to newspapers and magazines that I can view online.	1	2	3	4
18. I do not use a hair dryer.	1	2	3	4
19. I bring reusable bags to the grocery store.	1	2	3	4
20. I don't run water continuously when washing the dishes, shaving, or brushing my teeth.	1	2	3	4
21. I use unbleached or recycled paper.	1	2	3	4
22. I use both sides of printer paper and other paper when possible.	1	2	3	4
23. If I have items I do not want to use anymore, I donate them to charity so someone else can use them.	1	2	3	4
24. I carry a reusable mug for my coffee or tea and have it filled, rather than using a new paper cup each time I buy a hot beverage.	1	2	3	4
25. I carry and use a refillable water bottle rather than frequently buying bottled water.	1	2	3	4
26. I clean up after myself while enjoying the outdoors (picnicking, camping, etc.).	1	2	3	4
27. I volunteer for cleanup days in the community in which I live.	1	2	3	4
28. I consider candidates' positions on environmental issues before casting my vote.	1	2	3	4

For Further Thought

Review your scores. Are your responses mostly 1s and 2s? If not, what actions can you take to become more environmentally responsible? Are there ways to help the environment on this list that you had not thought of before? Are there behaviors not on the list that you are already doing?

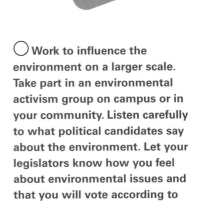

Your Plan for Change

The Assess Yourself activity gave you the chance to look at your behavior and consider ways to conserve energy, save water, reduce waste, and otherwise help protect the planet. Now that you have considered these results, you can take steps to become more environmentally responsible.

Today, you can:

◯ Find out how much energy you are using. Visit www .carbonfund.org, www .carbonoffsets.org, or www .greatestplanet.org to find out what your carbon footprint is and to learn about projects you can support to offset your own emissions and energy usage. New carbon offset programs and organizations are popping up all the time, so watch for other opportunities to counter your carbon usage.

◯ Reduce the amount of paper waste in your mailbox. You can stop junk mail, such as credit card offers and unwanted

catalogs, by visiting the Direct Marketing Association's Mail Preference Service site at www .dmachoice.org. You can also call 1-888-5 OPT OUT to put an end to unwanted mail. In addition, the website www.catalogchoice .org is a free service that lets you decline paper catalogs you no longer want to receive.

Within the next 2 weeks, you can:

◯ Look into joining a local environmental group, attending a campus environmental event, or taking an environmental science course.

◯ Take part in a local clean-up day or recycling drive. These can be fun opportunities to meet like-minded people while benefiting the planet.

By the end of the semester, you can:

◯ Interview and talk with your campus' dining hall director about initiating a compost recycling program. Check out other universities with policies and plans for minimizing their food waste through composting: www.grrn.org/campus/campus_ compost.html. The EPA provides information on setting up an indoor compost bin at www .epa.gov/epawaste/conserve/ rrr/composting/by_compost .htm.

◯ Make a habit of recycling everything you can. Find out what items can be recycled in your neighborhood and designate a box or bin to hold recyclable materials— cans, bottles, plastic, newspapers, junk mail, and so on—until you can transport them to a curbside bin or drop-off center.

◯ Work to influence the environment on a larger scale. Take part in an environmental activism group on campus or in your community. Listen carefully to what political candidates say about the environment. Let your legislators know how you feel about environmental issues and that you will vote according to their record on the issues.

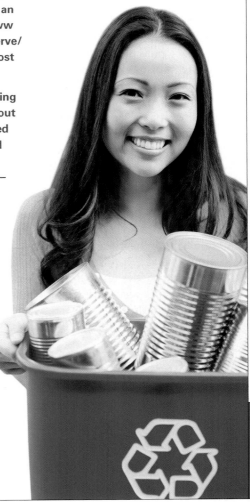

14.9 | Assess Yourself:
What Are You Doing to Preserve the Environment?

357

Summary

- Population growth is the single largest factor affecting the environment. Demand for more food, water, and energy—as well as places to dispose of waste—places great strain on Earth's resources. The United States is among the greatest consumers of natural resources per person of any nation in the world. We can do more to reduce, reuse, and recycle.

- The primary constituents of air pollution are sulfur dioxide, particulate matter, carbon monoxide, nitrogen dioxide, ground-level ozone, lead, carbon dioxide, and hydrocarbons. Indoor air pollution is caused primarily by tobacco smoke, woodstove smoke, furnace emissions, asbestos, formaldehyde, radon, lead, and mold. Pollution is depleting Earth's protective ozone layer and contributing to global warming by enhancing the greenhouse effect.

- Water pollution can be caused by either point sources (direct entry) or nonpoint sources (runoff or seepage). Major contributors to water pollution include petroleum products, organic solvents, polychlorinated biphenyls (PCBs), dioxins, pesticides, and lead. Solid waste pollution includes household trash, plastics, glass, metal products, and paper. Limited landfill space creates problems. Hazardous waste is toxic; improper disposal creates health hazards for people in surrounding communities.

- Nonionizing radiation comes from electromagnetic fields, such as those around power lines. Ionizing radiation results from the natural erosion of atomic nuclei. The disposal and storage of radioactive waste from nuclear power plants pose potential problems for public health.

Pop Quiz

1. The United States is responsible for what percentage of total global resource consumption?
   a. 10 percent
   b. 25 percent
   c. 50 percent
   d. 70 percent

2. Which of the following statements about population growth is *not* correct?
   a. Higher fertility rates and decreases in mortality rates are key factors in population growth.
   b. Populations of wealthier nations are static or declining overall.
   c. As education levels of women increase and women achieve equality in pay, job, and social status with men, fertility rates go down.
   d. Zero population growth has proved to be impossible; no countries of the world have been able to achieve it.

3. One possible source of indoor air pollution is a gas present in some carpets called
   a. lead.
   b. asbestos.
   c. radon.
   d. formaldehyde.

4. Which of the following substances separates into tiny fibers that can become embedded in the lungs?
   a. Asbestos
   b. Particulate matter
   c. Radon
   d. Formaldehyde

5. The terms *point source* and *nonpoint source* are used to describe the two general sources of
   a. water pollution.
   b. air pollution.
   c. noise pollution.
   d. ozone depletion.

6. The air pollutant that originates primarily from motor vehicle emissions is
   a. particulates.
   b. nitrogen dioxide.
   c. sulfur dioxide.
   d. carbon monoxide.

7. Which gas is considered radioactive and could become cancer causing when it seeps into a home?
   a. Carbon monoxide
   b. Radon
   c. Hydrogen sulfide
   d. Natural gas

8. The phenomenon that creates a barrier to protect us from the sun's harmful ultraviolet radiation rays is
   a. photochemical smog.
   b. the ozone layer.
   c. gray air smog.
   d. the greenhouse effect.

9. Your most recent DVD purchase came with less packaging than DVDs once had. This is an example of controlling municipal solid waste via
   a. source reduction.
   b. recycling.
   c. composting.
   d. incineration.

10. Some herbicides contain toxic substances called
    a. THMs.
    b. PCPs.
    c. dioxins.
    d. PCBs.

Answers to these questions can be found on page A-1.

Web Links

1. **Environmental Literacy Council.** An excellent source of information about environmental issues. Topics range from how the ozone layer works to why the rain forests are important. www.enviroliteracy.org

2. **Environmental Protection Agency (EPA).** The EPA is the government agency responsible for overseeing environmental regulation and protection issues in the United States. www.epa.gov

3. **National Center for Environmental Health (NCEH).** Information on a wide variety of environmental health issues; includes a series of helpful fact sheets. www.cdc.gov/nceh

4. **National Environmental Health Association (NEHA).** Educational resources and opportunities for environmental health professionals. www.neha.org

Consumerism and Complementary and Alternative Medicine

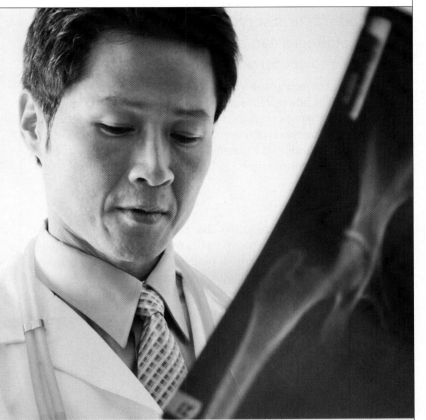

359

Have there been times when you wondered whether you were sick enough to go to your campus health clinic? Have you left medical visits feeling that you didn't get a thorough exam, or with more questions than when you arrived? Have you wondered about, or successfully used, alternative medical care? Have you ever had to help a loved one make health care decisions?

There are many reasons for you to learn to make better decisions about your health and health care. Most important, you only have one body. If you don't treat it with care, you will pay a major price in terms of monetary costs and consequences to your health. Doing everything you can to stay healthy and to recover rapidly when you do get sick will enhance every other part of your life. Throughout this book we have emphasized the importance of healthy preventive behaviors. Learning how to navigate the health care system is an important part of taking charge of your health.

- **Explain how to use the medical system and when to seek medical help.**

As the health care industry has become more sophisticated in seeking your business, so must you become more sophisticated in purchasing its products and services. Acting responsibly in times of illness can be difficult, but the person best able to act on your behalf is you.

If you are not feeling well, you must first decide whether you need to seek medical advice. Not seeking treatment, whether because of high costs or limited coverage, or trying to medicate yourself when more rigorous methods of treatment are needed is potentially dangerous. Understanding the benefits and limits of self-care is critical for responsible consumerism.

Self-Care

Individuals can practice behaviors that promote health, prevent disease, and minimize reliance on the formal medical system. Minor afflictions can often be treated without professional help. Self-care consists of knowing your body, paying attention to its signals, and taking appropriate action to stop the progression of illness or injury. Common forms of self-care include the following:

- Treating conditions that occur frequently but may not require physician visits (e.g., the common cold, minor abrasions)
- Using over-the-counter remedies to treat minor infrequent pains, scrapes, or symptoms
- Performing monthly breast or testicular self-examinations
- Learning first aid for common, uncomplicated injuries and conditions
- Checking blood pressure, pulse, and temperature
- Using home pregnancy tests and ovulation kits
- Using home HIV test kits
- Doing periodic checks for blood cholesterol level
- Learning from reliable self-help books, websites, and DVDs
- Benefiting from nutrition, rest, exercise, and meditation and other relaxation techniques

Using self-care methods appropriately takes education and effort. Taking prescription drugs used for a previous illness to treat your current illness, using unproven self-treatment methods, or using other people's medications are examples of inappropriate self-care.

When to Seek Help

With the vast array of home diagnostic products available, it seems relatively easy for most people to take care of themselves. But some caution is in order here: Although many home diagnostic kits and devices are valuable for making an initial diagnosis, home health tests are not substitutes for regular, complete examinations by a trained practitioner. Effective self-care also means paying attention to your body's warning signs and understanding when to seek medical attention. Deciding which conditions warrant professional advice is not always easy. Generally, you should consult a physician if you experience *any* of the following:

- A serious accident or injury
- Sudden or severe chest pains, especially if they cause breathing difficulties
- Trauma to the head or spine accompanied by persistent headache, blurred vision, loss of consciousness, vomiting, convulsions, or paralysis

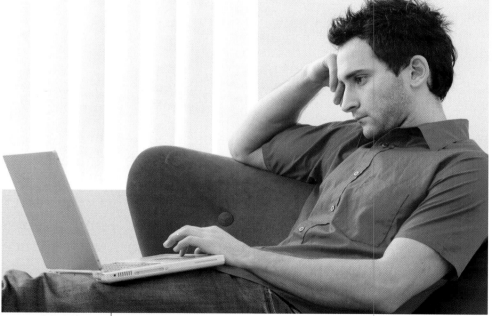

Deciding when to contact a physician can be difficult. Most people first research symptoms online and try to diagnose and treat a condition themselves.

- Sudden high fever or recurring high temperature (over 102 °F for children and 103 °F for adults) and/or sweats
- Tingling sensation in the arm accompanied by slurred speech or impaired thought processes
- Adverse reactions to a drug or insect bite (shortness of breath, severe swelling, dizziness)
- Unexplained bleeding or loss of fluid from any body opening
- Unexplained sudden weight loss
- Persistent or recurrent diarrhea or vomiting
- Blue-colored lips, eyelids, or nail beds
- Any lump, swelling, thickness, or sore that does not subside or that grows for over a month
- Any marked change or pain in bowel or bladder habits
- Yellowing of the skin or the whites of the eyes
- Any symptom that is unusual and recurs over time
- Pregnancy

The Placebo Effect

The *placebo effect* is an apparent cure or improved state of health brought about by a substance, product, or procedure that has no generally recognized therapeutic value. Patients often report improvements in a condition based on what they expect, desire, or were told would happen after receiving a treatment, even though that treatment was, for example, simple sugar pills instead of powerful drugs.

Researchers are investigating how and why placebos work on some people. One theory is that expecting a positive outcome activates the same natural pathways in the brain as some medications do. One study involved patients with Parkinson's disease. The patients who thought that they were receiving the real treatment but actually received a placebo had the same changes in their brains on positron-emission tomography (PET) scans as those who received the medication.[1] Similar chemical changes on brain imaging tests were seen with placebos in studies of pain, depression, and alcohol dependency treatment.[2]

People who unknowingly use placebos when medical treatment is needed increase their risk for health problems. However, what we learn from the ways in which placebos work may someday help us harness the mind's power to treat certain diseases and conditions.

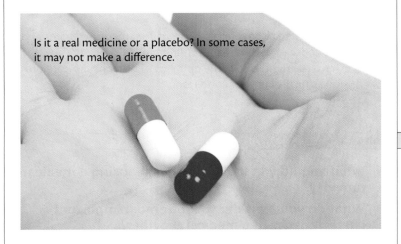

Is it a real medicine or a placebo? In some cases, it may not make a difference.

Skills for **Behavior Change**

BE PROACTIVE IN YOUR HEALTH CARE

Here are some tips for getting the most out of doctor visits and being proactive in your health care:

- Keep records of your own and your family's medical histories.
- Research your condition—causes, physiological effects, possible treatments, and prognosis. Don't rely on your health care provider for this information.
- If you use a complementary and alternative medicine (CAM) therapy such as acupuncture, choose a practitioner with care. Your insurer may also cover such services.
- Bring a friend or relative along to medical visits to help you review what the doctor says. If you go alone, take notes. Write down what happened and what was said.
- Ask the practitioner to explain the problem and possible treatments, tests, and drugs in a clear and understandable way. If you don't understand something, ask for clarification.
- If a health care provider prescribes any medications, ask whether you can take generic equivalents that cost less.
- Ask for a written summary of the results of your visit and any lab tests.
- Find out what studies have been done on the safety and effectiveness of any treatment in which you are interested. Consult only reliable sources—texts, journals, and government resources. Start with the websites listed at the end of this and every chapter.
- If you have any doubt about a recommended treatment, get a second opinion.
- Decisions regarding treatment should be made in consultation with your health care provider and based on your condition and needs.
- If you use any CAM therapy, inform your primary health care provider. It is particularly important to talk with your provider if you are thinking about replacing your prescribed treatment with one or more supplements, are currently taking a prescription drug, have a chronic medical condition, are planning to have surgery, are pregnant or nursing, or are thinking about giving supplements to children.
- When filling prescriptions, ask the pharmacist to show you the package inserts that list medical considerations. Request detailed information about potential drug and food interactions.
- Remember that *natural* and *safe* are not necessarily the same. You can become seriously ill from seemingly harmless "natural" products. Be cautious about combining herbal medications, just as you would about combining other drugs. Seek help if you notice any unusual side effects.

check yourself

- **What are four instances in which you should seek medical help?**

Assessing Health Professionals

■ **List factors to consider when choosing a medical provider.**

Selecting a medical professional may seem simple, yet many people have little idea how to assess the qualifications of a health care provider.[3]

Ask yourself the following questions when selecting a health care provider:

■ How are the provider's communication skills? The most satisfied patients are those who feel their health care providers explain diagnosis and treatment options thoroughly.

■ Does the provider listen to you, and give you time to ask questions? Does the provider return your calls? Is he or she available to answer questions between visits?

■ What professional education and training has the provider had? What license or board certification(s) does he or she hold? Note that *board-certified* indicates that a physician has passed the national board examination for his or her specialty (e.g., pediatrics) and has been certified as competent in that specialty; *board-eligible* means that the physician is eligible to take a specialty board's exam, but not necessarily that he or she has passed it.

■ Is the provider affiliated with an accredited medical facility or institution? The Joint Commission is an independent nonprofit organization that evaluates and accredits more than 15,000 health care organizations and programs in the United States. Accreditation requires that these institutions verify all education, licensing, and training claims of affiliated practitioners.

■ Is the provider open to complementary or alternative strategies? Would he or she refer you for different treatments if appropriate?

■ Does the provider indicate clearly how long a given treatment may last, what side effects you might expect, and what problems you should watch for?

■ Who will be responsible for your care when your provider is on vacation or off call?

■ Are professional reviews and information on any lawsuits involving the provider available online?

Ask yourself the following questions about the quality of care you are receiving:

■ Did your health care provider take a thorough health history and ask for any recent updates to it? Was your examination thorough?

■ Did your provider listen to you?

■ Did you feel comfortable asking questions? Did your provider answer thoroughly, in a way that was easy to understand?

Asking the right questions at the right time may save you suffering and expense. Many patients find that writing their questions down before an appointment helps.

Active participation in your treatment is the only sensible course in a health care environment that encourages **defensive medicine**, or the use of medical practices designed to avert the possibility of malpractice suits.[4] Unwarranted treatment such as the overuse of antibiotics and use of diagnostic tests to protect against malpractice exposure are driving up the cost of medicine.[5] Unnecessary drugs and procedures are unlikely to improve health outcomes and may create new problems.

In addition to asking the suggested questions above, being proactive in your health care also means that you should be aware of your rights as a patient:[6]

1. The right of informed consent means that before receiving any care you should be fully informed of what is planned, the risks and potential benefits, and possible alternative forms of treatment, including the option to refuse treatment. Your consent must be voluntary and without any form of coercion. It is critical that you read any consent forms carefully and amend them as necessary before signing.
2. You are entitled to know whether the treatment you are receiving is standard or experimental. In experimental conditions, you have the legal and ethical right to know if any drug is being used in the research project for a purpose not approved by the Food and Drug Administration (FDA), and whether the study is one in which some people receive treatment while others receive a placebo.
3. You have the right to privacy, which includes the source of payment for treatment and care. It also includes protecting your right to make personal decisions concerning all reproductive matters.
4. You have the right to receive care. You also have the legal right to refuse treatment at any time and to cease treatment at any time.
5. You are entitled to have access to all of your medical records and to have those records remain confidential.
6. You have the right to seek the opinions of other health care professionals regarding your condition.

■ **What should you look for when choosing a medical provider?**

■ **What do you consider the four most important characteristics in a medical provider?**

Types of Allopathic Health Care Providers

CONSUMERISM AND COMPLEMENTARY AND ALTERNATIVE MEDICINE

learning outcomes

■ **Identify the main types of allopathic health care providers.**

Conventional health care, also called **allopathic medicine**, mainstream medicine, or traditional Western medical practice, is based on the premises that illness is a result of exposure to pathogens, such as bacteria and viruses, or organic changes in the body and prevention of disease and restoration of health may involve vaccines, drugs, surgery, and other treatments.

Allopathic health care providers use **evidence-based medicine,** in which decisions regarding patient care are based on a combination of clinical expertise, patient values, and current best scientific evidence.

Selecting a **primary care practitioner (PCP)**—a medical practitioner you can visit for routine ailments, preventive care, general medical advice, and referrals—is not easy. The PCP for most people is a family practitioner, internist, pediatrician, or obstetrician-gynecologist (ob-gyn). Some people see nurse practitioners or physician assistants who work for individual doctors or medical groups, whereas others use nontraditional providers as their primary source of care. As a college student, you may opt to visit a PCP at your campus health center.

Doctors undergo rigorous training before they can begin practicing. After 4 years of undergraduate work, students typically spend 4 years studying for the medical degree (MD). Some students then choose a specialty, such as pediatrics, cardiology, or surgery, spending a 1-year internship and several years in residency with that emphasis.

Specialists include **osteopaths**, general practitioners who receive training similar to that of MDs, but who place special emphasis on the skeletal and muscular systems. Their treatments may involve manipulation of muscles and joints. Osteopaths receive the degree of doctor of osteopathy (DO) rather than MD.

Eye care specialists can be either ophthalmologists or optometrists. An **ophthalmologist** holds a medical degree and can perform surgery and prescribe medications. An **optometrist** typically evaluates visual problems and fits glasses but is not a trained physician. If you have an eye infection, glaucoma, or other eye condition that requires diagnosis and treatment, you need to see an ophthalmologist.

Dentists are specialists who diagnose and treat diseases of the teeth, gums, and oral cavity. They attend dental school for 4 years and receive the title of doctor of dental surgery (DDS) or doctor of

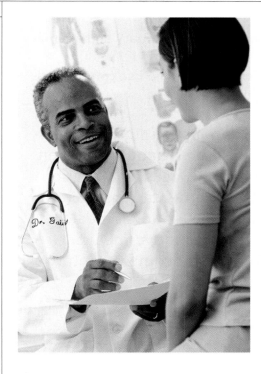

Understanding the differences among different types of health care providers is important. In some cases, you may need to see a doctor with a particular specialty; in other cases, a nurse practitioner or physician assistant may be satisfactory.

363

medical dentistry (DMD). *Orthodontists* specialize in the alignment of teeth. *Oral surgeons* perform surgical procedures to correct problems of the mouth, face, and jaw.

Nurses are highly trained and strictly regulated health professionals who provide a wide range of services, including patient education, counseling, community health and disease prevention information, and administration of medications. Registered nurses (RNs) in the United States complete either a 4-year program leading to a bachelor of science in nursing (BSN) degree or a 2-year associate degree program. Lower-level licensed practical or vocational nurses (LPNs or LVNs) complete a 1- to 2-year training program based in a community college or a hospital.

Nurse practitioners (NPs) are nurses with advanced training obtained through either a master's degree program or a specialized nurse practitioner program. Nurse practitioners have the training and authority to conduct diagnostic tests and prescribe medications (in some states).

Physician assistants (PAs) examine and diagnose patients, offer treatment, and write prescriptions under a physician's supervision. Unlike an NP, a PA must practice under a physician's supervision.

check yourself

■ **What is allopathic medicine?**

■ **What are some of the major types of allopathic health care providers?**

Complementary and Alternative Medicine (CAM)

learning **outcomes**

- **Distinguish between complementary and alternative medicine.**
- **List characteristics of those who use complementary and alternative medicine.**

Although the terms *complementary* and *alternative* are often used interchangeably when referring to therapies, there is a distinction between them. **Complementary medicine** is used *together with* conventional medicine as part of a modern integrative-medicine approach.[7] An example of complementary medicine is the use of massage therapy along with prescription medicine to treat anxiety. **Alternative medicine** has traditionally been used *in place of* conventional medicine—for example, following a special diet or using an herbal remedy to treat cancer *instead* of using radiation, surgery, or other conventional treatments.

Who Uses CAM and Why?

A survey conducted by the National Center for Complementary and Alternative Medicine (NCCAM; part of the National Institutes of Health) and the National Center of Health Statistics (NCHS; part of the Centers for Disease Control and Prevention) revealed that 38

36% of 18- to 29-year-olds report having used some form of CAM.

percent of adults use some form of CAM.[8] **Figure 15.1** shows more results from this study.

The list of practices considered CAM changes continually as therapies become accepted as mainstream. In general, CAM therapies serve as alternatives to the conventional Western system of medicine, which some people regard as too invasive, too high tech, and too toxic in terms of laboratory-produced medications. Complementary and alternative medical therapies incorporate a **holistic** approach to medicine that focuses on treating the mind and the whole body, rather than just an isolated part of the body. Often CAM users seek what they perceive as a more natural, gentle approach to healing. Other CAM patients distrust the traditional medical approach and believe that alternative practices will give them greater control over their own health care. Still others choose what works for them on a case-by-case basis, whether traditional or CAM. CAM therapies can vary greatly in terms of their acceptance in the mainstream medical community, with acceptance based largely on whether they have been scientifically studied and whether those studies have shown the therapies to be beneficial. Research has shown that many types of CAM, including acupuncture and massage therapy, are beneficial in treating conditions such as chronic back pain and cancer.[9]

As the NCCAM/NCHS survey indicates, more than one-third of adults in the United States have used CAM. Why do so many people seek alternative therapy? Distinct patterns of CAM use emerge from this survey.[10] The following groups are likely to use or have used CAM:

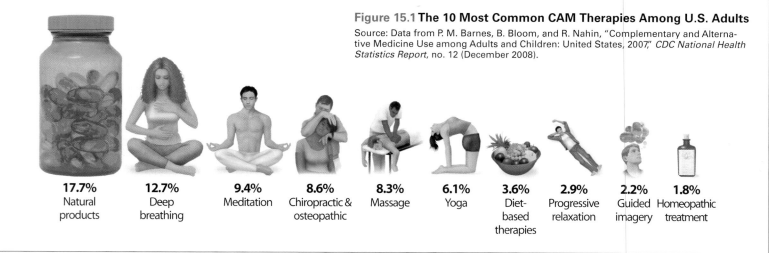

Figure 15.1 The 10 Most Common CAM Therapies Among U.S. Adults
Source: Data from P. M. Barnes, B. Bloom, and R. Nahin, "Complementary and Alternative Medicine Use among Adults and Children: United States, 2007," *CDC National Health Statistics Report*, no. 12 (December 2008).

17.7%	12.7%	9.4%	8.6%	8.3%	6.1%	3.6%	2.9%	2.2%	1.8%
Natural products	Deep breathing	Meditation	Chiropractic & osteopathic	Massage	Yoga	Diet-based therapies	Progressive relaxation	Guided imagery	Homeopathic treatment

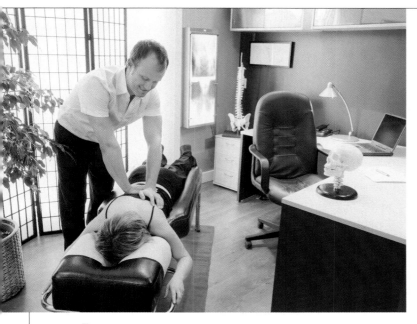

Why are so many people using alternative medicine?

People use alternative medicine for multiple reasons, and many treatments can benefit a variety of physical and mental ailments. For example, chiropractic medicine uses specialized techniques to manipulate the spine. The treatment has shown positive results among people with back and neck pain and headaches.

- More women than men
- People with higher educational levels
- People who have been hospitalized in the past year
- Former smokers (compared with current smokers or those who have never smoked)
- People with back, neck, head, or joint aches or other painful conditions
- People with gastrointestinal disorders or sleeping problems

Figure 15.2 summarizes the conditions for which respondents to the NCCAM/NCHS survey used CAM.

It is also interesting to note the results in the same survey regarding CAM use by children. According to adult respondents, about 12 percent of children use some sort of CAM. Use is greater among children whose parents used CAM (23.9 percent), adolescents aged 12–17 (16.4%) compared to younger children, and white children (12.8%) compared to Hispanic children (7.9%) and African American children (5.9%). The survey also found that 23.8 percent of children with six or more health conditions used CAM, as did 16.9 percent of children whose families delayed conventional care because of cost.[11]

Who Can Provide CAM Treatment?

As with traditional Western medicine, practitioners of most complementary and alternative therapies spend years learning their practice. Various forms of CAM are increasingly being taught in

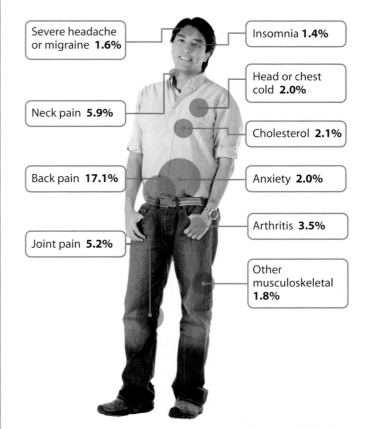

Figure 15.2 Diseases and Conditions for Which CAM Is Most Frequently Used among Adults

Source: Data from P. M. Barnes, B. Bloom, and R. Nahin, "Complementary and Alternative Medicine Use among Adults and Children: United States, 2007," *CDC National Health Statistics Report*, no. 12 (December 2008).

U.S. medical schools and are available to patients in some clinics and hospitals. Some, such as acupuncture, are even covered under many health insurance policies. However, it is important to note that complementary and alternative therapies vary widely in terms of the nature of treatment, extent of therapy, and types of problems for which they offer help. Most lack national training or licensure standards, and states differ in their practices (this latter situation is also true for conventional medicine). Whereas practitioners of conventional medicine have graduated from U.S.-sanctioned schools of medicine or are licensed medical practitioners recognized by the American Medical Association (AMA)—the governing body for all physicians—each CAM domain has its own set of training standards, guidelines for practice, and licensure procedures.

check yourself

- **What is the difference between complementary and alternative medicine?**
- **Who is most likely to use complementary and alternative medicine?**

Types of CAM and Alternative Medical Systems

learning outcomes

- **List the four categories of CAM.**
- **Describe the major alternative medical systems.**

Complementary and alternative medicine comprises four categories: manipulative and body-based practices, energy medicine, mind–body medicine, and natural products.

Major Categories of Complementary and Alternative Medicine

The U.S. government has created the National Center for Complementary and Alternative Medicine (NCCAM) within the National Institutes of Health (NIH) to provide a mechanism for reliable information about CAM practices. The NCCAM serves as a clearinghouse for CAM information and a focal point for research initiatives, policy development, and general recommendations. It has grouped the many varieties of CAM into four categories of practice **(Figure 15.3)**, recognizing that they may overlap and that aspects of them may be part of larger alternative medical systems.[12] Each category is described in greater detail in the following modules.

Alternative Medical Systems

Alternative (whole) medical systems are built on specific systems of theory and practice. Many alternative systems of medicine have been practiced by cultures throughout the world. Some have evolved from centuries-old practices, such as traditional Chinese medicine and Ayurveda, which are at the root of much of CAM thinking today. Other alternative medical systems include homeopathy and naturopathy.

Traditional Chinese Medicine **Traditional Chinese medicine (TCM)** emphasizes the proper balance or disturbances of *qi* (pronounced "chee"), or vital energy, in health and disease, respectively. Diagnosis is based on personal history, observation of the body (especially the tongue), palpation, and pulse diagnosis, an elaborate procedure requiring considerable skill and experience by the practitioner. Techniques such as acupuncture, herbal medicine, massage, and *qigong* (a form of energy therapy) are among the TCM approaches to health and healing.

Traditional Chinese medicine practitioners within the United States must complete a graduate program at a college or university approved by the Accreditation Commission for Acupuncture and Oriental Medicine (ACAOM). Graduate programs vary based on the specific area of concentration within TCM but usually involve

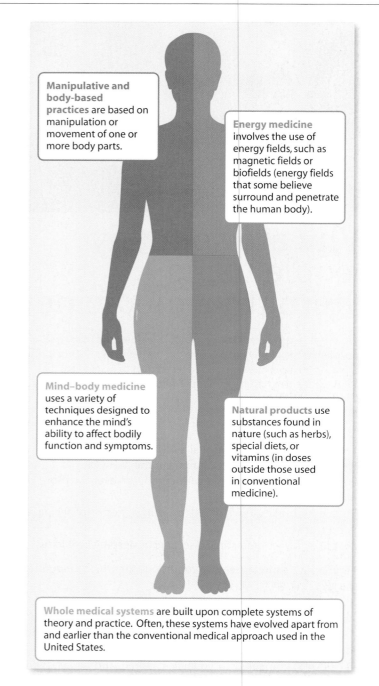

Manipulative and body-based practices are based on manipulation or movement of one or more body parts.

Energy medicine involves the use of energy fields, such as magnetic fields or biofields (energy fields that some believe surround and penetrate the human body).

Mind–body medicine uses a variety of techniques designed to enhance the mind's ability to affect bodily function and symptoms.

Natural products use substances found in nature (such as herbs), special diets, or vitamins (in doses outside those used in conventional medicine).

Whole medical systems are built upon complete systems of theory and practice. Often, these systems have evolved apart from and earlier than the conventional medical approach used in the United States.

Figure 15.3 The Categories of Complementary and Alternative Medicine (CAM)

NCCAM groups CAM practices into four types, recognizing that there can be some overlap. In addition, NCCAM studies entire CAM medical systems, which cut across all categories.

Source: National Center for Complementary and Alternative Medicine, "The Use of Complementary and Alternative Medicine in the United States," NCCAM Publication no. D434, 2010.

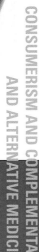

Shirodhara—a traditional Ayurvedic treatment in which warm herbalized oil is poured over the forehead in guided rhythmic patterns—is said to relieve stress and anxiety, treat insomnia and chronic headaches, and improve memory.

an extensive 3- or 4-year clinical internship. In addition, an examination by the National Commission for the Certification of Acupuncture and Oriental Medicine, a standard for licensing in the United States, must be completed. Specific practices incorporated in TCM are discussed later in this chapter under the individual CAM domains.

Ayurveda **Ayurveda (Ayurvedic medicine)** relates to the "science of life," an alternative medical system that began and evolved over thousands of years in India. Ayurveda seeks to integrate and balance the body, mind, and spirit and to restore harmony in the individual.[13] Ayurvedic practitioners use various techniques, including questioning, observing, and touching patients and classifying patients into one of three body types, or *doshas*, before establishing a treatment plan. The goals of Ayurvedic treatment are to eliminate impurities in the body and reduce symptoms. Dietary modification and herbal remedies drawn from the botanical wealth of the Indian subcontinent are common. Treatments may also include animal and mineral ingredients, powdered gemstones, yoga, stretching, meditation, massage, steam baths, exposure to the sun, and controlled breathing.

Training of Ayurvedic practitioners varies. At present, no national standard exists for certifying or training Ayurvedic practitioners, although professional groups are working toward creating licensing guidelines.

Naturopathy **Naturopathic medicine** views disease as a manifestation of an alteration in the processes by which the body naturally heals itself. Disease results from the body's effort to ward off impurities and harmful substances from the environment. Naturopathic physicians emphasize restoring health rather than curing disease. They employ an array of healing practices, including diet and clinical nutrition; homeopathy; acupuncture; herbal medicine; hydrotherapy (the use of water in a range of temperatures and methods of application); spinal and soft-tissue manipulation; physical

therapies involving electric currents, ultrasound, and light therapy; therapeutic counseling; and pharmacology.

Several major naturopathic schools in the United States and Canada provide training, conferring the *naturopathic doctor* (ND) degree on students who have completed a 4-year graduate program that emphasizes humanistically oriented family medicine.

Homeopathy **Homeopathic medicine** is an unconventional Western system based on the principle that "like cures like"—in other words, the same substance that in large doses produces the symptoms of an illness will in very small doses cure the illness. It was developed in the late 1700s by Samuel Hahnemann, a German physician, as an approach to medicine that was not as harsh as other treatments of the time, such as bloodletting and blistering.[14] Homeopathic physicians use herbal medicine, minerals, and chemicals in extremely diluted forms to kill infectious agents or to ward off illnesses that are caused by more potent forms or doses of those substances.

Homeopathic training varies considerably and is offered through diploma programs, certificate programs, short courses, and correspondence courses. Laws that detail requirements to practice vary from state to state.

Other Alternative Medical Systems Native American, Aboriginal, African, Middle Eastern, and South American cultures also have their own unique alternative systems. As the number of alternative therapists grows and systems become intertwined, so do the number of options available to consumers. Before considering any treatments, wise consumers will consult the most reliable resources to thoroughly evaluate risks, the scientific basis of claimed benefits, and any contraindications to using the CAM product or service. Tips to keep in mind include:

- Avoid practitioners who promote their treatments as a cure-all for every health problem.
- Reject practitioners who seem to promise remedies for ailments that have thus far defied the best scientific efforts of mainstream medicine.
- Apply the same strategies to researching CAM as you would to choosing allopathic care.

Very diluted plant essences are used in homeopathic medicine to treat a wide range of symptoms.

check yourself

- **What are the four categories of CAM?**
- **Describe three alternative medical systems.**

CAM: Manipulative and Body-Based Practices

- **Describe major manipulative and body-based CAM practices.**

The CAM category of **manipulative and body-based practices** includes methods based on manipulation or movement of the body.

Chiropractic Medicine **Chiropractic medicine** focuses on the relationship between the body's structures (primarily the spine) and their function and on how that relationship affects health. It has been practiced for more than 100 years.[15] Today, many health care organizations work closely with chiropractors, and many insurance companies pay for chiropractic treatment, particularly if it is recommended by an MD.

Chiropractic medicine is based on the idea that a life-giving energy flows through the spine by way of the nervous system. If the spine is partly misaligned, that force is disrupted. Chiropractors use a variety of techniques to manipulate the spine into proper alignment so energy can flow unimpeded. This treatment can be effective for back pain, neck pain, and headaches.

The average chiropractic training program requires 4 years of intensive courses in biochemistry, anatomy, physiology, diagnostics, pathology, nutrition, and related topics, plus hands-on clinical training. Many chiropractors then obtain certification in neurology, geriatrics, or pediatrics. Most state licensing boards require 4 years of study after at least a 2-year undergraduate program; many states require a 4-year undergraduate degree. Applicants must then pass an examination given by the National Board of Chiropractic Examiners. Chiropractic practice is licensed and regulated in all 50 states.[16]

Oh, my aching back? Try massage!

Massage Therapy *Massage therapy* is defined as soft-tissue manipulation by trained therapists for healing purposes.[17] Massage therapists use hand techniques to move muscles and soft tissues, releasing muscle tension and increasing the flow of blood and oxygen. Massage is used to treat painful conditions, relax tired and overworked muscles, reduce stress and anxiety, rehabilitate injuries, and promote general health.[18] There are many types of massage therapy; the following are some of the more popular:

- *Swedish massage* uses long strokes, kneading, and friction on the muscles, plus joint movement to aid flexibility.
- *Deep tissue massage* uses strokes and pressure on areas where muscles are tight or knotted, focusing on layers of muscle deep under the skin.
- *Trigger point massage* (or *pressure point massage*) applies deep, focused pressure on myofascial trigger points—"knots" that can form in the muscles, are painful when pressed, and can cause symptoms throughout the body.
- *Shiatsu massage* uses varying, rhythmic pressure on parts of the body believed important for the flow of vital energy.

There are about 1,500 massage therapy schools, college programs, and training programs in the United States.[19] They typically teach subjects such as anatomy and physiology; kinesiology; therapeutic evaluation; massage techniques; first aid; business, ethical, and legal issues; and hands-on practice. These educational programs vary in respect to length, quality, and accreditation. Many require 500 hours of training (the same number of hours many states require for certification). Some therapists also pursue specialty or advanced training. Massage therapists work in a variety of settings, including private offices, studios, hospitals, nursing homes, fitness centers, and sports medicine facilities.[20]

Bodywork Bodywork can take on several forms. The *Feldenkrais method* is a system of movements, floor exercises, and bodywork designed to retrain the nervous system to find new pathways around areas of blockage or damage. It is gentle and effective in rehabilitating trauma victims. *Rolfing* aims to restructure the musculoskeletal system and release repressed emotions by working on patterns of tension held in deep tissue via firm—sometimes painful—pressure. *Shiatsu* is a traditional healing art from Japan that applies pressure to specified points to increase the circulation of vital energy. *Trager bodywork* employs gentle, rhythmic shaking of the patient's limbs to induce states of deep, pleasant relaxation.[21]

- **What are two manipulative and body-based CAM practices? What treatments do they involve?**

CAM: Energy Medicine

learning outcomes

- **Describe major energy-based CAM practices.**

Energy medicine therapies focus either on energy fields thought to originate within the body (biofields) or on fields from other sources (electromagnetic fields). The existence of these fields has not been experimentally proven. Some forms of energy therapy manipulate biofields by applying pressure and/or manipulating the body by placing the hands in, or through, these fields.[22]

Popular examples of biofield therapy include qigong, Reiki, and therapeutic touch. *Qigong,* a component of traditional Chinese medicine, combines movement, meditation, and regulation of breathing to enhance the flow of vital energy (*qi*), improve blood circulation, and enhance immune function. *Reiki,* whose name derives from the Japanese word representing "universal life energy," is based on the belief that channeling spiritual energy through the practitioner heals the spirit, which heals the physical body. *Therapeutic touch* derives from the ancient technique of "laying on" of hands and is based on the premise that the healing force of the therapist brings about the patient's recovery and that healing is promoted when the body's energies are in balance. By passing the hands over the body, the healers identify bodily imbalances.

Bioelectromagnetic-based therapies involve the unconventional use of electromagnetic fields—such as pulsed fields, magnetic fields, or alternating current or direct current fields—to treat asthma, cancer, pain, migraines, and other conditions. There is little scientific documentation to support claims for energy field techniques at this point. However, two derivatives of energy medicine have gained much wider acceptance in recent years: acupuncture and acupressure.

Acupuncture

Acupuncture, one of the oldest forms of traditional Chinese medicine (and one of the most popular among Americans), is sought for a wide variety of health conditions, including musculoskeletal dysfunction, mood enhancement, and wellness promotion. It describes a family of procedures that involve stimulating anatomical points of the body with a series of precisely placed needles. The placement and manipulation of acupuncture needles is based on traditional Chinese theories of life-force energy (*qi*) flow through *meridians,* or energy pathways, in the body. Following acupuncture, most respondents and participants in clinical studies report high levels of satisfaction with the treatment, improved quality of life, improvement

in or cure of the condition, and reduced reliance on prescription drugs and surgery. In particular, results have been promising in the treatment of nausea associated with chemotherapy, dental pain, and knee pain.[23] Some Western researchers believe that acupuncture may work through stimulating or repressing the autonomic nervous system.[24]

Acupuncturists in the United States are state licensed, and each state has specific requirements regarding training programs. Most acupuncturists either have completed a 2- to 3-year postgraduate program to obtain a master of traditional Oriental medicine (MTOM) degree or have attended a shorter certification program in North America or Asia.

Acupressure

Acupressure is similar to acupuncture but does not use needles. Instead, the practitioner applies pressure to points critical to balancing *yin* and *yang,* the two Chinese principles that interact to influence overall harmony (health) of the body. Practitioners must have the same basic training and understanding of energy pathways as do acupuncturists.

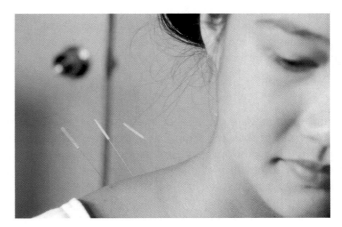

How does acupuncture work?

In acupuncture, long, thin needles are inserted into specific points along the body. This is thought to increase the flow of life-force energy, providing many physical and mental benefits.

check yourself

- **What are two energy-based CAM practices? What do their treatments involve?**

■ **Describe several mind–body and biologically based CAM practices.**

Mind–Body Medicine

Mind–body medicine employs a variety of techniques designed to facilitate the mind's capacity to affect bodily functions and symptoms. Some, such as biofeedback and cognitive-behavioral techniques, have been so well investigated that they are no longer considered alternative. Meditation; yoga; tai chi; certain uses of hypnosis; dance, music, and art therapies; prayer and mental healing; and several others are still categorized as complementary and alternative.

Psychoneuroimmunology (PNI) is defined as the "interaction of consciousness (*psycho*), the brain and central nervous system (*neuro*), and the body's defense against external infection and internal aberrant cell division (*immunology*)."[25] Scientists are exploring how relaxation, biofeedback, meditation, yoga, laughter, exercise, and activities that involve mind "quieting" may counteract negative stressors and increase immune function.

A classic study of PNI showed greatly improved immune system function in nursing home patients taught relaxation techniques. Other studies have shown positive effects of stress-reduction strategies for people with cancer or other health problems.[26]

Natural Products

Natural products are perhaps the most controversial domain of CAM because of their sheer number and limited FDA regulation. Natural products include natural treatments, interventions, and products, many of which overlap with conventional medicine's use of dietary supplements. The FDA defines a dietary supplement as a "product (other than tobacco) that is intended to supplement or add to the diet; contains one or more dietary ingredients (including vitamins, minerals, herbs or other botanicals, amino acids, and other substances) or their constituents; is intended to be taken by mouth as a pill, capsule, tablet, or liquid; and is labeled on the front panel as being a dietary supplement."[27] Typically, people take these—often without guidance from any CAM practitioner—to improve health, prevent disease, or enhance mood.

Dietary changes, which are often part of CAM therapies, commonly involve intake of *functional foods* designed to improve specific aspects of physical or mental functioning. Sometimes referred to as **nutraceuticals** for their combined nutritional and pharmaceutical benefit, they are believed to work in much the same way as pharmaceutical drugs in making a person well or in bolstering the immune system.

The following are some popular functional foods and their purported benefits, although research is mixed on their efficacy:

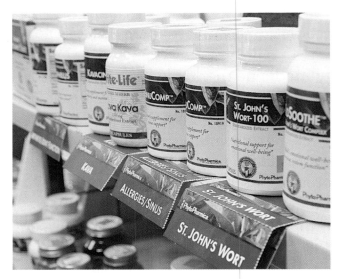

Do herbal remedies have any risks or side effects?

Herbs do have the potential to cause negative side effects. St. John's wort, for example, has potentially dangerous interactions with some prescription antidepressants and should never be taken with them. Other herbs, such as kava, can have negative effects even when taken alone.

■ **Antioxidants.** Chemicals that combat free radicals and oxidative damage in cells. Primary antioxidants include beta-carotene, selenium, vitamin C, and vitamin E.

■ **Plant stanols/sterols.** Can lower "bad" (low-density lipoprotein [LDL]) cholesterol.

■ **Oat fiber.** Can lower LDL cholesterol; serves as a natural soother of nerves; stabilizes blood sugar levels.

■ **Sunflower seeds and oil.** Can lower risk of heart disease; may prevent angina.

■ **Soy protein.** May lower heart disease risk by reducing LDL cholesterol and triglycerides.

■ **Garlic.** Lowers cholesterol and reduces clotting tendency of blood; lowers blood pressure; may serve as an antibiotic.

■ **Ginger.** May reduce motion sickness and stomach upset; discourages blood clots; may relieve rheumatism.

■ **Yogurt.** Yogurt labeled "Live Active Culture" contains friendly bacteria that can fight off infections.

■ **What are several mind–body practices used in complementary medicine?**

■ **What are functional foods?**

Making Choices about CAM Treatments and Over-the-Counter Drugs

learning outcomes

- **Explain how to evaluate the safety and efficacy of OTC drugs and CAM supplements and treatments.**

When you take any drug or supplement, you should be aware of the potential for interaction, with your individual body and particular medical issues, and with any other medicines, supplements, or practices that may affect your health.

With prescription drugs, you should discuss any potential side effects or interactions with your health care provider as well as with the pharmacist. But what about medical choices you make yourself—everything from over-the-counter (OTC) cold medicines and multivitamins to acupuncture and herbal remedies for occasional or chronic conditions? In these situations, your own ability to evaluate the drug or supplement's safety and efficacy becomes an even more important factor.

One way to think about these risks and benefits is by using the diagram in **Figure 15.4**; the figure presents CAM treatments, but its principles can be applied to OTC drugs or to almost any medical treatment or substance. The figure lays out a four-part matrix on which items are graphed according to safety (vertical axis) and effectiveness (horizontal axis).

Some medical choices can be placed firmly in the upper right quadrant, meaning that they are likely to be both safe and effective. For example, taking an OTC pain reliever a few times in as many days to reduce swelling and pain in a sprained ankle, in the absence of any known allergies or other drug interactions, is likely to be helpful and safe. Similarly, acupuncture for common symptoms such as headache or dental pain has little likelihood of negative interaction with drugs or other treatments and is supported as likely to be effective by both allopathic and complementary medical experts. Other choices may have less solid research showing their effectiveness, but offer little likelihood of danger if tried; you may want to see if they help you or not. Examples in this category include low-fat diets for cancer patients and homeopathic treatments such as pulsatilla for children's earache.

More caution is called for when using CAM or OTC products that have been shown effective in some cases but are contraindicated in others. Ginkgo biloba, for example, has shown promising results when used to treat dementia and may improve cognitive function in older adults, but it can affect the intensity with which a person's system responds to SSRIs taken for depression and other mood disorders, so the two should not be combined. Similarly, many common OTC pain relievers have blood-thinning effects—fine in most healthy people, but potentially dangerous in those taking prescription blood thinners.

Finally, choices that are of dubious effectiveness and have known dangers should be avoided entirely: for example, injections of unapproved substances that promise miraculous recovery from serious disease should be approached with great skepticism. If it sounds too good to be true, it very well may be—and possibly dangerous as well. Whatever the substance or treatment, always check it out with reliable sources—start with the websites suggested at the end of this chapter—and approach it with caution.

May be safe; efficacy unclear
Treatment examples: Acupuncture for chronic pain; homeopathy for seasonal allergies; low-fat diet for some cancers; massage therapy for low back pain; mind–body techniques for cancer
Advice: Physician monitoring recommended

MORE SAFE

Likely safe and effective
Treatment examples: Chiropractic care for acute low back pain; acupuncture for nausea from chemotherapy; acupuncture for dental pain; mind–body techniques for chronic pain and insomnia
Advice: Treatment is reasonable; physician monitoring advised

LESS EFFECTIVE ← → **MORE EFFECTIVE**

Dangerous or ineffective
Treatment examples: Injections of unapproved substances; use of toxic herbs; delaying essential medical treatments; taking herbs known to interact dangerously with conventional medications (e.g., St. John's wort and indinavir)
Advice: Avoid treatment

LESS SAFE

May work, but safety uncertain
Treatment examples: St. John's wort for depression; saw palmetto for an enlarged prostate; chondroitin sulfate for osteoarthritis; ginkgo biloba for improving cognitive function in dementia
Advice: Physician monitoring is important

Figure 15.4 Assessing the Risks and Benefits of CAM Treatments

Medical experts devised this chart to gauge the potential liability of recommending alternative treatments by categorizing treatments according to their relative safety and effectiveness. Patients and consumers can also use this chart to make appropriate choices.

Source: M. H. Cohen and D. M. Eisenberg, "Potential Physician Malpractice Liability Associated with Complementary and Integrative Medical Therapies," *Annals of Internal Medicine* 136, no. 8 (2002): 596–603. Copyright © 2002 American College of Physicians. Used with permission.

check yourself

- **What are some factors to consider when evaluating a drug or supplement?**

Choosing Health Products: Prescription and OTC Drugs

- **Explain how to determine the risks and benefits of prescription and over-the-counter medicines.**

Prescription drugs can be obtained only with a written prescription from a physician, whereas over-the-counter drugs can be purchased without a prescription. Just as making wise decisions about providers is an important aspect of responsible health care, so is making wise decisions about medications.

Prescription Drugs

In about two-thirds of doctor visits, the physician administers or prescribes at least one medication. In fact, prescription drug use has risen by 25 percent over the past decade. Even though these drugs are administered under medical supervision, the wise consumer still takes precautions. Hazards and complications arising from the use of prescription drugs are common.

Several resources can help you determine the risks of prescription medicines and to make educated decisions about whether to take a given drug. One of the best is the Center for Drug Evaluation and Research (www.fda.gov/drugs). This consumer-specific section of the FDA website provides current information on risks and benefits of prescription drugs.

Medications Online: Buyer Beware Consumers may choose to have prescriptions filled online for convenience and to save money. Although many websites operate legally and observe the traditional safeguards for dispensing drugs, be wary of rogue websites that sell unapproved or counterfeit drugs or that sidestep practices meant to protect consumers.

The Verified Internet Pharmacy Practice Sites (VIPPS) seal is given to online pharmacy sites that meet state licensure requirements. Follow these tips to protect yourself from fraudulent sites:[28]

- Buy only from state-licensed pharmacy sites based in the United States (preferably from VIPPS-certified sites).
- Don't buy from sites that sell prescription drugs without a prescription or that offer to prescribe a medication for the first time without a physical exam by your doctor.

Be very cautious if you consider ordering medications from an online pharmacy.

- Use legitimate websites that have a licensed pharmacist to answer your questions.
- Don't provide personal information, such as a Social Security number, credit card information, or medical or health history, unless you are sure the website will keep your information safe and private.

Generic drugs, medications sold under a chemical name rather than a brand name, contain the same active ingredients as brand-name drugs but are less expensive. If your doctor prescribes a drug, always ask if a generic equivalent exists and if it would be safe and effective for you to try.

There is some controversy about effectiveness of generic drugs: substitutions sometimes are made in minor ingredients that can affect the way the drug is absorbed, potentially causing discomfort or even allergic reactions in some patients. Tell your doctor about any reactions you have to medications.

45% of Americans report taking at least one prescription drug in the past month; 18% report taking three or more such drugs.

Over-the-Counter (OTC) Drugs

Over-the-counter (OTC) drugs are nonprescription substances used for self-medication. American consumers spend billions of dollars yearly on OTC preparations for relief of everything from runny noses to ingrown toenails. Despite a common belief that OTC products are safe and effective, indiscriminate use and abuse can occur with these drugs as with all others. For example, people who frequently drop medication into their eyes to "get the red out" or pop antacids after every meal are likely to become dependent on these remedies. Many experience adverse side effects because they ignore or don't read the warnings on OTC drug labels. The FDA has developed a standard label that appears on most OTC products (**Figure 15.5**).

Understanding the actions and side effects of OTC drugs is part of being a smart consumer. *Pain relievers* can be useful for counteracting localized or general pain and for reducing fever. They exist in several general formulations (common brand names follow each): *aspirin* (Bayer, Bufferin), *acetaminophen* (Tylenol), *ibuprofen* (Advil, Motrin), and

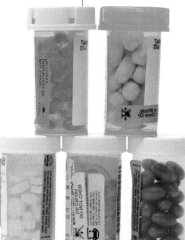

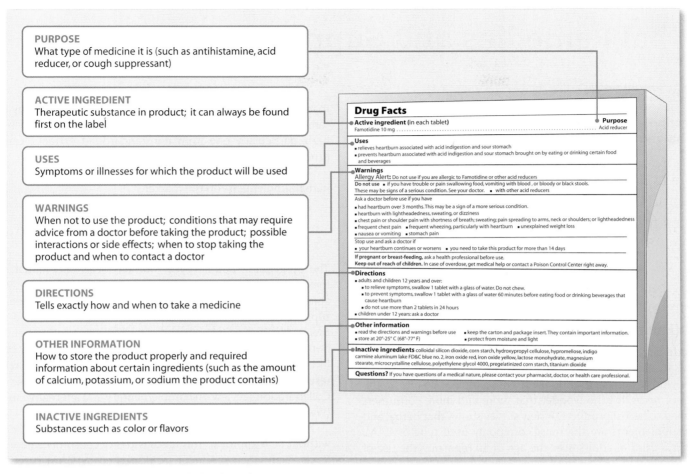

PURPOSE
What type of medicine it is (such as antihistamine, acid reducer, or cough suppressant)

ACTIVE INGREDIENT
Therapeutic substance in product; it can always be found first on the label

USES
Symptoms or illnesses for which the product will be used

WARNINGS
When not to use the product; conditions that may require advice from a doctor before taking the product; possible interactions or side effects; when to stop taking the product and when to contact a doctor

DIRECTIONS
Tells exactly how and when to take a medicine

OTHER INFORMATION
How to store the product properly and required information about certain ingredients (such as the amount of calcium, potassium, or sodium the product contains)

INACTIVE INGREDIENTS
Substances such as color or flavors

Drug Facts

Active ingredient (in each tablet)   **Purpose**
Famotidine 10 mg . . . . Acid reducer

Uses
- relieves heartburn associated with acid indigestion and sour stomach
- prevents heartburn associated with acid indigestion and sour stomach brought on by eating or drinking certain food and beverages

Warnings
Allergy Alert: Do not use if you are allergic to Famotidine or other acid reducers
Do not use ■ if you have trouble or pain swallowing food, vomiting with blood , or bloody or black stools. These may be signs of a serious condition. See your doctor. ■ with other acid reducers
Ask a doctor before use if you have
- had heartburn over 3 months. This may be a sign of a more serious condition.
- heartburn with lightheadedness, sweating, or dizziness
- chest pain or shoulder pain with shortness of breath; sweating; pain spreading to arms, neck or shoulders; or lightheadedness
- frequent chest pain ■ frequent wheezing, particularly with heartburn ■ unexplained weight loss
- nausea or vomiting ■ stomach pain
Stop use and ask a doctor if
- your heartburn continues or worsens ■ you need to take this product for more than 14 days
If pregnant or breast-feeding, ask a health professional before use.
Keep out of reach of children. In case of overdose, get medical help or contact a Poison Control Center right away.

Directions
- adults and children 12 years and over:
  - to relieve symptoms, swallow 1 tablet with a glass of water. Do not chew.
  - to prevent symptoms, swallow 1 tablet with a glass of water 60 minutes before eating food or drinking beverages that cause heartburn
  - do not use more than 2 tablets in 24 hours
- children under 12 years: ask a doctor

Other information
- read the directions and warnings before use ■ keep the carton and package insert. They contain important information.
- store at 20°-25° C (68°-77° F) ■ protect from moisture and light

Inactive ingredients colloidal silicon dioxide, corn starch, hydroxypropyl cellulose, hypromellose, indigo carmine aluminum lake FD&C blue no. 2, iron oxide red, iron oxide yellow, lactose monohydrate, magnesium stearate, microcrystalline cellulose, polyethylene glycol 4000, pregelatinized corn starch, titanium dioxide

Questions? If you have questions of a medical nature, please contact your pharmacist, doctor, or health care professional.

Figure 15.5 The Over-the-Counter Medicine Label
Source: Consumer Healthcare Products Association, OTC Label, www.otcsafety.org. Used with permission.

naproxen sodium (Aleve, Naprosyn). Possible side effects include stomach problems ranging from simple stomach upset to worsening of ulcers; overdose or prolonged overuse can cause liver damage. Aspirin and ibuprofen also reduce blood clotting ability (which can be a problem for those taking anticlotting medications) and, for a few users, can trigger severe allergic reactions. Finally, aspirin should not be taken by anyone under 18, because it has been associated with Reye's syndrome in children and teenagers.

Cold and allergy medicines mask (but don't eliminate) symptoms in a variety of ways. *Antihistamines* (Claritin, Benadryl, Xyzal) dry runny noses, clear postnasal drip and sinus congestion, and reduce tears. They are mild central nervous system depressants and, as such, can cause drowsiness, dizziness, and disturbed coordination in many people. *Decongestants* (Sudafed, DayQuil, Allermed) reduce nasal stuffiness due to colds. In terms of side effects, different people react differently to these medications: Some may exhibit nervousness, restlessness, and sleep problems, whereas others may feel drowsy or nauseated.

Antacids (Tums, Maalox) relieve "heartburn," usually by combating stomach acid with a chemical base such as calcium or aluminum. Occasional use is safe, but chronic use can lead to reduced mineral absorption from food; possible concealment of ulcer; reduced effectiveness of anticlotting medications; interference with

the function of certain antibiotics (for antacids that contain aluminum); worsened high blood pressure (for antacids that contain sodium); and aggravated kidney problems.

Laxatives (Ex-lax, Citrucel) are designed to relieve constipation. Although safe with limited and occasional use, long-term regular use can lead to reduced absorption of minerals from food, dehydration, and even dependency (the user's body becoming dependent on the drug for regular bowel movement).

Sleep aids and relaxants (Nytol, Sleep-Eze, Sominex) are designed to help relieve occasional sleeplessness. Short-term side effects include drowsiness and reduced mental alertness, dry mouth and throat, constipation, dizziness, and lack of coordination. Long-term use can lead to dependency.

check yourself

- **What factors should you consider when ordering prescription drugs online?**

- **What are the benefits and potential side effects for three OTC drugs that you use or might use in the future?**

Herbal Remedies and Supplements

- **Describe how to evaluate the safety and efficacy of herbal remedies and supplements.**

People have been using herbal remedies for thousands of years. Herbs were the original sources for compounds found in approximately 25 percent of the pharmaceutical drugs we use today, including aspirin (white willow bark), the heart medication digitalis (foxglove), and the cancer treatment paclitaxel (Pacific yew).

In addition, scientists continue to make pharmacological advances by studying the herbal remedies used in cultures throughout the world. With conventional scientists now recognizing the benefits of herbs, it is no wonder that more and more consumers are turning to herbal products. A new survey shows that herbal and dietary supplements are the most commonly used type of CAM, with over a third of adults over the age of 50 reporting the use of herbal supplements within the past year.[29]

However, herbal remedies are not to be taken lightly. Just because something is natural does not necessarily mean that it is safe for you, or anyone. For example, in recent years the FDA has warned that certain herbal products containing kava may be associated with severe liver damage.[30] Even rigorously tested products can be risky. Many plants are poisonous, and some can be toxic if ingested in high doses. Others may be dangerous when combined with particular prescription or over-the-counter drugs—they could disrupt the normal action of the drugs or could cause unusual side effects.[31] Properly trained herbalists and homeopaths receive graduate-level training in special programs such as herbal nutrition or traditional Chinese medicine. These practitioners are trained in diagnosis; in mixing herbs, titrations, and dosages; and in the follow-up care of patients.

Herbal remedies come in several different forms. **Tinctures** (extracts of fresh or dried plants) usually contain a high percentage of grain alcohol to prevent spoilage and are among the best herbal options. Freeze-dried extracts are very stable and offer good value for your money. Standardized extracts, often available in pill or capsule form, are also among the more reliable forms of herbal preparations.

In general, herbal medicines tend to be milder than chemical drugs and produce their effects more slowly; they also are much less likely to cause toxicity because they are diluted rather than concentrated forms of drugs. But diluted or not, and no matter how natural they are, herbs still contain many of the same chemicals as synthetic prescription drugs. Too much of any herb, particularly one from nonstandardized extracts, can cause problems.

Table 15.1 gives an overview of some of the most common herbal supplements on the market.

Strategies to Protect Supplement Consumers' Health

The burgeoning popularity of nutraceuticals and herbal supplements concerns many scientists. Although other alternative therapies have been widely studied, there is little quality research to support the many claims in the area of nutraceuticals and supplements. It is important to gather whatever information you can on both the safety and the efficacy of any CAM treatment you consider. In the case of herbal supplements or functional foods, start your research with NCCAM (www.nccam.nih.gov) and the Cochrane Collaboration's review on complementary and alternative medicine (www.cochrane.org).

Herbal supplements and functional foods can currently be sold without FDA approval. This raises issues of consumer safety to new levels. Even when products are dispensed by CAM practitioners, the situation can be risky. Some homeopaths and herbalists who mix their own tonics may not use standardized measures. The lack of standard regulation means that some unskilled and untrained people may be treating patients without fully understanding the potential chemical interactions of their preparations.

Pressure has mounted to establish consistent standards for herbal supplements and functional foods similar to those used in Germany and other countries, as well as a more stringent FDA approval process for supplements. As a result, the FDA has instituted new regulations to oversee the manufacture of dietary supplements, including herbal supplements. These require manufacturers to evaluate the identity, purity, strength, and composition of supplements to ensure they contain what the label claims.

The official public standards-setting authority for all medicines and supplements manufactured and sold in the United States is the U.S. Pharmacopeia, which tests select products, including herbal supplements, to ensure that they comply with safety and purity standards. Products that meet these standards display a "USP Dietary Supplement Verified" seal (Figure 15.6). In addition, dietary supplements are required to include specific information on their labels, as regulated by the Dietary Supplement Health and Education Act.

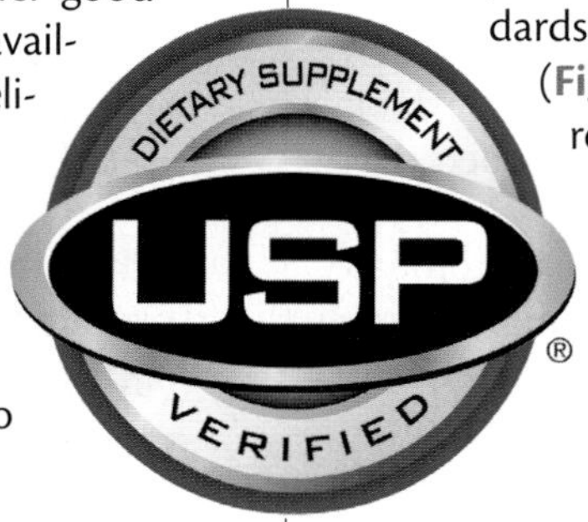

Figure 15.6 The U.S. Pharmacopeia Verified Mark
Source: Used with permission of The United States Pharmacopeial Convention, 12601 Twinbrook Parkway, Rockville, MD 20857.

TABLE

15.1

Common Herbs and Herbal Supplements: Benefits, Research, and Risks

Herb	Claims of Benefits	Research Findings	Potential Risks
Echinacea (purple coneflower, *Echinacea purpurea*, *E. angustifolia*, *E. pallida*)	Stimulates the immune system and increases the effectiveness of white blood cells that attack bacteria and viruses. Useful in preventing and treating colds or the flu.	Many studies in Europe have provided preliminary evidence of its effectiveness, but a recent controlled study in the United States indicated that it is no more effective than a placebo in preventing or treating a cold.	Allergic reactions, including rashes, increased asthma, gastrointestinal problems, and anaphylaxis (a life-threatening allergic reaction). Pregnant women and those with diabetes, autoimmune disorders, or multiple sclerosis should avoid it.
Ephedra (ma huang, Chinese ephedra, *Ephedra sinica*)	Useful for weight loss and athletic performance.	Comprehensive research has found that ephedra has only limited positive effects on weight loss and athletic performance, but has numerous adverse effects.	Heart attack, stroke, heart palpitations, psychiatric problems, upper gastrointestinal effects, tremor, insomnia, and death. The FDA has banned the sale of supplements containing ephedra.
Ginkgo (*Ginkgo biloba*)	Useful for depression, impotence, premenstrual syndrome, dementia and Alzheimer's disease, diseases of the eye, and general vascular disease.	Some promising results have been seen for Alzheimer's disease and dementia, and research continues on its ability to enhance memory and reduce the incidence of cardiovascular disease.	Gastric irritation, headache, nausea, dizziness, difficulty thinking, memory loss, and allergic reactions.
Ginseng (*Panax ginseng*)	Affects the pituitary gland, increasing resistance to stress, affecting metabolism, aiding skin, muscle tone, and sex drive; improves concentration and muscle strength.	Studies have raised questions about appropriate dosages. Because the potency of plants varies considerably, dosage is difficult to control and side effects are fairly common.	Nervousness, insomnia, high blood pressure, headaches, chest pain, depression, and abnormal vaginal bleeding.
Green tea (*Camellia sinensis*)	Useful for lowering cholesterol and risk of some cancers, protecting the skin from sun damage, bolstering mental alertness, and boosting heart health.	Although some studies have shown promising links between green and white tea consumption and cancer prevention, recent research questions the ability of tea to significantly reduce the risk of breast, lung, or prostate cancer.	Insomnia, liver problems, anxiety, irritability, upset stomach, nausea, diarrhea, or frequent urination.
Kava (*Piper methysticum*)	Useful for relaxation; relief of anxiety, insomnia, and menopausal symptoms; sometimes used topically as a numbing agent.	Scientific studies provide some evidence that kava may be beneficial for the management of anxiety.	Increases the effect of alcohol and other drugs; causes drowsiness; the FDA has issued a warning that using kava supplements has been linked to a risk of severe liver damage.
St. John's wort (SJW, Klamath weed, *Hypericum perforatum*)	Useful for depression, anxiety, and sleep disorders.	Some evidence suggests that SJW is useful for treating mild to moderate depression, but two large studies showed that it was no more effective than a placebo in treating major depression of moderate severity.	Gastrointestinal upset, fatigue, dry mouth, anxiety, sexual dysfunction, dizziness, skin rashes, itching, and extreme sensitivity to sunlight.
Valerian (*Valeriana officinalis*)	Useful for relaxation, sleep disorders, anxiety, headaches, depression, irregular heartbeat, and trembling.	Research suggests it may be helpful for insomnia, but there is not enough evidence to determine whether it works for anxiety, depression, or headaches.	Mild side effects, such as headaches, dizziness, upset stomach, and tiredness, occur the morning after use.

Source: National Center for Complementary and Alternative Medicine, "Herbs at a Glance," 2009, http://nccam.nih.gov/health/herbsataglance.htm; Office of Dietary Supplements, "Dietary Supplement Fact Sheets," 2009, http://ods.od.nih.gov/ Health_Information/Information_About_Individual_Dietary_Supplements.aspx; American Cancer Society, "Green Tea," 2008, www.cancer.org/docroot/ETO/content/ ETO_5_3x_Green_Tea.asp.

check yourself

■ **What factors should you consider when evaluating herbs or supplements?**

Health Insurance

- **Outline the structure of the U.S. health insurance system.**
- **Identify the challenges facing the U.S. health insurance system.**

Health insurance—who receives it and how to make it affordable—is one of the major issues of this decade.

The fundamental principle of insurance underwriting is that the cost of health care can be predicted for large populations, with the total resulting cost determining health care premiums (payments). Policyholders pay premiums into a pool, which is held in reserve until needed. When you are sick or injured, the insurance company pays out of the pool, regardless of your total contribution. Depending on circumstances, you may never pay for what your medical care costs, or you may pay much more. The idea is that you pay affordable premiums so that you never have to face catastrophic bills.

In today's profit-oriented system, insurers prefer to have healthy people in their plans who pour money into risk pools without taking money out. Unfortunately, not everyone has health insurance. Over 50 million Americans are uninsured—that is, they have no private health insurance and are not eligible for Medicare, Medicaid, or other government health programs.[32] Increasingly, those with "ordinary" chronic conditions such as migraine headaches and asthma are, like those with more serious preexisting conditions, turned down by private insurers even if they can afford to pay. Fewer and fewer small employers, too, can afford to offer health insurance to their employees, so even those employed by others may not have the opportunity for group coverage, whether affordable or not. And approximately 25 million more Americans between 19 and 64 are underinsured (at risk for spending more than 10% of their income on medical care because their insurance is inadequate).[33]

Lack of health insurance has been associated with delayed health care and increased mortality. *Underinsurance* (i.e., the inability to pay out-of-pocket expenses despite having insurance) also may result in adverse health consequences. People without coverage are less likely to have to get regular checkups, have their children immunized, seek prenatal care, and seek attention for serious symptoms. Experts believe that this ultimately leads to higher system costs, because conditions deteriorate to a more debilitating and costly stage before people are forced to seek help.

Contrary to the common belief that the uninsured are unemployed, 75 percent are either workers or the dependents of workers. One-quarter of the uninsured are children under age 16. Among young adults 18 to 24 years of age, 30 percent reported being uninsured at some point in time. This age group is more than twice as likely to be uninsured as are people 45 to 64 years of age. However,

college students fare much better. According to a recent survey, approximately 6 percent of college students report not having health insurance, and another 2 percent are unsure whether they have health insurance.[34]

Racial and ethnic minorities are more likely to be uninsured. Thirty-three percent of both Latinos and American Indian or Alaskan Natives are uninsured, as are 18.9 percent of African Americans, compared to 17.1 percent of whites.[35]

Private Health Insurance

Originally, health insurance consisted solely of coverage for hospital costs (it was called *major medical*), but gradually it was extended to cover routine treatment and other areas, such as dental services and pharmaceuticals. These payment mechanisms, which provided no incentive to contain costs, laid the groundwork for today's steadily rising health care costs. At the same time, because most insurance did not cover routine or preventive services, consumers were encouraged to use hospitals whenever possible (the coverage was better) and to wait until illness developed to seek care instead of seeking preventive care. Consumers were also free to choose any provider or service, including inappropriate—and often very expensive—care.

To limit losses, private insurance companies have employed several mechanisms. *Deductibles* are front-end payments (commonly $250 to $1,000) you must make to providers before your insurance company will start paying. *Co-payments* are set amounts paid per

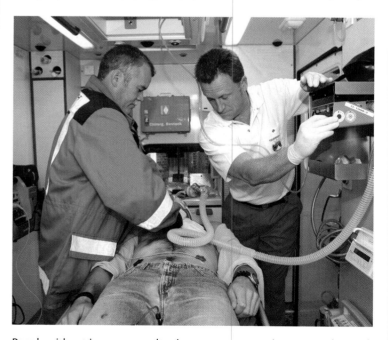

People without insurance can't gain access to preventive care, so they seek care only in an emergency or crisis. Because emergency care is extraordinarily expensive, they often are unable to pay, and the cost is absorbed by those who can pay—the insured or taxpayers.

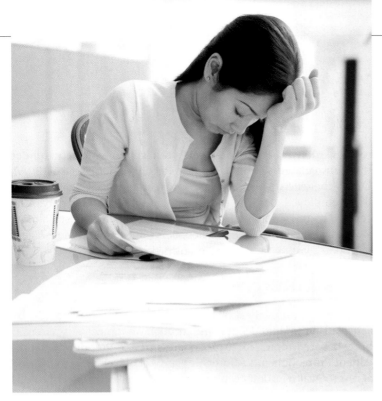

What should I consider when choosing health insurance?

Choosing a health insurance plan can be confusing. Some things to think about include how comprehensive your coverage needs to be, how convenient your care must be, how much you are willing to spend on premiums and co-payments, what the overall cost will be, and whether the services of the plan meet your needs.

service (e.g., $20 per doctor visit). *Coinsurance* is the percentage you must pay (e.g., 20% of the total bill). *Preexisting condition clauses* limit the insurance company's liability for medical conditions that a consumer had before obtaining coverage (i.e., if a woman takes out coverage while pregnant, the insurer may cover pregnancy complications and infant care but not charges related to "normal pregnancy").

Group plans of large employers generally do not have preexisting condition clauses in their plans, but smaller group plans often do. Some plans never cover preexisting conditions, whereas others specify a *waiting period* (e.g., 6 or 18 months) before they will cover them. All insurers set some limits on the services they cover (most exclude cosmetic surgery and experimental procedures). Some plans may also include an *upper* or *lifetime limit*. Although $250,000 may seem like an enormous sum, medical bills for a chronic disease can easily run this high within a few years.

Managed Care

Managed care describes a health care delivery system consisting of a network of providers and facilities linked contractually to deliver health benefits within a set annual budget, sharing economic risk,

with membership rules for participating patients. Approximately 68.2 million Americans are enrolled in HMOs, the most common type of managed care system.[36] Managed care plans have grown steadily over the past decade—indemnity insurance, which pays providers on a fee-for-service basis has become unaffordable or unavailable for most Americans.

Health maintenance organizations (HMOs) provide a range of covered benefits (e.g., checkups, surgery, lab tests) for a fixed pre-paid amount. This is both the least expensive form of managed care and the most restrictive—patients are typically required to use the plan's doctors and hospitals and to see a PCP for treatment and referrals.

Preferred provider organizations (PPOs) are networks of independent doctors and hospitals. Members may see doctors not on the preferred list, for an additional cost.

In point of service (POS) plans—offered by many HMOs—a patient selects a PCP from a list of participating providers; this physician becomes the patient's "point of service." If referrals are made outside the network, the patient is still partially covered.

Medicare and Medicaid

The government, through programs such as Medicare and Medicaid, currently funds 35 percent of total U.S. health spending. Under Medicare, the federal government pays 80 percent of most medical bills for people over 65.[37]

Medicare covers 99 percent of individuals over 65, all totally and permanently disabled people (after a waiting period), and all people with end-stage kidney failure—currently over 45 million people in all.[38] By 2030, an estimated 1 in 5—or 77 million—Americans will be insured by Medicare. As the costs of care have soared, Medicare has placed limits on provider reimbursements. As a result, some physicians and managed care programs have stopped accepting Medicare patients.

To control hospital costs, in 1983 the federal government set up a Medicare payment system based on **diagnosis-related groups (DRGs)**. Nearly 500 groupings of diagnoses were created to establish how much a hospital would be reimbursed for a particular patient. This gave hospitals the incentive to discharge patients quickly after doing as little as possible for them, to provide more ambulatory care, and to admit only patients in profitable DRGs. Many private health insurance companies have now adopted this type of reimbursement.

Medicaid is a federal–state welfare program for people who are defined as poor, including many who are blind, disabled, elderly, or receiving Aid to Families with Dependent Children—a total of about 36 million people.[39] Because each state determines eligibility and payments to providers, the way Medicaid operates from state to state varies widely.

check yourself

- **What are four common barriers to adequate health insurance?**
- **What structures and limits do private insurers use to control costs?**

Issues Facing the Health Care System

■ **Identify the major challenges facing the U.S. health care system.**

Cost

The United States spends more on health care than any other nation. Yet, unlike the rest of the industrialized world, we do not provide access for our entire population. We spend $2.3 trillion annually on health care—more than $7,500 for each person **(Figure 15.7)**, or 18.3 percent of GDP. Health care expenditures are projected to grow by 6.1 percent per year, reaching $4 trillion by 2019.[40]

Why do health care costs continue to skyrocket? Many factors are involved: a for-profit health industry; excess administrative costs; duplication of services; an aging population; growing rates of obesity, inactivity, and related health problems; demand for new medical technologies; an emphasis on crisis-oriented care instead of prevention; and inappropriate use of services.

Our system's more than 2,000 health insurance companies prevents *economies of scale* (bulk purchasing at a reduced cost) and administrative efficiency realized in countries with single-payer systems. Commercial insurance companies commonly have administrative costs greater than 10 percent of total premiums; the administrative costs of the government's Medicare program are less than 4 percent. These expenses contribute to the high cost of health care and are largely passed on to consumers.

Access

Over 133 million people in the United States suffer from at least one chronic health condition.[41] Their access to care is largely determined by whether they have health insurance. Catastrophic or chronic illness among only 10 percent of the population accounts for 75 percent of all health expenditures.[42] We cannot perfectly predict who will fall into that 10 percent—every American is potentially vulnerable to the high cost and devastating effects of such illnesses.

Access to care is determined by factors such as the supply of providers and facilities and a person's proximity to care, ability to maneuver in the health care system, health status, and insurance coverage. Although there are almost 700,000 physicians in the United States, many Americans lack adequate access to health services because of insurance barriers or maldistribution of providers.[43] There is an oversupply of higher-paid specialists and a shortage of lower-paid primary care physicians. Inner cities and some rural areas face constant physician shortages.

Until recently, employees lost insurance benefits when they changed jobs; this led the federal government to pass legislation mandating "portability" of health insurance benefits, guaranteeing coverage during the transition. Today, former employees (and retirees, spouses, and dependents) can continue benefits under the Consolidated Omnibus Budget Reconciliation Act (COBRA). COBRA beneficiaries usually pay a far greater amount than they did when employed, because they must cover the amount previously covered by the employer. However, COBRA benefits are still almost always less expensive than individual insurance. COBRA coverage is temporary, lasting for up to 18 months.

The Debate over Universal Coverage

Whether universal health care coverage will—or should—be achieved in the United States and through what mechanism remain hotly debated topics. In 2010, Congress passed President Obama's Patient Protection and Affordable Care Act, which aims to provide access to health insurance for more than 30 million previously uninsured individuals. The legislation achieves this by expanding Medicaid eligibility to include an additional 16 million people and by subsidizing private health insurance for low- and middle-income individuals. The law also bans or restricts practices such as denying coverage to people with preexisting conditions and imposing lifetime coverage limits. Reforms will be phased in over 4 years. Some changes are in effect now, such as allowing young adults to stay on their parents' health insurance plan up to age 26 if they do not have access to coverage through an employer.[44]

Debate continues over the goal of universal coverage. Arguments for national health insurance include the following:[45]

■ Health care is a human right. The United Nations Universal Declaration of Human Rights states that "everyone has the right to a standard of living adequate for the health and well-being of oneself and one's family, including . . . medical care."[46]

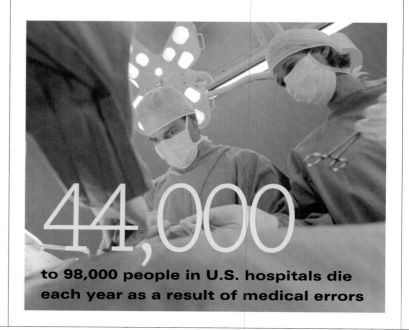

44,000 to 98,000 people in U.S. hospitals die each year as a result of medical errors

- Americans would be more likely to engage in preventive health behaviors and clinicians would be encouraged to practice preventive medicine; people without insurance often avoid preventive care checkups due to cost.
- Medical professionals could concentrate on patient care rather than on insurance procedures, malpractice liability, and other administrative issues.
- Taxes already pay for a substantial amount of our health care expenditures.
- Providing all citizens the right to health care is good for economic productivity because it allows people to live longer and healthier lives.

Arguments against national health insurance include the following:[47]

- Health care is not a right, because it is not in the Bill of Rights in the U.S. Constitution, which lists rights the government cannot infringe upon, not services the government must ensure.
- It is the individual's responsibility to ensure personal health. Diseases and health problems can often be prevented by choosing to live healthier lifestyles.
- Expenses for health care would have to be paid for with higher taxes or spending cuts in other areas.
- Profit motives, competition, and ingenuity lead to cost control and effectiveness. These concepts should be brought to health care reform.
- Providing a right to health care is bad for economic productivity.

Quality and Malpractice

The U.S. health care system has several mechanisms for ensuring quality: education, licensure, certification/registration, accreditation, peer review, and malpractice litigation. Some of these are mandatory before a professional or organization may provide care; others are voluntary. (Licensure, though mandated by the state for some practitioners and facilities, is only a minimum guarantee of quality.) Insurance companies and government payers may link payment to whether a practitioner is board certified or a facility is accredited by an appropriate agency. In addition, most insurance plans require prior authorization and/or second opinions, not only to reduce costs, but also to improve quality of care.

A new form of measurement uses "outcome" as the primary indicator for measuring health care quality at the individual level. Outcome measurements don't look just at what is done to the patient, but at the patient's subsequent health status—mortality and complication rates become important in assessing practitioners and facilities.

Medical Waste

The Medical Waste Tracking Act of 1988 defines medical waste as "any solid waste that is generated in the diagnosis, treatment, or immunization of human beings or animals, in research pertaining

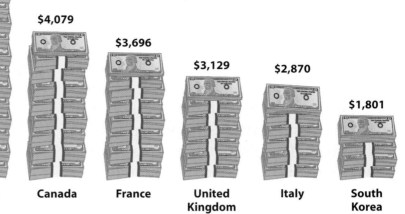

$7,538
United States

$4,079
Canada

$3,696
France

$3,129
United Kingdom

$2,870
Italy

$1,801
South Korea

Figure 15.7 Health Care Spending per Person, 2008 (in thousands of U.S. dollars)
Source: Data from Organisation for Economic Co-Operation and Development, *OECD Health Data 2010*, 2010, www.oecd.org/health.

thereto, or in the production or testing of biologicals." This includes, but is not limited to, culture dishes and other glassware; discarded surgical gloves, bandages, instruments, and needles; and removed body parts (e.g., tonsils, appendices, limbs).[48]

An estimated 2 million tons of medical waste is generated by hospitals each year. Much is disposed of in landfills, with the potential to contaminate groundwater and surface water. Currently, over 90 percent is incinerated, resulting in carbon emissions and other pollution.

In addition, both individuals and hospitals generate substantial pharmaceutical waste—mostly drugs that have been dispensed but not completely used. Nearly 54 percent of consumers put unwanted medications in the trash, and 35 percent flush them down the toilet. Drugs that are thrown away add waste to landfills, and those disposed of down a toilet or drain can end up back in our water supply, leading to high levels of chemicals that many water treatment facilities are unequipped to filter. A better way to manage unused medications is to seek out an organization that collects unused, unexpired medicine for donation.[49] Many states have passed legislation for recycling unused medications, but implementation has proven difficult.[50] Another option is to ask your pharmacy: Many accept unused prescription medicines and either return it to the manufacturer or destroy it safely.

check yourself

- **What are two arguments for, and two against, universal health care coverage?**
- **What are three challenges faced by the U.S. health care system?**

Advocating During a Health Care Crisis

learning outcomes

- **List strategies for helping loved ones in a health crisis.**

If you or a loved one faces a health care crisis, such as a heart attack, stroke, or unexpected surgery, it is important to act with knowledge, strength, and assertiveness. The following suggestions can help you deal with hospitals and health care providers:

1. **Know your rights as a patient.** Ask about the risks and costs of diagnostic tests. Some procedures may pose significant risks for older people and can be replaced or supplemented by less invasive tests. When you get test results, ask for an explanation of any abnormalities. If you still don't understand them, ask for further clarification.

2. **Find out about informed consent procedures, living wills, durable power of attorney, organ donation, and other legal issues before you, or any loved ones, become sick.** Having someone shove a clipboard in your face and ask if life support can be terminated in case of a problem is one of the great horrors of many people's hospital experiences. Be prepared by taking care of these issues well in advance. If your parents or loved ones have not done so, encourage them to think about these issues.

3. **Remain with your loved one as a personal advocate.** If your loved one is weak and unable to ask questions, ask the questions for him or her. Inquire about new medications, tests, and potentially risky procedures that may be undertaken during the course of treatment or recovery. If you feel that your loved one is being removed from intensive care or other closely monitored areas prematurely, ask if the hospital is taking this action to comply with DRGs and if this action is warranted.

4. **Check the credentials of the health care providers.** Find out if those staffing the surgery unit, giving anesthesia, and so on, are all part of your preferred provider insurance group. Many people are shocked to find that part-time staff members from unaffiliated hospitals are treating them, even in a preferred provider facility. When this happens, you may have to pay a much larger co-payment for out-of-group practitioners. Ask about the patient-to-staff ratio, and make sure that people monitoring you or your loved ones have appropriate credentials.

5. **Be considerate of the care providers.** One of the most stressful jobs is caring for critically ill people. Although questions are appropriate and your emotions are running high, be as considerate and tactful as possible. Nurses often carry a disproportionately large responsibility for patient care and have a higher-than-optimal patient load. Try to remain out of their way, ask questions as necessary, and report any problems to the supervisor.

6. **Be patient with the patient.** The pain, suffering, and fears associated with surgery or other major medical events can cause otherwise nice people to act in not-so-nice ways. Be patient and helpful, and allow time for the person to rest. Talk with the patient about his or her feelings, concerns, and fears. Do not ignore these concerns to ease your own anxieties. A wide range of psychological and physical problems, including severe depression, can occur in the aftermath of illness, as people struggle to deal with physical limitations, rehabilitation, lifestyle changes, and the recognition of their own vulnerability and mortality. Guilt and frustration can be challenges for survivors and their families.

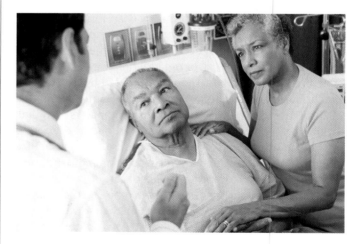

Facing a medical procedure is often frightening, but having a loved one present can help.

check yourself

- **What are three ways you can help a friend or family member going through a health crisis?**

Assessyourself

Are You a Smart Health Care Consumer?

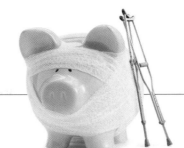

An interactive version of this assessment is available online. Download it from the Live It! section of www.pearsonhighered.com/donatelle.

Answer the following questions to determine what you might do to become a better health care consumer.

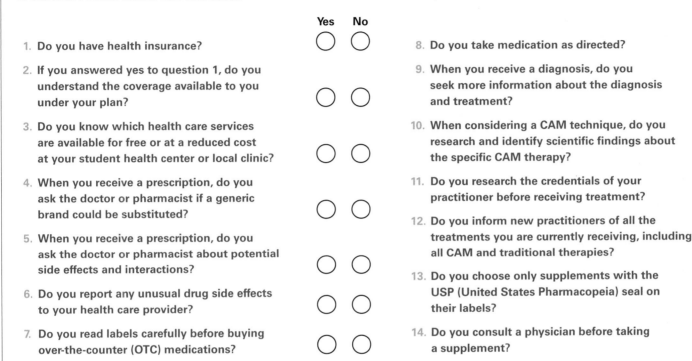

		Yes	No
1.	Do you have health insurance?	○	○
2.	If you answered yes to question 1, do you understand the coverage available to you under your plan?	○	○
3.	Do you know which health care services are available for free or at a reduced cost at your student health center or local clinic?	○	○
4.	When you receive a prescription, do you ask the doctor or pharmacist if a generic brand could be substituted?	○	○
5.	When you receive a prescription, do you ask the doctor or pharmacist about potential side effects and interactions?	○	○
6.	Do you report any unusual drug side effects to your health care provider?	○	○
7.	Do you read labels carefully before buying over-the-counter (OTC) medications?	○	○

		Yes	No
8.	Do you take medication as directed?	○	○
9.	When you receive a diagnosis, do you seek more information about the diagnosis and treatment?	○	○
10.	When considering a CAM technique, do you research and identify scientific findings about the specific CAM therapy?	○	○
11.	Do you research the credentials of your practitioner before receiving treatment?	○	○
12.	Do you inform new practitioners of all the treatments you are currently receiving, including all CAM and traditional therapies?	○	○
13.	Do you choose only supplements with the USP (United States Pharmacopeia) seal on their labels?	○	○
14.	Do you consult a physician before taking a supplement?	○	○

15.15 | Assess Yourself: Are You a Smart Health Care Consumer?

381

Your Plan for Change

Once you have considered your responses to the Assess Yourself questions, you may want to change or improve certain behaviors in order to get the best treatment from your health care provider and the health care system.

Today, you can:

○ Research your insurance plan. Find out which health care providers and hospitals you can visit, the amounts of co-payments and premiums you are responsible for, and the drug coverage offered.

○ Update your medicine cabinet. Dispose properly of any expired prescriptions or OTC medications. Keep on hand a supply of basic items, such as pain relievers, antiseptic cream, bandages, cough suppressants, and throat lozenges.

Within the next 2 weeks, you can:

○ Find a regular health care provider if you do not already have one and make an appointment for a general checkup.

○ Check with your insurance provider and see what CAM practitioners and therapies are covered.

○ Find out what alternative therapies your college's health clinic offers.

By the end of the semester, you can:

○ Become an advocate for others' health. Write to your congressperson or state legislature to express your interest in health care reform.

○ Make relaxation and mind–body stress-reducing techniques a part of your everyday life. This can simply mean practicing meditation, deep breathing, or even taking long walks in nature. You don't need to visit a CAM practitioner or follow a specific therapeutic practice to benefit from methods of relaxation, meditation, and spiritual awakening.

Summary

- Self-care and individual responsibility are key factors in reducing rising health care costs and improving health status. Planning can help you navigate health care treatment in unfamiliar situations or emergencies. Evaluate health professionals by considering their qualifications, their record of treating similar problems, and their ability to work with you.

- Conventional Western (allopathic) medicine is based on scientifically validated methods and procedures. Medical doctors, specialists of various kinds, nurses, and physician assistants practice allopathic medicine.

- People are using complementary and alternative medicine (CAM) in increasing numbers. Alternative medical systems include traditional Chinese medicine (TCM), Ayurveda, homeopathy, and naturopathy. CAM also includes manipulative and body-based practices, energy medicine, mind–body medicine, and biologically based practices.

- Consumers need to understand the risks and benefits of prescription drugs, over-the-counter (OTC) medications, and herbal products and supplements. Regulations governing drug labels help ensure that information about these products is available.

- Health insurance is based on the concept of spreading risk. Insurance is provided by private insurance companies (which charge premiums) and government Medicare and Medicaid programs (which are funded by taxes). Managed care attempts to control costs by streamlining administration and stressing preventive care.

- Concerns about the U.S. health care system include cost, access, choice of treatment, quality, and malpractice.

- You can support a loved one faced with a serious medical issue by accompanying him or her to appointments, asking and recording answers to questions, knowing about legal and medical issues, and offering emotional support.

Pop Quiz

1. Which of the following is *not* a condition that would indicate a visit to a physician is needed?
   a. Recurring high temperature (over 103 °F in adults)
   b. Persistent or recurrent diarrhea
   c. The common cold
   d. Yellowing of the skin or the whites of the eyes

2. What medical practice is based on procedures whose objective is to heal by countering the patient's symptoms?
   a. Allopathic medicine
   b. Nonallopathic medicine
   c. Osteopathic medicine
   d. Chiropractic medicine

3. What mechanism used by private insurance companies requires that the subscriber pay a certain amount directly to the provider before the insurance company will begin paying for services?
   a. Coinsurance
   b. Cost sharing
   c. Co-payments
   d. Deductibles

4. Deborah, 28, is a single parent on welfare. Her medical bills are paid by a federal health insurance program for the poor. This program is
   a. an HMO.
   b. Social Security.
   c. Medicaid.
   d. Medicare.

5. CAM therapies focus on treating both the mind and the whole body, which makes them part of a
   a. natural approach.
   b. psychological approach.
   c. holistic approach.
   d. gentle approach.

6. What type of medicine addresses imbalances of *qi*?
   a. Chiropractic medicine
   b. Naturopathic medicine
   c. Traditional Chinese medicine
   d. Homeopathic medicine

7. The alternative system of medicine based on the principle that "like cures like" is
   a. naturopathic medicine.
   b. homeopathic medicine.
   c. Ayurvedic medicine.
   d. chiropractic medicine.

8. The use of techniques to improve the psychoneuroimmunology of the human body is called
   a. acupressure.
   b. mind–body medicine.
   c. Reiki.
   d. bodywork.

9. What system places equal emphasis on body, mind, and spirit and strives to restore the innate harmony of the individual?
   a. Ayurvedic medicine
   b. Homeopathic medicine
   c. Naturopathic medicine
   d. Traditional Chinese medicine

10. The "USP Dietary Supplement Verified" seal indicates that a supplement is
    a. safe and pure.
    b. effective.
    c. low cost.
    d. child safe.

Answers to these questions can be found on page A-1.

Web Links

1. **Agency for Healthcare Research and Quality (AHRQ).** Links to sites that address health care concerns and provide information on making critical decisions about personal care. www.ahrq.gov

2. **Food and Drug Administration (FDA).** News on government-approved home health tests and other health-related products. www.fda.gov

3. **National Committee for Quality Assurance (NCQA).** Assessments and reports on managed care plans, including HMOs. www.ncqa.org

4. **HealthCare.Gov.** Information regarding the 2010 Patient Protection and Affordable Care Act. www.healthcare.gov

5. **National Center for Complementary and Alternative Medicine (NCCAM).** Information and research on complementary and alternative practices. http://nccam.nih.gov

Answers to Pop Quiz Questions

Chapter 1

1. d; 2. b; 3. a; 4. d; 5. a; 6. a; 7. c; 8. a; 9. c; 10. a

Chapter 2

1. a; 2. b; 3. a; 4. b; 5. c; 6. a; 7. b; 8. b; 9. c; 10. b

Chapter 3

1. c; 2. c; 3. d; 4. d; 5. c; 6. d; 7. c; 8. c; 9. c; 10. b

Chapter 4

1. b; 2. c; 3. c; 4. d; 5. d; 6. c; 7. c; 8. a; 9. b; 10. b

Chapter 5

1. b; 2. b; 3. a; 4. b; 5. b; 6. a; 7. c; 8. d; 9. c; 10. a

Chapter 6

1. b; 2. d; 3. c; 4. a; 5. c; 6. c; 7. c; 8. a; 9. c; 10. b

Chapter 7

1. d; 2. b; 3. c; 4. d; 5. a; 6. c; 7. a; 8. c; 9. b; 10. c

Chapter 8

1. d; 2. a; 3. a; 4. b; 5. b; 6. a; 7. b; 8. b; 9. c; 10. c

Chapter 9

1. c; 2. b; 3. b; 4. c; 5. b; 6. a; 7. a; 8. a; 9. b; 10. b

Chapter 10

1. c; 2. d; 3. d; 4. b; 5. a; 6. b; 7. d; 8. c; 9. b; 10. a

Chapter 11

1. a; 2. c; 3. b; 4. c; 5. b; 6. d; 7. a; 8. c; 9. b; 10. c

Chapter 12

1. a; 2. c; 3. c; 4. d; 5. a; 6. d; 7. c; 8. b; 9. c; 10. a

Chapter 13

1. b; 2. a; 3. c; 4. c; 5. a; 6. b; 7. c; 8. b; 9. b; 10. a

Chapter 14

1. b; 2. d; 3. d; 4. a; 5. a; 6. d; 7. b; 8. b; 9. a; 10. c

Chapter 15

1. c; 2. a; 3. d; 4. c; 5. c; 6. c; 7. b; 8. b; 9. a; 10. a

Glossary

abortion The termination of a pregnancy by expulsion or removal of an embryo or fetus from the uterus.

abstinence Refraining from a behavior.

accountability Accepting responsibility for personal decisions, choices, and actions.

acid deposition The acidification process that occurs when precipitation falls through air that contains molecules that turn to acid when mixed with water.

acquaintance rape A rape in which the rapist is known to the victim.

acquired immunodeficiency syndrome (AIDS) A disease caused by a retrovirus, the human immunodeficiency virus (HIV), that attacks the immune system, reducing the number of helper T cells and leaving the victim vulnerable to infections, malignancies, and neurological disorders.

acupressure Branch of traditional Chinese medicine related to acupuncture. Uses application of pressure to selected body points to balance energy.

acupuncture Branch of traditional Chinese medicine that uses the insertion of long, thin needles to affect flow of energy (*qi*) along pathways (meridians) within the body.

acute stress The short-term physiological response to an immediate perceived threat.

adaptive response Form of adjustment in which the body attempts to restore homeostasis.

adaptive thermogenesis Theoretical mechanism by which the brain regulates metabolic activity according to caloric intake.

addiction Persistent, compulsive dependence on a behavior or substance, including mood-altering behaviors or activities, despite ongoing negative consequences.

aerobic capacity (or power) The functional status of the cardiorespiratory system; refers specifically to the volume of oxygen the muscles consume during exercise.

aerobic exercise Any type of exercise that increases heart rate.

aggravated rape Rape that involves one or multiple attackers, strangers, weapons, or physical beating.

alcohol abuse Use of alcohol that interferes with work, school, or personal relationships or that entails violations of the law.

alcohol poisoning A potentially lethal blood alcohol concentration that inhibits the brain's ability to control consciousness, respiration, and heart rate; usually occurs as a result of drinking a large amount of alcohol in a short period of time. Also known as *acute alcohol intoxication*.

alcoholic hepatitis A condition resulting from prolonged use of alcohol in which the liver is inflamed; can be fatal.

Alcoholics Anonymous (AA) An organization whose goal is to help alcoholics stop drinking; includes auxiliary branches such as Al-Anon and Alateen.

alcoholism (alcohol dependency) Condition in which personal and health problems related to alcohol use are severe and stopping alcohol use results in withdrawal symptoms.

allele One of potentially several variants of the same gene.

allopathic medicine Conventional, Western medical practice; in theory, based on scientifically validated methods and procedures.

allostatic load Wear and tear on the body caused by prolonged or excessive stress responses.

alternative (whole) medical systems Complete systems of theory and practice that involve several types of CAM.

alternative insemination Fertilization accomplished by depositing a partner's or a donor's semen into a woman's vagina via a thin tube; almost always done in a doctor's office.

alternative medicine Treatment used in place of conventional medicine.

altruism The giving of oneself out of genuine concern for others.

Alzheimer's disease (AD) A chronic condition involving changes in nerve fibers of the brain that results in mental deterioration.

amino acids The nitrogen-containing building blocks of protein.

amniocentesis A medical test in which a small amount of fluid is drawn from the amniotic sac to test for Down syndrome and other genetic diseases.

amniotic sac The protective pouch surrounding the fetus.

amphetamines A large and varied group of synthetic agents that stimulate the central nervous system.

anabolic steroids Artificial forms of the hormone testosterone that promote muscle growth and strength.

anal intercourse The insertion of the penis into the anus.

androgyny High levels of traditional masculine and feminine traits in a single person.

aneurysm A weakened blood vessel that may bulge under pressure and, in severe cases, burst.

angina pectoris Chest pain occurring as a result of reduced oxygen flow to the heart.

angiography A technique for examining blockages in heart arteries.

angioplasty A technique in which a catheter with a balloon at the tip is inserted into a clogged artery; the balloon is inflated to flatten fatty deposits against artery walls and a stent is typically inserted to keep the artery open.

anorexia nervosa Eating disorder characterized by excessive preoccupation with food, self-starvation, or extreme exercising to achieve weight loss.

antagonism A drug interaction in which two drugs compete for the same available receptors, potentially blocking each other's actions.

antibiotic resistance The ability of bacteria or other microbes to withstand the effects of an antibiotic.

antibiotics Medicines used to kill microorganisms, such as bacteria.

antibodies Substances produced by the body that are individually matched to specific antigens.

antigen Substance capable of triggering an immune response.

antioxidants Substances believed to protect against oxidative stress and resultant tissue damage at the cellular level.

anxiety disorders Mental illnesses characterized by persistent feelings of threat and worry in coping with everyday problems.

appetite The desire to eat; normally accompanies hunger but is more psychological than physiological.

appraisal The interpretation and evaluation of information provided to the brain by the senses.

arrhythmia An irregularity in heartbeat.

arteries Vessels that carry blood away from the heart to other regions of the body.

arterioles Branches of the arteries.

asbestos A mineral compound that separates into stringy fibers and lodges in the lungs, where it can cause various diseases.

asthma A long-term, chronic inflammatory disorder that causes tiny airways in the lung to spasm in response to triggers. Many cases of asthma are triggered by environmental pollutants.

atherosclerosis Condition characterized by deposits of fatty substances (plaque) on the inner lining of an artery.

atria (singular: *atrium*) The heart's two upper chambers, which receive blood.

attention-deficit/hyperactivity disorder (ADHD) A neurobehavioral disorder characterized by hyperactivity and distraction.

autoerotic behaviors Sexual self-stimulation.

autoimmune disease Disease caused by an overactive immune response against the body's own cells.

autoinoculate Transmission of a pathogen from one part of your body to another part.

autonomic nervous system (ANS) The portion of the central nervous system regulating body functions that a person does not normally consciously control.

Ayurveda (Ayurvedic medicine) A comprehensive system of medicine, derived largely from ancient India, that places equal emphasis on the body, mind, and spirit, and strives to restore the body's innate harmony through diet, exercise, meditation, herbs, massage, exposure to sunlight, and controlled breathing.

background distressors Environmental stressors of which people are often unaware.

bacteria (singular: *bacterium*) Simple, single-celled microscopic organisms; about 100 known species of bacteria cause disease in humans.

barbiturates Drugs that depress the central nervous system and have sedating, hypnotic, and anesthetic effects.

barrier methods Contraceptive methods that block the meeting of egg and sperm by means of a physical barrier (such as condom, diaphragm, or cervical cap), a chemical barrier (such as spermicide), or both.

basal metabolic rate (BMR) The rate of energy expenditure by a body at complete rest in a neutral environment.

belief Appraisal of the relationship between some object, action, or idea and some attribute of that object, action, or idea.

benign Harmless; refers to a noncancerous tumor.

benzodiazepines A class of central nervous system depressant drugs with sedative, hypnotic, and muscle relaxant effects.

bereavement The loss or deprivation experienced by a survivor when a loved one dies.

bidis Hand-rolled flavored cigarettes.

binge-eating disorder A type of eating disorder characterized by binge eating once a week or more, but not typically followed by a compensatory behavior.

biofeedback A technique using a machine to self-monitor physical responses to stress.

biopsy Microscopic examination of tissue to determine if a cancer is present.

biopsychosocial model of addiction Theory of the relationship between an addict's biological (genetic) nature and psychological and environmental influences.

bipolar disorder A form of mood disorder characterized by alternating mania and depression; also called *manic depression*.

bisexual Experiencing attraction to and preference for sexual activity with people of both sexes.

blood alcohol concentration (BAC) The ratio of alcohol to total blood volume; the factor used to measure the physiological and behavioral effects of alcohol.

body composition Describes the relative proportions of fat and lean (muscle, bone, water, organs) tissues in the body.

body dysmorphic disorder (BDD) Psychological disorder characterized by an obsession with a minor or imagined flaw in appearance.

body image How you see yourself when you look in a mirror or picture yourself in your mind and how you feel about your body.

body mass index (BMI) A number calculated from a person's weight and height that is used to assess risk for possible present or future health problems.

bulimia nervosa Eating disorder characterized by binge eating followed by inappropriate measures, such as vomiting, to prevent weight gain.

calorie A unit of measure that indicates the amount of energy obtained from a particular food.

cancer A large group of diseases characterized by the uncontrolled growth and spread of abnormal cells.

candidiasis Yeastlike fungal infection often transmitted sexually; also called *moniliasis* or *yeast infection*.

capillaries Minute blood vessels that branch out from the arterioles and venules; their thin walls permit exchange of oxygen, carbon dioxide, nutrients, and waste products among body cells.

carbohydrates Basic nutrients that supply the body with glucose, the energy form most commonly used to sustain normal activity.

carbon dioxide (CO_2) Gas created by the combustion of fossil fuels, exhaled by animals, and used by plants for photosynthesis; the primary greenhouse gas in Earth's atmosphere.

carbon footprint The amount of greenhouse gases produced by an individual, nation, or other entity, usually expressed in equivalent tons of carbon dioxide emissions.

carbon monoxide A gas found in cigarette smoke that binds at oxygen receptor sites in the blood.

carcinogens Cancer-causing agents.

cardiometabolic risks Physical and biochemical changes that are risk factors for the development of cardiovascular disease and type 2 diabetes.

cardiorespiratory fitness The ability of the heart, lungs, and blood vessels to supply oxygen to skeletal muscles during sustained physical activity.

cardiovascular disease (CVD) Diseases of the heart and blood vessels.

cardiovascular system Organ system, consisting of the heart and blood vessels, that transports nutrients, oxygen, hormones, metabolic wastes, and enzymes throughout the body.

carotenoids Fat-soluble plant pigments with antioxidant properties.

carpal tunnel syndrome A common occupational injury in which the median nerve in the wrist becomes irritated, causing numbness, tingling, and pain in the fingers and hands.

celiac disease An inherited autoimmune disorder affecting the digestive process of the small intestine and triggered by the consumption of gluten.

celibacy State of abstaining from sexual activity.

cell-mediated immunity Aspect of immunity that is mediated by specialized white blood cells that attack pathogens and antigens directly.

cerebrospinal fluid Fluid within and surrounding the brain and spinal cord tissues.

cervical cap A small cup made of latex or silicone that is designed to fit snugly over the entire cervix.

cervix Lower end of the uterus that opens into the vagina.

cesarean section (C-section) A surgical birthing procedure in which a baby is removed through an incision made in the mother's abdominal and uterine walls.

chancre Sore often found at the site of syphilis infection.

chemotherapy The use of drugs to kill cancerous cells.

chewing tobacco A stringy type of tobacco that is placed in the mouth and then sucked or chewed.

chickenpox A highly infectious disease caused by the *herpes varicella zoster virus*.

child abuse The systematic harming of a child by a caregiver, typically a parent.

chiropractic medicine Manipulation of the spine to allow proper energy flow.

chlamydia Bacterially caused STI of the urogenital tract.

chlorofluorocarbons (CFCs) Chemicals that contribute to the depletion of the atmospheric ozone layer.

cholesterol A form of fat circulating in the blood that can accumulate on the inner walls of arteries, causing a narrowing of the channel through which blood flows.

chorionic villus sampling (CVS) A prenatal test that involves snipping tissue from the fetal sac to be analyzed for genetic defects.

chromosome Discrete bundle of DNA, 46 of which are present in the nucleus of almost all cells of the human body.

chromosome disorder A disorder arising from a missing or extra chromosome, or damage to part of a chromosome.

chronic disease A disease that typically begins slowly, progresses, and persists, with a variety of signs and symptoms that can be treated but not cured by medication.

chronic mood disorder Experience of persistent emotional states, such as sadness, despair, and hopelessness.

chronic stress An ongoing state of physiological arousal in response to ongoing or numerous perceived threats.

cirrhosis The last stage of liver disease associated with chronic heavy alcohol use during which liver cells die and damage becomes permanent.

clitoris A pea-sized nodule of tissue located at the top of the labia minora; central to sexual arousal in women.

club drugs Synthetic analogs (drugs that produce similar effects) of existing illicit drugs.

codependence A self-defeating relationship pattern in which a person is "addicted to the addict."

cognitive restructuring The modification of thoughts, ideas, and beliefs that contribute to stress.

cohabitation Living together without being married.

collateral circulation Adaptation of the heart to partial damage accomplished by rerouting needed blood through unused or underused blood vessels while the damaged heart muscle heals.

collective violence Violence perpetrated by groups against other groups.

common-law marriage Cohabitation lasting a designated period of time (usually 7 years) that is considered legally binding in some states.

comorbidities The presence of one or more diseases at the same time.

complementary medicine Treatment used in conjunction with conventional medicine.

complete (high-quality) proteins Proteins that contain all nine of the essential amino acids.

complex carbohydrates A major type of carbohydrate that provides sustained energy.

compulsion Preoccupation with a behavior and an overwhelming need to perform it.

compulsive exercise Disorder characterized by a compulsion to engage in excessive amounts of exercise and feelings of guilt and anxiety if the level of exercise is perceived as inadequate.

compulsive shoppers People who are preoccupied with shopping and spending.

computerized axial tomography (CAT) scan A scan by a machine that uses radiation to view internal organs not normally visible in X rays.

conception The fertilization of an ovum by a sperm.

conflict An emotional state that arises when the behavior of one person interferes with the behavior of another.

conflict resolution A concerted effort by all parties to constructively resolve points of contention.

congeners Forms of alcohol that are metabolized more slowly than ethanol and produce toxic byproducts.

congenital cardiovascular defect Cardiovascular problem that is present at birth.

congestive heart failure (CHF) An abnormal cardiovascular condition that reflects impaired cardiac pumping and blood flow; pooling blood leads to congestion in body tissues.

contemplation A practice of concentrating the mind on a spiritual or ethical question or subject, a view of the natural world, or an icon or other image representative of divinity.

contraception (birth control) Methods of preventing conception.

coping Managing events or conditions to lessen the physical or psychological effects of excess stress.

core strength Strength in the body's core muscles, including deep back and abdominal muscles that attach to the spine and pelvis.

coronary artery disease (CAD) A narrowing or blockage of coronary arteries, usually caused by atherosclerotic plaque buildup.

coronary bypass surgery A surgical technique whereby a blood vessel taken from another part of the body is implanted to bypass a clogged coronary artery.

coronary heart disease (CHD) A narrowing of the small blood vessels that supply blood to the heart.

coronary thrombosis A blood clot occurring in a coronary artery.

corpus luteum A body of cells that forms from the remains of the graafian follicle following ovulation; it secretes estrogen and progesterone during the second half of the menstrual cycle.

cortisol Hormone released by the adrenal glands that makes stored nutrients more readily available to meet energy demands.

countering Substituting a desired behavior for an undesirable one.

Cowper's glands Glands that secrete a fluid that lubricates the urethra and neutralizes any acid remaining in the urethra after urination.

cross-tolerance Development of a physiological tolerance to one drug that reduces the effects of another, similar drug.

cunnilingus Oral stimulation of a woman's genitals.

Daily Values (DVs) Percentages listed as "% DV" on food and supplement labels; made up of the RDIs and DRVs together.

defensive medicine The use of medical practices designed to avert the possibility of malpractice suits in the future.

dehydration Abnormal depletion of body fluids; a result of lack of water.

delirium tremens (DTs) A state of confusion brought on by withdrawal from alcohol; symptoms include hallucinations, anxiety, and trembling.

dementias Progressive brain impairments that interfere with memory and normal intellectual functioning.

denial Inability to perceive or accurately interpret the self-destructive effects of the addictive behavior.

dentist Specialist who diagnoses and treats diseases of the teeth, gums, and oral cavity.

Depo-Provera An injectable method of birth control that lasts for 3 months.

depressants Drugs that slow down the activity of the central nervous system.

determinants of health The array of critical influences that determine the health of individuals and communities.

detoxification The early abstinence period during which an addict adjusts physically and cognitively to being free from the influences of the addiction.

diabetes mellitus A group of diseases characterized by elevated blood glucose levels.

diagnosis-related groups (DRGs) Diagnostic categories established by the federal government to determine in advance how much hospitals will be reimbursed for the care of a particular Medicare patient.

diaphragm A latex, cup-shaped device designed to cover the cervix and block access to the uterus; should always be used with spermicide.

diastolic pressure The lower number in the fraction that measures blood pressure, indicating pressure on arterial walls during the relaxation phase of heart activity.

dietary supplements Vitamins and minerals taken by mouth that are intended to supplement existing diets.

digestive process The process by which the body breaks down foods and either absorbs or excretes them.

dilation and evacuation (D&E) An abortion technique that uses a combination of instruments and vacuum aspiration; fetal tissue is both sucked and scraped out of the uterus.

dioxins Highly toxic chlorinated hydrocarbons found in herbicides and produced during certain industrial processes.

dipping Placing a small amount of chewing tobacco between the front lip and teeth for rapid nicotine absorption.

disaccharides Combinations of two monosaccharides.

discrimination Actions that deny equal treatment or opportunities to a group, often based on prejudice.

disease prevention Actions or behaviors designed to keep people from getting sick.

disordered eating A pattern of atypical eating behaviors that is used to achieve or maintain a lower body weight.

disordered gambling Compulsive gambling that cannot be controlled.

distillation The process whereby mash is subjected to high temperatures to release alcohol vapors, which are then condensed and mixed with water to make the final product.

distress Stress that can have a detrimental effect on health; negative stress.

DNA (deoxyribonucleic acid) Acid molecule that resides in the nucleus of a cell and stores in its sequence of chemical subunits the instructions for assembling body proteins.

domestic violence The use of force to control and maintain power over another person in the home environment, including both actual harm and the threat of harm.

dominant Term describing an allele that is expressed even if there is only one copy in the pair.

drug abuse Excessive use of a drug.

drug misuse Use of a drug for a purpose for which it was not intended.

dysfunctional families Families in which there is violence; physical, emotional, or sexual abuse; parental discord; or other negative family interactions.

dysmenorrhea Condition of pain or discomfort in the lower abdomen just before or after menstruation.

dyspareunia Pain experienced by women during intercourse.

dysthymic disorder (dysthymia) A type of depression that is milder and harder to recognize than major depression; chronic; and often characterized by fatigue, pessimism, or a short temper.

eating disorder A psychiatric disorder characterized by severe disturbances in body image and eating behaviors.

eating disorders not otherwise specified (EDNOS) Eating disorders that are a true psychiatric illness but do not fit the strict diagnostic criteria for anorexia nervosa, bulimia nervosa, or binge-eating disorder.

ecological or public health model A view of health in which diseases and other negative health events are seen as the result of an individual's interaction with his or her social and physical environment.

ecosystem The collection of physical (nonliving) and biological (living) components of an environment and the relationships between them.

ectopic pregnancy Implantation of a fertilized egg outside the uterus, usually in a fallopian tube; a medical emergency that can end in death from hemorrhage or peritonitis.

ejaculation The propulsion of semen from the penis.

ejaculatory duct Tube formed by the junction of the seminal vesicle and the vas deferens that carries semen to the urethra.

electrocardiogram (ECG) A record of the electrical activity of the heart; may be measured during a stress test.

embolus A blood clot that becomes dislodged from a blood vessel wall and moves through the circulatory system.

embryo The fertilized egg from conception until the end of 2 months' development.

emergency contraceptive pills (ECPs) Drugs taken within 3 to 5 days after unprotected intercourse to prevent fertilization or implantation.

emotional health The feeling part of psychosocial health; includes your emotional reactions to life.

emotions Intensified feelings or complex patterns of feelings we constantly experience.

emphysema A chronic lung disease in which the tiny air sacs in the lungs are destroyed, making breathing difficult.

enablers People who knowingly or unknowingly protect addicts from the natural consequences of their behavior.

endemic Describing a disease that is always present to some degree.

endometriosis A disorder in which uterine lining tissue establishes itself outside the uterus; the leading cause of infertility in women in the United States.

endometrium Soft, spongy matter that makes up the uterine lining.

endorphins Opioid-like hormones that are manufactured in the human body and contribute to natural feelings of well-being.

energy medicine Therapies using energy fields, such as magnetic fields or biofields.

enhanced greenhouse effect The warming of Earth's surface as a direct result of human activities that release greenhouse gases into the atmosphere, trapping more of the sun's radiation than is normal.

environmental stewardship A responsibility for environmental quality shared by all those whose actions affect the environment.

environmental tobacco smoke (ETS) Smoke from tobacco products, including sidestream and mainstream smoke; commonly called *secondhand smoke*.

epidemic Disease outbreak that affects many people in a community or region at the same time.

epididymis The duct system atop the testis where sperm mature.

epinephrine Also called *adrenaline*, a hormone that stimulates body systems in response to stress.

erectile dysfunction (ED) Difficulty in achieving or maintaining a penile erection sufficient for intercourse.

ergogenic drug Substance believed to enhance athletic performance.

erogenous zones Areas of the body that, when touched, lead to sexual arousal.

essential amino acids Nine of the basic nitrogen-containing building blocks of protein, which must be obtained from foods to ensure health.

estrogens Hormones secreted by the ovaries that control the menstrual cycle.

ethnoviolence Violence directed at persons affiliated with a particular, usually ethnic, group.

ethyl alcohol (ethanol) An addictive drug produced by fermentation and found in many beverages.

eustress Stress that presents opportunities for personal growth; positive stress.

evidence-based practice Decisions regarding patient care based on clinical expertise, patient values, and current best scientific evidence.

exercise Planned, structured, and repetitive bodily movement done to improve or maintain one or more components of physical fitness.

exercise addicts People who exercise compulsively to try to meet needs of nurturance, intimacy, self-esteem, and self-competency.

exercise metabolic rate (EMR) The energy expenditure that occurs during exercise.

extensively drug-resistant TB (XDR-TB) Form of TB that is resistant to nearly all existing antibiotics.

fallopian tubes (oviducts) Tubes that extend from near the ovaries to the uterus; site of fertilization and passageway for fertilized eggs.

family of origin People present in the household during a child's first years of life—usually parents and siblings.

fats Basic nutrients composed of carbon and hydrogen atoms; needed for the proper functioning of cells, insulation of body organs against shock, maintenance of body temperature, and healthy skin and hair.

fellatio Oral stimulation of a man's genitals.

female athlete triad A syndrome of three interrelated health problems seen in some female athletes: disordered eating, amenorrhea, and poor bone density.

female condom A single-use polyurethane sheath for internal use during vaginal or anal intercourse to catch semen on ejaculation.

female orgasmic disorder A woman's inability to achieve orgasm.

fermentation The process whereby yeast organisms break down plant sugars to yield ethanol.

fertility A person's ability to reproduce.

fertility awareness methods (FAMs) Several types of birth control that require alteration of sexual behavior rather than chemical or physical intervention in the reproductive process.

fetal alcohol syndrome (FAS) A disorder involving physical and mental impairment that may affect the fetus when the mother consumes alcohol during pregnancy.

fetus The word for a developing baby from the third month of pregnancy until birth.

fiber The indigestible portion of plant foods that helps move food through the digestive system and softens stools by absorbing water.

fibrillation A sporadic, quivering pattern of heartbeat that results in extreme inefficiency in moving blood through the cardiovascular system.

fight-or-flight response Physiological arousal response in which the body prepares to combat or escape a real or perceived threat.

FITT Acronym for Frequency, Intensity, Time, and Type; the terms that describe the essential components of a program or plan to improve a component of physical fitness.

flexibility The range of motion, or the amount of movement possible, at a particular joint or series of joints.

food allergy Overreaction by the body to normally harmless proteins, which are perceived as allergens. In response, the body produces antibodies, triggering allergic symptoms.

food intolerance Adverse effects resulting when people who lack the digestive chemicals needed to break down certain substances eat those substances.

food irradiation Treating foods with gamma radiation from radioactive cobalt, cesium, or other sources of X rays to kill microorganisms.

formaldehyde A colorless, strong-smelling gas released through offgassing; causes respiratory and other health problems.

fossil fuels Carbon-based material used for energy; includes oil, coal, and natural gas.

frequency As part of the FITT prescription, refers to how many days per week a person should exercise to improve a component of physical fitness.

functional foods Foods believed to have specific health benefits and/or to prevent disease.

fungi A group of multicellular and unicellular organisms that obtain their food by infiltrating the bodies of other organisms, both living and dead; several microscopic varieties are pathogenic.

gay Sexual orientation involving primary attraction to people of the same sex.

gender The psychological condition of being feminine or masculine as defined by the society in which one lives.

gender identity Personal sense or awareness of being masculine or feminine, a male or a female.

gender roles Expressions of maleness or femaleness in everyday life.

gender-role stereotypes Generalizations concerning how men and women should express themselves and the characteristics each possesses.

gene Discrete segment of DNA in a chromosome that stores the code for assembling a particular body protein.

general adaptation syndrome (GAS) The pattern followed in the physiological response to stress, consisting of the alarm, resistance, and exhaustion phases.

generalized anxiety disorder (GAD) A constant sense of worry that may cause restlessness, difficulty in concentrating, tension, and other symptoms.

generic drugs Medications marketed by chemical names rather than brand names.

genetically modified (GM) foods Foods derived from organisms whose DNA has been altered using genetic engineering techniques.

genital herpes STI caused by the herpes simplex virus.

genital warts Warts that appear in the genital area or the anus; caused by the human papillomavirus (HPV).

genome All of the genetic information an organism possesses.

gestational diabetes Form of diabetes mellitus in which women who have never had diabetes before have high blood sugar (glucose) levels during pregnancy.

glycogen The polysaccharide form in which glucose is stored in the liver and, to a lesser extent, in muscles.

gonads The reproductive organs in a male (testes) or female (ovaries) that produce sperm (male), eggs (female), and sex hormones.

gonorrhea Second most common bacterial STI in the United States; if untreated, may cause sterility.

graafian follicle Mature ovarian follicle that contains a fully developed ovum, or egg.

greenhouse gases Gases that accumulate in the atmosphere, where they contribute to global warming by trapping heat near Earth's surface.

grief An individual's reaction to significant loss, including one's own impending death, the death of a loved one, or a quasi-death experience; grief can involve mental, physical, social, or emotional responses.

habit A repeated behavior in which the repetition may be unconscious.

hallucinogens Substances capable of creating auditory or visual distortions and heightened states.

hangover The physiological reaction to excessive drinking, including headache, upset stomach, anxiety, depression, diarrhea, and thirst.

hate crime A crime targeted against a particular societal group and motivated by bias against that group.

hazardous waste Waste that, due to its toxic properties, poses a hazard to humans or to the environment.

health The ever-changing process of achieving individual potential in the physical, social, emotional, mental, spiritual, and environmental dimensions.

health belief model (HBM) Model for explaining how beliefs may influence behaviors.

health disparities Differences in the incidence, prevalence, mortality, and burden of diseases and other health conditions among specific population groups.

health promotion The combined educational, organizational, procedural, environmental, social, and financial supports that help individuals and groups reduce negative health behaviors and promote positive change.

healthy life expectancy Expected number of years of full health remaining at a given age, such as at birth.

heat cramps Involuntary and forcible muscle contractions that occur during or following exercise in hot and/or humid weather.

heat exhaustion A heat stress illness caused by significant dehydration resulting from exercise in hot and/or humid conditions.

heatstroke A deadly heat stress illness resulting from dehydration and overexertion in hot and/or humid conditions.

heavy episodic (binge) drinking A *binge* is a pattern of drinking alcohol that brings blood alcohol concentration (BAC) to 0.08 gram-percent or above; for a typical adult, this pattern corresponds to consuming five or more drinks (male) or four or more drinks (female) in about 2 hours.

hepatitis A viral disease in which the liver becomes inflamed, producing symptoms such as fever, headache, and possibly jaundice.

herpes A general term for infections characterized by sores or eruptions on the skin caused by the herpes simplex virus.

herpes gladiatorum A skin infection caused by the herpes simplex type 1 virus and seen among athletes participating in contact sports.

heterosexual Experiencing primary attraction to and preference for sexual activity with people of the opposite sex.

high-density lipoproteins (HDLs) Compounds that facilitate the transport of cholesterol in the blood to the liver for metabolism and elimination from the body.

holistic Relating to or concerned with the whole body and the interactions of systems, rather than treatment of individual parts.

homeopathic medicine Unconventional Western system of medicine based on the principle that "like cures like."

homeostasis A balanced physiological state in which all the body's systems function smoothly.

homicide Death that results from intent to injure or kill.

homosexual Experiencing primary attraction to and preference for sexual activity with people of the same sex.

hormonal contraception Contraceptive methods that introduce synthetic hormones into the woman's system to prevent ovulation, thicken cervical mucus, or prevent a fertilized egg from implanting.

hormone replacement therapy or **menopausal hormone therapy** Use of synthetic or animal estrogens and progesterone to compensate for decreases in estrogens in a woman's body during menopause.

hostility Cognitive, affective, and behavioral tendencies toward anger and cynicism.

human chorionic gonadotropin (HCG) Hormone detectable in blood or urine samples of a mother within the first few weeks of pregnancy.

human immunodeficiency virus (HIV) The virus that causes AIDS by infecting helper T cells.

human papillomavirus (HPV) A group of viruses, many of which are transmitted sexually; some types of HPV can cause genital warts or cervical cancer.

humoral immunity Aspect of immunity that is mediated by antibodies secreted by white blood cells.

hunger The physiological impulse to seek food, prompted by the lack or shortage of basic foods needed to provide the energy and nutrients that support health.

hymen Thin tissue covering the vaginal opening in some women.

hyperglycemia Elevated blood glucose level.

hyperplasia A condition characterized by an excessive number of fat cells.

hypertension Sustained elevated blood pressure.

hypertrophy The act of swelling or increasing in size, as with cells.

hypnosis A trancelike state that allows people to become unusually responsive to suggestion.

hyponatremia or **water intoxication** The overconsumption of water, which leads to a dilution of sodium concentration in the blood with potentially fatal results.

hypothalamus An area of the brain located near the pituitary gland; works in conjunction with the pituitary gland to control reproductive functions. It also controls the sympathetic nervous system and directs the stress response.

hypothermia Potentially fatal condition caused by abnormally low body core temperature.

hysterectomy Surgical removal of the uterus.

hysterotomy The surgical removal of the fetus from the uterus.

imagined rehearsal Practicing, through mental imagery, to become better able to perform an event in actuality.

immunocompetence The ability of the immune system to respond to attack.

immunocompromised Having an immune system that is impaired.

Implanon A small plastic progestin-releasing implant under the skin of a woman's upper underarm that lasts for up to 3 years.

in vitro fertilization Fertilization of an egg in a nutrient medium and subsequent transfer back to the mother's body.

incomplete proteins Proteins that lack one or more of the essential amino acids.

incubation period The time between exposure to a disease and the appearance of symptoms.

induction abortion An abortion technique in which chemicals are injected into the uterus through the uterine wall; labor begins, and the woman delivers a dead fetus.

infection The state of pathogens being established in or on a host and causing disease.

infertility Inability to conceive after a year or more of trying.

influenza A common viral disease of the respiratory tract.

inhalants Products that are sniffed or inhaled in order to produce highs.

inhalation The introduction of drugs through breathing into the lungs.

inheritance Process by which physical and biological characteristics—called traits—are transmitted from parents to their offspring.

inhibited sexual desire Lack of sexual appetite or lack of interest and pleasure in sexual activity.

inhibition A drug interaction in which the effects of one drug are eliminated or reduced by the presence of another drug at the same receptor site.

injection The introduction of drugs into the body via a hypodermic needle.

insulin Hormone secreted by the pancreas and required by body cells for the uptake and storage of glucose.

insulin resistance State in which body cells fail to respond to the effects of insulin; obesity increases the risk that cells will become insulin resistant.

intact dilation and extraction (D&X) A late-term abortion procedure in which the body of the fetus is extracted up to the head and then the contents of the cranium are aspirated.

intensity As part of the FITT prescription, refers to how hard or how much effort is needed when a person exercises to improve a component of physical fitness.

intentional injuries Injury, death, psychological harm, maldevelopment, or deprivation that involves intentional use of physical force or power, threatened or actual, against oneself, another person, or a group or community.

Internet addiction Compulsive use of the computer, PDA, cell phone, or other forms of technology to access the Internet for activities such as e-mail, games, shopping, or blogging.

interpersonal violence Violence inflicted against one individual by another, or by a small group of others.

intersex General term for a variety of conditions in which a person is born with reproductive or sexual anatomy that doesn't seem to fit the typical definitions of female or male. Also termed disorders of sexual development (DSDs).

intervention A planned process of confronting an addict; carried out by close family, friends, and a professional counselor.

intimate partner violence (IPV) Violent behavior, including physical violence, sexual violence, threats, and emotional abuse, occurring between current or former spouses or dating partners.

intimate relationships Relationships with family members, friends, and romantic partners, characterized by behavioral interdependence, need fulfillment, emotional attachment, and emotional availability.

intolerance A drug interaction in which the combination of two or more drugs in the body produces extremely uncomfortable symptoms.

intrauterine device (IUD) A device, often T-shaped, that is implanted in the uterus to prevent pregnancy.

ionizing radiation Electromagnetic waves and particles having short wavelengths and energy high enough to ionize atoms.

ischemia Reduced oxygen supply to a body part or organ.

jealousy An aversive reaction evoked by a real or imagined relationship involving a person's partner and a third person.

labia majora "Outer lips," or folds of tissue covering the female sexual organs.

labia minora "Inner lips," or folds of tissue just inside the labia majora.

leach To dissolve and filter through soil.

lead A highly toxic metal found in emissions from lead smelters and processing plants; also sometimes found in pipes or paint in older houses.

learned helplessness Pattern of responding to situations by giving up because of repeated failure in the past.

learned optimism Teaching oneself to think positively.

lesbian Sexual orientation involving attraction of women to other women.

leukoplakia A condition characterized by leathery white patches inside the mouth; produced by contact with irritants in tobacco juice.

libido Sexual drive or desire.

life expectancy Expected number of years of life remaining at a given age, such as at birth.

locavore A person who primarily eats food grown or produced locally.

locus of control The location, *external* (outside oneself) or *internal* (within oneself), that an individual perceives as the source and underlying cause of events in his or her life.

loss of control Inability to reliably predict whether a particular instance of involvement with the addictive substance or behavior will be healthy or damaging.

low-density lipoproteins (LDLs) Compounds that facilitate the transport of cholesterol in the blood to the body's cells and cause the cholesterol to build up on artery walls.

low sperm count A sperm count below 20 million sperm per milliliter of semen; the leading cause of infertility in men.

lymphocyte A type of white blood cell involved in the immune response.

macrominerals Minerals that the body needs in fairly large amounts.

macrophage A type of white blood cell that ingests foreign material.

magnetic resonance imaging (MRI) A device that uses magnetic fields, radio waves, and computers to generate an image of internal tissues of the body for diagnostic purposes without the use of radiation.

mainstream smoke Smoke that is drawn through tobacco while inhaling.

major depression Severe depressive disorder that entails chronic mood disorder, physical effects such as sleep disturbance and exhaustion, and mental effects such as the inability to concentrate; also called *clinical depression*.

male condom A single-use sheath of thin latex or other material designed to fit over an erect penis and to catch semen upon ejaculation.

malignant Very dangerous or harmful; refers to a cancerous tumor.

malignant melanoma A virulent cancer of the melanocytes (pigment-producing cells) of the skin.

managed care Cost-control procedures used by health insurers to coordinate treatment.

manipulative and body-based practices Treatments involving manipulation or movement of one or more body parts.

marijuana Chopped leaves and flowers of *Cannabis indica* or *Cannabis sativa* (hemp); a psychoactive stimulant.

marital rape Any unwanted intercourse or penetration obtained by force, threat of force, or when the spouse is unable to consent.

masturbation Self-stimulation of genitals.

medical abortion The termination of a pregnancy during its first 9 weeks using hormonal medications that cause the embryo to be expelled from the uterus.

medical model A view of health in which health status focuses primarily on the individual and a biological or diseased organ perspective.

meditation A relaxation technique that involves deep breathing and concentration.

menarche The first menstrual period.

meningitis An infection of the meninges, the membranes that surround the brain and spinal cord.

menopause The permanent cessation of menstruation, generally between the ages of 40 and 60.

mental health The thinking part of psychosocial health; includes your values, attitudes, and beliefs.

mental illnesses Disorders that disrupt thinking, feeling, moods, and behaviors, and that impair daily functioning.

metabolic syndrome (MetS) A group of metabolic conditions occurring together that increase a person's risk of heart disease, stroke, and diabetes.

metastasis Process by which cancer spreads from one area to different areas of the body.

methicillin-resistant *Staphylococcus aureus* (MRSA) Highly resistant form of staph infection that is growing in international prevalence.

migraine A condition characterized by localized headaches that possibly result from alternating dilation and constriction of blood vessels.

mind–body medicine Techniques designed to enhance the mind's ability to affect bodily functions and symptoms.

mindfulness A practice of purposeful, nonjudgmental observation in which we are fully present in the moment.

minerals Inorganic, indestructible elements that aid physiological processes.

miscarriage Loss of the fetus before it is viable; also called *spontaneous abortion*.

modeling Learning specific behaviors by watching others perform them.

monogamy Exclusive sexual involvement with one partner.

mononucleosis A viral disease that causes pervasive fatigue and other long-lasting symptoms.

monosaccharides Simple sugars that contain only one molecule of sugar.

mons pubis Fatty tissue covering the pubic bone in females; in physically mature women, the mons is covered with coarse hair.

morbidly obese Having a body weight 100 percent or more above healthy recommended levels; in an adult, having a BMI of 40 or more.

mortality The proportion of deaths to the total population, within a given period of time.

motivation A social, cognitive, and emotional force that directs human behavior.

multidrug-resistant TB (MDR-TB) Form of TB that is resistant to at least two of the best antibiotics available.

multifactorial disease Disease caused by interactions of several factors.

multifactorial disorder A disorder attributable to more than one of a variety of factors.

municipal solid waste (MSW) Solid wastes such as durable goods; nondurable goods; containers and packaging; food waste; yard waste; and miscellaneous wastes from residential, commercial, institutional, and industrial sources.

muscle dysmorphia Body image disorder in which men believe that their body is insufficiently lean or muscular.

muscular endurance A muscle's ability to exert force repeatedly without fatiguing or the ability to sustain a muscular contraction for a length of time.

muscular strength The amount of force that a muscle is capable of exerting in one contraction.

mutant cells Cells that differ in form, quality, or function from normal cells.

myocardial infarction (MI) or **heart attack** A blockage of normal blood supply to an area in the heart.

natural products Treatments using substances found in nature, such as herbs, special diets, or vitamin megadoses.

naturopathic medicine System of medicine originating from Europe that views disease as a manifestation of alterations in the body's natural self-healing processes, and that emphasizes health restoration as well as disease treatment.

negative consequences Severe problems associated with addiction, such as physical damage, legal trouble, financial problems, academic failure, or family dissolution.

neglect Failure to provide for a child's basic needs such as food, shelter, medical care, and clothing.

neoplasm A new growth of tissue that serves no physiological function and results from uncontrolled, abnormal cellular development.

neurotransmitters Biochemical messengers that bind to specific receptor sites on nerve cells.

nicotine The primary stimulant chemical in tobacco products; nicotine is highly addictive.

nicotine poisoning Symptoms often experienced by beginning smokers, including dizziness, diarrhea, lightheadedness, rapid and erratic pulse, clammy skin, nausea, and vomiting.

nicotine withdrawal Symptoms, including nausea, headaches, irritability, and intense tobacco cravings, suffered by addicted smokers who stop using tobacco.

nonionizing radiation Electromagnetic waves having relatively long wavelengths and enough energy to move atoms around or cause them to vibrate.

nonpoint source pollutants Pollutants that run off or seep into waterways from broad areas of land.

nonverbal communication All unwritten and unspoken messages, both intentional and unintentional.

nuclear meltdown An accident that results when the temperature in the core of a nuclear reactor increases enough to melt the nuclear fuel and the containment vessel housing it.

nurse Health professional who provides many services for patients and who may work in a variety of settings.

nurse practitioner (NP) Professional nurse with advanced training obtained through either a master's degree program or a specialized nurse practitioner program.

nutraceuticals Term often used interchangeably with *functional foods*; refers to the combined nutritional and pharmaceutical benefit derived through use of foods or food supplements.

nutrients The constituents of food that sustain humans physiologically: proteins, carbohydrates, fats, vitamins, minerals, and water.

nutrition The science that investigates the relationship between physiological function and the essential elements of foods eaten.

NuvaRing A soft, flexible ring inserted into the vagina that releases hormones, preventing pregnancy.

obesity A body weight more than 20 percent above healthy recommended levels; in an adult, a BMI of 30 or more.

obesogenic Characterized by environments that promote increased food intake, nonhealthful foods, and physical inactivity; refers to conditions that lead people to become excessively fat.

obsession Excessive preoccupation with an addictive object or behavior.

obsessive-compulsive disorder (OCD) A form of anxiety disorder characterized by recurrent, unwanted thoughts and repetitive behaviors.

oncogenes Suspected cancer-causing genes present on chromosomes.

one repetition maximum (1 RM) The amount of weight or resistance that can be lifted or moved only once.

open relationship A relationship in which partners agree that sexual involvement can occur outside the relationship.

ophthalmologist Physician who specializes in the medical and surgical care of the eyes, including prescriptions for glasses.

opioids Drugs that induce sleep and relieve pain; includes derivatives of opium and synthetics with similar chemical properties; also called *narcotics*.

opium The parent drug of the opioids; made from the seedpod resin of the opium poppy.

opportunistic infections Infections that occur when the immune system is weakened or compromised.

optometrist Eye specialist whose practice is limited to prescribing and fitting lenses.

oral contraceptives Pills containing synthetic hormones that prevent ovulation by regulating hormones.

oral ingestion Intake of drugs through the mouth.

organic Grown without use of pesticides, chemicals, or hormones.

Ortho Evra A patch that releases hormones similar to those in oral contraceptives; each patch is worn for 1 week.

osteopath General practitioner who receives training similar to a medical doctor's but with an emphasis on the skeletal and muscular systems; often uses spinal manipulation as part of treatment.

ovarian follicles Areas within the ovary in which individual eggs develop.

ovaries Almond-sized organs that house developing eggs and produce hormones.

overload A condition in which a person feels overly pressured by demands.

overuse injuries Injuries that result from the cumulative effects of day-after-day stresses placed on tendons, muscles, and joints.

overweight Having a body weight more than 10 percent above healthy recommended levels; in an adult, having a BMI of 25 to 29.

ovulation The point of the menstrual cycle at which a mature egg ruptures through the ovarian wall.

ovum A single mature egg cell.

pancreas Organ that secretes digestive enzymes into the small intestine, and hormones, including insulin, into the bloodstream.

pandemic Global epidemic of a disease.

panic attack Severe anxiety reaction in which a particular situation, often for unknown reasons, causes terror.

Pap test A procedure in which cells taken from the cervical region are examined for abnormal cellular activity.

parasitic worms The largest of the pathogens, most of which are more a nuisance than they are a threat.

parasympathetic nervous system Branch of the autonomic nervous system responsible for slowing systems stimulated by the stress response.

pathogen A disease-causing agent.

pelvic inflammatory disease (PID) An infection that scars the fallopian tubes and consequently blocks sperm migration, causing infertility.

penis Male sexual organ that releases sperm into the vagina.

peptic ulcer Damage to the stomach or intestinal lining, usually caused by digestive juices; most ulcers result from infection by the bacterium *Helicobacter pylori*.

perfect-use failure rate The number of pregnancies (per 100 users) that are likely to occur in the first year of use of a particular birth control method if the method is used consistently and correctly.

perineum Tissue that forms the "floor" of the pelvic region in both men and women.

peripheral artery disease (PAD) Atherosclerosis occurring in the lower extremities, such as in the feet, calves, or legs, or in the arms.

personal flotation device A device worn to provide buoyancy and keep the wearer, conscious or unconscious, afloat with the nose and mouth out of the water; also known as a life jacket.

personality disorders A class of mental disorders that are characterized by inflexible patterns of thought and beliefs that lead to socially distressing behavior.

pesticides Chemicals that kill pests such as insects, weeds, and rodents.

phobia A deep and persistent fear of a specific object, activity, or situation that results in a compelling desire to avoid the source of the fear.

photochemical smog The brownish yellow haze resulting from the combination of hydrocarbons and nitrogen oxides.

physical activity Refers to all body movements produced by skeletal muscles resulting in substantial increases in energy expenditure.

physical fitness Refers to a set of attributes that allow you to perform moderate- to vigorous-intensity physical activities on a regular basis without getting too tired and with energy left over to handle physical or mental emergencies.

physician assistant (PA) A midlevel practitioner trained to handle most standard cases of care under the supervision of a physician.

physiological dependence The adaptive state that occurs with regular addictive behavior and results in withdrawal syndrome.

pituitary gland The endocrine gland that controls the release of hormones from the gonads.

placenta The network of blood vessels connected to the umbilical cord that carries nutrients, oxygen, and wastes between the developing infant and the mother.

plant sterols Essential components of plant membranes that, when consumed in the diet, appear to help lower cholesterol levels.

plaque Buildup of deposits in the arteries.

platelet adhesiveness Stickiness of red blood cells associated with blood clots.

pneumonia Inflammatory disease of the lungs characterized by chronic cough, chest pain, chills, high fever, and fluid accumulation; may be caused by bacteria, viruses, fungi, chemicals, or other substances.

point source pollutants Pollutants that enter waterways at a specific location.

poison Any substance harmful to the body when ingested, inhaled, injected, or absorbed through the skin.

pollutant A substance that contaminates some aspect of the environment and causes potential harm to living organisms.

polychlorinated biphenyls (PCBs) Toxic chemicals that were once used as insulating materials in high-voltage electrical equipment.

polydrug use Taking several medications, vitamins, recreational drugs, or illegal drugs simultaneously.

polysaccharides Complex carbohydrates formed by the combination of long chains of monosaccharides.

positive reinforcement Presenting something positive following a behavior that is being reinforced.

positron emission tomography (PET) scan Method for measuring heart activity by injecting a patient with a radioactive tracer that is scanned electronically to produce a three-dimensional image of the heart and arteries.

postpartum depression Energy depletion, anxiety, mood swings, and depression that women may feel during the postpartum period.

post-traumatic stress disorder (PTSD) A collection of symptoms that may occur as a delayed response to a serious trauma.

power The ability to make and implement decisions.

prayer Communication with a transcendent Presence.

preconception care Medical care received prior to becoming pregnant that helps a woman assess and address potential maternal health issues.

pre-diabetes Condition in which blood glucose levels are higher than normal, but not high enough to be classified as diabetes.

preeclampsia A complication in pregnancy characterized by high blood pressure, protein in the urine, and edema.

pre-gaming A strategy of drinking heavily at home before going out to an event or other location.

prejudice A negative evaluation of an entire group of people that is typically based on unfavorable and often wrong ideas about the group.

premature ejaculation Ejaculation that occurs prior to or almost immediately following penile penetration of the vagina.

premenstrual dysphoric disorder (PMDD) Collective name for a group of negative symptoms similar to but more severe than PMS, including severe mood disturbances.

premenstrual syndrome (PMS) Comprises the mood changes and physical symptoms that occur in some women during the 1 or 2 weeks prior to menstruation.

primary aggression Goal-directed, hostile self-assertion that is destructive in character.

primary care practitioner (PCP) A medical practitioner who treats routine ailments, advises on preventive care, gives general medical advice, and makes appropriate referrals when necessary.

prion A recently identified self-replicating, protein-based pathogen.

process addictions Behaviors such as disordered gambling, compulsive buying, compulsive Internet or technology use, work addiction, compulsive exercise, and sexual addiction that are known to be addictive because they are mood altering.

procrastinate To intentionally put off doing something.

progesterone Hormone secreted by the ovaries; helps the endometrium develop and helps maintain pregnancy.

proof A measure of the percentage of alcohol in a beverage.

prostate gland Gland that secretes nutrients and neutralizing fluids into the semen.

prostate-specific antigen (PSA) An antigen found in prostate cancer patients.

proteins The essential constituents of nearly all body cells; necessary for the development and repair of bone, muscle, skin, and blood; the key elements of antibodies, enzymes, and hormones.

protozoans Microscopic single-celled organisms that can be pathogenic.

psychoactive drugs Drugs that have the potential to alter mood or behavior.

psychological hardiness A personality trait characterized by control, commitment, and the embrace of challenge.

psychological health The mental, emotional, social, and spiritual dimensions of health.

psychoneuroimmunology (PNI) The science that examines the relationship between the brain and behavior and how this affects the body's immune system.

puberty The period of sexual maturation.

pubic lice Parasitic insects that can inhabit various body areas, especially the genitals.

qi Element of traditional Chinese medicine that refers to the vital energy force that courses through the body; when *qi* is in balance, health is restored.

radiation absorbed doses (rads) Units that measure exposure to radiation.

radiotherapy The use of radiation to kill cancerous cells.

radon A naturally occurring radioactive gas resulting from the decay of certain radioactive elements.

rape Sexual penetration without the victim's consent.

reactive aggression Hostile emotional reaction brought about by frustrating life experiences.

receptor sites Specialized areas of cells and organs where chemicals, enzymes, and other substances interact.

recessive Term describing an allele that is expressed only in the absence of a dominant allele; that is, if both alleles are recessive or if the recessive gene is on the X chromosome of the twenty-third pair.

relapse The tendency to return to the addictive behavior after a period of abstinence.

religion A system of beliefs, practices, rituals, and symbols designed to facilitate closeness to the sacred or transcendent.

repetitive motion disorder (RMD) An injury to soft tissue, tendons, muscles, nerves, or joints due to the physical stress of repeated motions.

resting metabolic rate (RMR) The energy expenditure of the body under BMR conditions plus other daily sedentary activities.

rheumatic heart disease A heart disease caused by untreated streptococcal infection of the throat.

RICE Acronym for the standard first aid treatment for virtually all traumatic and overuse injuries: **r**est, **i**ce, **c**ompression, and **e**levation.

rickettsia A small form of bacteria that live inside other living cells.

risk behaviors Actions that increase susceptibility to negative health outcomes.

satiety The feeling of fullness or satisfaction at the end of a meal.

saturated fats Fats that are unable to hold any more hydrogen in their chemical structure; derived mostly from animal sources; solid at room temperature.

schizophrenia A mental illness with biological origins that is characterized by irrational behavior, severe alterations of the senses, and often an inability to function in society.

scrotum External sac of tissue that encloses the testes.

seasonal affective disorder (SAD) A type of depression that occurs in the winter months, when sunlight levels are low.

secondary sex characteristics Characteristics associated with sex but not directly related to reproduction, such as vocal pitch, degree of body hair, and location of fat deposits.

self-disclosure Sharing personal feelings or information with others.

self-efficacy Belief in one's ability to perform a task successfully.

self-injury Intentionally causing injury to one's own body in an attempt to cope with overwhelming negative emotions; also called *self-mutilation, self-harm,* or *nonsuicidal self-injury* (NSSI).

self-nurturance Developing individual potential through a balanced and realistic appreciation of self-worth and ability.

self-talk The customary manner of thinking and talking to yourself, which can affect your self-image.

semen Fluid containing sperm and nutrients that increase sperm viability and neutralize vaginal acid.

seminal vesicles Glandular ducts that secrete nutrients for the semen.

serial monogamy A series of monogamous sexual relationships.

set point theory Theory that a form of internal thermostat controls our weight and fights to maintain this weight around a narrowly set range.

sexual abuse of children Sexual interaction between a child and an adult or older child.

sexual addiction Compulsive involvement in sexual activity.

sexual assault Any act in which one person is sexually intimate with another without that person's consent.

sexual aversion disorder Desire dysfunction characterized by sexual phobias and anxiety about sexual contact.

sexual dysfunction Problems associated with achieving sexual satisfaction.

sexual fantasies Sexually arousing thoughts and dreams.

sexual harassment Any form of unwanted sexual attention related to any condition of employment or performance evaluation.

sexual identity Recognition of oneself as a sexual being; a composite of biological sex characteristics, gender identity, gender roles, and sexual orientation.

sexual orientation A person's enduring emotional, romantic, sexual, or affectionate attraction to other persons.

sexual performance anxiety A condition of sexual difficulties caused by anticipating some sort of problem with the sex act.

sexual prejudice Negative attitudes and hostile actions directed at sexually identified social groups; also referred to as sexual bias.

sexuality All the thoughts, feelings, and behaviors associated with being male or female, experiencing attraction, being in love, and being in relationships that include sexual intimacy and activity.

sexually transmitted infections (STIs) Infectious diseases caused by pathogens transmitted through some form of intimate, usually sexual, contact.

shaping Using a series of small steps to gradually achieve a particular goal.

shingles A disease characterized by a painful rash that occurs when the chickenpox virus is reactivated.

sick building syndrome (SBS) Problem that exists when 80 percent of a building's occupants report maladies that tend to lessen or vanish when they leave the building.

sidestream smoke The cigarette, pipe, or cigar smoke breathed by nonsmokers.

simple carbohydrates A major type of carbohydrate that provides short-term energy; also called *simple sugars.*

simple rape Rape by one person, usually known to the victim, that does not involve physical beating or use of a weapon.

single-gene disorder A disorder characterized by structural and/or functional impairments resulting from a defect involving only one gene.

sinoatrial node (SA node) Cluster of electric pulse-generating cells that serves as a natural pacemaker for the heart.

situational inducement Attempt to influence a behavior through situations and occasions that are structured to exert control over that behavior.

sleep debt The difference between the number of hours of sleep an individual needed in a given time period and the number of hours he or she actually slept.

snuff A powdered form of tobacco that is sniffed or absorbed through the mucous membranes in the nose or placed inside the cheek and sucked.

social bonds Degree and nature of interpersonal contacts.

social cognitive model Model of behavior change emphasizing the role of social factors and thought processes (cognition) in behavior change.

social health Aspect of psychosocial health that includes interactions with others, ability to use social supports, and ability to adapt to various situations.

social learning theory Theory that people learn behaviors by watching role models—parents, caregivers, and significant others.

social phobia A phobia characterized by fear and avoidance of social situations; also called *social anxiety disorder.*

social physique anxiety (SPA) A desire to look good that has a destructive effect on a person's ability to function well in social interactions and relationships.

social support Network of people and services with whom you share ties and from whom you get support.

socialization Process by which a society communicates behavioral expectations to its individual members.

spermatogenesis The development of sperm.

spermicides Substances designed to kill sperm.

spiritual health The aspect of psychosocial health that relates to having a sense of meaning and purpose to one's life, as well as a feeling of connection with others and with nature.

spiritual intelligence (SI) The intelligence of the deep self; a capacity to live in alignment with our inner wisdom, values, and vision.

spirituality An individual's sense of purpose and meaning in life, beyond material values.

stalking The willful, repeated, and malicious following, harassing, or threatening of another person.

standard drink The amount of any beverage that contains about 14 grams of pure alcohol (about 0.6 fluid ounce or 1.2 tablespoons).

staphylococci A group of round bacteria, usually found in clusters, that cause a variety of diseases in humans and other animals.

starch Polysaccharide that is the storage form of glucose in plants.

static stretching Stretching techniques that slowly and gradually lengthen a muscle or group of muscles and their tendons.

stent A stainless steel, meshlike tube that is inserted to prop open the artery.

sterilization Permanent fertility control achieved through surgical procedures.

stillbirth The birth of a dead baby.

stimulants Drugs that increase activity of the central nervous system.

Streptococcus A round bacterium, usually found in chain formation.

stress A series of physiological responses and adaptations in response to a real or imagined threat to one's well-being.

stress inoculation Stress-management technique in which a person consciously tries to prepare ahead of time for potential stressors.

stressor A physical, social, or psychological event or condition that upsets homeostasis and produces a stress response.

stroke A condition occurring when the brain is damaged by disrupted blood supply; also called *cerebrovascular accident.*

subjective well-being An uplifting feeling of inner peace.

suction curettage An abortion technique that uses gentle suction to remove fetal tissue from the uterus.

sudden cardiac death Death that occurs as a result of abrupt, profound loss of heart function.

sudden infant death syndrome (SIDS) The sudden death of an infant under 1 year of age for no apparent reason.

suicidal ideation A desire to die and thoughts about suicide.

Superfund Fund established under the Comprehensive Environmental Response, Compensation, and Liability Act to be used for cleaning up toxic waste dumps.

suppositories Mixtures of drugs and a waxy medium (designed to melt at body temperature) that are inserted into the anus or vagina.

sympathetic nervous system Branch of the autonomic nervous system responsible for stress arousal.

sympathomimetics Food substances that can produce stresslike physiological responses.

synergism The interaction of two or more drugs that produces more profound effects than would be expected if the drugs were taken separately; also called *potentiation*.

syphilis One of the most widespread bacterial STIs; characterized by distinct phases and potentially serious results.

systolic pressure The upper number in the fraction that measures blood pressure, indicating pressure on arterial walls when the heart contracts.

tar A thick, brownish substance condensed from particulate matter in smoked tobacco.

target heart rate The heart rate range of aerobic exercise that leads to improved cardiorespiratory fitness (i.e., 70% to 90% of maximal heart rate).

temperature inversion A weather condition occurring when a layer of cool air is trapped under a layer of warmer air.

teratogenic Causing birth defects; may refer to drugs, environmental chemicals, X rays, or diseases.

terrorism The unlawful use of force or violence against persons or property to intimidate or coerce a government, the civilian population, or any segment thereof in furtherance of political or social objectives.

testes Male sex organs that manufacture sperm and produce hormones.

testosterone The male sex hormone manufactured in the testes.

tetrahydrocannabinol (THC) The chemical name for the active ingredient in marijuana.

thrombolysis Injection of an agent to dissolve clots and restore some blood flow, thereby reducing the amount of tissue that dies from ischemia.

thrombus Blood clot attached to a blood vessel's wall.

time As part of the FITT prescription, refers to how long a person needs to exercise each time to improve a component of physical fitness.

tinctures Herbal extracts usually combined with grain alcohol to prevent spoilage.

Today sponge A contraceptive device, made of polyurethane foam and containing nonoxynol-9, that fits over the cervix to create a barrier against sperm.

tolerance Phenomenon in which progressively larger doses of a drug or more intense involvement in a behavior is needed to produce the desired effects.

total fertility rate The hypothetical average number of children born to women during their lifetime, given prevailing fertility and mortality rates.

toxic shock syndrome (TSS) A potentially life-threatening disease that occurs when specific bacterial toxins multiply and spread to the bloodstream, most commonly through improper use of tampons or diaphragms.

toxins Poisonous substances produced by certain microorganisms that cause various diseases.

toxoplasmosis A disease caused by an organism found in cat feces that, when contracted by a pregnant woman, may result in stillbirth or an infant with mental retardation or birth defects.

trace minerals Minerals that the body needs in only very small amounts.

traditional Chinese medicine (TCM) Ancient comprehensive system of healing that uses herbs, acupuncture, and massage to bring the body into balance and to remove blockages of vital energy flow that lead to disease.

***trans* fats (*trans* fatty acids)** Fatty acids that are produced when polyunsaturated oils are hydrogenated to make them more solid.

transdermal The introduction of drugs through the skin.

transgendered Having a gender identity that does not match one's biological sex.

transient ischemic attack (TIA) Brief interruption of the blood supply to the brain that causes only temporary impairment; often an indicator of impending major stroke.

transsexual A person who is psychologically of one sex but physically of the other.

transtheoretical model Model of behavior change that identifies six distinct stages people go through in altering behavior patterns; also called the *stages of change model*.

traumatic injuries Injuries that are accidental and occur suddenly and violently.

trichomoniasis Protozoan STI characterized by foamy, yellowish discharge and unpleasant odor.

triglycerides The most common form of fat in the body; excess calories consumed are converted into triglycerides and stored as body fat.

trimester A 3-month segment of pregnancy; used to describe specific developmental changes that occur in the embryo or fetus.

triple marker screen (TMS) A maternal blood test that can be used to help identify fetuses with certain birth defects and genetic abnormalities.

tubal ligation Sterilization of the woman that involves the cutting and tying off or cauterizing of the fallopian tubes.

tuberculosis (TB) A disease caused by bacterial infiltration of the respiratory system.

tumor A neoplasmic mass that grows more rapidly than surrounding tissue.

type As part of the FITT prescription, refers to what kind of exercises a person needs to do to improve a component of physical fitness.

type 1 diabetes Form of diabetes mellitus in which the pancreas is not able to make insulin and therefore blood glucose cannot enter the cells to be used for energy.

type 2 diabetes Form of diabetes mellitus in which the pancreas does not make enough insulin or the body is unable to use insulin correctly.

typical-use failure rate The number of pregnancies (per 100 users) that are likely to occur in the first year of use of a particular birth control method if the method's use is not consistent or always correct.

ultrasonography (ultrasound) A common prenatal test that uses high-frequency sound waves to create a visual image of the fetus.

underweight Having a body weight more than 10 percent below healthy recommended levels; in an adult, having a BMI below 18.5.

unintentional injuries Injury, death, or harm that involves accidents committed without intent to harm, often as a result of circumstances, or without premeditation.

unsaturated fats Fats that have room for more hydrogen in their chemical structure; derived mostly from plants; liquid at room temperature.

urethral opening The opening through which urine is expelled.

uterus (womb) Hollow, pear-shaped muscular organ whose function is to contain the developing fetus.

vaccination Inoculation with killed or weakened pathogens or similar, less dangerous antigens in order to prevent or lessen the effects of a disease.

vagina The passage in females leading from the vulva into the uterus.

vaginal intercourse The insertion of the penis into the vagina.

vaginismus A state in which the vaginal muscles contract so forcefully that penetration cannot occur.

values Principles that influence our thoughts and emotions, and guide the choices we make in our lives.

variant sexual behavior A sexual behavior that is not practiced by most people.

vas deferens Tube that transports sperm from the epididymis to the ejaculatory duct.

vasectomy Sterilization of the man that involves the cutting and tying off of both vasa deferentia.

vasocongestion The engorgement of the genital organs with blood.

vegetarian A person who follows a diet that excludes some or all animal products.

veins Vessels that transport waste and carry blood back to the heart from other regions of the body.

ventricles The heart's two lower chambers, which pump blood through the blood vessels.

venules Branches of the veins.

very-low-calorie diets (VLCDs) Diets with a daily caloric value of 400 to 700 calories.

violence A set of behaviors that produces injuries, as well as the outcomes of these behaviors (the injuries themselves).

virulent Strong enough to overcome host resistance and cause disease.

viruses Minute microbes consisting of DNA or RNA that invade a host cell and use the cell's resources to reproduce themselves.

visualization The creation of mental images to promote relaxation.

vitamins Essential organic compounds that promote growth and reproduction and help maintain life and health.

vulva Collective term for the external female genitalia.

waist-to-hip ratio Waist circumference divided by hip circumference; a high ratio indicates increased health risks due to unhealthy fat distribution.

wellness The achievement of the highest level of health possible in each of several dimensions.

whole grains Grains that are milled in their complete form, and so include the bran, germ, and endosperm, with only the husk removed.

withdrawal 1 A method of contraception that involves withdrawing the penis from the vagina before ejaculation; also called coitus interruptus.

withdrawal 2 A series of temporary physical and biopsychosocial symptoms that occurs when an addict abruptly abstains from an addictive chemical or behavior.

work addiction The compulsive use of work and the work persona to fulfill needs for intimacy, power, and success.

yoga A system of physical and mental training involving controlled breathing, physical postures (*asanas*), meditation, chanting, and other practices that are believed to cultivate unity with the *Atman*, or Absolute.

yo-yo diets Cycles in which people diet and regain weight.

References

Chapter 1

1. World Health Organization (WHO), "Constitution of the World Health Organization," *Chronicles of the World Health Organization* (Geneva: WHO, 1947), Available at www.who.int/governance/eb/constitution/en/index.html.
2. R. Dubos, *So Human an Animal: How We Are Shaped by Surroundings and Events* (New York: Scribner, 1968), 15.
3. E. A. Finkelstein et al., "Annual Medical Spending Attributable to Obesity: Payer- and Service-Specific Estimates," *Health Affairs* 28, no. 5 (2009): w822–31.
4. U.S. Census Bureau, *The 2010 Statistical Abstract of the United States: Births, Deaths, Marriages, and Divorces*, "Table 102 Expectations of Life at Birth, 1970 to 2006, and Projections 2010 and 2020," 2010, Available at www.census.gov/compendia/statab/cats/births_deaths_marriages_divorces.html.
5. Centers for Disease Control and Prevention, "Achievements in Public Health, 1900–1999: Control of Infectious Diseases," *MMWR* 48, no. 29 (1999): 621–29, Available at www.cdc.gov/mmwr/preview/mmwrhtml/mm4829a1.htm.
6. G. Danaei et al., "The Promise of Prevention: The Effects of Four Preventable Risk Factors on National Life Expectancy and Life Expectancy Disparities by Race and County in the United States," *PLoS Medicine* 7, no. 3 (2010): e1000248, Available at www.plosmedicine.org/article/info%3Adoi%2F10.1371%2Fjournal.pmed.1000248.
7. K. D. Kochanek, et al., "Deaths: Preliminary Data for 2009," *National Vital Statistics Reports* 59, no. 4 (2011), Available at www.cdc.gov/nchs/data/nvsr/nvsr59/nvsr59_04.pdf.
8. U.S. Department of Health and Human Services, "*Healthy People 2020*: The Road Ahead," Revised 2011, Available at www.healthypeople.gov/HP2020.
9. Ibid.
10. U.S. Department of Health and Human Services, "*Healthy People 2020*: Foundation Health Measures," Available at http://healthypeople.gov/2020/about/tracking.aspx.
11. U.S. Department of Health and Human Services, "*Healthy People 2020*: Topics and Objectives," Available at http://healthypeople.gov/2020/topicsobjectives2020/default.aspx.
12. Ibid.
13. U.S. Department of Health and Human Services, *Healthy People 2010* (Washington, DC: U.S. Government Printing Office, 2000).
14. K. Kochanek et al., "Deaths, Preliminary Data for 2009," (2011).
15. G. Danaei et al., "The Preventable Causes of Death in the United States: Comparative Risk Assessment of Dietary, Lifestyle, and Metabolic Risk Factors," *PLoS Medicine* 6, no. 4 (2009): e1000058, Available at www.plosmedicine.org/article/info:doi/10.1371/journal.pmed.1000058; Centers for Disease Control and Prevention, Chronic Disease and Health Promotion, *Chronic Disease Overview*, December 17, 2009, Available at www.cdc.gov/chronicdisease/overview/index.htm#2.
16. U.S. Department of Health and Human Services, *Healthy People 2020*, 2010.
17. R. Wilkinson and M. Marmot, eds., *Social Determinants of Health: The Solid Facts*, 2nd ed. (Geneva: World Health Organization, 2003), Available at www.euro.who.int/en/what-we-publish/abstracts/social-determinants-of-health.-the-solid-facts.
18. Prevention Institute, *The Built Environment and Health: 11 Profiles of Neighborhood Transformation*, July 2004, Available at www.preventioninstitute.org/index.php?option=com_jlibrary&view=article&id=114&Itemid=127.
19. W. C. Willett and A. Underwood, "Crimes of the Heart," *Newsweek*, February 5, 2010, Available at www.newsweek.com/id/233006.
20. Centers for Disease Control and Prevention. (2011). "CDC Health Disparities and Inequalities Report." *Morbidity and Mortality Weekly Report. Supplement.* 60: 1–116. January 14, 2011. Available at www.cdc.gov/mmwr/preview/ind2011_su.html; H. Mead, et al., Racial and Ethnic Disparities in U.S. Health Care: A Chartbook, The Commonwealth Fund, March 2008.
21. U.S. Department of Health and Human Services, *Healthy People 2020*, 2010.
22. I. Rosenstock, "Historical Origins of the Health Belief Model," *Health Education Monographs* 2, no. 4 (1974): 328–35.
23. J. O. Prochaska and C. C. DiClemente, "Stages and Processes of Self-Change of Smoking: Toward an Integrative Model of Change," *Journal of Consulting and Clinical Psychology* 51 (1983): 390–95.
24. M. Hesse, "The Readiness Ruler as a Measure of Readiness to Change Polydrug Use in Drug Abusers," *Journal of Harm Reduction* 3, no. 3 (2006): 1477–81; M. Cismaru, "Using Protection Motivation Theory to Increase the Persuasiveness of Public Service Communications," The Saskatchewan Institute of Public Policy, Public Policy Series paper no. 40 (February 2006); E. A. Fallon, S. Wilcox, and M. Laken, "Health Care Provider Advice for African American Adults Not Meeting Health Behavior Recommendations," *Preventing Chronic Disease* 3, no. 2 (2006): A45; M. R. Chacko et al., "New Sexual Partners and Readiness to Seek Screening for Chlamydia and Gonorrhea: Predictors among Minority Young Women," *Sexually Transmitted Infections* 82 (2006): 75–79.
25. J. M. Twenge, Z. Liqing, and C. Im, "It's Beyond My Control: A Cross-Temporal Meta-Analysis of Increasing Externality in Locus of Control, 1960–2002," *Personality and Social Psychology Review* 8 (2004): 308–20.
26. A. Ellis and M. Benard, *Clinical Application of Rational Emotive Therapy* (New York: Plenum, 1985).

Chapter 2

1. A. H. *Maslow, Motivation and Personality*, 2nd ed. (New York: Harper and Row, 1970).
2. U.S. Department of Health and Human Services, *Mental Health: A Report of the Surgeon General—Executive Summary* (Rockville, MD: U.S. Department of Health and Human Services, Substance Abuse and Mental Health Services Administration, National Institute of Mental Health, 1999), Available at www.surgeongeneral.gov/library/mentalhealth/summary.html.
3. T. M. Chaplin, "Anger, Happiness, and Sadness: Association with Depressive Symptoms in Late Adolescence," *Journal of Youth and Adolescence* 35, no. 6 (2006): 977–86.
4. S. Braithwaite, et al., "Romantic Relationships and Physical and Mental Health of College Students," *Personal Relationships* 17, no. 1 (2010): 1–12; J. Holt-Lunstad, et al., (2010) "Social Relationships and Mortality Risks: A Meta-Analytic Review" *PLoS Med* 7(7): e1000316. doi: 10.1371/journal.pmed.1000316; S. Haslam et al., "When Other People Are Heaven/When Other People Are Hell," in J. Jetten et al., (eds.) *The Social Cure: Identity, Health, and Well-Being* (New York: Psychology Press, 2010).
5. K. Karren et al., *Mind/Body Health*, 4th ed. (San Francisco: Benjamin Cummings, 2010).
6. National Center for Complementary and Alternative Medicine (NCCAM), "Prayer and Spirituality in Health: Ancient Practices, Modern Science," *CAM at the NIH: Focus on Complementary and Alternative Medicine* 12, no. 1 (2005), Updated October 2007, Available at http://nccam.nih.gov/news/newsletter/archive.htm.
7. W. Schneider and L. Davidson, "Physical Health and Adult Well-Being," in *Well-Being: Positive Development across the Life Course*, eds. M. H. Bornstein, L. Davidson, and C. Keyes (Mahwah, NJ: Lawrence Erlbaum Associates, 2003), 407–23.
8. J. Hefner and D. Eisenberg, "Social Support and Mental Health among College Students," *American Journal of Orthopsychiatry* 79, no. 4 (2009): 491–499.
9. K. S. Berger, *The Developing Person through the Life Span*, 8th ed. (New York: Worth, 2011), 9–10.
10. M. Seligman and C. Peterson, "Learned Helplessness," in *International Encyclopedia for the Social and Behavioral Sciences*, vol. 13, ed. N. Smelser (New York: Elsevier, 2002), 8583–866.
11. M. Seligman, *Learned Optimism: How to Change Your Mind and Your Life* (New York: Free Press, 1998); J. H. Martin, "Motivation Processes and Performance: The Role of Global and Facet Personality," PhD dissertation, University of North Carolina at Chapel Hill, 2002.
12. K. Davidson, et al., "Don't Worry, Be Happy: Positive Affect and Reduced 10-year Incident Coronary Heart Disease: The Canadian Nova Scotia Health Survey," *European Heart Journal* 31, no. 9 (2010): 1065–1070; B. Krijthe, et al. "Is Positive Affect Associated with Survival? A Population-based Study of Elderly Persons," *American Journal of Epidemiology* 173, no. 11 (2011): 1298–1307.
13. R. Mora-Ripoli, "The Therapeutic Value of Laughter in Medicine," *Alternative Therapy Medicine* 16, no. 6 (2010): 56–64; M. Miller and W. F. Fry, "The effect of mirthful laughter on the human cardiovascular system," *Medical Hypotheses* 73, no. 5 (2009): 636–39; S. Horowitz, "The Effect of Positive Emotions on Health: Hope and Humor," *Alternative and Complementary Therapies* 15, no. 4 (2009): 196–202.
14. Ibid.

15. R. Davidson et al., "The Privileged Status of Emotion in the Brain," *Proceedings of the National Academy of Sciences of the United States of America* 101, no. 33 (2004).

16. E. Diener and M. E. P. Seligman, "Beyond Money: Toward an Economy of Well-Being," *Psychological Science in the Public Interest* 5 (2004): 1–31; C. Peterson and M. Seligman, *Character Strengths and Virtues* (London: Oxford University Press, 2004).

17. Higher Education Research Institute, "Press Release: Students Experience Spiritual Growth During College: UCLA Study Reveals Significant Changes in Undergraduates' Values and Beliefs," December 18, 2007, Available at http://spirituality.ucla.edu/publications/news.

18. NCCAM, "Prayer and Spirituality in Health," 2005.

19. H. G. Koenig, M. McCullough, and D. B. Larson, *Handbook of Religion and Health: A Century of Research Reviewed* (New York: Oxford University Press, 2001).

20. Ibid.

21. Pew Forum on Religion & Public Life, *U.S. Religious Landscape Survey Religious Beliefs and Practices: Diverse and Politically Relevant* (Washington, DC: Pew Research Center, 2008), Available at http://religions.pewforum.org/reports.

22. B. L. Seaward, *Health of the Human Spirit: Spiritual Dimensions for Personal Health* (Boston: Allyn & Bacon, 2001), 85–90; B. L. Seaward, *Managing Stress: Principles and Strategies for Health and Well Being*, 6th ed. (Sudbury, MA: Jones and Bartlett, 2009).

23. D. Zohar, *ReWiring the Corporate Brain: Using the New Science to Rethink How We Structure and Lead Organizations* (San Francisco: Berrett Koehler, 1997); D. B. King and T. L. DeCicco, "A Viable Model and Self-Report Measure of Spiritual Intelligence," *The International Journal of Transpersonal Studies* 28 (2009): 68–85.

24. A. Moreira-Almeida and H. G. Koenig, "Retaining the Meaning of the Words Religiousness and Spirituality," *Social Science and Medicine* 63, no. 4 (2006): 843–45.

25. NCCAM, "Prayer and Spirituality in Health," 2005.

26. A. J. Weaver and H. G. Koenig, "Religion, Spirituality, and Their Relevance to Medicine: An Update," *American Family Physician* 73, no. 8 (2006): 1336–37; R. F. Gillum, D. E. King, T. O. Obisesan, and H. G. Koenig, "Frequency of Attendance at Religious Services and Mortality in a U.S. National Cohort," *Annals of Epidemiology* 18, no. 2 (2008): 124–29.

27. M. E. McCullough and B. L. B. Willoughby, "Religion, Self-Regulation, and Self-Control: Associations, Explanations, and Implications," *Psychological Bulletin* 135, no. 1 (2009): 69–93.

28. National Cancer Institute (NCI), "Spirituality in Cancer Care," Modified March 6, 2009, www.cancer.gov/cancertopics/pdq/supportivecare/spirituality/patient.

29. F. A. Curlin, S. A. Sellergren, J. D. Lantos, and M. H. Chin, "Physicians' Observations and Interpretations of the Influence of Religion and Spirituality on Health," *Archives of Internal Medicine* 167, no. 7 (2007): 649–54.

30. M. Baetz and R. Bowen, "Chronic Pain and Fatigue: Associations with Religion and Spirituality," *Pain Research & Management* 13, no. 5 (2008): 383–88.

31. G. Ironson, R. Stuetzle, and M. A. Fletcher, "An Increase in Religiousness/Spirituality Occurs after HIV Diagnosis and Predicts Slower Disease Progression over 4 Years in People with HIV," *Journal of General Internal Medicine* 21, no. 5 (2006): S62–S68.

32. A. Moreira-Almeida and H. G. Koenig, "Religiousness and Spirituality in Fibromyalgia and Chronic Pain Patients," *Current Pain and Headache Reports* 12, no. 5 (2008): 327–32; B. R. Doolittle and M. Farrell, "The Association between Spirituality and Depression in an Urban Clinic," *Primary Care Companion to the Journal of Clinical Psychiatry* 6, no. 3 (2004): 114–18; NCI, "Spirituality in Cancer Care," 2009; I. Olver and H. Whitford, "Prayer Improves Spiritual Wellbeing in a Randomized Controlled Trial in Patients with Cancer," *Asia-Pacific Journal of Clinical Oncology* 5 (2009): A172.

33. M. Javnbakht, R. Hejazi Kenari, and M. Ghasemi, "Effects of Yoga on Depression and Anxiety of Women," *Complementary Therapies in Clinical Practice* 15, no. 2 (2009): 102–04; A. Woolery, H. Myers, B. Sternlieb, and L. Zeltzer, "A Yoga Intervention for Young Adults with Elevated Symptoms of Depression," *Alternative Therapies in Health and Medicine* 10, no. 2 (2004): 60–63.

34. K. Master and G. Spielman, "Prayer and Health: Review, Meta-analysis, and Research Agenda," *Journal of Behavioral Medicine* 30 (2007): 329–338.

35. D. Ledesma and H. Dumano, "Mindfulness-based Stress Reduction and Cancer: A Meta-analysis," *Psychooncology* 18 (2009): 571–579; U. Winter, D. Hauri, S. Huber, J. Jenewein, U. Schnyder, and B. Kraemer, "The Psychological Outcome of Religious Coping with Stressful Life Events in a Swiss Sample of Church Attendees," *Psychotherapy and Psychosomatics* 78, no. 4 (2009): 240–44.

36. A. Chiesa and A. Serretti, "Mindfulness-Based Stress Reduction for Stress Management in Healthy People: A Review and Meta-Analysis," *Journal of Alternative and Complementary Medicine* 15, no. 5 (2009): 593–600.

37. G. R. Sharplin et al., "Mindfulness-based Cognitive Therapy: An Efficacious Community-based Group Intervention for Depression and Anxiety in a Sample of Cancer Patients," *The Medical Journal of Australia* 193 (2010): S79.

38. J. Kabat-Zinn, *Coming to Our Senses: Healing Ourselves and the World through Mindfulness* (New York: Hyperion, 2005).

39. National Center for Complementary and Alternative Medicine (NCCAM), "Research Spotlight: Meditation May Increase Empathy," Modified October 2009, http://nccam.nih.gov/research/results/spotlight/060608.htm.

40. D. Oman, S. Shapiro, C. Thoreson, T. Plante, and T. Flinders, "Meditation Lowers Stress and Supports Forgiveness among College Students: A Randomized Controlled Trial," *Journal of American College Health* 56, no. 5 (2008): 425–31.

41. National Center for Complementary and Alternative Medicine (NCCAM), "Research Spotlight: Meditation May Make Information Processing in the Brain More Efficient," Modified October 2009, http://nccam.nih.gov/research/results/spotlight/082307.htm; A. Chiesa and A. Serretti, "Mindfulness-Based Stress Reduction for Stress Management in Healthy People," 2009; N. Y. Winbush, C. R. Gross, and M. J. Kreitzer, "The Effects of Mindfulness-Based Stress Reduction on Sleep Disturbance: A Systematic Review. *EXPLORE: The Journal of Science and Healing* 3, no. 6 (2007): 585–91; N. E. Morone, C. S. Lynch, C. M. Greco, H. A. Tindle, and D. K. Weiner, "'I Felt Like a New Person.' The Effects of Mindfulness Meditation on Older Adults with Chronic Pain: Qualitative Narrative Analysis of Diary Entries," *Journal of Pain*, no. 9 (2008): 841–48.

42. Environmental Protection Agency (EPA), "Environmental Stewardship," Updated January 6, 2010, www.epa.gov/stewardship.

43. Mayo Clinic Staff, MayoClinic.com, "Mental Illness: Causes," 2008, www.mayoclinic.com/health/mental-illness/DS01104/DSECTION=causes.

44. Ibid.

45. R. C. Kessler, et al, "Prevalence, Severity, and Comorbidity of 12-month DSM-IV Disorders in the National Comorbidity Survey Replication," *Archives of General Psychiatry* 62, no. 6 (2005): 617–27.

46. Ibid.

47. J. Hunt and D. Eisenberg, "Mental Health Problems and Help-Seeking Behavior among College Students," *Journal of Adolescent Health* 46, no. 1 (2010): 3–10.

48. American College Health Association, *American College Health Association–National College Health Assessment II (ACHA–NCHA II): Reference Group Data Report Fall 2010* (Baltimore: American College Health Association, 2011), Available at www.acha-ncha.org/reports_ACHA-NCHAII.html.

49. C. Blanco et al., "Mental Health of College Students and Their Non-College Attending Peers: Results from the National Epidemiologic Study on Alcohol and Related Conditions," *Archives of General Psychiatry* 65, 12 (2008): 1429–37.

50. J. Hunt and D. Eisenberg, "Mental Health Problems and Help-Seeking Behavior among College Students," 2010.

51. R. C. Kessler, et al, "Prevalence, Severity, and Comorbidity of 12-month DSM-IV Disorders," 2005.

52. American College Health Association, *ACHA–NCHA II: Reference Group Data Report Fall 2010*, 2011.

53. National Institute of Mental Health, "Generalized Anxiety Disorder, GAD," Reviewed July 7, 2009, www.nimh.nih.gov/health/publications/anxiety-disorders/generalized-anxiety-disorder-gad.shtml.

54. R. C. Kessler, et al, "Prevalence, Severity, and Comorbidity of 12-month DSM-IV Disorders," 2005.

55. Mayo Clinic Staff, MayoClinic.com, "Panic Attacks and Panic Disorder: Symptoms," 2010, www.mayoclinic.com/health/panic-attacks/DS00338/DSECTION=symptoms.

56. R. C. Kessler, et al, "Prevalence, Severity, and Comorbidity of 12-month DSM-IV Disorders," 2005.

57. Ibid.

58. Ibid.

59. C. W. Hoge et al., "Combat Duty in Iraq and Afghanistan, Mental Health Problems, and Barriers to Care," *New England Journal of Medicine* 351 (2004): 13–22.

60. National Institute of Mental Health, "Generalized Anxiety Disorder, GAD," 2009.

61. R. C. Kessler, et al, "Prevalence, Severity, and Comorbidity of 12-month DSM-IV Disorders," 2005.

62. Ibid.

63. National Institute of Mental Health, "Depression," 2009, www.nimh.nih.gov/publicat/depression.cfm.

64. American College Health Association, *ACHA–NCHA II: Reference Group Data Report Fall 2010*, 2011.

65. R. C. Kessler, et al, "Prevalence, Severity, and Comorbidity of 12-month DSM-IV Disorders," 2005.

66. Ibid.
67. American Psychiatric Association, Healthy Minds. Healthy Lives, "Seasonal Affective Disorder," 2010, www.healthyminds.org/Main-Topic/Seasonal-Affective-Disorder.aspx.
68. Mayo Clinic Staff, MayoClinic.com, "Depression: Causes," 2010, www.mayoclinic.com/health/depression/DS00175/DSECTION=causes.
69. National Institute of Mental Health (NIMH), *Women and Depression: Discovering Hope,* NIH Publication no. 09-4779, revised 2009, Available at www.nimh.nih.gov/health/publications/women-and-depression-discovering-hope/index.shtml.
70. NIMH, "Real Men. Real Depression." NIH Publication no. 03-5300, March 2003, Available at www.nimh.nih.gov/health/publications/real-men-real-depression-easy-to-read/index.shtml.
71. American Psychiatric Association (APA), Healthy Minds. Healthy Lives, "Children," 2010, www.healthyminds.org/More-Info-For/Children.aspx.
72. APA, Healthy Minds. Healthy Lives, "Seniors," 2010, www.healthyminds.org/More-Info-For/Seniors.aspx.
73. H. Kannan, S. Bolge, and S. Wagner, "Depression: Ethnic Differences in Prevalence, Diagnosis, and Symptoms" (Princeton, NJ: Consumer Health Sciences, 2009), Poster presented at the International Society of Pharmacoeconomics and Outcomes Research (ISPOR) 14th Annual International Meeting, May 2009, Available at www.chsinternational.com/Resources/2009_05_20_ISPOR_Poster_no3_Depression-Ethnicity.pdf.
74. W. T. O'Donohue, K. A. Fowler, and S. O. Lilienfeld, *Personality Disorders: Toward the DSM-V* (Thousand Oaks, CA: Sage Publications, 2007).
75. National Institute of Mental Health, "National Survey Tracks Prevalence of Personality Disorders in U.S. Population," October 18, 2007, www.nimh.nih.gov/science-news/2007/national-survey-tracks-prevalence-of-personality-disorders-in-us-population.shtml.
76. Mayo Clinic Staff, MayoClinic.com, "Borderline Personality Disorder," 2010, www.mayoclinic.com/health/borderline-personality-disorder/DS00442.
77. J. Cole, "Facts," BPDWORLD, 2010, www.bpdworld.org/demo-category/106-facts.
78. J. Bennett, "Why She Cuts," *Newsweek* Web Exclusive, December 29, 2008, www.newsweek.com/id/177135; M. J. Prinstein, "Introduction to the Special Section on Suicide and Nonsuicidal Self-Injury: A Review of Unique Challenges and Important Directions for Self-Injury Science," *Journal of Consulting and Clinical Psychology* 76, no. 1 (2008): 1–8; Mayo Clinic Staff, MayoClinic.com, "Self-Injury/Cutting," August 2008, www.mayoclinic.com/health/self-injury/DS00775.
79. National Institute of Mental Health, "The Numbers Count: Mental Disorders in America," Reviewed September 2010, www.nimh.nih.gov/health/publications/the-numbers-count-mental-disorders-in-america.shtml.
80. National Institute of Mental Health, "Schizophrenia," Reviewed March 2010, www.nimh.nih.gov/health/topics/schizophrenia/index.shtml.
81. Ibid.
82. Centers for Disease Control and Prevention, "Attention-Deficit Hyperactivity Disorder," www.cdc.gov/ncbddd/adhd, Updated October 2009; Helpguide.org, "Adult ADD/ADHD: Signs, Symptoms, Effects, and Treatment," Reviewed November 2010, www.helpguide.org/mental/adhd_add_adult_symptoms.htm; National Institute of Mental Health, "The Numbers Count,"

www.nimh.nih.gov/health/publications/the-numbers-count-mental-disorders-in-america/index.shtml, 2008; H. R. Searight, J. M. Burke, and F. Rottnek, "Adult ADHD: Evaluation and Treatment in Family Medicine," *American Family Physician* 62, no. 9 (2000): 2091–92; T. Brown, *Attention Deficit Disorder: The Unfocused Mind in Children and Adults* (New Haven, CT: Yale University Press, 2005).
83. Alzheimer's Association, *2011 Alzheimer's Disease Facts and Figures* (Chicago: Alzheimer's Association, 2011), Available at www.alz.org/alzheimers_disease_facts_figures.asp.
84. Alzheimer's Association, "What is Alzheimer's," 2011, www.alz.org/alzheimers_disease_what_is_alzheimers.asp
85. Ibid.
86. National Institute of Mental Health, "Suicide in the U.S.: Statistics and Prevention," NIH Publication no. 06-4594, Reviewed September 2010, www.nimh.nih.gov/health/publications/suicide-in-the-us-statistics-and-prevention/index.shtml.
87. Ibid.
88. Ibid.
89. Crisis Link, "Suicide Myths (Adult)," 2009, www.crisislink.org/resources/suicide/suicide_myths_adult.html.
90. National Institute of Mental Health, "Suicide in the U.S.: Statistics and Prevention," 2010.
91. American Association of Suicidology, "Understanding and Helping the Suicidal Individual," Accessed May 2011, www.suicidology.org/web/guest/how-can-you-help.
92. Mayo Clinic Staff, MayoClinic.com, "Mental Health: Overcoming the Stigma of Mental Illness," 2009, www.mayoclinic.com/health/mental-health/MH00076; P. Corrigan and R. Lundin, *Don't Call Me Nuts: Coping with the Stigma of Mental Illness* (Tinley Park, IL: Recovery Press, 2001).
93. U.S. Food and Drug Administration, "New Warnings Proposed for Antidepressants," May 2007, www.fda.gov/ForConsumers/ConsumerUpdates/ucm048950.htm.

Chapter 3

1. American Psychological Association, *Stress in America 2010, Key Findings,* 2010, Available at www.apa.org/news/press/releases/stress/key-findings.pdf.
2. K. Glanz and M. Schwartz, "Stress, Coping and Health Behavior," in *Health Behavior and Health Education: Theory, Research and Practice,* 4th ed., eds. K. Glanz, B. Rimer, and K. Viswanath (San Francisco: Jossey Bass, 2008), 210–236.
3. B. L. Seaward, *Managing Stress: Principles and Strategies for Health and Well-Being,* 6th ed. (Sudbury, MA: Jones and Bartlett, 2009), 8.
4. American Psychological Association, *Stress in America 2010, Key Findings,* 2010.
5. H. Selye, *Stress without Distress* (New York: Lippincott, 1974), 28–29.
6. W. B. Cannon, *The Wisdom of the Body* (New York: Norton, 1932).
7. B. S. McEwen, "Mood Disorders and Allostatic Load," *Biological Psychiatry* 54 (2003): 200–207.
8. A. Mokdad et al., "Actual Causes of Death in the United States, 2000," *Journal of the American Medical Association* 291 (2004): 1238–45.
9. S. Cohen, D. Janicki-Deverts, and G. Miller, "Psychological Stress and Cardiovascular Disease," *Journal of the American Medical Association* 298, no. 14 (2007): 1685–87; A. Väänänen et al., "Lack of Predictability at Work and Risk

of Acute Myocardial Infarction: An 18-Year Prospective Study of Industrial Employees," *American Journal of Public Health* 98, no. 12 (2008): 2264–71; J. Bremner et al., *Stress and Health: Effects of a Cognitive Stress Challenge on Myocardial Perfusion and Plasma Cortisol in Coronary Heart Disease Patients with Depression* (San Francisco: John Wiley & Sons, 2009); A. Sgoifo, N. Montano, C. Shively, J. Thayer, and A. Steptoe, "The Inevitable Link between Heart and Behavior: New Insights from Biomedical Research and Implications for Practice," *Neuroscience and Biobehavioral Reviews* 33, no. 2 (2008): 61–67; K. Monyeki and H. Kemper, "The Risk Factors for Elevated Blood Pressure and How to Address Cardiovascular Risk Factors: A Review in Pediatric Populations," *Journal of Human Hypertension* 22 (2008): 450–59; F. Sparrenberger et al., "Does Psychological Stress Cause Hypertension? A Systematic Review of Observational Studies," *Journal of Human Hypertension* 23 (2009): 12–19; M. Hamer, G. Molloy, and E. Stamatakis, "Psychological Distress as a Risk Factor for Cardiovascular Events," *Journal of the American College of Cardiology* 52 (2008): 2156–62.
10. S. Yusef et al., "Effect of Potentially Modifiable Risk Factors Associated with Myocardial Infarction in 52 Countries (The INTERHEART Study): Case-Control Study," *Lancet* 364, no. 9438 (2004): 937–52.
11. J. Dimsdale, "Psychological Stress and Cardiovascular Disease," *Journal of the American College of Cardiology* 51 (2008): 1237–46.
12. B. Aggarwart, M. Liao, A. Christian, and L. Mosca, "Influence of Care-Giving on Lifestyle and Psychosocial Risk Factors among Family Members of Patients Hospitalized with Cardiovascular Disease," *Journal of General Internal Medicine* 24, no. 1 (2009): 1497–1525; F. Sparrenberger et al., "Does Psychological Stress Cause Hypertension?" 2009; M. Kivimäki et al., "Socioeconomic Position, Psychosocial Work Environment, and Cerebrovascular Disease among Women: The Finnish Public Sector Study," *International Journal of Epidemiology* (January 20, 2009); A. Väänänen et al., "Lack of Predictability at Work and Risk of Acute Myocardial Infarction," 2008; A. Miller and B. Arquilla, "Chronic Disease and Natural Hazards: Impact of Disasters on Diabetes, Renal and Cardiac Patients," *Prehospital Disaster Medicine* 23, no. 2 (2008): 185–94; I. Weissbecker, S. Sephton, M. Martin, and D. Simpson, "Psychological and Physiological Correlates of Stress in Children Exposed to Disaster: Current Research and Recommendations for Intervention," *Children, Youth and Environments* 18, no. 1 (2008): 30–70.
13. V. Vicennati et al., "Stress-Related Development of Obesity and Cortisol in Women," *Obesity* 17, no. 19 (2009): 1678–83; C. Shively, T. Register, and T. Clarkson, "Social Stress, Visceral Obesity and Coronary Atherosclerosis in Female Primates," Obesity 17, no. 8 (2009): 1513–20; L. Brydon et al., "Stress-Induced Cytokine Responses and Central Adiposity in Young Women," *International Journal of Obesity* 32, no. 3 (2008): 443–50; R. Pasquali et al., "Sex Dependent Role of Glucocorticoids and Androgens in the Pathophysiology of Human Obesity," *International Journal of Obesity* 32 (2008): 1764–79.
14. D. K. Hall-Flavin, "Stress and Hair Loss: Are They Related?" Mayo Clinic.com, 2008, www.mayoclinic.com/health/stress-and-hair-loss/AN01442.

15. M. Scollan-Koliopoulos, "Managing Stress Response to Control Hypertension in Type 2 Diabetes," *Nurse Practitioner* 30, no. 2 (2005): 46–49.

16. University of Maryland Medical Center, "Digestive Disorders: Irritable Bowel Syndrome," March 2009, www.umm.edu/digest/ibs.htm; National Digestive Diseases Information Clearinghouse (NDDIC), "Irritable Bowel Syndrome," NIH Publication no. 07-693, September 2007; Johns Hopkins Health Alerts, "Four Relaxation Techniques to Soothe Your Digestive Discomfort," 2008, www.johnshopkinshealthalerts.com/reports/digestive_health/2683-1.html?ty.

17. S. Lightman, "Chronic Stress Can Significantly Damage Health," *Discovery Health* (2008), http://health.discovery.com/centers/stress/interviews/liteman_int.html; J. Walburn et al., "Psychological Stress and Wound Healing in Humans: A Systematic Review and Meta-Analysis," *Journal of Psychosomatic Research* 67, no. 3 (2009): 253–71; T. Denson, M. Spanovic, and N. Miller, "Cognitive Appraisals and Emotions Predict Cortisol and Immune Responses: A Meta-Analysis of Acute Laboratory Social Stressors and Emotion Inductions," *Psychological Bulletin* 135, no. 6 (2009): 823–53; S. Seagerstrom and G. Miller, "Psychological Stress and the Human Immune System: A Meta-Analytic Study of 30 Years of Inquiry," *Psychological Bulletin* 130, no. 4 (2004) 601–30; E. R. Volkmann and N. Y. Weekes, "Basal SigA and Cortisol Levels Predict Stress-Related Health Outcomes," *Stress and Health* 22 (2006): 11–23.

18. G. Miller, N. Rohleder, and S. Cole, "Chronic Interpersonal Stress Predicts Activation of Pro- and Anti-Inflammatory Signaling 6 Months Later," *Psychosomatic Medicine* 71, no. 1 (2009): 57–62.

19. S. Seagerstrom and G. Miller, "Psychological Stress and the Human Immune System: A Meta-Analytic Study of 30 Years of Inquiry," *Psychological Bulletin* 130, no. 4 (2004): 601–30.

20. V. Bitsika, C. Sharpley, and R. Bell, "The Contribution of Anxiety and Depression to Fatigue among a Sample of Australian University Students: Suggestions for University Counselors," *Counseling Psychology Quarterly* 22, no. 2 (2009): 243–53; A. Katz, "'Not Tonight, Dear': The Elusive Female Libido," *AJN, American Journal of Nursing* 107, no. 12 (2007): 32–34.

21. American College Health Association (ACHA), *American College Health Association—National College Health Assessment II (ACHA-NCHA II) Reference Group Data Report Fall 2010*, (Baltimore: ACHA, 2011), Available at www.acha-ncha.org/reports_ACHA-NCHAII.html.

22. L. Schwabe, T. Wolf, and M. Oitzi. "Memory Formation under Stress: Quantity and Quality," *Neuroscience and Biobehavioral Reviews* 34, no. 4 (2009): 584–91.

23. E. Dias-Ferreira et al., "Chronic Stress Causes Frontostriatal Reorganization and Affects Decision-Making," *Science* 325, no. 5940 (2009): 621–25; D. de Quervan et al., "Glucocorticoids and the Regulation of Memory in Health and Disease," *Frontiers in Neuroendocrinology* 30, no. 3 (2009): 358–70.

24. D. A. Katerndahl and M. Parchman, "The Ability of the Stress Process Model to Explain Mental Health Outcomes," *Comprehensive Psychiatry* 43 (2002): 351–60; R. C. Kessler et al., "The Epidemiology of Major Depressive Disorder," *Journal of the American Medical Association* 289 (2003): 3095–105.

25. R. L. Turner and D. A. Lloyd, "Stress Burden and the Lifetime Incidence of Psychiatric Disorder in Young Adults: Racial and Ethnic Contrasts," *Archives of General Psychiatry* 61 (2004): 481–88; A. Väänänen et al., "Sources of Social Support as Determinants of Psychiatric Morbidity after Severe Life Events: Prospective Cohort Study of Female Employees," *Journal of Psychosomatic Research* 58 (2005): 459–67.

26. V. R. Wilburn and D. E. Smith, "Stress, Self-Esteem, and Suicidal Ideation in Late *Adolescence*," *Adolescence* 40 (2005): 33–46.

27. National Headache Foundation, "Press Kits: Categories of Headache," 2010. www.headaches.org/press/NHF_Press_Kits/Press_Kits_-_Categories_of_Headache.

28. Mayo Clinic, "Tension Headache: Symptoms," February 2009, www.mayoclinic.com/health/tension-headache/ds00304/dsection=symptoms.

29. Mayo Clinic, "Migraine: Symptoms," June 2009, www.mayoclinic.com/health/migraine-headache/DS00120/DSECTION=symptoms.

30. National Headache Foundation, "The Complete Guide to Headache: Migraine," 2010, www.headaches.org/educational_modules/completeguide/migrindex.html.

31. Ibid.

32. Mayo Clinic, "Migraine: Risk Factors," June 2009, www.mayoclinic.com/health/migraine-headache/DS00120/DSECTION=risk-factors.

33. National Headache Foundation, "The Complete Guide to Headache: Migraine," 2010.

34. American College Health Association, *American College Health Association–National College Health Assessment II (ACHA–NCHA II): Reference Group Data Report Fall 2010* (Baltimore: American College Health Association, 2010), Available at www.achancha.org/reports_ACHA-NCHAII.html.

35. S. Cohen et al., "Sleep Habits and Susceptibility to the Common Cold," *Archives of Internal Medicine* 169, no. 1 (2009): 62–67. D. J. Gottlieb et al., "Association of Usual Sleep Duration with Hypertension: The Sleep Heart Health Study," *Sleep* 29, no. 8 (2006): 1009–14. S. R. Patel et al., "Sleep Duration and Biomarkers of Inflammation," *Sleep* 32, no. 2 (2009): 200–04; M. L. Okun, M. Coussons-Read, and M. Hall, "Disturbed Sleep Is Associated with Increased C-Reactive Protein in Young Women," *Brain, Behavior, and Immunity* 23, no. 3 (2009): 351–54.

36. S. Banks and D. F. Dinges, "Behavioral and Physiological Consequences of Sleep Restriction," *Journal of Clinical Sleep Medicine* 3, no. 5 (2007): 519–28.

37. H. Eichenbaum, "To Sleep, Perchance to Integrate," *Proceedings of the National Academy of Sciences of the United States of America* 104, no. 18 (2007): 7317–18; J. M. Ellenbogen, P. T. Hu, D. Titone, and M. P. Walker, "Human Relational Memory Requires Time and Sleep," *Proceedings of the National Academy of Sciences of the United States of America* 104, no. 18 (2007): 7723–28; J. M. Ellenbogen, J. C. Hulbert, Y. Jiang, and R. Stickgold, "The Sleeping Brain's Influence on Verbal Memory: Boosting Resistance to Interference," *PLoS ONE* 4, no. 1 (2009): e4117.

38. B. R. Sheth, D. Janvelyan, and M. Khan, "Practice Makes Imperfect: Restorative Effects of Sleep on Motor Learning," *PLoS ONE* 3, no. 9 (2008): e3190.

39. T. Jan, "Colleges Calling Sleep a Success Prerequisite," *Boston Globe* (September 30, 2008), www.boston.com/news/education/higher/articles/2008/09/30/colleges_calling_sleep_a_success_prerequisite.

40. National Sleep Foundation, "Depression and Sleep," www.sleepfoundation.org/article/sleep-topics/depression-and-sleep., Accessed March 2009; T. Roth, "Expert Column-Stress, Anxiety, and Insomnia: What Every PCP Should Know," *Current Perspectives in Insomnia* 4 (2004), Available at http://cme.medscape.com; A. Gregory et al., "The Direction of Longitudinal Associations between Sleep Problems and Depression Symptoms: A Study of Twins Aged 8 and 10 Years," *Sleep* 32, no. 2 (2009): 189–99.

41. J. Ferrie et al., "A Prospective Study of Change in Sleep Duration: Associations with Mortality in the Whitehall II Cohort," *Sleep* 30, no. 12 (2007): 1659–66; C. Hublin et al., "Sleep and Mortality: A Population-Based 22-Year Follow-up Study," *Sleep* 30, no. 12 (2007): 1614–15.

42. National Sleep Foundation, "Caffeine and Sleep," 2009, www.sleepfoundation.org/article/sleep-topics/caffeine-and-sleep.

43. R. Lazarus, "The Trivialization of Distress," in *Preventing Health Risk Behaviors and Promoting Coping with Illness*, eds. J. Rosen and L. Solomon (Hanover, NH: University Press of New England, 1985), 279–98.

44. D. J. Maybery and D. Graham, "Hassles and Uplifts: Including Interpersonal Events," *Stress and Health* 17 (2001): 91–104; R. Blonna, *Coping with Stress in a Changing World*, 4th ed. (New York: McGraw-Hill, 2006).

45. M. Weil and L. Rosen, "Technostress: Are You a Victim?" 2007, www.technostress.com.

46. American Psychological Association, *Stress in America 2010, Key Findings*, 2010.

47. C. L. Park, S. Armeli, and H. Tennen, "The Daily Stress and Coping Process and Alcohol Use among College Students," *Journal of Studies on Alcohol* 65, no. 1 (2004): 126–30; B. E. Miller et al., "Alcohol Misuse among College Athletes: Self-Medication for Psychiatric Symptoms?" *Journal of Drug Education* 32 (2002): 41–52.

48. S. Sumer, "International Students' Psychological and Sociocultural Adaptation in the United States," Georgia State University, Doctoral Dissertation, 2009, http://digitalarchive.gsu.edu/cps_diss/34; L. Johnson and D. Sandhu, "Isolation, Adjustment and Acculturation Issues of International Students: Intervention Strategies for Counselors," in *A Handbook for Counseling International Students in the U.S.*, eds. S. Singaravelu and M. Pope (Alexandria, VA: American Counseling Association, 2007), 13–36.

49. Z. Djuric et al., "Biomarkers of Psychological Stress in Health Disparities Research," *The Open Biomarkers Journal* 1 (2008): 7–19; J. Watson, H. Logan, and S. Tomar, "The Influence of Active Coping and Perceived Stress on Health Disparities in a Multi-Ethnic Low Income Sample," *BMC Public Health* 8 (2008): 41; C. M. Arthur, "A Little Bit of Rain Each Day: Psychological Stress and Health Disparities," *California Journal of Health Promotion* 5, Special Edition (2007): 58–67.

50. N. Buchanan et al., "Unique and Joint Effects of Sexual and Racial Harassment on College Students' Well-Being," Basic and *Applied Social Psychology* 31, no. 3 (2009): 267–85.

51. S. Sumer, "International Students' Psychological and Sociocultural Adaptation," 2009; Institute of International Education, "Open Doors Data," 2010, www.iie.org/en/Research-and-Publications/Open-Doors/Data; S. T. Mortenson,

"Cultural Differences and Similarities in Seeking Social Support as a Response to Academic Failure: A Comparison of American and Chinese College Students," *Communication Education* 55 no. 2 (2006): 127–46.

52. D. Stang, "Calming Down: An Introduction to Stress and Some Stress Solutions," HealthVideo.com, Accessed May 2011, www.healthvideo.com/article.php?id=1174.

53. K. Karren et al., *Mind/Body Health: The Effects of Attitudes, Emotions, and Relationships,* 4th ed. (San Francisco: Benjamin Cummings, 2010).

54. K. Karren et al., *Mind/Body Health,* 2010; B. L. Seaward, *Managing Stress,* 2009; V. R. Wilburn and D. E. Smith, "Stress, Self-Esteem, and Suicidal Ideation," 2005.

55. V. R. Wilburn and D. E. Smith, "Stress, Self-Esteem, and Suicidal Ideation," 2005; D. Robotham and C. Julian, "Stress and the Higher Education Student: A Critical Review of the Literature," *Journal of Further and Higher Education* 30, no. 2 (2006): 107–17.

56. K. Glanz, B. Rimer, and F. Levis, eds., *Health Behavior and Health Education: Theory, Research, and Practice,* 3rd ed. (San Francisco: Jossey-Bass, 2002).

57. A. D. Von et al., "Predictors of Health Behaviors in College Students," *Journal of Advanced Nursing* 48, no. 5 (2004): 463–74.

58. M. Friedman and R. H. Rosenman, *Type A Behavior and Your Heart* (New York: Knopf, 1974).

59. K. Karren et al., *Mind/Body Health,* 2010; R. Niaura et al., "Hostility, Metabolic Syndrome, and Incident Coronary Heart Disease," *Health Psychology* 21, no. 6 (2002): 588–93.

60. M. Jawer and M. Micozzi, *The Spiritual Anatomy of Emotion: How Feelings Link the Brain, the Body, and the Sixth Sense* (Rochester, VT: Park Street Press, 2009).

61. J. Denollet, "Prognostic Value of Type D Personality Compared with Depressive Symptoms," *Archives of Internal Medicine* 168, no. 4 (2008): 431–35; N. Kupper and J. Denollet, "Type D Personalities as a Prognostic Factor in Heart Disease: Assessment and Mediating Mechanisms," *Journal of Personality Assessment* 89, no. 3 (2007): 265–66; L. Williams et al., "Type D Personality Mechanisms of Effect: The Role of Health-Related Behavior and Social Support," *Journal of Psychosomatic Research* 64, no. 1 (2008): 63–68.

62. S. Kobasa, "Stressful Life Events, Personality, and Health: An Inquiry into Hardiness," *Journal of Personality and Social Psychology* 37 (1979): 1–11.

63. B. J. Crowley, B. Hayslip, and J. Hobdy, "Psychological Hardiness and Adjustment to Life Events in Adulthood," *Journal of Adult Development* 10 (2003): 237–48; S. R. Maddi, "The Story of Hardiness: Twenty Years of Theorizing, Research, and Practice," *Consulting Psychology Journal: Practice and Research* 54 (2002): 173–86.

64. K. Glanz and M. Schwartz, "Stress, Coping and Health Behavior," 2008.

65. B. L. Seaward, *Managing Stress,* 2009.

66. D. A. Girdano, D. E. Dusek, and G. S. Everly, *Controlling Stress and Tension,* 8th ed. (San Francisco: Benjamin Cummings, 2009), 375.

67. M. Bennett and C. Lengacher, "Humor and Laughter May Influence Health IV: Humor and Immune Function," *Evidence-Based Complementary and Alternative Medicine* 6, no. 2 (2009): 159–64.

68. P. Holmes, "Managing Anger," 2004; B. L. Seaward, *Managing Stress,* 2009.

69. J. Graham et al., "Cognitive Word Use during Marital Conflict and Increases in Pro-inflammatory Cytokines," *Health Psychology* 28, no. 5 (2009): 621–30.

70. P. Steel, "The Nature of Procrastination: A Meta-Analytic and Theoretical Review of Quintessential Self-Regulatory Failure," *Psychological Review* 133, no. 1 (2007): 65–94.

71. T. Gura, "Procrastinating Again? How to Kick the Habit," *Scientific American Mind,* December 2008, www.sciam.com/article.cfm?id=procrastinating-again.

72. Ibid.

73. J. H. Pryor et al., *The American Freshman: National Norms Fall 2010* (Los Angeles: Higher Education Research Institute, 2011).

Chapter 4

1. J. Snelgrove, P. Hynek, and M. Stafford, "A Multi-Level Analysis of Social Capital and Self-Rated Health: Evidence from the British Household Panel Survey," *Social Science and Medicine* 68, no. 11 (2009): 1993–2001; C. J. Hale, J. W. Hannum, and D. L. Espelage, "Social Support and Physical Health: The Importance of Belonging," *Journal of American College Health* 53 (2005): 276–84; S. Braithwaite, R. Delevi, and F. Fincham, "Romantic Relationships and the Physical and Mental Health of College Students," *Personal Relationships* 17, no. 1 (2010): 1–12; E. Cornwell and L. Waite, "Social Disconnectedness, Perceived Isolation, and Health among Older Adults," *Journal of Health and Social Behavior* 50, no. 11 (2009): 31–48.

2. E. Hatfield, J. T. Pillemer, M. U. O'Brien, and Y. L. Le, "The Endurance of Love: Passionate and Companionate Love in Newlywed and Long-Term Marriages," *Interpersona: An International Journal of Personal Relationships* 2 (June 2008): 35–64; E. Hatfield and R. L. Rapson, *Love, Sex, and Intimacy: Their Psychology, Biology, and History* (New York: Harper Collins, 1993).

3. R. Sternberg, "Construct Validation of a Triangular Love Scale," *European Journal of Social Psychology* 27 (1997): 313–35.

4. H. Fisher, *Why We Love* (New York: Henry Holt, 2004); H. Fisher, A. Aron, D. Mashek, H. Li, and L. L. Brown, "Defining the Brain System of Lust, Romantic Attraction, and Attachment," *Archives of Sexual Behavior* 31, no. 5 (2002): 413–19.

5. Ibid.

6. M. Gatzeva and A. Paik, "Emotional and Physical Satisfaction in Noncohabiting, Cohabiting, and Marital Relationships: The Importance of Jealous Conflict," *Journal of Sex Research* 25 (2009): 1–14; D. Nannini and L. Mayers, "Jealousy in Sexual and Emotional Infidelity: An Alternative to the Evolutionary Explanation," *Journal of Sex Research* 37, no. 2 (2000): 117–22.

7. C. R. Rogers, "Interpersonal Relationship: The Core of Guidance" in *Person to Person: The Problem of Being Human,* eds. C. R. Rogers and B. Stevens (Lafayette, CA: Real People Press, 1967).

8. C. Burggraf Torppa, Family and Consumer Sciences, Ohio State University Extension, "Gender Issues: Communication Differences in Interpersonal Relationships," 2010, Available at http://ohioline.osu.edu/flm02/pdf/fs04.pdf.

9. J. Wood, *Gendered Lives: Communication, Gender, and Culture,* 8th ed. (Belmont, CA: Cengage, 2010); M. L. Knapp and A. L. Vangelisti, *Interpersonal Communication and Human Relationships,* 5th ed. (Boston: Allyn & Bacon, 2004).

10. J. Wood, *Interpersonal Communication: Everyday Encounters* (Belmont, CA: Cengage, 2010); J. K. Burgoon, C. Segrin, and N. E. Dunbar, "Nonverbal Communication and Social Influence," in *Persuasion: Developments in Theory and Practice,* eds. J. P. Dillard and M. Pfau (Thousand Oaks, CA: Sage, 2002), 445–76.

11. R. S. Miller, D. Perlman, and S. S. Brehm, *Intimate Relationships,* 4th ed. (New York: McGraw-Hill, 2007), 150–56.

12. The National Marriage Project, University of Virginia, *The State of Our Unions: Marriage in America, 2010: When Marriage Disappears: The New Middle America* (Charlottesville, VA: National Marriage Project and the Institute for American Values, 2010), Available at www.stateofourunions.org.

13. U.S. Census Bureau News, "Press Release: March 2009 Current Population Survey: Census Bureau Reports Families with Children Increasingly Face Unemployment," January 15, 2010, Available at www.census.gov/newsroom/releases/archives/families_households/cb10-08.html.

14. K. McCoy, "Can Marriage Help You Live Longer?" HealthLibrary, EBSCO Publishing, Updated April 2010, Available at http://healthlibrary.epnet.com/GetContent.aspx?token=af362d97-4f80-4453-a175-02cc6220a387&chunkiid=43793.

15. C. A. Schoenborn, "Marital Status and Health: United States, 1999–2002," *Advance Data from Vital and Health Statistics,* no. 351, DHHS Publication No. 2005-1250 (Hyattsville, MD: National Center for Health Statistics, 2004), Available at www.cdc.gov/nchs/products/ad.htm.

16. U.S. Census Bureau, Housing and Household Economic Statistics Division, Fertility & Family Statistics Branch, "America's Families and Living Arrangements: 2009," 2010, Available at www.census.gov/population/www/socdemo/hh-fam/cps2009.html.

17. Ibid.

18. M. Lino, *Expenditures on Children by Families, 2009* (Alexandria, VA: U.S. Department of Agriculture, Center for Nutrition Policy and Promotion, 2010), Available at www.cnpp.usda.gov/ExpendituresonChildrenbyFamilies.htm.

19. P. Y. Goodwin, W. D. Mosher, and A. Chandra, "Marriage and Cohabitation in the United States: A Statistical Portrait Based on Cycle 6 (2002) of the National Survey of Family Growth, National Center for Health Statistics," *Vital Health Statistics* 23, no. 28 (2010), Available at www.cdc.gov/nchs/nsfg/nsfg_products.htm.

20. Ibid.

21. G. J. Gates, "Same-Sex Spouses and Unmarried Partners in the American Community Survey, 2008" (Los Angeles: The Williams Institute, UCLA School of Law, 2009), Available at www.law.ucla.edu/williamsinstitute/publications/Policy-Census-index.html.

22. National Gay and Lesbian Task Force, "Relationship Recognition Map for Same-Sex Couples in the U.S.," June 2011, Available at www.thetaskforce.org/reports_and_research/relationship_recognition.

23. U.S. Census Bureau, "2005–2009 American Community Survey 5-Year Estimates," table S1201, 2009, Available at http://factfinder.census.gov/servlet/STTable?_bm=y&-geo_id=01000US&-qr_name=ACS_2009_5YR_G00_S1201&-ds_name=ACS_2009_5YR_G00_&-_lang=en&-_caller=geoselect&-state=st&-format=.

24. A. Cherlin, "Between Poor and Prosperous: Do Family Patterns of Moderately Educated Americans Deserve a Closer Look?" in *Social Class and Changing Families in an Unequal America*, eds. M. Carlson and P. England (Palo Alto, CA: Stanford University Press, 2011).

25. Ibid.

26. Federal Bureau of Investigation, "Hate Crime Statistics, 2009," November 2010, Available at www2.fbi .gov/ucr/hc2009/documents/incidentsandoffenses .pdf.

27. Consortium on the Management of Disorders of Sexual Development, *Handbook for Parents* (Rohnert Park, CA: Intersex Society of North America, 2006), Available at http://dsdguidelines.org.

28. "Consensus Statement on Management of Intersex Disorders," *Pediatrics* 118 (2006): e488–e500.

29. S. E. Anderson, G. E. Dallal, and A. Must, "Relative Weight and Race Influence Average Age at Menarche: Results from Two Nationally Representative Surveys of U.S. Girls Studied 25 Years Apart," *Pediatrics* 111, no. 4 (2003): 844–50; H. Baer, G. Colditz, W. Willet, and J. Dorgan, "Adiposity and Sex Hormones in Girls," *Cancer Epidemiology Biomarkers Preview* 16, no. 9 (2007): 1880–08; L. Shi, S. Wudy, A. Buyken, M. Hartmann, and T. Remer, "Body Fat and Animal Protein Intakes Are Associated with Adrenal Androgen Secretion in Children," *American Journal of Clinical Nutrition* 90, no. 5 (2009): 1321–28; K. K. Ong et al., "Infancy Weight Gain Predicts Childhood Body Fat and Age at Menarche in Girls," *Journal of Clinical Endocrinology & Metabolism* 94 (2009): 1527–32.

30. Mayo Clinic Staff, "Menstrual Cramps," 2007, Available at www.mayoclinic.com/Health/ Menstrual-Cramps/DS00506.

31. National Institutes of Health, *Facts about Menopausal Hormone Therapy* (NIH Publication no. 05-5200: 2005), Available at www.nhlbi.nih.gov/ health/women/pht_facts.htm.

32. M. Moreno, "Advice for Patients: Male Circumcision," *Archives of Pediatrics & Adolescent Medicine* 164, no. 1 (2010): 104; Centers for Disease Control and Prevention; Mayo Clinic Staff, "Circumcision (male): Why It's Done," February 2010, Available at www.mayoclinic.com/health/circumcision/ MY01023/DSECTION=why-its-done.

33. Mayo Clinic Staff, "Male Menopause: Myth or Reality?" July 23, 2011, Available at www.mayoclinic .com/health/male-menopause/MC00058.

34. Ibid.

35. G. F. Kelly, "Sexual Individuality and Sexual Values," in *Sexuality Today: The Human Perspective*, 9th ed. (New York: McGraw-Hill, 2008).

36. Ibid.

37. J. A. Higgins, J. Trussell, N. B. Moore, and J. K. Davidson, "Young Adult Sexual Health: Current and Prior Sexual Behaviours among Non-Hispanic White U.S. College Students," *Sexual Health* 7, no. 1 (2010): 35–43.

38. American College Health Association, *American College Health Association—National College Health Assessment II (ACHA-NCHA II) Reference Group Data Report Fall 2010* (Baltimore: American College Health Association, 2011), Available at www.acha-ncha.org/reports_ACHA-NCHAII .html.

39. Ibid.

40. Ibid.

41. G. F. Kelly, "Sexual Individuality and Sexual Values," 2008.

42. Medline Plus, "Sexual Problems Overview: Medline Plus," Updated May 2010, Available at www .nlm.nih.gov/medlineplus/ency/article/001951.htm.

43. Mayo Clinic Staff, "Erectile Dysfunction," January 2010, Available at www.mayoclinic.com/health/ erectile-dysfunction/DS00162.

44. National Kidney and Urological Diseases Information Clearinghouse, "Erectile Dysfunction," 2009, Available at http://kidney.niddk.nih.gov/ kudiseases/pubs/impotence/index.htm.

45. Medline Plus, "Sexual Problems Overview: Medline Plus," Updated May 2010.

46. K. M. Smith and F. Romanelli, "Recreational Use and Misuse of Phosphodiesterase 5 Inhibitors," *Journal of the American Pharmacists Association* 45, no. 1 (2005): 63–75; R. Kloner, "Erectile Dysfunction and Hypertension," *International Journal of Impotence Research* 19, no. 3 (2007): 296–302.

Chapter 5

1. American College Health Association, *American College Health Association—National College Health Assessment II: Fall 2010 Reference Group Data Report* (Baltimore: American College Health Association, 2011), Available at www.acha-ncha .org/reports_ACHA-NCHAII.html.

2. R. A. Hatcher et al., *Contraceptive Technology*, 19th rev. ed. (New York: Ardent Media, 2007), 299.

3. American College Health Association, *American College Health Association—National College Health Assessment II*, 2011.

4. Drugs.com, "Seasonale," Available at www.drugs .com/seasonale.html.

5. R. A. Hatcher et al., *Contraceptive Technology*, 2007.

6. Ibid.

7. Food and Drug Administration, "Safety Labeling Changes Approved by FDA Center for Drug Evaluation and Research (CDER)—April 2010: Ortho Evra (Norelgestromin/Ethinyl Estradiol) Transdermal System," Updated May 2010, Available at www.fda.gov/Safety/MedWatch/ SafetyInformation/ucm211821.htm.

8. Office of Population Research & Association of Reproductive Health Professionals, "Answers to Frequently Asked Questions about Effectiveness," Updated March 2010, Available at http:// ec.princeton.edu/questions/eceffect.html.

9. Guttmacher Institute, "State Policies in Brief: As of May 1, 2010: Emergency Contraception," May 2010, Available at www.guttmacher.org/ statecenter/spibs.

10. American College Health Association, *American College Health Association—National College Health Assessment II*, 2011.

11. Ibid.

12. Guttmacher Institute, "Facts on Contraceptive Use in the United States," June 2010, Available at www.guttmacher.org/pubs/fb_contr_use.html.

13. R. A. Hatcher et al., *Contraceptive Technology*, 2007.

14. Guttmacher Institute, "Facts on Induced Abortion in the United States," January 2011, Available at www.guttmacher.org/pubs/fb_induced_abortion .html.

15. American Psychological Association, Task Force on Mental Health and Abortion, *Report of the Task Force on Mental Health and Abortion* (Washington, DC: American Psychological Association, 2008), Available at www.apa.org/pi/wpo/ mental-health-abortion-report.pdf.

16. Boston Women's Health Collective, *Our Bodies, Ourselves: A New Edition for a New Era* (New York: Simon & Schuster, 2005).

17. Guttmacher Institute, "Facts on Induced Abortion in the United States," 2011.

18. NARAL, Pro Choice America, "The Bush Administration's Federal Abortion Ban," January 2010, Available at www.prochoiceamerica.org/issues/ abortion/abortion-bans/federal-abortion-ban .html.

19. Guttmacher Institute, "Supreme Court Upholds Federal Abortion Ban, Opens Door for Further Restrictions by States," *Guttmacher Policy Review* 10, no. 2 (2007): 19.

20. American Psychological Association, Task Force on Mental Health and Abortion, *Report of the Task Force on Mental Health and Abortion* (Washington, DC: Author, 2008).

21. Ibid.

22. Ibid.

23. Guttmacher Institute, "Facts on Induced Abortions in the United States," 2011.

24. Ibid.

25. Planned Parenthood, "The Abortion Pill (Medical Abortion)," May 2010, Available at www .plannedparenthood.org/health-topics/abortion/ abortion-pill-medication-abortion-4354.asp.

26. Ibid.

27. Donald Wigle et al., "Epidemiologic Evidence of Relationships between Reproductive and Child Health Outcomes and Environmental Chemical Contaminants," *Journal of Toxicology* 11, no. 5–6 (2008): 373–517.

28. M. Lino and A. Carlson, *Expenditures on Children by Families, 2008*, U.S. Department of Agriculture, Center for Nutrition Policy and Promotion. Miscellaneous Publication no. 1528-2008 (2009), Available at www.cnpp.usda.gov/Publications/ CRC/crc2008.pdf.

29. National Association of Child Care Resource and Referral Agencies, *Parents and the High Price of Childcare, 2009 Update*, 2009, Available at www .naccrra.org/publications/naccrra-publications/ publications/665-0410_PriceReport_ FINAL_051409.kv.pdf.

30. Centers for Disease Control and Prevention, "Preconception Care Questions and Answers," April 2006, Available at www.cdc.gov/ncbddd/ preconception/QandA.htm.

31. Ibid.

32. National Center for Chronic Disease Prevention and Health Promotion, "Tobacco Use and Pregnancy," Modified May 2009, Available at www .cdc.gov/reproductivehealth/TobaccoUse Pregnancy/index.htm; U.S. Department of Health and Human Services, *How Tobacco Smoke Causes Disease: The Biology and Behavioral Basis for Smoking-Attributable Disease: A Report of the Surgeon General* (Atlanta, GA: U.S. Department of Health and Human Services, Centers for Disease Control and Prevention, National Center for Chronic Disease Prevention and Health Promotion, Office on Smoking and Health, 2010).

33. M. Kharrazi et al., "Environmental Tobacco Smoke and Pregnancy Outcome," *Epidemiology* 15, no. 6 (November 2006): 660–70.

34. E. Puscheck, "Early Pregnancy Loss," eMedicine from WebMD, Updated February 2010, Available at http://emedicine.medscape.com/ article/266317-overview.

35. March of Dimes, "Stillbirth Fact Sheet," February 2010, Available at www.marchofdimes.com/ professionals/14332_1198.asp.

36. U.S. Department of Health and Human Services, Health Resources and Services Administration, Maternal and Child Health Bureau, *Child Health USA 2010* (Rockville, MD: U.S. Department of Health and Human Services, 2010), Available at http://mchb.hrsa.gov/chusa10/popchar/ pages/109ma.html.

37. F. Menacker and B. Hamilton, "Recent Trends in Cesarean Delivery in the United States," NCHS Data Brief no. 35 (Hyattsville, MD: National Center for Health Statistics, 2010), DHHS Publication no. (PHS) 2010–1209, Available at www.cdc.gov/nchs/data/databriefs/db35.htm.

38. U.S. Department of Health and Human Services, Office on Women's Health, "Frequently Asked Questions: Depression During and After Pregnancy," Updated March 2009, Available at www.womenshealth.gov/faq/depression-pregnancy.cfm.

39. American Academy of Pediatrics, "Benefits of Breastfeeding for Mom," Updated April 2010, Available at www.healthychildren.org/English/ages-stages/baby/breastfeeding/pages/Benefits-of-Breastfeeding-for-Mom.aspx.

40. A. Gardner, "Report Shows Dangerous Chemical Can Leach from Baby Bottles," U.S. News & World Report, February 7, 2008.

41. National Institute on Child and Human Development, "Research on Sudden Infant Death Syndrome," Updated October 2009, Available at www.nichd.nih.gov/womenshealth/research/pregbirth/sids.cfm.

42. Ibid.

43. Mayo Clinic Staff, MayoClinic.com, "Infertility: Causes," June 2009, Available at www.mayoclinic.com/health/infertility/DS00310/DSECTION=causes.

44. U.S. Department of Health and Human Services, Office on Women's Health, "Frequently Asked Questions: Polycystic Ovary Syndrome (PCOS)," Updated March 2010, Available at www.womenshealth.gov/faq/polycystic-ovary-syndrome.cfm.

45. Centers for Disease Control and Prevention (CDC), "Pelvic Inflammatory Disease CDC Fact Sheet," Modified April 2008, Available at www.cdc.gov/std/PID/STDFact-PID.htm.

46. Centers for Disease Control and Prevention (CDC), "Assisted Reproductive Technology Home," Reviewed November 2009, Available at www.cdc.gov/ART.

47. Ibid.

48. WebMD Medical Reference, "Fertility Drugs," Reviewed February 2010, Available at www.webmd.com/infertility-and-reproduction/guide/fertility-drugs.

49. J. Jones, "Who Adopts? Characteristics of Women and Men Who Have Adopted Children," NCHS Data Brief no. 12 (Hyattsville, MD: National Center for Health Statistics, 2009) DHHS Publication No. (PHS) 2009–1209, Available at www.cdc.gov/nchs/data/databriefs/db12.htm.

Chapter 6

1. Substance Abuse and Mental Health Services Administration, Office of Applied Studies, Results from the 2009 National Survey on Drug Use and Health: Volume I. Summary of National Findings, NSDUH Series H-38A, HHS Publication No. SMA 10-4856 Findings, 2010, Available at www.oas.samhsa.gov/nsduh/2k8nsduh/2k8Results.cfm.

2. National Drug Intelligence Center, "National Drug Threat Assessment 2010," 2010, Available at www.justice.gov/ndic/pubs38/38661/drugImpact.htm; Centers for Disease Control and Prevention, "CDC Statement Regarding the Misuse of Prescription Drugs," June 2010, Available at www.cdc.gov/media/pressrel/2010/s100603.htm.

3. R. Goldberg, Drugs across the Spectrum, 6th ed. (Belmont, CA: Brooks/Cole, 2009).

4. R. McHugh, et al., "The Serotonin Transporter Gene and Risk for Alcohol Dependence: A Meta-Analytical Review." Drug and Alcohol Dependence 108, nos. 1–2 (2010): 1–6.

5. A. Agrawal et al., "Linkage Scan for Quantitative Traits Identifies New Regions of Interest for Substance Dependence in the Collaborative Study on the Genetics of Alcoholism (COGA) Sample," Drug and Alcohol Dependence 93, no. 1–2 (2008): 12–20.

6. J. Kinney, Loosening the Grip: A Handbook of Alcohol Information (New York: McGraw-Hill, 2009), 106.

7. G. Hansen and P. Venturelli, Drugs and Society, 10th ed. (Sudbury, MA: Jones and Bartlett, 2009), 49.

8. Ibid, 4.

9. National Institute on Drug Abuse, National Institutes of Health, U.S. Department of Health and Human Services, Drugs, Brains, and Behavior: The Science of Addiction, NIH Publication no. 07-5605 (Bethesda, MD: National Institute on Drug Abuse, 2007), Available at www.nida.nih.gov/scienceofaddiction.

10. National Council on Problem Gambling, "FAQs—Problem Gamblers," Available at www.ncpgambling.org/i4a/pages/index.cfm?pageid=3390.

11. H. Bowden-Jones and L. Clark, "Pathological Gambling: A Neurobiological and Clinical Update," British Journal of Psychiatry 199 (2011): 87–89; W. Brink, "Pathological Gambling: Impulse Control Disorder or Addiction?" European Psychiatry 26, no.1 (2011): 1767.

12. Ibid.

13. J. W. Welte et al., "Gambling Participation and Pathology in the United States: A Sociodemographic Analysis Using Classification Trees," Addictive Behaviors 29, no. 5 (2004): 983–89.

14. L. M. Koran et al., "Estimated Prevalence of Compulsive Buying Behavior in the United States," American Journal of Psychiatry 163, no. 10 (2006): 1806–12.

15. H. Tavares et al., "Compulsive Buying Disorder: A Review and Case Vignette." Brazilian Journal of Psychiatry 30, suppl. 1 (2008): S16–23; R. Engs, "How Can I Manage Compulsive Shopping and Spending Addiction (Shopoholism)?" Updated December 2006, Available at www.indiana.edu/~engs/hints/shop.html.

16. K. Young, X. Yue, and L. Ying, "Prevalence Estimates and Etiological Models of Internet Addiction" in (eds.) Young, K., and C. Abreu, Internet Addiction: A Handbook and Guide to Evaluation and Treatment (New York: John Wiley and Sons, 2011).

17. American College Health Association, American College Health Association—National College Health Assessment II: Reference Group Executive Summary Fall 2010 (Baltimore: American College Health Association, 2011), Available at www.acha-ncha.org/reports_ACHA-NCHAII.html.

18. C. Chamberlin and N. Zhang, "Workaholism, Health and Self-Acceptance," Journal of Counseling and Development 87, no. 2 (2009): 159–69.

19. Ibid.

20. J. F. Morgan, The Invisible Man: A Self-Help Guide for Men with Eating Disorders, Compulsive Exercise and Bigorexia (New York: Routledge, 2008), 36.

21. MedicineNet, " Sexual Addiction," 2010, Available at www.medicinenet.com/sexual_addiction/article.htm.

22. P. Kittenger and D. Herrick, "Patient Power: Over-the-Counter Drugs," National Center for Policy Analysis, Brief Analysis, no. 524, August 2005, Available at www.ncpa.org/pub/ba/ba524.

23. Consumer Healthcare Products Association, "OTC Medicines Serve an Important Health Care Need," 2009, Available at www.chpa-info.org/media/resources/r_4862.pdf.

24. L. D. Johnston et al., Monitoring the Future: National Survey Results on Drug Use, 1975–2010, Volume I, Secondary School Students, (Bethesda, MD: National Institute on Drug Abuse, 2011), Available at http://monitoringthefuture.org/pubs.html.

25. U.S. Department of Justice's National Drug Intelligence Center, Intelligence Bulletin: DXM (Dextromethorphan), DOJ Publication no. 2004-L0424-029 (Johnstown, PA: National Drug Intelligence Center, 2004), Available at www.justice.gov/ndic/pubs11/11563/index.htm.

26. U.S. Food and Drug Administration, "Legal Requirements for the Sale and Purchase of Drug Products Containing Pseudoephedrine, Ephedrine, and Phenylpropanolamine," Updated July 2009, Available at www.fda.gov/Drugs/DrugSafety/InformationbyDrugClass/ucm072423.htm.

27. National Youth Anti-Drug Media Campaign, "Prescription Drug (Rx) Abuse," 2010, Available at www.theantidrug.com/drug-information/otc-prescription-drug-abuse/prescription-drug-rx-abuse/default.aspx.

28. National Institute on Drug Abuse, Research Report Series: Prescription Drugs: Abuse and Addiction, NIH Publication no. 05-4881 (Bethesda, MD: National Institute on Drug Abuse, 2005), Available at www.nida.nih.gov/researchreports/prescription/prescription.html.

29. Substance Abuse and Mental Health Services Administration, Results from the 2008 National Survey on Drug Use and Health, 2009; Office of National Drug Control Policy, "Prescription Opioid-Related Deaths Increased 114 Percent from 2001 to 2005," 2009, Available at www.ondcp.gov/news/press09/052009.html.

30. Ibid.

31. National Center on Addiction and Substance Abuse at Columbia University, Wasting the Best and the Brightest: Substance Abuse at America's Colleges and Universities (New York: National Center on Addiction and Substance Abuse at Columbia University, 2007), Available at www.casacolumbia.org/templates/publications_reports.aspx.

32. Ibid.

33. D. L. Rabiner et al., "Motives and Perceived Consequences of Nonmedical ADHD Medication Use by College Students: Are Students Treating Themselves for Attention Problems?" Journal of Attention Disorders 13, no. 3 (2009): 259–70.

34. T. E. Wilens et al., "Misuse and Diversion of Stimulants Prescribed for ADHD: A Systematic Review of the Literature," Journal of the American Academy of Child and Adolescent Psychiatry 47, no. 1 (2008): 21–31.

35. Substance Abuse and Mental Health Services Administration, Results from the 2009 National Survey on Drug Use and Health: Volume I. Summary of National Findings, 2010.

36. L. D. Johnston et al., Monitoring the Future National Survey Results on Drug Use, 1975–2008, Volume II, College Students and Adults Ages 19–50, NIH Publication no. 09-7403 (Bethesda, MD: National Institute on Drug Abuse, 2009), Available at http://monitoringthefuture.org/pubs.html.

37. National Center on Addiction and Substance Abuse at Columbia University, Wasting the Best and the Brightest, 2007.

38. Ibid.

39. Ibid.
40. L. D. Johnston et al., *Monitoring the Future: National Survey Results on Drug Use, 1975–2010, Volume I,* 2011.
41. D. Schardt, "Caffeine: The Good, the Bad, and the Maybe," *Nutrition Action Healthletter* (March 2008): 1–7, Available at http://cspinet.org/nah/archives.html.
42. Office of National Drug Control Policy, "Marijuana Facts and Figures," 2010, Available at www.whitehousedrugpolicy.gov/drugfact/marijuana/marijuana_ff.html.
43. L. D. Johnston, et al., *Monitoring the Future: National Results on Adolescent Drug Use, Overview of Key Findings, 2010* (Ann Arbor, MI: Institute for Social Research, 2011).
44. U.S. Department of Health and Human Services, "Marijuana: Facts for Teens," 2010, Available at http://teens.drugabuse.gov/facts/facts_mj2.php.
45. National Institute on Drug Abuse, *Research Report: Marijuana Abuse,* NIH Publication no. 05-3859, 2005, Available at www.drugabuse.gov/ResearchReports/Marijuana; National Institute on Drug Abuse, "NIDA InfoFacts: Drugged Driving," 2009, Available at www.nida.nih.gov/infofacts/driving.html.
46. National Highway Traffic Safety Administration, "Drugs and Human Performance Fact Sheets: Cannabis/Marijuana," 2004, Available at www.nhtsa.gov/people/injury/research/job185drugs/cannabis.htm.
47. National Institute on Drug Abuse, "NIDA InfoFacts: Marijuana," Revised July 2009, Available at http://drugabuse.gov/infofacts/marijuana.html.
48. J. R. Daling et al., "Association of Marijuana Use and the Incidence of Testicular Germ Cell Tumors," *Cancer* 115, no. 6 (2009): 1215–23.
49. Ibid.
50. W. Hall and L. Degenhardt, "Adverse Health Effects of Non-Medical Cannabis Use," *The Lancet* 374, no. 9698 (2009): 1383–91.
51. Substance Abuse and Mental Health Services Administration, *Results from the 2009 National Survey on Drug Use and Health: National Findings,* 2010.
52. National Institute on Drug Abuse, *Marijuana: Facts Parents Need to Know,* NIH Publication no. 07-4036 (Rockville, MD: National Institutes of Health, 2007), Revised August 2007, Available at www.nida.nih.gov/marijbroch/marijparentsN.html.
53. Marijuana Policy Project, *State by State Medical Marijuana Laws: How to Remove the Threat of Arrest* (Washington, DC: Author, 2008).
54. Marijuana Policy Project, "Medical Marijuana Overview," 2009, Available at www.mpp.org/library/research/medical-marijuana-overview.html; ProCon.org, "Medical Marijuana," 2009, Available at http://medicalmarijuana.procon.org.
55. Substance Abuse and Mental Health Services Administration, *Results from the 2009 National Survey on Drug Use and Health: Volume I. Summary of National Findings,* 2010.
56. National Institute on Drug Abuse, "NIDA InfoFacts: Club Drugs (GHB, Ketamine, and Rohypnol)," Revised July 2010, Available at www.drugabuse.gov/infofacts/clubdrugs.html.
57. Substance Abuse and Mental Health Services Administration, *Results from the 2009 National Survey on Drug Use and Health: Volume I. Summary of National Findings,* 2010.
58. L. D. Johnston et al., *Monitoring the Future: National Survey Results on Drug Use, 1975–2008, Volume II, College Students and Adults Ages 19–50,* 2009.
59. National Institute on Drug Abuse, "NIDA InfoFacts: MDMA (Ecstasy)," Revised March 2010, Available at www.drugabuse.gov/infofacts/ecstasy.html.
60. National Collegiate Athletic Association, *NCAA Study of Substance Use of College Student-Athletes* (Indianapolis, IN: National College Athletic Association, 2006), Available at www.ncaa.org/wps/portal/ncaahome?WCM_GLOBAL_CONTEXT=/ncaa/ncaa/research/student-athlete+well-being/sa_substance_use.html.
61. Office of National Drug Control Policy, "Steroids Facts & Figures," 2010, Available at www.whitehousedrugpolicy.gov/drugfact/steroids/steroids_ff.html.
62. National Institute on Drug Abuse, NIDA for Teens, "Anabolic Steroids," 2010, Available at http://teens.drugabuse.gov/drnida/drnida_ster1.php.
63. Substance Abuse and Mental Health Services Administration, *Results from the 2009 National Survey on Drug Use and Health: Volume I. Summary of National Findings,* 2010.
64. U.S. Department of Justice, National Drug Intelligence Center, *National Drug Threat Assessment 2010,* 2010, Available at http://www.justice.gov/ndic/pubs38/38661/index.htm.
65. Butler Center for Research, *Research Update: Substance Use in the Workplace* (Center City, MN: Hazelden Foundation, 2009), Available at www.hazelden.org/web/public/researchupdates.page.
66. Ibid.

Chapter 7

1. Centers for Disease Control and Prevention, National Center for Health Statistics, *Health, United States, 2008, with Special Feature on the Health of Young Adults* (Hyattsville, MD: National Center for Health Statistics, 2009), Available at www.cdc.gov/nchs/data/hus/hus08.pdf; J. R. Pleis, J. W. Lucas, and B. W. Ward, "Summary Health Statistics for U.S. Adults: National Health Interview Survey, 2009, National Center for Health Statistics," *Vital and Health Statistics* 10, no. 242 (2010), Available at www.cdc.gov/nchs/products/series.htm.
2. R. LaVallee and H. Yi, "Apparent per Capita Alcohol Consumption: National, State, and Regional Trends, 1977–2008," Surveillance Report #90 (Bethesda, MD: National Institute on Alcohol Abuse and Alcoholism, 2010), Available at http://pubs.niaaa.nih.gov/publications/Surveillance90/CONS08.htm.
3. Committee on Reducing Tobacco Use: Strategies, Barriers, and Consequences, R. Bonnie, K. Stratton, and R. Wallace, eds., *Ending the Tobacco Problem, A Blueprint for the Nation* (Washington, DC: The National Academies of Press, 2007), Available at www.nap.edu/catalog.php?record_id=11795.
4. Centers for Disease Control and Prevention, *Tobacco Control State Highlights, 2010* (Atlanta: U.S. Department of Health and Human Services, Centers for Disease Control and Prevention, National Center for Chronic Disease Prevention and Health Promotion, Office on Smoking and Health, 2010), Available at www.cdc.gov/tobacco/data_statistics/state_data/state_highlights/2010/index.htm.
5. American Cancer Society, "Cigarette Smoking," Revised November 2010, Available at www.cancer.org/docroot/ped/content/ped_10_2x_cigarette_smoking.asp.
6. American College Health Association, *American College Health Association—National College Health Assessment II: Reference Group Executive Summary Fall 2010* (Linthicum, MD: American College Health Association, 2011), Available at www.acha-ncha.org/reports_ACHA-NCHAII.html.
7. U.S. Department of Health and Human Services, National Institute on Alcohol Abuse and Alcoholism, "What Colleges Need to Know: An Update on College Drinking Research," NIH Publication no. 07-5010, November 2007, Available at www.collegedrinkingprevention.gov.
8. American College Health Association, *American College Health Association—National College Health Assessment II: Reference Group Executive Summary Fall 2010,* 2011.
9. Ibid.
10. R. Hingson et al., "Magnitude of Alcohol-Related Mortality and Morbidity among U.S. College Students Ages 18–24: Changes from 1998 to 2005," *Journal of Studies on Alcohol and Drugs* (2009): 12–20.
11. R. R. Wetherill et al., "Perceived Awareness and Caring Influences Alcohol Use by High School and College Students," *Psychology of Addictive Behaviors* 21, no. 2 (2007): 147–54.
12. L. D. Johnston, et al., *Monitoring the Future National Survey Results on Drug Use 1975–2010 Volume II: College Students and Adults Ages 19–50* (Ann Arbor, MI: Institute for Social Research, 2011).
13. J. W. Labrie et al., "What Men Want: The Role of Reflective Opposite-Sex Normative Preferences in Alcohol Use among College Women," *Psychology of Addictive Behavior* 23, no. 1 (2009): 157–62.
14. J. Reingle et al., "An Exploratory Study of Bar and Nightclub Expectancies," *Journal of American College Health* 57, no. 6 (2009): 629–38.
15. E. Allen and M. Madden, *Hazing in View: College Students at Risk* (Orono, ME: National Collaborative for Hazing Research and Prevention, 2008), Available at www.hazingstudy.org.
16. R. J. O'Mara et al., "Alcohol Price and Intoxication in College Bars," *Journal on Studies of Alcohol* 33, no. 11 (2009): 1973–80.
17. National Center on Addiction and Substance Abuse at Columbia University, *Wasting the Best and the Brightest: Substance Abuse at America's Colleges and Universities* (New York: National Center on Addiction and Substance Abuse at Columbia University, March 2007), Available at www.casacolumbia.org/templates/publications_reports.aspx.
18. S. Wells et al., "Policy Implications of the Widespread Practice of 'Pre-drinking' or 'Pre-gaming' before Going to Public Drinking Establishments—Are Current Prevention Strategies Backfiring?" *Addiction* 104 (2008): 4–9.
19. National Institute on Alcohol Abuse and Alcoholism, "College Drinking: A Snapshot of Annual High-Risk College Drinking Consequences," Reviewed July 2010, Available at www.collegedrinkingprevention.gov/StatsSummaries/snapshot.aspx.
20. R. Hingson et al., "Magnitude of Alcohol-Related Mortality and Morbidity," 2008.
21. The Higher Education Center for Alcohol, Drug Abuse, and Violence Prevention, *Sexual Violence and Alcohol and Other Drug Use on Campus* (Newton, MA: The Higher Education Center for Alcohol, Drug Abuse, and Violence Prevention, 2008), Available at www.higheredcenter.org/services/publications/sexual-violence-and-alcohol-and-other-drug-use-campus.
22. U.S. Department of Health and Human Services, National Institute on Alcohol Abuse and Alcoholism, "What Colleges Need to Know," 2007; T. Nelson, et al., "Implementation of NIAAA College Drinking Task Force Recommendations: How Are

Colleges Doing 6 Years Later?" *Alcoholism: Clinical and Experimental Research* 34, no. 10 (2010): 1–7.

23. American College Health Association, *American College Health Association—National College Health Assessment II: Reference Group Executive Summary Fall 2010*, 2011.

24. D. L. Thombs et al., "Event-level Analyses of Energy Drink Consumption and Alcohol Intoxication in Bar Patrons," *Addictive Behaviors* 35, no. 4 (2010): 325–30.

25. Center for Science in the Public Interest, "Alcohol Policies Project Fact Sheet: Alcoholic Energy Drinks," Updated September 2008, Available at www.cspinet.org/booze/fctindex.htm.

26. M. C. O'Brien et al., "Caffeinated Cocktails: Energy Drink Consumption, High-Risk Drinking, and Alcohol-Related Consequences among College Students," *Society for Academic Emergency Medicine* 15 (2008): 1–8.

27. Substance Abuse and Mental Health Services Administration (SAMHSA), *Drug Abuse Warning Network, 2009: Selected Tables of National Estimates of Drug-Related Emergency Department Visits* (Rockville, MD: Office of Applied Studies, SAMHSA, 2010), Available at https://dawninfo.samhsa.gov/data.

28. J. Turner et al., "Serious Health Consequences Associated with Alcohol Use among College Students: Demographic and Clinical Characteristics of Patients Seen in the Emergency Department," *Journal of Studies on Alcohol* 65, no. 2 (2004): 179.

29. S. MacDonald, "The Criteria for Causation of Alcohol in Violent Injuries in Six Countries," *Addictive Behaviors* 30, no. 1 (2005): 103–13.

30. Turner et al., "Serious Health Consequences Associated with Alcohol Use among College Students," 2004.

31. Centers for Disease Control and Prevention, "Injury Prevention and Control: Home and Recreational Safety: Unintentional Drowning: Fact Sheet," Updated June 2010, Available at www.cdc.gov/HomeandRecreationalSafety/Water-Safety/waterinjuries-factsheet.html; Centers for Disease Control and Prevention, "Injury Prevention and Control: Home and Recreational Safety: Fire Deaths and Injuries: Fact Sheet," Updated October 2009, Available at www.cdc.gov/HomeandRecreationalSafety/Fire-Prevention/fires-factsheet.html.

32. L. Sher, "Alcohol Consumption and Suicide," *QJM: An International Journal of Medicine* 99, no. 1 (2006): 57–61; Bureau of Justice Statistics, "Criminal Victimization in the United States, Table 32, Percent Distribution of victimizations by perceived drug or alcohol use by offender, 2007," Accessed June 2010, Available at http://bjs.ojp.usdoj.gov/content/pub/html/cvus/alcohol.cfm.

33. K. Butler, "The Grim Neurology of Teenage Drinking," *New York Times* (July 4, 2006).

34. R. W. Hingson et al., "Age at Drinking Onset and Alcohol Dependence," *Archives of Pediatric and Adolescent Medicine* 160 (2006): 739–46.

35. J. Theruvathu et al., "Polyamines Stimulate the Formation of Mutagenic 1, N2-Propanodeoxyguanosine Adducts from Acetaldehyde," *Nucleic Acids Research* 33, no. 11 (2005): 3513–20.

36. American Association for Cancer Research, "Excessive Alcohol Drinking Can Lead to Increased Risk of Breast Cancer, Study Suggests," *Science Daily*, April 14, 2008, Available at www.sciencedaily.com/releases/2008/04/080413173510

.htm; National Institute on Alcohol Abuse and Alcoholism, *Alcohol: A Women's Health Issue,* NIH Publication no. 03-4956 (Bethesda, MD: National Institutes of Health, revised 2008), Available at www.niaaa.nih.gov/Publications/PamphletsBrochuresPosters/English/Pages/default.aspx.

37. C. S. Berkey et al., "Prospective Study of Adolescent Alcohol Consumption and Risk of Benign Breast Disease in Young Women," *Pediatrics* 125, no. 5 (2010): e1081–e1087.

38. Centers for Disease Control and Prevention, "Alcohol Use among Pregnant and Nonpregnant Women of Childbearing Age—United States, 1991–2005," *Morbidity and Mortality Weekly* 58, no. 19 (2009): 529–32.

39. Centers for Disease Control and Prevention, "Fetal Alcohol Spectrum Disorders (FASDs) Data and Statistics," Updated May 2010, Available at www.cdc.gov/ncbddd/fasd/data.html.

40. Ibid.

41. Centers for Disease Control and Prevention, "Injury Mortality: Unintentional Injury: US 2001–2006," 2009, Available at http://205.207.175.93/HDI/TableViewer/tableView.aspx?ReportId=71.

42. National Highway Traffic Safety Administration, "Traffic Safety Facts Annual Report 2009 Early Edition," DOT HS 811 402, 2009, Available at www-nrd.nhtsa.dot.gov/CATS/index.aspx.

43. American College Health Association, *American College Health Association—National College Health Assessment II: Reference Group Data Report Fall 2010*, 2011.

44. Ibid.

45. A. Quinn-Zobeck, *Screening and Brief Intervention Tool Kit for College and University Campuses,* (U.S. Department of Transportation, National Highway Traffic Safety Administration [NHTSA] with The BACCHUS Network: Washington, DC, 2007) DOT HS 810 751, page 14, Available at www.stopimpaireddriving.org/3672Toolkit/index.htm.

46. Insurance Institute for Highway Safety, "Fatality Facts 2009: Alcohol," 2010, Available at www.iihs.org/research/fatality_facts_2009/alcohol.html.

47. Ibid.

48. Ibid.

49. National Institutes of Health, Medline Plus, "Alcoholism and Alcohol Abuse," Updated April 2010, Available at www.nlm.nih.gov/medlineplus/ency/article/000944.htm.

50. J. Knight et al., "Alcohol Abuse and Dependence among U.S. College Students," *Journal of Studies on Alcohol* 63, no. 3 (2002): 263–70.

51. C. A. Presley et al., "The Introduction of the Heavy and Frequent Drinker: A Proposed Classification to Increase Accuracy of Alcohol Assessments in Postsecondary Education Settings," *Journal of Alcohol Studies on Alcohol* 67 (2006): 324–31.

52. W. R. Lovallo et al., "Working Memory and Decision-Making Biases in Young Adults with a Family History of Alcoholism: Studies from the Oklahoma Family Health Patterns Project," *Alcoholism: Clinical & Experimental Research* 30, no. 5 (2006): 763–73; National Institute on Alcohol Abuse and Alcoholism, U.S. Department of Health and Human Services, *A Family History of Alcoholism: Are You at Risk?* NIH Publication no. 03–5340 (Bethesda, MD: National Institute on Alcohol Abuse and Alcoholism, 2007), Available at www.niaaa.nih.gov/Publications/PamphletsBrochuresPosters/English/Pages/default.aspx.

53. C. Wilson and J. Knight, "When Parents Have a Drinking Problem," *Contemporary Pediatrics* 18, no. 1 (January 2001): 67.

54. A. Agrawal and M. T. Lynskey, "Are There Genetic Influences on Addiction? Evidence from Family, Adoption and Twin Studies," *Addiction* 103 (2008): 1069–81.

55. C. Wilson and J. Knight, "When Parents Have a Drinking Problem," 2001.

56. J. Niels Rosenquist et al., "The Spread of Alcohol Consumption Behavior in a Large Social Network," *Annals of Internal Medicine* 152, no. 7 (2010): 426–33.

57. Claudia Black, "Children of Addiction," The Many Faces of Addiction Blog, *Psychology Today*, February 8, 2010, Available at www.psychologytoday.com/blog/the-many-faces-addiction/201002/children-addiction.

58. Ensuring Solutions to Alcohol Problems, *Workplace Screening & Brief Intervention: What Employers Can and Should Do about Excessive Alcohol Use* (The George Washington University Medical Center: Washington, DC, March 2008), Available at www.jointogether.org/resources/2008/workplace-sbi.html.

59. Ibid.

60. Pacific Institute of Research and Evaluation, Underage Drinking Costs," 2009, Available at www.udetc.org/UnderageDrinkingCosts.asp.

61. Ibid.

62. National Institute on Alcohol Abuse and Alcoholism, *Alcohol: A Women's Health Issue,* 2008.

63. National Institute on Drug Abuse, "Info Facts: Treatment Methods for Women," Updated 2009, Available at www.drugabuse.gov/infofacts/treatwomen.html.

64. E. Cohen et al., "Alcohol Treatment Utilization: Findings from the National Epidemiologic Survey on Alcohol and Related Conditions," *Drug and Alcohol Dependence* 86, nos. 2–3 (2007): 214–21.

65. Substance Abuse and Mental Health Administration (SAMHSA), *Results from the 2009 National Survey on Drug Use and Health* (Rockville, MD: Office of Applied Studies, 2010), Available at http://oas.samhsa.gov/NSDUH/2k9NSDUH/2k9Results.htm.

66. Centers for Disease Control and Prevention, "Cigarette Smoking among Adults and Trends in Smoking Cessation—United States 2008," *Morbidity and Mortality Weekly Report* 58, no. 44 (2009): 1227–32.

67. Centers for Disease Control and Prevention, *Tobacco Control State Highlights, 2010* (Atlanta: U.S. Department of Health and Human Services, Centers for Disease Control and Prevention, National Center for Chronic Disease Prevention and Health Promotion, Office on Smoking and Health, 2010), Available at www.cdc.gov/tobacco/data_statistics/state_data/state_highlights/2010/index.htm.

68. A. Agrawal et al., "Are There Genetic Influences on Addiction? Evidence from Family, Adoption and Twin Studies," *Addiction* 103, no. 7 (2008): 1069–81.

69. W. Hall, "Will Nicotine Genetics and a Nicotine Vaccine Prevent Cigarette Smoking and Smoking-Related Diseases?" *PLoS Med* 2, no. 9 (2005): e266.

70. National Institute on Drug Abuse, "Topics in Brief: Tobacco and Nicotine Research," Updated August 2008, Available at www.drugabuse.gov/tib/tobnico.html.

71. G. Gutierrez, "Nicotine Creates Stronger Memories, Cues to Drug Use," Modified September

2009, Available at www.bcm.edu/news/packages/nicotine.cfm.

72. Campaign for Tobacco-Free Kids, "Tobacco Company Marketing to Kids," 2010, Available at www.tobaccofreekids.org/research/factsheets.

73. Centers for Disease Control and Prevention, "Cigarette Brand Preference among Middle and High School Students Who Are Established Smokers—United States, 2004 and 2006," *Morbidity and Mortality Weekly* 58, no. 5 (2009): 112–15.

74. Campaign for Tobacco-Free Kids, "Toll of Tobacco in the United States of America," January 2010, Available at www.tobaccofreekids.org/research/factsheets.

75. Campaign for Tobacco-Free Kids, *Big Tobacco's Guinea Pigs: How an Unregulated Industry Experiments on America's Kids and Consumers* (Washington, DC: Campaign for Tobacco-Free Kids, 2008), Available at www.tobaccofreekids.org/reports/products.

76. Centers for Disease Control and Prevention, *Tobacco Control State Highlights, 2010,* 2010; Centers for Disease Control and Prevention, "Smoking-Attributable Mortality, Years of Potential Life Lost, and Productivity Losses, 2000–2004," *Morbidity and Mortality Weekly Report* 57, no. 45 (2008): 1226–28.

77. Reuters, "U.S. Would Reap Billions from $1 Cigarette Tax Hike," February 10, 2010, Available at www.reuters.com/article/idUSTRE6194SD20100210.

78. American College Health Association, *American College Health Association–National College Health Assessment II: Reference Group Data Report, Fall 2010,* 2011.

79. National Center on Addiction and Substance Abuse at Columbia University, *Wasting the Best and the Brightest,* 2007.

80. American College Health Association, *American College Health Association–National College Health Assessment II: Reference Group Data Report, Fall 2010,* 2011.

81. National Center on Addiction and Substance Abuse at Columbia University, *Wasting the Best and the Brightest,* 2007.

82. Ibid.

83. Ibid.

84. L. Stoner et al., "Occasional Cigarette Smoking Chronically Affects Arterial Function," *Ultrasound in Medicine and Biology* 34, no. 12 (2008): 1885–92.

85. L. An et al., "Symptoms of Cough and Shortness of Breath among Occasional Young Adult Smokers," *Nicotine & Tobacco Research* 11, no. 2 (2009): 126–33.

86. Stop Smoking! "Smoking and Birth Control Pills Are Not Made for Each Other," May 8, 2010, Available at www.stop-smoking-updates.com/quitsmoking/smoking-factsheet/facts/smoking-and-birth-control-pills-are-not-made-for-each-other.htm.

87. National Center on Addiction and Substance Abuse at Columbia University, *Wasting the Best and the Brightest,* 2007.

88. Ibid.

89. N. Rigotti et al., "U.S. College Students' Exposure to Tobacco Promotions: Prevalence and Association with Tobacco Use," *American Journal of Public Health* 94, no. 12 (2004): 1–7.

90. U.S. Department of Health and Human Services, *The Health Consequences of Involuntary Exposure to Tobacco Smoke: A Report of the Surgeon General* (Atlanta, GA: U.S. Department of Health and Human Services, Centers for Disease Control and Prevention, Coordinating Center for Health Promotion, National Center for Chronic Disease Prevention and Health Promotion, Office on Smoking and Health, 2006), Available at www.surgeongeneral.gov/library/secondhandsmoke; National Toxicology Program, *Report on Carcinogens,* 11th ed. (Rockville, MD: U.S. Department of Health and Human Services, Public Health Service, National Toxicology Program, 2005).

91. American Cancer Society, "Cigar Smoking: Who Smokes Cigars?" Revised July 2010, Available at www.cancer.org/Cancer/CancerCauses/TobaccoCancer/CigarSmoking/cigar-smoking-who-smokes-cigars.

92. Ibid.

93. American Cancer Society, "Questions about Smoking, Tobacco, and Health: What about More Exotic Forms of Smoking Tobacco, Such as Clove Cigarettes, Bidis, and Hookahs?" Revised July 2010, Available at www.cancer.org/Cancer/CancerCauses/TobaccoCancer/QuestionsaboutSmokingTobaccoandHealth/questions-about-smoking-tobacco-and-health-other-forms-of-smoking.

94. Centers for Disease Control and Prevention, "Smoking and Tobacco Use: Bidis and Kreteks," Updated May 2009, Available at www.cdc.gov/tobacco/data_statistics/fact_sheets/tobacco_industry/bidis_kreteks.

95. Ibid.

96. Centers for Disease Control and Prevention, "Smoking and Tobacco Use: Smokeless Tobacco Facts," March 2011, Available at www.cdc.gov/tobacco/data_statistics/fact_sheets/smokeless/smokeless_facts/index.htm.

97. American College Health Association, *American College Health Association–National College Health Assessment II: Reference Group Data Report 2010,* 2011.

98. W. Dunham, "Chewing Tobacco Use Surges among Boys," Reuters, March 25, 2009, Available at www.reuters.com/article/idUSTRE5240WJ20090305.

99. Centers for Disease Control and Prevention, "Smoking-Attributable Mortality, Years of Potential Life Lost, and Productivity Losses, 2000–2004," *Morbidity and Mortality Weekly Report* 57, no. 45 (2008):1226–1228.

100. American Cancer Society, *Cancer Facts & Figures 2010,* 2010.

101. Ibid.

102. Ibid.

103. Ibid.

104. Ibid.

105. American Heart Association, *Heart Disease and Stroke Statistics—2010 Update* (Dallas: American Heart Association, 2010), Available at www.americanheart.org/presenter.jhtml?identifier=3000090.

106. Ibid.

107. American Heart Association, "Stroke Risk Factors," 2010, Available at www.americanheart.org/presenter.jhtml?identifier=4716.

108. American Lung Association, "Benefits of Quitting," Available at www.lungusa.org/stop-smoking/how-to-quit/why-quit/benefits-of-quitting.

109. American Cancer Society, *Cancer Facts & Figures, 2010,* 2010.

110. John Hopkins Health Alerts, "Emphysema: Symptoms and Remedies," Available at www.johnshopkinshealthalerts.com/symptoms_remedies/emphysema/96-1.html.

111. National Kidney and Neurological Diseases Information Clearing House, "Erectile Dysfunction," NIH Publication no. 06–3923, December 2005, Available at http://kidney.niddk.nih.gov/kudiseases/pubs/impotence.

112. Centers for Disease Control and Prevention, "Pregnant? Don't Smoke!" Updated March 2011, Available at www.cdc.gov/Features/PregnantDontSmoke.

113. Centers for Disease Control and Prevention, "Tobacco Use and Pregnancy," Modified January 2011, Available at www.cdc.gov/reproductivehealth/TobaccoUsePregnancy/index.htm.

114. American Academy of Periodontology, "Tobacco Use and Periodontal Disease," 2010, Available at www.perio.org/consumer/smoking.htm.

115. American Academy of Neurology, "Alzheimer's Starts Earlier for Heavy Drinkers, Smokers," Press Release, April 16, 2008, Available at www.aan.com/press/index.cfm?fuseaction=release.view&release=594.

116. American Cancer Society, "Secondhand Smoke," Revised November 2010, Available at www.cancer.org/docroot/ped/content/ped_10_2x_secondhand_smoke-clean_indoor_air.asp.

117. Centers for Disease Control and Prevention, "Smoking and Tobacco Use Fact Sheet: Secondhand Smoke," Updated March 2011, Available at www.cdc.gov/tobacco/data_statistics/fact_sheets/secondhand_smoke/general_facts/index.htm.

118. Ibid.

119. Ibid.

120. U.S. Department of Health and Human Services, *The Health Consequences of Involuntary Exposure to Tobacco Smoke,* 2006; American Cancer Society, "Secondhand Smoke," 2010.

121. Ibid.

122. Ibid.

123. Ibid.

124. S. Leatherdale et al., "Second-Hand Exposure in Homes and in Cars among Canadian Youth: Current Prevalence, Beliefs about Exposure, and Changes between 2004–2006," *Cancer Causes & Control* 20, no. 6 (2009): 1573–1625.

125. K. Yolton et al., "Exposure to Environmental Tobacco Smoke and Cognitive Abilities among U.S. Children and Adolescents," *Environmental Health Perspectives* 113, no. 1 (2005): 9–103.

126. M. R. Becklake et al., "Childhood Predictors of Smoking in Adolescence: A Follow-Up Study of Montreal School Children," *Canadian Medical Association Journal* 173, no. 4 (2005): 377–79.

127. O. Shafey, M. Eriksen, H. Ross, and J. Mackay, "Secondhand Smoking," chap. 9 in *The Tobacco Atlas,* 3d ed. (Atlanta: American Cancer Society, 2009), Available at www.cancer.org/aboutus/GlobalHealth/CancerandTobaccoControlResources/the-tobacco-atlas-3rd-edition.

128. Centers for Disease Control and Prevention, *Tobacco Control State Highlights, 2010,* 2010.

129. M. Fogarty, "Public Health and Smoking Cessation," *Scientist* 17, no. 6 (2003): 23.

130. *Family Smoking Prevention and Tobacco Control Act of 2009,* HR 1256, 111th Congress of the United States of America, Available at www.govtrack.us/congress/billtext.xpd?bill=h111-1256.

131. M. C. Fiore et al., *Treating Tobacco Use and Dependence: 2008 Update. Clinical Practice Guideline* (Rockville, MD: U.S. Department of Health and Human Services. Public Health Service, May 2008), Available at www.surgeongeneral.gov/tobacco; U.S. Department of Health and Human Services, "Effective Strategies for Tobacco Cessation Underused, Panel Says," National Institutes of Health News Press Release, June 2006, Available at www.nih.gov/news/pr/jun2006/od-14.htm.

132. American Cancer Society, "Guide to Quitting Smoking: A Word about Quitting Success Rates," Revised July 2010, Available at www .cancer.org/Healthy/StayAwayfromTobacco/ GuidetoQuittingSmoking/guide-to-quitting- smoking-success-rates.

133. V. Willingham, "Nicotine Vaccine Effective in Early Tests," CNN Health, April 22, 2010, Avail- able at www.cnn.com/2010/HEALTH/04/21/ nicotine.vaccine.nicvax/index.html.

Chapter 8

1. U.S. Department of Agriculture and U.S. Depart- ment of Health and Human Services, *Dietary Guidelines for Americans, 2010*, 7th ed. (Wash- ington, DC: U.S. Government Printing Office, December 2010).

2. D. Negoianu and S. Goldfarb, "Just Add Water," *Journal of the American Society of Nephrology* 19, no. 6 (2008): 1041–43; E. Jéquier and F. Constant, "Water as an Essential Nutrient: The Physiological Basis of Hydration," *European Journal of Clinical Nutrition* 64, no. 2 (2010): 115–23.

3. Institute of Medicine of the National Academies, Food and Nutrition Board, *Dietary Reference Intakes for Water, Potassium, Sodium, Chloride, and Sulfate* (Washington, DC: The National Acad- emies Press, 2004), Available at http://iom.edu/ Reports/2004/Dietary-Reference-Intakes-Water- Potassium-Sodium-Chloride-and-Sulfate.aspx.

4. ACSM, "Exercise and Fluid Replacement," *Medi- cine and Science in Sports and Exercise* 39, no. 2 (2007): 377–90.

5. Sierra Club, "Bottled Water: Learning the Facts and Taking Action," 2008, Available at www .sierraclub.org/committees/cac/water/bottled_ water/bottled_water.pdf.

6. Oregon State University, "Bottled Water Boom Has Environmental Drawbacks," Media release, 2007, Available at http://oregonstate.edu/dept/ ncs/newsarch/2007/May07/bottledwater.html; J. Rodwan Jr., "Bottled Water Statistic 2009: Challenging Circumstances Persist: U.S. and In- ternational Developments and Statistics," *Bottled Water Reporter* 50, no. 3 (2010): 10–16, Available at www.bottledwater.org/content/455/bottled- water-reporter.

7. Sierra Club, "Bottled Water," 2008.

8. U.S. Department of Agriculture, Agricultural Research Service, Beltsville Human Nutrition Research Center, Food Surveys Research Group (Beltsville, MD) and U.S. Department of Health and Human Services, Centers for Disease Control and Prevention, National Center for Health Statistics (Hyattsville, MD), *What We Eat in America, NHANES 2007–2008, Data: Table 1. Nutrient Intakes from Food: Mean Amounts Con- sumed per Individual by Gender and Age, in the United States, 2007–2008*, Revised August 2010, Available at www.ars.usda.gov/Services/docs .htm?docid=18349.

9. Institute of Medicine of the National Academies, "Dietary, Functional, and Total Fiber," in *Dietary Reference Intakes for Energy, Carbohydrate, Fiber, Fat, Fatty Acids, Cholesterol, Protein, and Amino Acids* (Washington, DC: The National Academies Press, 2005), 339–421, Available at www.nap.edu/ openbook.php?isbn=0309085373.

10. L. Hanson, et al., "Intake of Dietary Fiber, Especially from Cereal Foods, Is Associated with Lower Incidence of Colon Cancer in the HELGA Cohort," *International Journal of Cancer* (2011) DOI: 10.1002/ijc.26381.

11. K. Maki et al., "Whole-Grain Ready-to-Eat Oat Cereal, as Part of a Dietary Program for Weight Loss, Reduces Low-Density Lipoprotein Cho- lesterol in Adults with Overweight an d Obesity More than a Dietary Program Including Low-Fiber Control Foods," *Journal of the American Dietetic Association* 110, no. 2 (2010): 205–14.

12. P. Nijjar, et al., "Role of Dietary Supplements in Lowering Low-Density Lipoprotein Cholesterol: A Review," *Journal of Clinical Lipidology* 4, no. 4 (2010): 248–258.

13. E. J. Brunner et al., "Dietary Patterns and 15 Year Risks of Major Coronary Events, Diabetes and Mortality," *American Journal of Clinical Nutrition* 87, no. 5 (2008): 1414–21.

14. P. Newby et al., "Intake of Whole Grains, Refined Grains and Cereal Fiber Measured with 7-d Diet Records and Associations with Risk Factors for Chronic Disease," *American Journal of Clinical Nutrition* 86, no. 6 (2007): 1745–53.

15. D. Mozaffarian et al., "Effects on Coronary Heart Disease of Increasing Polyunsaturated Fat in Place of Saturated Fat: A Systematic Review and Meta- Analysis of Randomized Controlled Trials," *PLoS Med* 7, no. 3 (2010): e1000252; N. D. Riediger et al., "A Systemic Review of the Roles of n-3 Fatty Acids in Health and Disease," *Journal of the American Dietetic Association* 109 (2009): 668–79; B. McKevith, "Review: Nutritional Aspects of Oil- seeds," *Nutrition Bulletin* 30, no. 1 (2005): 13–14.

16. P. M. Kris-Etherton, W. S. Harris, and L. J. Appel, "Fish Consumption, Fish Oil, Omega-3 Fatty Acids, and Cardiovascular Disease," *Circulation* 106, no. 21 (2002): 2747–57.

17. W. Harris et al., "Omega-6 Fatty Acids and Risk for Cardiovascular Disease," *Circulation* 119 (2009): 902–907.

18. P. McKeigue, "*Trans* Fatty Acids and Coronary Heart Disease: Weighing the Evidence against Hardened Fat," *Lancet* 345, no. 8945 (1995): 269–70; W. C. Willwett et al., "Intake of *Trans* Fatty Acids and Risk of Coronary Heart Disease among Women," *Lancet* 341, no. 8845 (1993): 581–85.

19. W. Willett and D. Mozaffarian, "*Trans* Fats in Cardiac and Diabetes Risk: An Overview," *Cur- rent Cardiovascular Risk Reports* 1, no. 1 (2007): 16–23; S. E. Chiuve et al., "Intake of Total *Trans*, *Trans*-18:1, and *Trans*-18:2 Fatty Acids and Risk of Sudden Cardiac Death in Women," *American Heart Journal* 158, no. 5 (2009): 761–67; D. Mo- zaffarian et al., "*Trans* Fatty Acids and Cardiovas- cular Disease," *New England Journal of Medicine* 354 (2006): 1601–13.

20. C. Scott-Thomas, "Californian Trans Fat Ban Takes Effect," FoodNavigator-USA.com, January 4, 2010, Available at www.foodnavigator-usa.com/ Legislation/Californian-trans-fat-ban-takes-effect.

21. F. Sacks et al., "Comparison of Weight-Loss Diets with Different Compositions of Fat, Protein, and Carbohydrates," *New England Journal of Medicine* 360, no. 9 (2009): 859–73; M. Hession et al., "Systematic Review of Randomized Controlled Trials of Low-Carbohydrate vs. Low-fat/Low-cal- orie Diets in the Management of Obesity and its Comorbidities," *Obesity Reviews* 10, no. 1 (2008): 36–50.

22. U.S. Department of Agriculture, Economic Research Service, "U.S. Per Capita Loss-Adjusted Food Availability: Total Calories," Updated Febru- ary 2010, Available at www.ers.usda.gov/Data/ FoodConsumption/app/reports/displayCom- modities.aspx?reportName=Total+Calories&id= 36#startForm.

23. U.S. Department of Agriculture, Center for Nutrition Policy and Promotion, "Development of the 2010 *Dietary Guidelines*," Modified July 2010, Available at www.cnpp.usda.gov/ DietaryGuidelines.htm.

24. U.S. Department of Agriculture, "Dietary Guide- lines for Americans 2010, " Available at www .cnpp.usda.gov/dietaryguidelines.htm.

25. U.S. Department of Agriculture, Center for Nutri- tion Policy and Promotion, "10 Tips to a Great Plate," June 2011, Available at www.choosemyplate .gov/downloads/. TenTips/DGTipsheet1ChooseMyPlate.pdf.

26. B. Black, "Health Library: Just How Much Food Is on That Plate? Understanding Portion Control," Last reviewed February 2009, EBSCO Publishing, Available at www.ebscohost.com/healthLibrary.

27. "How Many Vegetarians Are There?" Vegetarian Resource Group, Press release, May 15, 2009, Available at www.vrg.org/press/2009poll.htm.

28. "Vegetarian Times Study Shows 7.3 Million Americans Are Vegetarians," *Vegetarian Times*, Press release, April 15, 2008, Available at www .vegetariantimes.com/features/667.

29. American Dietetic Association, "Position of the American Dietetic Association: Vegetarian Diets," *Journal of the American Dietetic Association* 109, no. 7 (2009): 1266–82.

30. K. M. Fairfield and R. H. Fletcher, "Vitamins for Chronic Disease Prevention in Adults: Scientific Review," *Journal of the American Medical Associa- tion* 287, no. 23 (2001): 3116–26.

31. "NIH State-of-the-Science Conference Statement on Multivitamin/Mineral Supplements and Chronic Disease Prevention," *Annals of Internal Medicine* 145, no. 5 (2006): 364–71.

32. A. L. Rogovik, S. Vohra, and R. D. Goldman, "Safety Considerations and Potential Interactions of Vitamins: Should Vitamins Be Considered Drugs?" *Annals of Pharmacotherapy* 44, no. 2 (2010): 311–24.

33. U.S. Department of Agriculture, Economic Research Services, "Organic Agriculture: Organic Market Overview," 2009, Available at www .ers.usda.gov/briefing/organic/demand.htm.

34. Iowa State University, "Food Irradiation: What Is It?" *Iowa State University Extension Newsletter*, Revised August 2006, Available at www.extension .iastate.edu/foodsafety/irradiation.

35. U.S. Department of Agriculture, Economic Research Service, "Adoption of Genetically Engineered Crops in the U.S.," Updated July 2010, Available at www.ers.usda.gov/Data/BiotechCrops.

36. Ibid.

37. A. Coghlan, "Engineered Maize Toxicity Claims Roundly Rebuffed," *New Scientist* 2744 (January 22, 2010).

38. A. Bakshi, "Potential Adverse Health Effects of Genetically Modified Crops," *Journal of Toxicology and Environmental Health Part B: Critical Reviews* 6, no. 3 (2003): 211–25.

39. World Health Organization, "20 Questions on Genetically Modified Foods," Accessed April 2010, Available at www.who.int/foodsafety/ publications/biotech/20questions/en.

40. A. M. Branum and S. L. Lukacs, "Food Allergy among U.S. Children: Trends in Prevalence and Hospitalizations," *National Center for Health Statistics Data Brief*, no 10. (Hyattsville, MD: National Center for Health Statistics, 2008).

41. Food Allergy and Anaphylaxis Network, "Food Allergy Facts and Statistics," 2008, Available at www.foodallergy.org/section/helpful-information.

42. Food Allergy and Anaphylaxis Network, "Advocacy: FALCPA FAQ," 2010, Available at www.foodallergy.org/page/falcpa-faq.

43. University of Chicago Celiac Disease Center, "Celiac Disease Facts and Figures," 2010, Available at www.celiacdisease.net/factsheets.

44. National Center for Infectious Diseases, Division of Bacterial and Mycotic Diseases, "Food-Borne Illnesses," Updated December 2010, Available at www.cdc.gov/ncidod/dbmd/diseaseinfo/foodborneinfections_g.htm.

45. Centers for Disease Control and Prevention, "Preliminary FoodNet Data on the Incidence of Infection with Pathogens Transmitted Commonly through Food—10 States, 2008," *Morbidity and Mortality Weekly Report* 58, no. 13 (April 10, 2009): 333–37.

46. National Center for Infectious Diseases, Division of Bacterial and Mycotic Diseases, "Food-Borne Illnesses," 2010.

47. Centers for Disease Control and Prevention, "Preliminary FoodNet Data on the Incidence of Infection with Pathogens Transmitted Commonly Through Food," 2009.

48. National Center for Infectious Diseases, Division of Bacterial and Mycotic Diseases, "E. Coli," Modified March 2010, Available at www.cdc.gov/ecoli; Centers for Disease Control and Prevention, "Preliminary FoodNet Data on the Incidence of Infection with Pathogens Transmitted Commonly through Food," 2009.

Chapter 9

1. U.S. Department of Health and Human Services, *Surgeon General's Call to Action to Prevent and Decrease Overweight and Obesity* (Washington, DC: USOHHS, 2005), Available at www.surgeongeneral.gov/topics/obesity/calltoaction/toc.htm.

2. J. Spence et al., "Relation between Local Food Environments and Obesity among Adults," *BMC Public Health* 9, no. 1 (2009): 192.

3. Centers for Disease Control and Prevention, "Obesity: Halting the Epidemic by Making Health Easier," 2009, Available at www.cdc.gov/chronicdisease/resources/publications/aag/pdf/obesity.pdf.

4. U.S. Department of Health and Human Services, *The Surgeon General's Vision for a Healthy and Fit Nation* (Rockville, MD: U.S. Department of Health and Human Services, Office of the Surgeon General, 2010), Available at www.surgeongeneral.gov/library/obesityvision.

5. K. M. Flegal et al., "Prevalence and Trends in Obesity among U.S. Adults, 1999–2008," *Journal of the American Medical Association* 303, no. 3 (2010): 235–41.

6. Ibid.

7. S. Steward et al., "Forecasting the Effects of Obesity and Smoking on U.S. Life Expectancy," *New England Journal of Medicine* 361, no. 23 (2009): 2252–60.

8. S. Anderson and R. Whitaker, "Prevalence of Obesity among U.S. Preschool Children in Different Racial and Ethnic Groups," *Archives of Pediatrics and Adolescent Medicine* 163, no. 4 (2009): 344–48.

9. C. Ogden, "Disparities in Obesity Prevalence in the United States: Black Women at Risk," *American Journal of Clinical Nutrition* 89, no. 4 (2009): 1001–02.

10. C. Ogden et al., "Prevalence of High Body Mass Index in U.S. Children and Adolescents, 2007–2008," *JAMA: The Journal of the American Medical Association* 303, no. 3 (2010): 242–49.

11. World Health Organization, *The World Health Report 2006: Working Together for Health* (Geneva, World Health Organization, 2006).

12. K. M. Flegal and B. I. Graubard, "Estimates of Excess Deaths Associated with Body Mass Index and Other Anthropometric Variables," *American Journal of Clinical Nutrition* 89, no. 4 (2009): 1213–19; J. P. Reis et al., "Comparison of Overall Obesity and Body Fat Distribution in Predicting Risk of Mortality," *Obesity* 17, no. 6 (2009): 1232–39; J. P. Reis et al., "Overall Obesity and Abdominal Adiposity as Predictors of Mortality in U.S. White and Black Adults," *Annals of Epidemiology* 19, no. 2 (2009): 2134–42.

13. J. P. Boyle, et al., "Projection of the Year 2050 Burden of Diabetes in the U.S. Adult Population: Dynamic Modeling of Incidence, Mortality, and Prediabetes Prevalence," *Population Health Metrics* 2010, Available at www.pophealthmetrics.com/content/8/1/29.

14. E. Finkelstein et al., "Annual Medical Spending Attributable to Obesity: Payer- and Service-Specific Estimates," *Health Affairs* 28, no. 5 (2009): w822–w831.

15. J. Bhattacharya and K. Bundorf, "The Incidence of the Healthcare Costs of Obesity," *Journal of Health Economics* 28, no. 3 (2009): 649–58.

16. C. Murtaugh, et al., "Lifetime Risk and Duration of Chronic Diseases and Disability," *Journal of Aging and Health* 23, no. 3 (2011): 554–577.

17. D. Cummings and M. Schwartz, "Genetics and Pathophysiology of Human Obesity," *Annual Review of Medicine* 54 (2003): 453–71.

18. K. Silventoinen et al., "The Genetic and Environmental Influences on Childhood Obesity: A Systematic Review of Twin and Adoption Studies," *International Journal of Obesity* 34, no. 1 (2010): 29–40.

19. S. Li et al., "Cumulative and Predictive Value of Common Obesity—Susceptibility Variants Identified by Genome-wide Association Studies," *American Journal of Clinical Nutrition* 91, no. 1 (2010): 184–90.

20. H. Chang, "Scientists Probe the Role of the Brain in Obesity," *Journal of the American Medical Association* 303, no. 1 (2010): 19–20.

21. C. Bouchard, "Defining the Genetic Architecture of the Predisposition to Obesity: A Challenging but Not Insurmountable Task," *American Journal of Clinical Nutrition* 91, no. 1 (2010): 5–6.

22. C. Bouchard, "Thrifty Gene Hypothesis: Maybe Everyone Is Right?" *International Journal of Obesity* 32, no. 4 (2008): 25–27; R. Stoger, "The Thrifty Epigenotype: An Acquired and Heritable Predisposition for Obesity and Diabetes?" *Bioessays* 30, no. 2 (2008): 156–66.

23. C. Bouchard, "Defining the Genetic Architecture of the Predisposition to Obesity," 2010; S. Li et al., "Cumulative and Predictive Value of Common Obesity," 2010.

24. E. Schuer et al., "Activation in Brain Energy Regulation and Reward Centers by Food Cues Varies with Choice of Visual Stimulation," *International Journal of Obesity* 33, no. 6 (2009): 653–61.

25. T. Reinehr et al., "Thyroid Hormones and Their Relation to Weight Status," *Hormone Research* 70, no. 1 (2008): 51–57.

26. D. E. Cummings et al., "Plasma Ghrelin Levels after Diet-Induced Weight Loss or Gastric Bypass Surgery," *New England Journal of Medicine* 346, no. 21 (2002): 1623–30.

27. C. DeVriese et al., "Focus on the Short- and Long-Term Effects of Ghrelin on Energy Homeostasis," *Nutrition* 26, no. 6 (2010): 579–84; T. Castaneda et al., "Ghrelin in the Regulation of Body Weight and Metabolism," *Frontiers in Neuroendocrinology* 31, no. 1 (2010): 44–60.

28. V. Paracchini et al., "Genetics of Leptin and Obesity: A HuGE Review," *American Journal of Epidemiology* 162, no. 2 (2005): 101–14; Y. Friedlander et al., "Leptin, Insulin, and Obesity-Related Phenotypes: Genetic Influences on Levels and Longitudinal Changes," *Obesity* 17, no. 7 (2009): 1458–60.

29. K. L. Spalding et al., "Dynamics of Fat Cell Turnover in Humans," *Nature* 453 (2008): 783–787.

30. J. Spence et al., "Relation between Local Food Environments and Obesity among Adults," 2009; T. Harder et al., "Duration of Breast Feeding and Risk of Overweight," *American Journal of Epidemiology* 162, no. 5 (2005): 397–403; M. Wang et al., "Changes in Neighbourhood Food Store Environment, Food Behaviour, and Body Mass Index, 1981–1990," *Public Health Nutrition* 11, no. 9 (2008): 963–70; R. Havermans et al., "Food Liking, Food Wanting, and Sensory Specific Satiety," *Appetite* 52, no. 1 (2009): 222–25; J. Smith and T. Ditschun, "Controlling Satiety: How Environmental Factors Influence Food Intake," *Trends in Food Science and Technology* 20, nos. 6–7 (2009): 271–77.

31. M. Treuth et al., "A Longitudinal Study of Sedentary Behavior and Overweight in Adolescent Girls," *Obesity* 17, no. 5 (2009): 1003–08.

32. B. Levin, "Synergy of Nurture and Nature in the Development of Childhood Obesity," *International Journal of Obesity* 33, Suppl 1 (2009): S53–S56.

33. S. Anderson and R. Whitaker, "Prevalence of Obesity among U.S. Preschool Children in Different Racial and Ethnic Groups," 2009.

34. M. Beydoun et al., "The Association of Fast Food, Fruit, and Vegetable Prices with Dietary Intakes among U.S. Adults: Is There Modification by Family Income?" *Social Science and Medicine* 66, no. 11 (2008): 2218–29; J. Tillotson, "Americans' Food Shopping in Today's Lousy Economy," *Nutrition Today* 44, no. 5 (2009): 218–21.

35. F. Li et al., "Built Environment, Adiposity, and Physical Activity in Adults Aged 50–75," *American Journal of Preventive Medicine* 35, no. 1 (2008): 38–46.

36. A. Roskam et al., "Comparative Appraisal of Educational Inequalities in Overweight and Obesity among Adults in 19 European Countries," *International Journal of Epidemiology* 39, no. 2 (2010): 392–404.

37. Centers for Disease Control and Prevention, "U.S. Physical Activity Statistics," Updated February 2010, Available at www.cdc.gov/nccdphp/dnpa/physical/stats/index.htm; National Center for Health Statistics, "Prevalence of Sedentary Leisure Time Behavior among Adults in the United States," Updated February 2010, Available at www.cdc.gov/nchs/data/hestat/sedentary/sedentary.htm.

38. C. Schoenborn and P. Adams, "Health Behaviors of Adults, United States: 2005–2007," National Center for Health Statistics, *Vital Health Statistics* 10, no. 245 (2010).

39. D. Dunstan et al., "Television Viewing Time and Mortality: The Australian Diabetes, Obesity and Lifestyle Study (AusDiab)," *Circulation* 121 (2010): 384–91; G. Duntun et al., "Joint Associations of Physical Activity and Sedentary Behaviors with Body Mass Index: Results from a Time Use Survey of U.S. Adults," *International Journal of Obesity* 33 (2010): 1427–36; N. Owen, A. Bauman, and W. Brown, "Too Much Sitting: A Novel and Important Predictor of Chronic Disease Risk?" *British Journal of Sports Medicine* 43, no. 2

(2009): 81–83; S. A. Anderssen et al., "Changes in Physical Activity Behavior and the Development of Body Mass Index during the Last 30 Years in Norway," *Scandinavian Journal of Medicine and Science in Sports* 18, no. 3 (2008): 309–17; P. Katzmarzyk et al., "Sitting Time and Mortality from All Causes, Cardiovascular Diseases, and Cancer," *Medicine and Science in Sports and Exercise* 41, no. 5 (2009): 998–1005; 2655–67.

40. American Heart Association, "Body Composition Tests," 2010, Available at www.americanheart.org/presenter.jhtml?identifier=4489.

41. Obesity Society, "What Is Obesity?" Accessed June 2011, Available at http://www.obesity.org/resources-for/what-is-obesity.htm?qh=YToxOnt pOjA7czoxNToid2hhdCBpcyBvYmVzaXR5Ijt9.

42. Centers for Disease Control and Prevention, "Defining Overweight and Obesity," Updated June 2010, Available at www.cdc.gov/obesity/defining.html.

43. K. Flegal et al., "Prevalence and Trends in Obesity among U.S. Adults, 1999–2008," 2010.

44. J. Hill and H. Wyatt, "Is It OK to Call Children Obese?" *Obesity Management* 2, no. 4 (2006): 131–32.

45. Centers for Disease Control and Prevention, "About BMI for Children and Teens," Updated February 2011, Available at www.cdc.gov/healthyweight/assessing/bmi/childrens_BMI/about_childrens_BMI.html.

46. The National Heart, Lung, and Blood Institute (NHLBI), "Classification of Overweight and Obesity by BMI, Waist Circumference and Associated Disease Risks," 2011, Available at www.nhlbi.nih.gov/health/public/heart/obesity/lose_wt/bmi_dis.htm.

47. Rush University, "Waist to Hip Ratio Calculator," Accessed May 2010, Available at www.rush.edu/itools/hip/hipcalc.html.

48. E. Stice et al., "Risk Factors and Prodomal Eating Pathology," *Journal of Child Psychology and Psychiatry* 51, no. 4 (2010): 518–525.

49. J. Thompson and M. Manore, *Nutrition: An Applied Approach*, 2d ed. (San Francisco: Benjamin Cummings, 2009), 126.

50. D. Rucker et al., "Long-Term Pharmacotherapy for Obesity and Overweight: Updated Meta-Analysis," *British Medical Journal* 335, no. 7631 (2007): 1194–99.

51. U.S. Food and Drug Administration, "Fen-Phen Safety Update Information," Updated September 2009, Available at www.fda.gov/Drugs/DrugSafety/PostmarketDrugSafetyInformationforPatientsandProviders/ucm072820.htm.

52. U.S. Food and Drug Administration, "Follow-Up to the November 2009 Early Communication about an Ongoing Safety Review of Sibutramine, Marketed as Meridia," January 2010, Available at www.fda.gov/Drugs/DrugSafety/PostmarketDrugSafetyInformationforPatientsandProviders/DrugSafetyInformationforHeathcareProfessionals/ucm198206.htm.

53. ConsumerSearch, "Diet Pills: Reviews," 2011, Available at www.consumersearch.com/diet-pills.

54. F. Rubino et al., "Metabolic Surgery to Treat Type 2 Diabetes: Clinical Outcomes and Mechanisms of Action," *Annual Review of Medicine* 61 (2010): 393–411; E. Karra et al., "Mechanisms Facilitating Weight Loss and Resolution of Type 2 Diabetes Following Bariatric Surgery," *Trends in Endocrinology and Metabolism* 21, no. 6 (2010): 227–344.

55. C. Mottin et al., "Behavior of Type 2 Diabetes Mellitus in Morbid Obese Patients Submitted to Gastric Bypass," *Obesity Surgery* 18, no. 2 (2008): 179–82.

56. J. S. Blake, *Nutrition and You*, 2nd ed. (San Francisco, Pearson Education, 2011).

57. V. Swami et al., "The Attractive Female Body Weight and Female Body Dissatisfaction in 26 Countries Across 10 World Regions—Results of the International Body Project I," *Personality and Social Psychology Bulletin* 36, no. 3 (2010): 309–325.

58. National Eating Disorders Association, "Body Image," 2005, Available at www.nationaleatingdisorders.org/information-resources/general-information.php#body-image-issues.

59. Centers for Disease Control and Prevention, "U.S. Obesity Trends 1985 to 2009," Updated March 2011, Available at www.cdc.gov/obesity/data/trends.html.

60. National Eating Disorders Association, "The Media, Body Image, and Eating Disorders," 2005, Available at www.nationaleatingdisorders.org/information-resources/general-information.php#body-image-issues.

61. S. Grogan, *Body Image: Understanding Body Dissatisfaction in Men, Women, and Children*, 2nd ed. (New York: Psychology Press, 2008), 159–61.

62. Mayo Clinic Staff, "Body Dysmorphic Disorder," 2010, Available at www.mayoclinic.com/health/body-dysmorphic-disorder/DS00559.

63. J. D. Feusner et al., "Visual Information Processing of Faces in Body Dysmorphic Disorder," *Archives of General Psychiatry* 64, no. 12 (2007): 1417–25.

64. K. Kater, "Building Healthy Body Esteem," *Healthy Body Image: Teaching Kids to Eat and Love Their Bodies Too* (Seattle: National Eating Disorders Association, 2005), Available at www.bodyimagehealth.org.

65. Mayo Clinic Staff, "Body Dysmorphic Disorder," 2010.

66. Mayo Clinic Staff, "Body Dysmorphic Disorder," 2010; KidsHealth, "Body Dysmorphic Disorder," 2007, Available at http://kidshealth.org/parent/emotions/feelings/bdd.html.

67. Mayo Clinic Staff, "Body Dysmorphic Disorder," 2010.

68. G. Flett and P. Hewitt, "The Perils of Perfectionism in Sports and Exercise," *Current Directions in Psychological Science* 14, no. 1 (2005): 14–22; P. Crocker et al., "Examining Current Ideal Discrepancy Scores and Exercise Motivations as Predictors of Social Physique Anxiety in Exercising Females," *Journal of Sport Behavior* 28 (2005): 63–72.

69. Disordered Eating, UK, "Eating Disorders Statistics (U.S.)," 2010, Available at www.disordered-eating.co.uk/eating-disorders-statistics/eating-disorders-statistics-us.html; National Eating Disorder Association, "Statistics: Eating Disorders and Their Precursors," 2005, Available at www.nationaleatingdisorders.org/information-resources/general-information.php#facts-statistics.

70. American College Health Association, *National College Health Assessment II: Reference Group Executive Summary Spring 2010* (Linthicum, MD: American College Health Association, 2010), Available at www.acha-ncha.org/reports_ACHA-NCHAII.html.

71. K. Beals and A. Hill, "The Prevalence of Disordered Eating, Menstrual Dysfunction, and Low Bone Mineral Density among U.S. Collegiate Athletes," *International Journal of Sport Nutrition and Exercise Metabolism* 16, no. 3 (2006): 1–23; L. Ronco, "The Female Athlete Triad: When Women Push Their Limits in High-Performance Sports," *American Fitness* 25, no. 2 (2007): 22–24.

72. E. Bernstein, "Men, Boys Lack Options to Treat Eating Disorders," *Wall Street Journal* (April 17, 2007): D1–D2.

73. S. Forsberg and J. Lock, "The Relationship between Perfectionism, Eating Disorders and Athletes: A Review," *Minerva Pediatrica* 58, no. 6 (2006): 525–34.

74. K. Beals and A. Hill, "The Prevalence of Disordered Eating," 2006.

75. American Psychiatric Association, "DSM-5 Development: Proposed Revision: 307.1 Anorexia Nervosa," Updated October 2010, Available at www.dsm5.org/ProposedRevisions/Pages/proposedrevision.aspx?rid=24.

76. A. L. Ahern et al., "Internalization of the Ultra-Thin Ideal: Positive Implicit Associations with Underweight Fashion Models Are Associated with Drive for Thinness in Young Women," *Eating Disorders* 16, no. 4 (2008): 294–307; M. Eisenberg and D. Neumark-Sztainer, "Peer Harassment and Disordered Eating," *International Journal of Adolescent Medicine and Health* 20, no. 2 (2008): 155–64.

77. National Eating Disorders Association, "Factors That May Contribute to Eating Disorders," 2004, Available at www.nationaleatingdisorders.org/information-resources/general-information.php#causes-eating-disorders.

78. National Alliance on Mental Illness, "Bulimia Nervosa," 2010, Available at www.nami.org/template.cfm?Section=by_illness&template=/ContentManagement/ContentDisplay.cfm&ContentID=65839.

79. American Psychiatric Association, "DSM-5 Development: Proposed Revision: 307.51 Bulimia Nervosa," Updated October 2010, Available at www.dsm5.org/ProposedRevisions/Pages/proposedrevision.aspx?rid=25.

80. National Alliance on Mental Illness, "Bulimia Nervosa," 2010.

81. R. Marsh et al, "Deficient Activity in the Neural Systems That Mediate Self-Regulatory Control in Bulimia Nervosa," *Archives of General Psychiatry* 66, no. 1 (2009): 51–63.

82. J. Manwaring et al., "Risk Factors and Patterns of Onset in Binge Eating Disorder," *International Journal of Eating Disorders* 39, no. 2 (2005): 101–07.

83. J. Hudson et al., "The Prevalence and Correlates of Eating Disorders in the National Comorbidity Survey Replication," *Biological Psychiatry* 61, no. 3 (2007): 348–58.

84. American Psychiatric Association, "DSM-5 Development: Proposed Revision: Binge Eating Disorder," Updated October 2010, Available at www.dsm5.org/ProposedRevisions/Pages/proposedrevision.aspx?rid=372.

85. K. N. Franco, Cleveland Clinic Center for Continuing Education, "Eating Disorders," Accessed June 2011, Available at www.clevelandclinicmeded.com/medicalpubs/diseasemanagement/psychiatry-psychology/eating-disorders.

86. J. Guidi et al., "The Prevalence of Compulsive Eating and Exercise among College Students: An Exploratory Study," *Psychiatry Research* 165, nos. 1–2 (2009): 154–62.

87. C. G. Pope et al., "Clinical Features of Muscle Dysmorphia among Males with Body Dysmorphic Disorder," *Body Image* 2, no. 4 (2005): 395–400.

88. Ibid.

89. A. Nattiv et al., "American College of Sports Medicine Position Stand: The Female Athlete Triad," *Medicine and Science in Sports and Exercise* 39, no. 10 (2007): 1867–82.

Chapter 10

1. D. E. R. Warburton, C. Whitney Nicol, and S. S. D. Bredin, "Prescribing Exercise as Preventive Therapy," *Canadian Medical Association Journal,* 174, no. 7 (2006): 961–74. Erratum, 178, no. 6 (2008): 731–32.

2. Centers for Disease Control and Prevention, "Physical Activity Statistics," Updated February 2010, Available at http://www.cdc.gov/nccdphp/dnpa/physical/stats; Centers for Disease Control and Prevention, "QuickStats: Percentage of Adults Aged >18 Years Who Engaged in Leisure Time Strengthening Activities, by Age Group and Sex— National Health Interview Survey, United States, 2008," *Morbidity and Mortality Weekly Report* 58, no. 34 (2009): 955.

3. Office of Disease Prevention and Health Promotion, U.S. Department of Health and Human Services, *2008 Physical Activity Guidelines for Americans: Be Active, Healthy, and Happy!* ODPHP Publication no. U0036 (Washington, DC: U.S. Department of Health and Human Services, 2008), Available at www.health.gov/paguidelines; Centers for Disease Control and Prevention, "Physical Activity Statistics: Definitions," Updated May 2007, Available at www.cdc.gov/nccdphp/dnpa/physical/stats/definitions.htm; Centers for Disease Control and Prevention, "Physical Activity for Everyone: Physical Activity and Health," Updated February 2011, Available at www.cdc.gov/nccdphp/dnpa/physical/everyone/health.

4. American College Health Association, *American College Health Association-National College Health Assessment II (ACHA-NCHA II) Reference Group Executive Summary Fall 2010* (Linthicum, MD: American College Health Association, 2011), Available at www.achancha.org/reports_ACHA-NCHAII.html.

5. American College Health Association, *American College Health Association-National College Health Assessment II (ACHA-NCHA II) Reference Group Data Report Fall 2010* (Linthicum, MD: American College Health Association, 2011), Available at www.achancha.org/reports_ACHA-NCHAII.html.

6. W. L. Haskell et al., "Physical Activity and Public Health: Updated Recommendation for Adults from the American College of Sports Medicine and the American Heart Association," *Medicine and Science in Sports and Exercise* 39, no. 8 (2007): 1423–34; Office of Disease Prevention and Health Promotion, U.S. Department of Health and Human Services, *2008 Physical Activity Guidelines for Americans,* 2008.

7. W. L. Haskell et al., "Physical Activity and Public Health," 2007.

8. D. E. R. Warburton, C. Whitney Nicol, and S. S. D. Bredin, "Health Benefits of Physical Activity: The Evidence," *Canadian Medical Association Journal,* 174, no. 6 (2006): 801–09.

9. D. E. R. Warburton et al., "Evidence-Informed Physical Activity Guidelines for Canadian Adults," *Canadian Journal of Public Health* 98, Suppl. 2 (2007): S16–S68.

10. S. Plowman and D. Smith, *Exercise Physiology for Health, Fitness, and Performance.* 3rd ed. (Philadelphia: Lippincott Williams & Wilkins, 2011).

11. W. L. Haskell et al., "Cardiovascular Benefits and Assessment of Physical Activity and Physical Fitness in Adults," *Medicine and Science in Sports and Exercise* 24, Suppl. 6 (1992): S201–S220.

12. American Heart Association, "About Cholesterol," Updated July 2010, Available at www.heart.org/HEARTORG/Conditions/Cholesterol/AboutCholesterol/About-Cholesterol_UCM_001220_Article.jsp.

13. A. Mehta, "Management of Cardiovascular Risk Associated with Insulin Resistance, Diabetes, and the Metabolic Syndrome," *Postgraduate Medicine* 122, no. 3 (2010) 61–70.

14. Ibid.

15. U.S. Department of Health and Human Services, *2008 Physical Activity Guidelines for Americans: Be Active, Healthy, and Happy!* 2008.

16. C. E. Tudor-Locke, R. C. Bell, and A. M. Meters, "Revisiting the Role of Physical Activity and Exercise in the Treatment of Type 2 Diabetes," *Canadian Journal of Applied Physiology* 25, no. 6 (2000): 466–92.

17. National Diabetes Information Clearinghouse, U.S. Department of Health and Human Services, *Diabetes Prevention Program (DPP),* NIH Publication no. 09–5099 (Bethesda, MD: National Diabetes Information Clearinghouse, 2008), Available at http://diabetes.niddk.nih.gov/dm/pubs/preventionprogram.

18. J. Peto, "Cancer Epidemiology in the Last Century and the Next Decade," *Nature* 411 (2001): 390–95.

19. World Cancer Research Fund/American Institute for Cancer Research, *Policy and Action for Cancer Prevention. Food, Nutrition, and Physical Activity: A Global Perspective* (Washington, DC: American Institute for Cancer Research, 2009), Available at www.dietandcancerreport.org/downloads/Policy_Report.pdf.

20. C. M. Friedenreich and A. E. Cust, "Physical Activity and Breast Cancer Risk: Impact of Timing, Type, and Dose of Activity and Population Subgroup Effects," *British Journal of Sports Medicine* 42, no. 8 (2008): 636–47.

21. World Cancer Research Fund/American Institute for Cancer Research, *Policy and Action for Cancer Prevention,* 2009; A. Shibata, K. Ishii, and K. Oka, "Psychological, Social, and Environmental Factors of Meeting Recommended Physical Activity Levels for Colon Cancer Prevention among Japanese Adults," *Journal of Science and Medicine in Sport* 12, no. 2 (2010): e155–e156; K. Y. Wolin et al., "Physical Activity and Colon Cancer Prevention: A Meta-Analysis," *British Journal of Cancer* 100, no. 4 (2009): 611–16.

22. S. Tolomio et al., "Short-Term Adapted Physical Activity Program Improves Bone Quality in Osteopenic/Osteoporotic Postmenopausal Women," *Journal of Physical Activity and Health,* 5, no. 6 (2008): 844–53.

23. T. Post et al., "Bone Physiology, Disease and Treatment: Towards Disease System Analysis in Osteoporosis," *Clinical Pharmacokinetics,* 49, no. 2 (2010): 89–118.

24. A. Koch, "Immune Response to Resistance Exercise," *American Journal of Lifestyle Medicine* 4, no. 3 (2010): 244–52.

25. MedLine Plus, National Institutes of Health, "Exercise and Immunity," Updated May 2010, Available at www.nlm.nih.gov/medlineplus/ency/article/007165.htm.

26. N. P. Walsh et al., "Position Statement. Part Two: Maintaining Immune Health," *Exercise and Immunology Review* 17 (2011): 64–103.

27. M. Gleeson, "Immune Function in Sport and Exercise," *Journal of Applied Physiology* 103, no. 2 (2007): 693–99.

28. M. Cardinale et al., "Hormonal Responses to a Single Session of Wholebody Vibration Exercise in Older Individuals," *British Journal of Sports Medicine,* 44, no. 4 (2010): 284–88.

29. O. H. Franco et al., "Effects of Physical Activity on Life Expectancy with Cardiovascular Disease," *Archives of Internal Medicine* 165, no. 20 (2005): 2355–60.

30. J. G. Thomas and R. R. Wing, "Maintenance of Long-Term Weight Loss," *Medicine & Health Rhode Island* 92, no. 2 (2009): 56–57.

31. W. L. Haskell et al., "Physical Activity and Public Health," 2007.

32. B. Stamford, "Tracking Your Heart Rate for Fitness," *The Physician and Sports Medicine* 21, no. 3 (1993): 227–28.

33. W. L. Haskell et al., "Physical Activity and Public Health," 2007.

34. Ibid.

35. S. A. Herring et al., "The Team Physician and Conditioning of Athletes for Sports: A Consensus Statement," *Medicine and Science in Sports and Exercise* 33, 10 (2001): 1789–93.

36. N. A. Ratamess et al., "American College of Sports Medicine Position Stand: Progression Models in Resistance Training for Healthy Adults," *Medicine and Science in Sports and Exercise* 41, no. 3 (2009): 687–708.

37. L. Y. Lee, D. T. Lee, and J. Woo, "Tai Chi and Health-Related Quality of Life in Nursing Home Residents," *Journal of Nursing Scholarship* 41, no. 1 (2009): 35–43.

38. Arthritis Foundation, "Exercise and Arthritis: Introduction to Exercise," 2010, Available at www.arthritis.org/conditions/exercise.

39. M. L. Pollack et al., "American College of Sports Medicine Position Stand: The Recommended Quantity and Quality of Exercise for Developing and Maintaining Cardiorespiratory and Muscular Fitness, and Flexibility in Healthy Adults," *Medicine & Science in Sports & Exercise* 30, no. 6 (1998): 975–91.

40. Ibid.

41. D. G. Behm and A. Chaouachi, "A Review of the Acute Effects of Static and Dynamic Stretching on Performance," *European Journal of Applied Physiology* Published on-line March 4 (2011): 21373870.

42. K. Small, L. McNaughton, and M. Matthews, "A Systematic Review into the Efficacy of Static Stretching as Part of a Warm-Up for the Prevention of Exercise-Related Injury," *Research in Sports Medicine* 16, no. 3 (2008): 213–31.

43. V. Baltzpoulos, "Isokinetic Dynamometry," in *Biomechanical Evaluation of Movement in Sport and Exercise: The British Association of Sport and Exercise Sciences Guidelines,* eds. C. Payton and R. Bartlett (New York: Routledge, 2008), 105.

44. J. R. Fowles, "What I Always Wanted to Know about Instability Training," *Applied Physiology, Nutrition, and Metabolism* 35, no. 1 (2010): 89–90; D. G. Behm et al., "The Use of Instability to Train the Core Musculature," *Applied Physiology, Nutrition, and Metabolism* 35, no. 1 (2010): 91–108.

45. J. R. Fowles, "What I Always Wanted to Know about Instability Training," 2010.

46. M. N. Sawka et al., "American College of Sports Medicine Position Stand: Exercise and Fluid Replacement," *Medicine and Science in Sports and Exercise* 39, no. 2 (2007): 377–90.

47. Ibid.

48. D. Ritchie, "Plantar Fasciitis: Treatment Pearls," American Academy of Podiatric Sports Medicine, Accessed June 2011, www.aapsm.org/plantar_fasciitis.html.

49. M. H. Moen et al., "Medial Tibial Stress Syndrome: A Critical Review," *Sports Medicine* 39, no. 7 (2009): 523–46.

50. D. M. Brody, "Running Injuries: Prevention and Management," *Clinical Symposia* 39, no. 3 (1987): 1–36.

51. M. A. Schiff, D. J. Caine, and R. O'Halloran, "Injury Prevention in Sport," *American Journal of Lifestyle Medicine* 4, no. 1 (2010): 42–64.

52. U. G. Kersting and G. P. Brüggemann, "Midsole Material-Related Force Control During Heel-Toe Running," *Research in Sports Medicine* 14, no. 1 (2006): 1–17.

53. American Academy of Ophthalmology, "Protective Eyewear," 2011, Available at www.aao.org/eyesmart/injuries/eyewear.cfm.

54. American College Health Association, *American College Health Association-National College Health Assessment II (ACHA-NCHA II) Reference Group Executive Summary Fall 2010*, 2010.

55. Bicycle Helmet Safety Institute, "Helmet-Related Statistics from Many Sources," Revised July 2010, www.helmets.org/stats.htm.

56. N. G. Nelson et al., "Exertional Heat-Related Injuries Treated in Emergency Departments in the U.S., 1997–2006" *American Journal of Preventive Medicine* 40, no. 1 (2011): 54–60.

57. L. E. Armstrong et al., "The American Football Uniform: Uncompensable Heat Stress and Hyperthermic Exhaustion," *Journal of Athletic Training* 45, no. 2 (2010): 117–27.

58. E. E. Turk, "Hypothermia" *Forensic Science Medical Pathology* 6, no. 2 (2010): 106–115.

59. American Council on Exercise, "Exercising in the Cold," 2011, Available at www.acefitness.org/fitfacts/fitfacts_display.aspx?itemid=24.

60. The Canadian Lung Association, "Asthma: Exercise and Asthma," Updated April 2010, Available at www.lung.ca/diseases-maladies/asthma-asthme/exercise-exercice/index_e.php.

61. J. E. Donnelly et al., "American College of Sports Medicine Position Stand: Appropriate Physical Activity Intervention Strategies for Weight Loss, and Prevention of Weight Regain for Adults," *Medicine and Science in Sports and Exercise* 41, no. 2 (2009): 459–71.

62. B. A. Franklin et al., "American College of Sports Medicine and American Heart Association Joint Position Stand: Exercise and Acute Cardiovascular Events: Placing the Risks into Perspective, *Medicine and Science in Sports and Exercise* 39, no. 5 (2007): 886–97.

63. L. S. Pescatello et al., "American College of Sports Medicine Position Stand: Exercise and Hypertension," *Medicine and Science in Sports and Exercise* 36, no. 3 (2004): 533–53.

64. W. J. Chodzko-Zajko et al., "American College of Sports Medicine Position Stand: Exercise and Physical Activity for Older Adults," *Medicine and Science in Sports and Exercise* 41, no. 7 (2009): 1510–30.

65. M. L. Pollack et al., "American College of Sports Medicine Position Stand: The Recommended Quantity and Quality of Exercise for Developing and Maintaining Cardiorespiratory and Muscular Fitness, and Flexibility in Healthy Adults," 1998.

Chapter 11

1. American Heart Association, "Heart Disease and Stroke Statistics—2011 Update: A Report from the American Heart Association," *Circulation* 123 (2011): e18–e209, Available at http://circ.ahajournals.org/content/123/4.toc.

2. National Diabetes Information Clearinghouse, National Institute of Diabetes and Digestive and Kidney Diseases (NIDDK), *National Diabetes Statistics, 2011* (Bethesda, MD: National Institutes of Health, 2011) NIH Publication no. 08-3892, Available at http://diabetes.niddk.nih.gov/dm/pubs/statistics.

3. Ibid.

4. Centers for Disease Control and Prevention, "Diabetes Data & Trends," 2011, Available at http://apps.nccd.cdc.gov/ddtstrs.

5. Centers for Disease Control and Prevention, "Childhood Overweight and Obesity," Updated March 2010, Available at www.cdc.gov/obesity/childhood/index.html.

6. Centers for Disease Control and Prevention, "Diabetes Data & Trends," 2011.

7. American Heart Association, "Heart Disease and Stroke Statistics—2011 Update," 2011.

8. Ibid.

9. Ibid.

10. Ibid.

11. American Heart Association, "Statistical Fact Sheet—Populations 2009 Update: International Cardiovascular Disease Statistics," 2009, Available at www.americanheart.org/presenter.jhtml?identifier=3001008.

12. American Heart Association, "Heart Disease and Stroke Statistics—2011 Update," 2011.

13. Ibid.

14. Ibid.

15. Ibid.

16. Ibid.

17. National Heart, Lung and Blood Institute. "Angina: What Is Angina?" Revised March 2010, Available at www.nhlbi.nih.gov/health/dci/Diseases/Angina/Angina_WhatIs.html.

18. American Heart Association, "Heart Disease and Stroke Statistics—2011 Update," 2011.

19. Ibid.

20. Ibid.

21. J. Arnlov et al., "Impact of Body Mass Index and the Metabolic Syndrome on the Risks of CVD and Death in Middle-aged Men," *Circulation* 121, no. 2 (2010): 230–36; D. Conen et al., "Metabolic Syndrome, Inflammation, and Risk of Symptomatic Peripheral Artery Disease in Women: A Prospective Study," *Circulation* 120, no. 12 (2009): 1041–47; J. Després et al., "Abdominal Obesity and Metabolic Syndrome: Contribution to Global Cardiometabolic Risk," *Arteriosclerosis, Thrombosis, and Vascular Biology* 28, no. 6 (2008): 1039–49; S. Haffner, "Epidemiology of Cardiometabolic Diseases," *Mechanisms and Syndromes of Cardiometabolic Disease: Emerging Science in Atherosclerosis Hypertension and Diabetes*, 2008, Medscape CME, http://cme.medscape.com/viewprogram/8704; American Heart Association, "Heart Disease and Stroke Statistics," 2010; J. Rosenzwigg et al., "Primary Prevention of Cardiovascular Disease and Type 2 Diabetes in Patients at Metabolic Risk: An Endocrine Society Clinical Practice Guideline," *Journal of Clinical Endocrinology and Metabolism* 93, no. 10 (2008): 3671–89.

22. S. Haffner, "Epidemiology of Cardiometabolic Diseases," 2009; J. Després et al., "Abdominal Obesity and Metabolic Syndrome," 2008; A. Gami et al., "Metabolic Syndrome and Risk of Incident Cardiovascular Events and Death: A Systematic Review and Meta-Analysis of Longitudinal Studies," *Journal of the American College of Cardiology* 49, no. 4 (2007): 403–14; T. Horwich and G. Fonarow, "Glucose, Obesity, Metabolic Syndrome, and Diabetes: Relevance to Incidence of Heart Failure," *Journal of the American College of Cardiology* 55, no. 4 (2010): 283–93.

23. National Heart, Lung, and Blood Institute, "Metabolic Syndrome: What Is Metabolic Syndrome?" Revised April 2011, Available at www.nhlbi.nih.gov/health/dci/Diseases/ms/ms_whatis.html.

24. Ibid.

25. B. Brummett et al., "Systolic Blood Pressure, Socioeconomic Status, and Biobehavioral Risk Factors in a Nationally Representative U.S. Young Adult Sample," *Hypertension* 58 (2011): 161–166; T. Huang et al., "Metabolic Syndrome and Related Disorders in College Students: Prevalence and Gender Differences," *Metabolic Syndrome and Related Disorders* 5, no. 4 (2007): 365–72.

26. American Heart Association, "Heart Disease and Stroke Statistics," 2010.

27. U.S. Department of Health and Human Services, *The Health Consequences of Smoking: A Report of the Surgeon General* (Atlanta: U.S. Department of Health and Human Services, Centers for Disease Control and Prevention, National Center for Chronic Disease Prevention and Health Promotion, Office on Smoking and Health, 2004), Available at www.surgeongeneral.gov/library/smokingconsequences/index.html.

28. American Heart Association, "Heart Disease and Stroke Statistics—2011 Update," 2011; B. Howard et al., "Low-Fat Dietary Pattern and Risk of Cardiovascular Disease: The Women's Health Initiative Randomized Controlled Dietary Modification Trial," *Journal of the American Medical Association* 295, no. 6 (2006): 655–66.

29. C. A. Garza et al., "The Association between Lipoprotein-Associated Phospholipase A_2 and Cardiovascular Disease: A Systematic Review," *Mayo Clinic Proceedings* 82, no. 2 (2007): 159–65.

30. P. J. Barter et al., "Apo B versus Cholesterol in Estimating Cardiovascular Risk and in Guiding Therapy: Report of the Thirty-Person/Ten-Country Panel," *Journal of Internal Medicine* 259, no. 3 (2006): 247–58; E. Ingelsson et al., "Clinical Utility of Different Lipid Measures for Prediction of Coronary Heart Disease in Men and Women," *JAMA: The Journal of the American Medical Association* 298, no. 7 (2007): 776–85; M. McQueen et al., "Lipids, Lipoproteins and Apolipoproteins as Risk Markers of Myocardial Infarction in 52 Countries (The INTERHEART Study): A Case-Control Study," *Lancet* 372, no. 9634 (2008): 244–33.

31. The Linus Pauling Institute, "Micronutrient Information Center," Available at http://lpi.oregonstate.edu/infocenter; Office of Dietary Supplements, *Annual Bibliography of Significant Advances in Dietary Supplement Research 2007* (Bethesda, MD: U.S. Department of Health and Human Services, National Institutes of Health, 2008), NIH Publication no. 08-6456, Available at http://ods.od.nih.gov/Research/Annual_Bibliographies.aspx

32. U.S. Food and Drug Administration, "Food Labeling: Health Claims; Plant Sterol/Stanol Esters and Coronary Heart Disease; Interim Final Rule," 2000, Available at www.fda.gov/Food/LabelingNutrition/LabelClaims/HealthClaims-MeetingSignificantScientificAgreementSSA/ucm074747.htm; International Food Information Council Foundation, "Functional Food Fact Sheet: Plant Stanols and Sterols," 2007, Available at www.foodinsight.org/Resources/Detail.aspx?topic=Functional_Foods_Fact_Sheet_Plant_Stanols_and_Sterols.

33. American Heart Association, "Heart Disease and Stroke Statistics—2011 Update," 2011.

34. C. H. Saely, P. Rein, and H. Drexel, "The Metabolic Syndrome and Risk of Cardiovascular Disease and Diabetes: Experiences with the New Diagnostic Criteria from the International Diabetes Federation," *Hormone and Metabolic Research* 39, no. 9 (2007): 642–50; K. Galassi, K. Reynolds, and J. He, "Metabolic Syndrome and Risk of Cardiovascular Disease: A Meta-Analysis," *American Journal of Medicine* 119, no. 10 (2007): 812–19.

35. W. Lovello, "Cardiovascular Responses to Stress and Disease Outcomes: A Test of the Reactivity Hypothesis," *Hypertension* 55, no. 4 (2010): 842–43; Y. Chida and A. Steptoe, "Greater Cardiovascular Responses to Laboratory Mental Stress Are Associated with Poor Subsequent Cardiovascular Risk Status: A Meta-Analysis of Prospective Evidence," *Hypertension* 55, no. 4 (2010): 1026–32; M. Esler et al., "Chronic Mental Stress Is a Cause of Essential Hypertension: Presence of Biological Markers of Stress," *Clinical and Experimental Pharmacology and Physiology* 35, no. 4 (2008): 498–502; A. Flaa et al., "Sympathoadrenal Stress Reactivity Is a Predictor of Future Blood Pressure: An 18 Year Follow-Up Study," *Hypertension* 52, no. 2 (2008): 336–41; T. Chadola et al., "Work Stress and Coronary Heart Disease: What Are the Mechanisms?" *European Heart Journal* 29, no. 5 (2008): 640–48; P. Surtees et al., "Psychological Distress, Major Depressive Disorder, and Risk of Stroke," *Neurology* 70, no. 10 (2008): 788–94; J. Dimsdale, "Psychological Stress and Cardiovascular Disease," *Journal of the American College of Cardiology* 51, no. 13 (2008): 1237–46.

36. D. Buckley et al., "C-Reactive Protein as a Risk Factor for Coronary Heart Diseases: A Systematic Review and Meta-Analyses for the U.S. Preventive Services Task Force," *Annals of Internal Medicine* 151, no. 7 (2009): 483–95.

37. Ibid.

38. D. Buckley et al., "C-Reactive Protein as a Risk Factor for Coronary Heart Diseases," 2009; O. Ben-Yehuda, "High-Sensitivity C-Reactive Protein in Every Chart? The Use of Biomarkers in Individual Patients," *Journal of the American College of Cardiology* 49, no. 21 (2007): 2139–41; D. D. Sin and S. F. P. Man, "Biomarkers in COPD: Are We There Yet?" *Chest* 133, no. 6 (2008): 1296–98.

39. Wald, D., Morris, J and Wald, N. "Reconciling the Evidence on Serum Homocysteine and Ischemic Heart Disease: A Meta-Analysis," *PLoS ONE* 6(2): e16473. doi:10.1371/journal.pone.0016473; Abraham, J., and L. Cho. "The Homocysteine Hypothesis: Still Relevant to the Prevention and Treatment of Cardiovascular Disease?" Cleveland Clinic Journal of Medicine. 77, no. 12 (2010): 911–918.

40. Heartsite, "Coronary Stents," Available at www.heartsite.com/html/stent.html.

41. C. Cannon et al., "Current Use of Aspirin and Antithrombotic Agents in the United States among Outpatients with Atherothrombotic Disease (from the REduction of Atherothrombosis for Continued Health [REACH] Registry),"*American Journal of Cardiology* 105, no. 4 (2010): 445–52; G. Biondi-Zoccai et al., "A Systematic Review and Meta-Analysis on the Hazards of Discontinuing or Not Adhering to Aspirin among 50,279 Patients at Risk for Coronary Artery Disease," *European Heart Journal* 27, no. 22 (2006): 2667–74; C. Campbell et al., "Aspirin Dose for the Prevention of Cardiovascular Disease: A Systematic Review," *Journal of the American Medical Association* 297, no. 18 (2007): 2018–24; A. Mathews, "The Danger of Daily Aspirin," *Wall Street Journal,* February 23, 2010, Available at http://online.wsj.com/article/SB10001424052748704511304575075701363436686.html.

42. American Heart Association, "Heart Attack Treatments," 2011, Available at www.americanheart.org/presenter.jhtml?identifier=4601.

43. American Heart Association, "Heart Disease and Stroke Statistics—2011 Update," 2011.

44. American Cancer Society, *Cancer Facts & Figures 2011* (Atlanta: American Cancer Society, 2010), Available at www.cancer.org/Research/Cancer-FactsFigures.

45. Ibid.

46. Ibid.

47. Ibid.

48. V. Bagnardi et al., "Alcohol Consumption and the Risk of Cancer: A Meta-Analysis," *Alcohol Research and Health* 25, no. 4 (2001): 263–70.

49. N. Allen et al., "Moderate Alcohol Intake and Cancer Incidence in Women," *Journal of the National Cancer Institute* 101, no. 5 (2009): 296–305.

50. S. Gupta et al., "Risk of Pancreatic Cancer by Alcohol Dose, Duration, and Pattern of Consumption, Including Binge Drinking: A Population-Based Study," *Cancer Causes & Control* 21, no. 7 (2010): 1047–59.

51. A. Benedetti et al., "Lifetime Consumption of Alcoholic Beverages and Risk of 13 Types of Cancer in Men: Results from a Case-Control Study in Montreal," *Cancer Epidemiology* 32, no. 5 (2009): 352–62.

52. American Cancer Society, *Cancer Facts & Figures 2011,* 2010.

53. D. Guh et al., "The Incidence of Co-Morbidities Related to Obesity and Overweight: A Systematic Review and Meta-Analysis," *BMC Public Health* 9, no. 88 (2009).

54. Kay, T., Spencer, E. and G. Reeves. "Overnutrition: Consequences and Solutions--Obesity and Cancer Risks." *Proceedings of the Nutrition Society* 69 (2010): 86–90.

55. E. Reiche, H. Morimoto, and S. Nunes, "Stress and Depression-Induced Immune Dysfunction: Implications for the Development and Progression of Cancer," *International Review of Psychiatry* 17, no. 6 (2005): 515–27; K. Ross, "Mapping Pathways from Stress to Cancer Progression," *Journal of the National Cancer Institute* 100, no. 13 (2008): 914–15, 17; Tel Aviv University, "Stress and Fear Can Affect Cancer's Recurrence," *Science Daily* (February 29, 2008), Available at www.sciencedaily.com/releases/2008/02/080227142656.htm.

56. American Cancer Society, *Cancer Facts & Figures 2011,* 2010.

57. American Cancer Society, "Breast Cancer Overview: What Causes Breast Cancer?" Revised September 2010, Available at www.cancer.org/Cancer/BreastCancer/OverviewGuide/breast-cancer-overview-what-causes.

58. L. Hines et al., "Comparative Analysis of Breast Cancer Risk Factors among Hispanic and Non-Hispanic White Women," *Cancer* 116, no. 13 (2010): 3215–23.

59. B. Binukumar and A. Mathew, "Dietary Fat and Risk of Breast Cancer," Would *Journal of Surgical Oncology* 3, no. 45 (2005): 1477.

60. J. Schüz et al., "Cellular Telephone Use and Cancer Risk: Update of a Nationwide Danish Cohort," *Journal of the National Cancer Institute* 98, no. 23 (2006): 1707–13.

61. J. Parsonnet, "Infectious Disease: A Surprising Cause of Cancer," *Stanford Medicine News,* (Spring 2008): 4–5, Available at www.stanfordmedicine.org/communitynews/2008spring/infectiousdisease.html.

62. American Cancer Society, *Cancer Facts & Figures 2011,* 2010.

63. J. Parsonnet, "Infectious Disease: A Surprising Cause of Cancer," 2008.

64. A. Jemal et al., "Cancer Statistics," *CA: A Cancer Journal for Clinicians* 2009, 59 (4): 225–49.

65. American Cancer Society, *Cancer Facts and Figures 2011,* 2010.

66. Ibid.

67. J. Samet et al., "Lung Cancer in Never Smokers: Clinical Epidemiology and Environmental Risk Factors," *Clinical Cancer Research* 15, no. 18 (2009): 5626–45; C. Rudin et al., "Lung Cancer in Never Smokers: A Call to Action," *Clinical Cancer Research* 15, no. 18 (2009): 5622–25.

68. J. Samet et al., "Lung Cancer in Never Smokers," 2009.

69. American Cancer Society, *Cancer Facts & Figures 2011,* 2010.

70. Ibid.

71. S. A. Kenfield et al., "Smoking and Smoking Cessation in Relation to Mortality in Women," *Journal of the American Medical Association* 299, no. 17 (2008): 2037–47.

72. American Cancer Society, *Cancer Facts & Figures 2011,* 2010.

73. B. K. Edwards et al., "Annual Report to the Nation on the Status of Cancer, 1975–2006. Featuring Colorectal Cancer Trends and Impact of Interventions (Risk Factors, Screenings, and Treatment) to Reduce Future Rates," *Cancer* 2009, 16, no. 3 (2009): 544–73.

74. American Cancer Society, *Cancer Facts & Figures 2011,* 2010.

75. American Cancer Society, *Colorectal Cancer Facts & Figures 2008–2010* (Atlanta: American Cancer Society, 2010), Available at www.cancer.org/Research/CancerFactsFigures/ColorectalCancerFactsFigures/colorectal-cancer-facts--figures-2008-2010.

76. Ibid.

77. American Cancer Society, *Cancer Facts & Figures 2011,* 2010.

78. B. K. Edwards et al., "Annual Report to the Nation on the Status of Cancer, 1975–2006 (2009).

79. American Cancer Society, *Cancer Facts & Figures 2011,* 2010.

80. Ibid.

81. Ibid.

82. T. M. Peters et al., "Physical Activity and Postmenopausal Breast Cancer Risk in the NIH-AARP Diet and Health Study," *Cancer Epidemiology, Biomarkers, and Prevention* 18, no. 1 (2009): 289–96; American Cancer Society, *Cancer Facts & Figures 2011,* 2010.

83. Susan G. Komen for the Cure, "Table 11: *BRCA1* and *BRCA2* Gene Mutations and Cancer Risk," 2009, Available at ww5.komen.org/BreastCancer/Table11BRCA1or2genemutationsandcancerrisk.html.

84. Susan G. Komen for the Cure, "Table 4: Physical Activity and Breast Cancer Risk," 2009, Available at ww5.komen.org/BreastCancer/Table4Recreationalphysicalactivityandbreastcancerrisk.html; C. M. Dallal et al., "Long-Term Recreational Physical Activity and Risk of Invasive and in situ Breast Cancer: The California Teachers Study," *Archives of Internal Medicine* 167, no. 4 (2007): 408–16.

85. X. Shu et al., "Soy Food Intake and Breast Cancer Survival," *Journal of the American Medical Association* 302, no. 22 (2009): 2437–43; R. Ballard-Barbash and M. Neuhouser, "Challenges in Design and Interpretation of Observational Research on Health Behaviors and Cancer Survival," *Journal of the American Medical Association* 302, no. 22 (2009): 2483–84.

86. Adapted from "Breast Awareness and Self-Examination." Reprinted by the permission of the American Cancer Society, Inc., from www.cancer.org. All rights reserved.

87. American Cancer Society, *Cancer Facts & Figures 2011,* 2010.

88. Ibid.

89. U.S. Food and Drug Administration, "The Risk of Tanning," Revised March 2010, Available at

www.fda.gov/Radiation-EmittingProducts/ RadiationEmittingProductsandProcedures/ Tanning/ucm116432.htm; S. Danoff-Berg and C. E. Mosher,"Prediction of Tanning Salon Use: Behavioral Alternatives for Enhancing Appearance, Relaxing and Socializing," *Journal of Health Psychology* 11, no. 3 (2006): 511–18; Skin Cancer Foundation, "Skin Cancer Facts," 2010, Available at www.skincancer .org/Skin-Cancer/Skin-Cancer-Facts.

90. American Cancer Society, *Cancer Facts & Figures 2011*, 2010.

91. Ibid.

92. American Cancer Society, "Prostate Cancer: What Causes Prostate Cancer?" Revised December 2010, Available at www.cancer.org/Cancer/ ProstateCancer/OverviewGuide/prostate-cancer-overview-what-causes.

93. American Cancer Society, *Cancer Facts & Figures 2011*, 2010.

94. S. M. Lippman et al., "Effect of Selenium and Vitamin E on Risk of Prostate Cancer and Other Cancers: The Selenium and Vitamin E Cancer Prevention Trial (SELECT)," *Journal of the American Medical Association* 301, no. 1 (2009): 39–51.

95. National Cancer Institute, "Testicular Cancer," 2010, Available at www.cancer.gov/cancertopics/ types/testicular.

96. Adapted from "Do I Have Testicular Cancer? Testicular Self-Exam." Reprinted by the permission of the American Cancer Society, Inc. from www.cancer.org. All rights reserved.

97. American Cancer Society, *Cancer Facts & Figures 2011*, 2010.

98. Ibid.

99. Ibid.

100. National Cancer Institute, "Ovarian Cancer Screening (PDQ)," 2010, Available at www .cancer.gov/cancertopics/pdq/screening/ovarian/ Patient.

101. American Cancer Society, *Cancer Facts & Figures 2011*, 2010.

102. Ibid.

103. National Cancer Institute, "Endometrial Cancer," 2010, Available at www.cancer.gov/cancertopics/ types/endometrial.

104. American Cancer Society, *Cancer Facts & Figures 2011*, 2010.

105. Ibid.

106. American Diabetes Association, "Diabetes Basics: Type 1," 2011, Available at www.diabetes .org/diabetes-basics/type-1.

107. The World Health Organization, "Diabetes," Fact Sheet #312, January 2011, Available at www.who .int/mediacentre/factsheets/fs312/en/index.html.

108. H. Rodbard, "Diabetes Screening, Diagnosis, and Therapy in Pediatric Patients with Type 2 Diabetes," *Medscape Journal of Medicine* 10, no. 8 (2008): 184.

109. American Diabetes Association, "Diabetes Statistics," 2011, Available at www.diabetes.org/ diabetes-basics/diabetes-statistics.

110. G. Dedoussis et al., "Genes, Diet, and Type 2 Diabetes Mellitus: A Review," *Review of Diabetic Studies* 4, no. 1 (2007): 13–24; U. Das and A. Rao, "Gene Expression Profile in Obesity and Type 2 Diabetes Mellitus," *Lipids in Health and Disease* 6 (2007): 35.

111. New Mexico Health Care Takes on Diabetes, "Pre-Diabetes Is a Precursor to Diabetes," *Diabetes Resources* 10, no. 2 (2008), Available at http:// nmtod.com/diabetesresources.html.

112. American Diabetes Association, "Top 10 Benefits of Being Active," 2011, Available at www.diabetes .org/food-nutrition-lifestyle/fitness/fitness-management/top-10-benefits-being-active.jsp.

113. F. Cappuccio et al., "Quantity and Quality of Sleep and Incidence of Type 2 Diabetes: A Systematic Review and Meta-Analysis," *Diabetes Care* 33, no. 2 (2010): 414–20; R. Aronsohn et al., "Diabetes, Sleep Apnea, and Glucose Control," *American Journal of Respiratory and Critical Care Medicine* 182, no. 2 (2010): 287–89; K. Knutson et al., "The Metabolic Consequences of Sleep Deprivation," *Sleep Medicine Reviews* 11, no. 3 (2007): 163–78.

114. F. Pouwer et al., "Does Emotional Stress Cause Type 2 Diabetes Mellitus? A Review from the European Depression In Diabetes (EDID) Research Consortium," *Discovery Medicine* 9, no. 45 (2010) 112–18; Y. Fan et al., "Dynamic Changes in Salivary Cortisol and Secretory Immuno-globulin A Response to Acute Stress," *Stress and Health* 25, no. 2 (2009): 189–94.

115. American Diabetes Association, "Diabetes Statistics," 2011.

116. American Heart Association, "Metabolic Syndrome," 2011, Available at www.americanheart .org/presenter.jhtml?identifier=4756.

117. National Heart Lung and Blood Institute, "Metabolic Syndrome: What Is Metabolic Syndrome?" Revised April 2011, Available at www.nhlbi.nih .gov/health/dci/Diseases/ms/ms_whatis.html.

118. American Diabetes Association, "Diabetes Basics: What Is Gestational Diabetes?" 2011, Available at www.diabetes.org/diabetes-basics/ gestational/what-is-gestational-diabetes.html.

119. L. Bellamy et al., "Type 2 Diabetes Mellitus after Gestational Diabetes: A Systematic Review and Meta-Analysis," *The Lancet* 373, no. 9677 (2009): 1773–1779.

120. American Diabetes Association, "Diabetes Statistics," 2011.

121. National Diabetes Education Program, *Small Steps, Big Rewards: Your GAME PLAN to Prevent Type 2 Diabetes* (Bethesda, MD: National Institutes of Health, 2006) NIH Publication no. 06-5334, Available at http://ndep.nih.gov/ publications/PublicationDetail.aspx?PubId=71.

122. American Diabetes Association, "Living with Diabetes: A1C," 2011, Available at www.diabetes .org/living-with-diabetes/treatment-and-care/ blood-glucose-control/a1c.

123. American Diabetes Association, "Diabetes Basics: Pre-Diabetes FAQs," 2011, Available at www.diabetes.org/diabetes-basics/prevention/ pre-diabetes/pre-diabetes-faqs.html.

124. National Diabetes Education Program, *Small Steps, Big Rewards*, 2006.

125. J. de Munter et al., "Whole Grain, Bran, and Germ Intake and Risk of Type 2 Diabetes: A Prospective Cohort Study and Systematic Review," *PLoS Medicine* 4, no. 8 (2007): e261.

126. J. Anderson et al., "Health Benefits of Dietary Fiber," *Nutrition Reviews* 67, no. 4 (2009): 188–205.

127. B. Hopping et al., "Dietary Fiber, Magnesium, and Glycemic Load Alter Risk of Type 2 Diabetes in a Multiethnic Cohort in Hawaii," *Journal of Nutrition* 140, no. 1 (2010): 68–74.

128. M. Lankinen et al., "Fatty Fish Intake Decreases Lipids Related to Inflammation and Insulin Signaling—a Lipidomics Approach," *PLoS One* 4, no. 4 (2009): e5258; G. Dedoussis et al., "Genes, Diet, and Type 2 Diabetes Mellitus: A Review," 2007.

129. National Diabetes Education Program, *Small Steps, Big Rewards*, 2006.

130. W. Bennett et al., "Fatness and Fitness: How Do They Influence Health-Related Quality of Life in Type 2 Diabetes Mellitus?" *Health and Quality of Life Outcomes* 6 (2008): 110.

131. G. Gillies et al., "Pharmacological and Lifestyle Interventions to Prevent or Delay Type 2 Diabetes in People with Impaired Glucose Tolerance: Systematic Review and Meta-analysis," *British Medical Association Journal* 334 (2007): 299.

132. National Diabetes Information Clearinghouse, National Institute of Diabetes and Digestive and Kidney Diseases, "Alternative Devices for Taking Insulin," NIH Publication no. 09-4643. May 2009, Available at http://diabetes.niddk.nih.gov/ dm/pubs/insulin/index.htm.

133. J. L. Thompson and M. M. Manore, *Nutrition: An Applied Approach,* 3rd ed. (San Francisco: Benjamin Cummings, 2011).

134. March of Dimes, "Birth Defects: Chromosomal Abnormalities," December 2009, Available at www.marchofdimes.com/Baby/birthdefects_ chromo somal.html.

135. Genetics Home Reference, "Mutations and Health," June 2011, Available at http://ghr.nlm .nih.gov/handbook/mutationsanddisorders.

136. Genetics Home Reference, "Inheriting Genetic Conditions," June 2011, Available at http:// ghr.nlm.nih.gov/handbook/inheritance.

137. American Cancer Society, *Cancer Facts & Figures 2011*, 2010.

138. Human Genome Project, "Genetic Counseling," September 2008, Available at www.ornl.gov/sci/ techresources/Human_Genome/medicine/ genecounseling.shtml.

139. Human Genome Project, "Gene Testing," September 2010, Available at www.ornl.gov/sci/ techresources/Human_Genome/medicine/ genetest.shtml.

Chapter 12

1. Environmental Protection Agency, "Climate Change—Health and Environmental Effects," Updated April 2011, Available at www.epa.gov/ climatechange/effects/health.html; A. Greer et al., "Climate Change and Infectious Diseases in North America: The Road Ahead," *Canadian Medical Association Journal* 178, no. 6 (2008): 715–22.

2. B. Feingold et al., "A Niche for Infectious Disease in Environmental Health: Rethinking the Toxicological Paradigm," *Environmental Health Perspectives* 118, no. 8 (2010): 1165–72; L. Martin et al., "The Effects of Anthropogenic Global Changes on Immune Functions and Disease Resistance," *Annals of the New York Academy of Sciences* 1195, no. 1 (2010): 129–48.

3. American Autoimmune Related Diseases Association, "Autoimmune Statistics," 2011, Available at www.aarda.org/autoimmune_statistics.php.

4. M. R. Klevens et al., "Invasive Methicillin-Resistant *Staphylococcus aureus* Infections in the United States," *Journal of the American Medical Association* 298, no. 15 (2007): 1763–71.

5. W. Jarvis, "Prevention and Control of Methicillin-Resistant *Staphylococcus aureus*: Dealing with Reality, Resistance, and Resistance to Reality," *Clinical Infectious Diseases* 50, no. 2 (2010): 218–20.

6. Centers for Disease Control and Prevention, "Group A Streptococcal (GAS) Disease," April 2008, Available at www.cdc.gov/ncidod/dbmd/ diseaseinfo/groupastreptococcal_g.htm.

7. Ibid.

8. Centers for Disease Control and Prevention, "About Group B Strep," Modified November 2010, Available at www.cdc.gov/groupbstrep/about/ index.html.

9. Centers for Disease Control and Prevention, "Meningitis Questions and Answers," Updated March 2011, Available at www.cdc.gov/meningitis/about/faq.html; J. Tully et al., "Risk and Protective Factors for Meningococcal Disease in Adolescents: Matched Cohort Study," *British Medical Journal* 332, no. 7539 (2006): 445–50.

10. Centers for Disease Control and Prevention, *Reported Tuberculosis in the United States, 2009* (Atlanta, GA: U.S. Department of Health and Human Services, 2010), Available at www.cdc.gov/tb/statistics/reports/2009/default.htm.

11. World Health Organization, *Global Tuberculosis Control 2010* (Geneva: World Health Organization, 2011), Available at www.who.int/tb/publications/global_report/2010/en/index.html.

12. T. H. Le and G. T. Fantry, eMedicine from WebMD, "Peptic Ulcer Disease," Updated June 2011, Available at http://emedicine.medscape.com/article/181753-overview.

13. Ibid.

14. WebMD, "Cold Guide: Understanding Common Cold—Basics," July 2011, Available at www.webmd.com/cold-and-flu/cold-guide/understanding-common-cold-basics.

15. Linus Pauling Institute Micronutrient Information Center, "Micronutrient Center: Vitamin C: Common Cold," Updated November 2009, Available at http://lpi.oregonstate.edu/infocenter/vitamins/vitaminC/index.html#cold; National Center for Complementary and Alternative Medicine, "Herbs at a Glance: Echinacea," NCCAM Publication no. D271, Updated July 2010, Available at http://nccam.nih.gov/health/echinacea/ataglance.htm.

16. Centers for Disease Control and Prevention, "Seasonal Influenza: Key Facts about Influenza (Flu) and Flu Vaccine," Updated July 2011, Available at www.cdc.gov/flu/keyfacts.htm.

17. Centers for Disease Control and Prevention, "Hepatitis A FAQs for Health Professionals," Updated June 2009, Available at www.cdc.gov/hepatitis/HAV/HAVfaq.htm.

18. A. Wasley et al., "The Prevalence of Hepatitis B Virus in the United States in the Era of Vaccination," *Journal of Infectious Diseases* 202, no. 2 (2010): 192–201; Centers for Disease Control and Prevention, "Hepatitis A FAQs for Health Professionals," 2009.

19. Centers for Disease Control and Prevention. "Hepatitis B FAQs for the Public," 2009, Available at www.cdc.gov/hepatitis/B/bFAQ.htm#overview.

20. Centers for Disease Control and Prevention, "Hepatitis C FAQs for Health Professionals," Updated December 2010, Available at www.cdc.gov/hepatitis/HCV/HCVfaq.htm.

21. S. Rajaguru and M. Nettleman, "Hepatitis C," MedicineNet.com, 2011, Available at www.medicinenet.com/hepatitis_c/article.htm.

22. Centers for Disease Control and Prevention, "Prevention of Herpes Zoster: Recommendations of the Advisory Committee on Immunization Practices (ACIP)," *MMWR Recommendations and Reports* 57, no. 5 (2008) 1–30.

23. Centers for Disease Control and Prevention, "vCJD (Variant Creutzfeldt-Jakob Disease)," August 2010, Available at www.cdc.gov/ncidod/dvrd/vcjd/index.htm.

24. Centers for Disease Control and Prevention, "Get Smart: Know When Antibiotics Work: Fast Facts," Updated January 2011, Available at www.cdc.gov/getsmart/antibiotic-use/fast-facts.html; J. Ritterman, "Preventing Antibiotic Resistance: The Next Step," *Permanente Journal* 10, no. 3 (2006): 22–24.

25. Centers for Disease Control and Prevention, "Dengue: Epidemiology," Updated October 2010, Available at www.cdc.gov/Dengue/epidemiology.

26. Ibid.

27. Centers for Disease Control and Prevention, "West Nile Virus: What You Need to Know," Modified April 2011, Available at www.cdc.gov/ncidod/dvbid/westnile/wnv_factsheet.htm.

28. Centers for Disease Control and Prevention, "West Nile Virus: Updated Information Regarding Insect Repellents," Modified October 2009, Available at www.cdc.gov/ncidod/dvbid/westnile/RepellentUpdates.htm.

29. World Health Organization, "Confirmed Human Cases of Avian Influenza A (H5N1)," 2011, Available at www.who.int/csr/disease/avian_influenza/country/en.

30. World Health Organization, "Cumulative Number of Confirmed Human Cases of Avian Influenza A/(H5N1) Reported to WHO," Updated August 2010, Available at www.who.int/csr/disease/avian_influenza/country/cases_table_2010_08_03/en/index.html.

31. R. Snow et al., "International Funding for Malaria Control in Relation to Populations at Risk of Stable *Plasmodium falciparum* Transmission," *PLoS Medicine* 5, no. 7 (2008): e142; World Health Organization, "Malaria," Fact Sheet no. 94, April 2010, Available at www.who.int/mediacentre/factsheets/fs094/en.

32. World Health Organization, "Malaria," 2010.

33. Centers for Disease Control and Prevention, National Center for Emerging and Zoonotic Infectious Diseases, Division of Healthcare Quality Promotion, "Diseases/Pathogens Associated with Antimicrobial Resistance," Updated July 2010, Available at www.cdc.gov/drugresistance/DiseasesConnectedAR.html; Centers for Disease Control and Prevention, National Center for Immunization and Respiratory Diseases, Division of Bacterial Diseases, "Antibiotic Resistance Questions & Answers," Updated June 2009, Available at www.cdc.gov/getsmart/antibiotic-use/antibiotic-resistance-faqs.html; H. Boucher et al., "Bad Bugs, No Drugs: No ESKAPE! An Update from the Infectious Diseases Society of America," *Clinical Infectious Diseases* 48, no. 1 (2009): 1–12; Global Health Council, "The Impact of Infectious Diseases," 2011, Available at www.globalhealth.org/infectious_diseases.

34. Centers for Disease Control and Prevention, *Sexually Transmitted Diseases Surveillance* 2009 (Atlanta: U.S. Department of Health and Human Services, 2010), Available at www.cdc.gov/std/stats09/default.htm.

35. Ibid.

36. Joint United Nations Programme on HIV/AIDS (UNAIDS) and World Health Organization (WHO), *UNAIDS Report on the Global AIDS Epidemic* (Geneva: UNAIDS, 2010), Available at www.unaids.org/globalreport/Global_report.htm.

37. Centers for Disease Control and Prevention, *HIV Surveillance Report: Diagnoses of HIV Infection and AIDS in the United States and Dependent Areas, 2009*, 2010, Available at www.cdc.gov/hiv/surveillance/resources/reports/2009report.

38. Centers for Disease Control and Prevention, *HIV Surveillance Report 2009*, 2010; H. I. Hall et al., "Estimation of HIV Incidence in the United States," *Journal of the American Medical Association* 300, no. 5 (2008): 520–29.

39. AVERT, "Can You Get HIV From . . . ?" Updated July 2010, Available at www.avert.org/can-you-get-hiv-aids.htm.

40. Ibid.

41. Centers for Disease Control and Prevention, "Mother-to-Child (Perinatal) HIV Transmission and Prevention," October 2007, Available at www.cdc.gov/hiv/topics/perinatal/resources/factsheets/perinatal.htm; AVERT, "Preventing Mother-to-Child Transmission of HIV (PMTCT)," Updated July 2010, Available at www.avert.org/motherchild.htm.

42. Mayo Clinic Staff, "Tattoos: Understand Risks and Precautions," June 2011, Available at www.mayoclinic.com/health/tattoos-and-piercings/MC00020.

43. Centers for Disease Control and Prevention, *Sexually Transmitted Diseases Surveillance, 2009*, 2010.

44. Center for Young Women's Health, "Chlamydia," Updated January 2010, Available at www.youngwomenshealth.org/chlamydia.html.

45. National Institute of Allergy and Infectious Diseases, "Chlamydia: Complications," Updated August 2010, Available at www.niaid.nih.gov/topics/chlamydia/understanding/pages/complications.aspx.

46. Centers for Disease Control and Prevention, *Sexually Transmitted Diseases Surveillance, 2009*, 2010.

47. MedlinePlus, U.S. National Library of Medicine, "Gonorrhea," Updated May 2009, Available at www.nlm.nih.gov/medlineplus/ency/article/007267.htm.

48. Centers for Disease Control and Prevention, "Gonorrhea: CDC Fact Sheet," Updated June 2011, Available at www.cdc.gov/std/gonorrhea/stdfact-gonorrhea.htm.

49. National Institute of Allergy and Infectious Diseases, "Gonorrhea: Treatment," Updated January 2011, Available at www.niaid.nih.gov/topics/gonorrhea/understanding/pages/treatment.aspx.

50. Centers for Disease Control and Prevention, *Sexually Transmitted Diseases Surveillance, 2009*, 2010.

51. MedlinePlus, "Pelvic Inflammatory Disease (PID)," Updated September 2009, Available at www.nlm.nih.gov/medlineplus/ency/article/000888.htm.

52. Mayo Clinic Staff, "Urinary Tract Infection: Risk Factors," June 2010, Available at www.mayoclinic.com/health/urinary-tract-infection/DS00286/DSECTION=risk-factors.

53. Centers for Disease Control and Prevention, *Sexually Transmitted Diseases Surveillance, 2009*, 2010.

54. National Institute of Allergy and Infectious Diseases, "Syphilis: Symptoms," Updated December 2010, Available at www.niaid.nih.gov/topics/syphilis/understanding/Pages/symptoms.aspx.

55. Centers for Disease Control and Prevention, "Genital Herpes—CDC Fact Sheet," Modified July 2010, Available at www.cdc.gov/std/herpes/stdfact-herpes.htm.

56. Centers for Disease Control and Prevention, "Genital Herpes—CDC Fact Sheet," 2010; American Social Health Association, "Learn about Herpes: Fast Facts," 2011, Available at www.ashastd.org/herpes/herpes_learn.cfm.

57. Centers for Disease Control and Prevention, "Genital Herpes—CDC Fact Sheet," 2010.

58. Centers for Disease Control and Prevention, "Genital HPV Infection—CDC Fact Sheet," Modified November 2009, Available at www.cdc.gov/std/HPV/STDFact-HPV.htm.

59. Centers for Disease Control and Prevention, "Cervical Cancer," Updated June 2011, Available at www.cdc.gov/cancer/cervical.

60. Centers for Disease Control and Prevention, "Vaccines and Preventable Diseases: HPV Vaccine—Questions & Answers," Reviewed April 2011, Available at www.cdc.gov/vaccines/vpd-vac/hpv/vac-faqs.htm; American Cancer Society, 2009, "Human Papillomavirus (HPV), Cancer and HPV Vaccines—Frequently Asked Questions," Revised October 2009, Available at www.cancer.org/Cancer/CancerCauses/OtherCarcinogens/InfectiousAgents/HPV/HumanPapillomaVirusandHPVVaccinesFAQ/hpv-faq.

61. National Institute of Allergy and Infectious Diseases, "Vaginal Yeast Infection: Symptoms," Updated August 2008, Available at www.niaid.nih.gov/topics/vaginalYeast/Pages/symptoms.aspx.

62. Centers for Disease Control and Prevention, "Trichomoniasis: CDC Fact Sheet," Modified December 2007, Available at www.cdc.gov/std/trichomonas/STDFact-Trichomoniasis.htm.

63. National Institute of Allergy and Infectious Diseases, "Trichomoniasis: Symptoms," Updated March 2009, Available at www.niaid.nih.gov/TOPICS/TRICHOMONIASIS/UNDERSTANDING/Pages/symptoms.aspx.

Chapter 13

1. World Health Organization, *World Report on Violence and Health* (Geneva: World Health Organization, 2002), Available at www.who.int/violence_injury_prevention/violence/world_report/en.

2. Ibid.

3. U.S. Department of Justice, Federal Bureau of Investigation, *Crime in the United States, Preliminary Semiannual Uniform Crime Report*, 2010, Available at www.fbi.gov/-us/cjis/ucr/crime-in-the-us/2010/preliminary-cri.

4. American College Health Association, *American College Health Association—National College Health Assessment II: Reference Group Data Report Fall 2010* (Baltimore: American College Health Association, 2010), Available at www.acha-ncha.org/reports_ACHA-NCHAII.html.

5. Center for Public Integrity, "Sexual Assault on Campus: A Frustrating Search for Justice," Updated February 2010, Available at www.publicintegrity.org/investigations/campus_assault.

6. World Health Organization Violence Prevention Alliance, "The Ecological Framework," 2010, Available at www.who.int/violenceprevention/approach/ecology/en/index.html; Centers for Disease Control and Prevention, National Center for Injury Prevention and Control, "Understanding Youth Violence," 2009, Available at www.cdc.gov/violenceprevention/youthviolence.

7. U.S. Department of Justice, National Institute of Justice, "Economic Distress and Intimate Partner Violence," 2009, Available at www.ojp.usdoj.gov/nij/topics/crime/intimate-partner-violence/economic-distress.htm.

8. J. H. Derzon, "The Correspondence of Family Features with Problem, Aggressive, Criminal and Violent Behaviors: A Meta-Analysis," *Journal of Experimental Criminology* 6, no. 3 (2010): 263–92; C. Ferguson, C. San Miguel, and R. Hartley, "A Multivariate Analysis of Youth Violence and Aggression: The Influences of Family, Peers, Depression, and Media Violence," *Journal of Pediatrics* 155, no. 6 (2009): 904–08.

9. M. Flood and B. Pease, "Factors Influencing Attitudes to Violence against Women," *Trauma, Violence and Abuse* 10, no. 2 (2009): 125–42.

10. Centers for Disease Control and Prevention. "Understanding Intimate Partner Violence. CDC Fact Sheet, 2011," Available at www.cdc.gov/violenceprevention/ pdf/IPV factsheet-a-pdf.

11. G. Stuart et al., "Examining the Interface between Substance Misuse and Intimate Partner Violence," *Substance Abuse Research and Treatment* 3 (2009): 25–29.

12. M. Teicher et al., "Sticks, Stones and Hurtful Words: Relative Effects of Various Forms of Childhood Maltreatment," *American Journal of Psychiatry* 163 (2006): 993–1000; C. Cook et al. "Predictors of Bullying and Victimization in Childhood and Adolescence: A Meta-Analytic Investigation." *School Psychology Quarterly* 25, no. 2 (2010): 65–83.

13. M. Teicher et al., "Sticks, Stones and Hurtful Words: Relative Effects of Various Forms of Childhood Maltreatment," 2006.

14. M. Randolph et al., "Alcohol Use and Sexual Risk Behavior among College Students: Understanding Gender and Ethnic Differences," *American Journal of Drug & Alcohol Abuse* 35, no. 2 (2009): 80–84; E. Reed et al., "The Relation between Interpersonal Violence and Substance Use among a Sample of University Students: Examination of the Role of Victim and Perpetrator Substance Use," *Addictive Behaviors* 34, no. 3 (2009): 316–18; T. Messman-Moore, R. Ward, and A. Brown, "Substance Use and PTSD Symptoms Impact the Likelihood of Rape and Revictimization in College Women," *Journal of Interpersonal Violence* 24, no. 3 (2009): 499–521; P. Giancola et al., "Men and Women, Alcohol and Aggression," *Experimental and Clinical Psychopharmacology* 17, no. 3 (2009): 154–64; J. McCauley, K. Calhoun, and C. Gidycz, "Binge Drinking and Rape: A Prospective Examination of College Women with a History of Previous Sexual Victimization," *Journal of Interpersonal Violence* 25, no. 9 (2010): 1655–68.

15. M. Ybares et al., "Linkages between Internet and Other Media Violence with Serious Violent Behavior by Youth," *Pediatrics* 122, no. 5 (2008): 929–37; C. Anderson et al., "Longitudinal Effects of Violent Video Games on Aggression in Japan and the United States," *Pediatrics* 122 (2008): e1067–e1072; J. Savage, "The Effects of Media Violence Exposure on Criminal Aggression," *Criminal Justice and Behavior* 35, no. 6 (2008): 772–91.

16. M. Ferguson, "Weak Results: Misleading Conclusions—Response to Anderson Article," *Pediatrics*, "eLetters," Available at http://pediatrics.aappublications.org/cgi/eletters/122/5/e1067, 2008; C. Ferguson et al., "Personality, Parental and Media Influences on Aggressive Personality and Violent Crime in Youth," *Journal of Aggression, Maltreatment and Trauma* 17, no. 4 (2008): 395–414; B. Wilson, "Media and Children's Aggression, Fear, and Altruism," *The Future of Children* 18, no. 1 (2008): 1550–54; L. Price and V. Maholmes, "Understanding the Nature and Consequences of Children's Exposure to Violence: Research Perspectives," *Clinical Child and Family Psychology Review* 12, no. 2 (2009): 65–70.

17. U.S. Department of Justice, Office of Justice Programs, Bureau of Justice Statistics, *National Crime Victimization Survey: Criminal Victimization*, 2009 (Washington, DC: Bureau of Justice Statistics, 2010) NCJ 227777, Available at http://bjs.ojp.usdoj.gov/index.cfm?ty=pbdetail&iid=2217.

18. J. Savage and C. Yancey, "The Effects of Media Violence Exposure on Criminal Aggression: A Meta-Analysis," *Criminal Justice and Behavior* 35, no. 6 (2008): 772–91.

19. C. Ferguson, *Violent Crime: Clinical and Social Implications* (Thousand Oaks, CA: Sage, 2010).

20. World Health Organization, *World Report on Violence and Health*, 2002.

21. K. Kochanek et al., "Deaths: Preliminary Data for 2009," *National Vital Statistics Reports* 59, no. 4 (2011).

22. U.S. Department of Justice, Federal Bureau of Investigation, *Crime in the United States 2009*, 2010, Available at www2.fbi.gov/ucr/cius2009.

23. J. Fox and M. Swatt, *The Recent Surge in Homicides Involving Young Black Males and Guns: Time to Reinvest in Prevention and Crime Control* (Alexandria, VA: American Statistical Association, 2008), Available at www.ncjrs.gov/App/publications/abstract.aspx?ID=248092.

24. Centers for Disease Control and Prevention, "FastStats: Assault or Homicide," 2009, Available at www.cdc.gov/nchs/FASTATS/homicide.htm.

25. U.S. Department of Justice, Office of Justice Programs, Bureau of Justice Statistics, *National Crime Victimization Survey: Criminal Victimization*, 2009. 2010.

26. L. Hepburn, M. Miller, and D. Hemenway, "The U.S. Gun Stock: Results from the 2004 National Firearms Survey," *Injury Prevention* 13 (2007): 15–19.

27. National Center for Injury Prevention and Control, "WISQARS Fatal Injury Reports 1999–2007," Updated 2010, Available at www.cdc.gov/injury/wisqars/fatal.html; Statistics Canada, "CANSIM," Updated 2010, Available at http://cansim2.statcan.gc.ca.

28. Federal Bureau of Investigation, "Hate Crime Statistics, 2009," 2011, Available at www.fbi.gov/ucr/hc2009/index.html.

29. Ibid.

30. Ibid.

31. J. Carr, *American College Health Association Campus Violence White Paper* (Baltimore: American College Health Association, 2005), Available at www.acha.org/Publications/Guidelines_WhitePapers.cfm.

32. Centers for Disease Control and Prevention, National Center for Injury Prevention and Control, Division of Violence Prevention, "Understanding Intimate Partner Violence Fact Sheet, 2011," Available at www.cdc.gov/violenceprevention/pdf/IPV_factsheet-a.pdf .

33. P. Lin and J. Gill, "Homicides of Pregnant Women," *American Journal of Forensic Medicine and Pathology* 32, no. 2 (2011): 161–3.

34. Violence Policy Center, *American Roulette: Murder-Suicide in the United States*, 3rd ed. (Washington, DC: Violence Policy Center, 2008), Available at www.vpc.org/studies/amroul2006.pdf.

35. L. Walker, *The Battered Woman* (New York: Harper and Row, 1979).

36. L. Walker, *The Battered Woman Syndrome*, 3rd ed. (New York: Springer, 2009).

37. L. Rosen and J. Fontaine, *Compendium of Research on Violence against Women, 1993–Present* (Washington, DC: National Institute of Justice, 2009), DOJ (US) NCJ223572, Available at www.ojp.usdoj.gov/nij/pubs-sum/vaw-compendium.htm.

38. A. J. Sedlak et al., *Fourth National Incidence Study of Child Abuse and Neglect (NIS-4): Report to Congress, Executive Summary* (Washington, DC: U.S. Department of Health and Human Services, Administration for Children and Families, 2010), Available at www.acf.hhs.gov/programs/opre/abuse_neglect/natl_incid/index.html.

39. L. P. Chen et al., "Sexual Abuse and Lifetime Diagnosis of Psychiatric Disorders: Systematic Review and Meta-Analysis," 2010.

40. Childhelp, "National Child Abuse Statistics," 2011, Available at www.childhelp.org/pages/statistics#stats-sources.

41. L. P. Chen et al., "Sexual Abuse and Lifetime Diagnosis of Psychiatric Disorders: Systematic Review and Meta-Analysis," 2010; R. Gilbert et al. "Burden and Consequences of Child Maltreatment in High-Income Countries," *Lancet* 373, no. 3 (2009): 68–81; T. Hilberg et al., "Review of Meta-Analyses on the Association between Child Sexual Abuse and Adult Mental Health Difficulties: A Systematic Approach," 2011.

42. Childhelp, "National Child Abuse Statistics," 2011.

43. L. P. Chen et al., "Sexual Abuse and Lifetime Diagnosis of Psychiatric Disorders: Systematic Review and Meta-Analysis," *Mayo Clinic Proceedings* 85, no. 7 (2010): 618–29; R. Gilbert et al. "Burden and Consequences of Child Maltreatment in High-Income Countries," *Lancet* 373, no. 3 (2009): 68–81; T. Hilberg, C. Hamilton-Giachrtsis, and L. Dixon. "Review of Meta-Analyses on the Association between Child Sexual Abuse and Adult Mental Health Difficulties: A Systematic Approach," *Trauma, Violence, Abuse* 12, no. 1 (2011): 38–49.

44. C. Cooper, A. Selwood, and G. Livingston, "The Prevalence of Elder Abuse and Neglect: A Systematic Review," *Age and Ageing* 37, no. 2 (2008): 151–60; National Center on Elder Abuse, "Fact Sheet: Elder Abuse Prevalence and Incidence," 2005, Available at www.ncea.aoa.gov/ncearoot/main_site/library/statistics_research/abuse_statistics/statistics_at_glance.aspx.

45. Centers for Disease Control and Prevention, National Center for Injury Prevention and Control, "Sexual Violence: Facts at a Glance," 2008, Available at www.cdc.gov/violenceprevention/sexualviolence/index.html.

46. D. Kilpatrick et al., "Drug-Facilitated, Incapacitated, and Forcible Rape: A National Study," National Crime Victims Research and Treatment Center, February 1, 2007, Available at www.ncjrs.gov/pdffiles1/nij/grants/219181.pdf.

47. Centers for Disease Control and Prevention, National Center for Injury Prevention and Control, "Sexual Violence: Facts at a Glance," 2008.

48. M. Rand, *National Crime Victimization Survey: Criminal Victimization, 2009* (Washington, DC: Bureau of Justice Statistics, 2010) NCJ 231239. Available at http://bjs.ojp.usdoj.gov/index.cfm?ty=pbdetail&iid=2217.

49. Centers for Disease Control and Prevention, National Center for Injury Prevention and Control, "Understanding Sexual Violence Fact Sheet," 2009.

50. M. Rand, *National Crime Victimization Survey,* 2010.

51. Centers for Disease Control and Prevention, "Sexual Violence: Facts at a Glance," 2008; L. Schneider et al., "The Role of Gender and Ethnicity in Perceptions of Rape and Its Aftereffects," *Sex Roles* 60, no. 5/6 (2009): 410–21.

52. D. Kilpatrick et al., "Drug-Facilitated, Incapacitated, and Forcible Rape," 2007.

53. J. Carr, *American College Health Association Campus Violence White Paper,* 2005.

54. D. Kilpatrick et al., "Drug-Facilitated, Incapacitated, and Forcible Rape," 2007.

55. Centers for Disease Control and Prevention, National Center for Injury Prevention and Control, Understanding Sexual Violence Fact Sheet," 2009.

56. University of Illinois at Chicago, "Most Sexual Assaults Drug Facilitated, Study Claims," ScienceDaily, May 13, 2006, Available at www.sciencedaily.com/releases/2006/05/060513122928.htm.

57. R. Bergen and E. Barnhill, "Marital Rape: New Research and Directions," National Online Resource Center on Violence against Women, 2006, Available at http://new.vawnet.org/category/Main_Doc.php?docid=248.

58. Ibid.

59. CDC Injury Center, "Preventing Intimate Partner Violence, Sexual Violence and Child Maltreatment," 2006, Available at www.cdc.gov/ncipc/pub-res/research_agenda/07_violence.htm; P. York, "Traditional Gender Role Attitudes and Violence against Women: A Test of Feminist Theory," Paper presented at the annual meeting of the American Society of Criminology, November 13, 2007, Available at www.allacademic.com/meta/p200649_index.html.

60. Ibid.

61. Ibid.

62. K. Baum et al., *National Crime Victimization Survey: Stalking Victimization in the United States* (Bureau of Justice Statistics: Washington, DC, 2009), NCJ 224527, Available at http://bjs.ojp.usdoj.gov/index.cfm?ty=pbdetail&iid=1211.

63. U.S. Code of Federal Regulations, Title 28CFR0.85.

64. U.S. Department of Justice, National Drug Intelligence Center, *National Gang Threat Assessment 2009* (Washington, DC: National Drug Intelligence Center, 2009), 2009-M0335-001, Available at www.justice.gov/ndic/pubs32/32146/index.htm.

65. National Youth Violence Prevention Resource Center, "Youth Gangs and Violence," Updated January 4, 2008, Available at www.safeyouth.org/scripts/faq/youthgang.asp.

66. J. Carr, *American College Health Association Campus Violence White Paper,* 2005.

67. Adapted from E. Allan and M. Madden, *Hazing in View: College Students at Risk* (Orono, ME: National Collaborative for Hazing Research and Prevention, 2008), Available at www.hazingstudy.org.

68. Ibid.

69. National Highway Traffic Safety Administration, "Traffic Safety Facts: Early Estimate of Motor Vehicle Traffic Fatalities in 2009," DOT HS 811 291, 2010, Available at www-nrd.nhtsa.dot.gov/Pubs/811291.PDF.

70. National Safety Council, "Driver Safety," 2010, Available at www.nsc.org/safety_road/DriverSafety/Pages/driver_safety.aspx.

71. Governors Highway Safety Association, "Cell Phone and Texting Laws: May 2011," 2011, Available at www.ghsa.org/html/stateinfo/laws/cellphone_laws.html; Distraction.gov, "U.S. Department of Transportation. Statistics and Facts about Distracted Driving," 2011, Available at www.distraction.gov/stats-and-facts/index.html; M. Reardon, "Study: Distractions, Not Phones, Cause Car Crashes," CNET.com, 2010, Available at http://news.cnet.com/8301-30686_3-10444717-266.html.

72. Centers for Disease Control and Prevention, "Parents Are the Key: Eight Danger Zones," Updated October 2009, Available at www.cdc.gov/parentsarethekey/danger/index.html.

73. National Highway Traffic Safety Administration, *Traffic Safety Facts 2008 Data: Alcohol-Impaired Driving* (Washington, DC: NHTSA's National Center for Statistics and Analysis, 2009), DOT HS 811 155, Available at www-nrd.nhtsa.dot.gov/cats/listpublications.aspx?Id=A&ShowBy=DocType.

74. National Institute on Drug Abuse, "NIDA InfoFacts: Drugged Driving," Revised September 2009, Available at http://drugabuse.gov/infofacts/driving.html.

75. National Safety Council, "Speeding," 2010, Available at www.nsc.org/safety_road/DriverSafety/Pages/speeding.aspx.

76. Centers for Disease Control and Prevention, "Parents Are the Key: Eight Danger Zones," 2009.

77. Insurance Institute for Highway Safety, "New Crash Tests Demonstrate the Influence of Vehicle Size and Weight on Safety in Crashes; Results Are Relevant to Fuel Economy Policies," April 2009, Available at www.iihs.org/news/rss/pr041409.html.

78. National Highway Traffic Safety Administration, *Traffic Safety Facts 2008 Data: Motorcycles* (Washington, DC: NHTSA's National Center for Statistics and Analysis, 2009), DOT HS 811 159, Available at www-nrd.nhtsa.dot.gov/cats/listpublications.aspx?Id=A&ShowBy=DocType.

79. Centers for Disease Control and Prevention, "Parents Are the Key: Eight Danger Zones," 2009.

80. A. Williams and R. Shults, "Graduated Driver Licensing Research, 2007–Present: A Review and Commentary," *Journal of Safety Research* 41, no. 2 (2010): 77–84.

81. National Safety Council, "Graduated Driver Licensing," 2010, Available at www.nsc.org/safety_road/TeenDriving/ GDL/Pages/GraduatedDriverLicensing.aspx.

82. National Highway Traffic Safety Administration, "Aggressive Driving Enforcement," 2004, Available at www.nhtsa.gov/people/injury/research/AggDrivingEnf.

83. National Highway Traffic Safety Administration, "Traffic Safety Facts 2009: Bicyclists and Other Cyclists," 2010, Available at www-nrd.nhtsa.dot.gov/Pubs/811386.pdf.

84. Ibid.

85. Consumer Product Safety Commission, "Fact Sheet: Skateboards," 2009, Available at www.cpsc.gov/cpscpub/pubs/rec_sfy.html.

86. National Ski Areas Association, "Facts about Skiing/Snowboarding Safety," 2010, Available at www.nsaa.org/nsaa/press/facts-ski-snbd-safety.asp.

87. Centers for Disease Control and Prevention, "Unintentional Drowning: Fact Sheet," June 2010, Available at www.cdc.gov/HomeandRecreationalSafety/Water-Safety/waterinjuries-factsheet.html.

88. Ibid.

89. American Red Cross, "Summer Water Safety Guide," March 2009, Available at http://american.redcross.org/site/DocServer/watersafety0609.pdf?docID=735.

90. Centers for Disease Control and Prevention, "Unintentional Drowning: Fact Sheet," 2010.

91. Ibid.

92. U. S. Coast Guard, "Boating Safety Resource Center: Boating under the Influence Initiatives," 2009, Available at www.uscgboating.org/safety/boating_under_the_influence_initiatives.aspx.

93. American Boating Association, "Boating Safety—It Could Mean Your Life," 2010, Available at www.americanboating.org/safety.asp.

94. National Institute on Deafness and Other Communication Disorders, "Quick Statistics," 2010, Available at www.nidcd.nih.gov/health/statistics/quick.htm.

95. V. Rawool and L. Colligon-Wayne, "Auditory Lifestyles and Beliefs Related to Hearing Loss among College Students in the USA," *Noise and Health* 10, no. 38 (January–March 2008): 1–10.

96. Mayo Clinic, "Hearing Loss: MP3 Players Can Pose Risk," 2006, Available at www.riversideonline.com/health_reference/Ear-Nose-Throat/GA00046.cfm.

97. H. Keppler et al., "Short-Term Auditory Effects of Listening to an MP3 Player," *Archives of Otolaryngology—Head & Neck Surgery* 136, no. 6 (2010): 538–48.

98. Centers for Disease Control and Prevention, "Poisoning in the United States: Fact Sheet," 2010, Available at www.cdc.gov/HomeandRecreationalSafety/Poisoning/poisoning-factsheet.htm.

99. Centers for Disease Control and Prevention, "Falls among Older Adults: An Overview," 2009, Available at www.cdc.gov/HomeandRecreationalSafety/Falls/adultfalls.html.

100. Fire Safety Council, "Home Fires: The Big Picture," 2007, Available at www.firesafety.gov/media/overview/index.shtm.

101. Fire Safety Council, "Campus Fire Safety," 2008, Available at www.firesafety.gov/citizens/firesafety/college.shtm.

102. U.S. Bureau of Labor Statistics, "Census of Fatal Occupational Injuries (CFOI)—Current and Revised Data," 2010, Available at www.bls.gov/iif/oshcfoi1.htm.

103. National Institute of Neurological Disorders and Stroke, "Low Back Pain Fact Sheet," June 2010, Available at www.ninds.nih.gov/disorders/backpain/detail_backpain.htm.

104. National Institute of Neurological Disorders and Stroke, "NINDS Repetitive Motion Disorders Information Page," 2007, Available at www.ninds.nih.gov/disorders/repetitive_motion/repetitive_motion.htm.

105. Mayo Clinic, "Carpal Tunnel Syndrome: Prevention," 2011, www.mayoclinic.com/health/carpal-tunnel-syndrome/DS00326/DSECTION=prevention.

Chapter 14

1. R. Caplan, *Our Earth, Ourselves* (New York: Bantam, 1990), 247.

2. R. H. Friis, *Essentials of Environmental Health* (Boston: Jones and Bartlett, 2007), 7; R. Engelman, "Population Growth Steady in Recent Years," 2009, Available at http://vitalsigns.worldwatch.org/vs-trend/population-growth-steady-recent-years.

3. United Nations, "World Population to Reach 10 billion by 2100 if Fertility in all Countries Converges to Replacement Level," 2011, Available at http://esa.un.org/unpd/wpp/index.htm.

4. United Nations Environment Programme, *Global Environment Outlook: Environment for Development (GEO-4)* (Valletta, Malta: United Nations Environment Programme, 2007), Available at www.unep.org/geo/geo4.asp.

5. Ibid.

6. N. Eberstadt, "Born in the USA," American Enterprise Institute for Public Research, 2007, Available at www.aei.org/article/25988.

7. Central Intelligence Agency, "The World Factbook: Country Comparison: Total Fertility Rate," Updated August 2010, Available at www.cia.gov/library/publications/the-world-factbook/rankorder/2127rank.html.

8. U.S. Census Bureau, Population Division, "International Data Base Country Rankings," 2010, Available at http://sasweb.ssd.census.gov/idb/ranks.html.

9. U.S. Census Bureau, U.S. and World Population Clocks, "U.S. POPClock Projection," 2010, Available at www.census.gov/population/www/popclockus.html.

10. Central Intelligence Agency, "The World Factbook: United States," Updated August 2010, Available at www.cia.gov/library/publications/the-world-factbook/geos/us.html.

11. V. Markham, *U.S. National Report on Population and the Environment* (New Canaan, CT: Center for Environment and Population, 2006), Available at www.cepnet.org.

12. C. Flavin et al., *State of the World 2008: Innovations for a Sustainable Economy* (Washington, DC: Worldwatch Institute, 2008), Available at www.worldwatch.org/node/5560.

13. Ibid.

14. Ibid.

15. Population Reference Bureau, "World Population Growth, 1950–2050," 2010, Available at www.prb.org/educators/teachersguides/humanpopulation/populationgrowth.aspx?p=1; M. Rosenberg, "Negative Population Growth," 2010, Available at http://geography.about.com/od/populationgeography/a/zero.htm.

16. R. H. Friis, *Essentials of Environmental Health,* 2007, 232.

17. U.S. Environmental Protection Agency, "Air Pollution Control Orientation Course: Criteria Pollutants," Updated January 2010, Available at www.epa.gov/apti/course422/ap5.html.

18. Ibid.

19. American Lung Association, "Health Effects of Ozone and Particle Pollution," in *State of the Air 2010* (Washington, DC: American Lung Association, 2010), Available at www.stateoftheair.org/2010/health-risks.

20. Ibid.

21. U.S. Environmental Protection Agency, "Acid Rain: What Is Acid Rain?" Updated June 2007, Available at www.epa.gov/acidrain/what/index.html.

22. U.S. Environmental Protection Agency, "Acid Rain: Effects of Acid Rain—Surface Waters and Aquatic Animals," Updated December 2008, Available at www.epa.gov/acidrain/effects/surface_water.html.

23. U.S. Environmental Protection Agency, "Acid Rain: Effects of Acid Rain—Forests," Updated June 2007, Available at www.epa.gov/acidrain/effects/forests.html.

24. U.S. Environmental Protection Agency, "Acid Rain: Effects of Acid Rain—Human Health," Updated May 2009, Available at www.epa.gov/acidrain/effects/health.html.

25. U.S. Environmental Protection Agency, "Ozone Layer Depletion: Ozone Science: Brief Questions and Answers on Ozone Depletion," Updated February 2010, Available at www.epa.gov/ozone/science/q_a.html.

26. U.S. Environmental Protection Agency, "An Introduction to Indoor Air Quality," Updated April 2010, Available at www.epa.gov/iaq/ia-intro.html.

27. Ibid.

28. U.S. Environmental Protection Agency, "Indoor Air Quality: Radon: Health Risks," Updated March 2010, Available at www.epa.gov/radon/healthrisks.html.

29. U.S. Environmental Protection Agency, "U.S. Homes above EPA's Radon Action Level," Updated June 2010, Available at http://cfpub.epa.gov/eroe/index.cfm?fuseaction=detail.viewInd&lv=list.listByAlpha&r=201747.

30. Centers for Disease Control and Prevention, "Lead," Updated July 2010, Available at www.cdc.gov/nceh/lead.

31. North Carolina Department of Health and Human Services, Epidemiology, "Indoor Air Quality: Schools," Updated July 2010, Available at www.epi.state.nc.us/epi/air/schools.html.

32. U.S. Environmental Protection Agency, "IAQ Tools for Schools: Improved Academic Performance: Evidence from Scientific Literature," Updated May 2010, Available at www.epa.gov/iaq/schools/student_performance/evidence.html.

33. National Center for Health Statistics, "FASTSTATS Asthma," Updated May 2009, Available at www.cdc.gov/nchs/fastats/asthma.htm; American Lung Association, "About Asthma," 2010, Available at www.lungusa.org/lung-disease/asthma/about-asthma.

34. American Lung Association, "About Asthma," 2010.

35. Ibid.

36. S. Arrhenius, "On the Influence of Carbonic Acid in the Air upon the Temperature of the Ground," *Philosophical Magazine and Journal of Science* (fifth series) 41 (1896): 237–75.

37. U.S. Environmental Protection Agency, "Climate Change: Basic Information," Updated May 2010, Available at www.epa.gov/climatechange/basicinfo.html.

38. U.S. Government Accountability Office, "Climate Change: Trends in Greenhouse Gas Emissions and Emissions Intensity in the United States and Other High-Emitting Nations," GAO-04-146R, October 2003, Available at www.gao.gov/products/GAO-04-146R.

39. United Nations Framework Convention on Climate Change, "Kyoto Protocol," 2010, Available at http://unfccc.int/kyoto_protocol/items/2830.php.

40. D. Malakoff and E. M. Williams, "Q & A: An Examination of the Kyoto Protocol," June 2007, Available at www.npr.org/templates/story/story.php?storyId=5042766.

41. "Cancun Climate Conference: What It All Means," *The Telegraph,* December 11, 2010, Available at www.telegraph.co.uk/earth/environment/climatechange/8196246/Cancun-Climate-Conference-what-it-all-means.html.

42. U.S. Geological Survey, "Water Science for Schools: Where Is Earth's Water Located?" Modified July 2010, Available at http://ga.water.usgs.gov/edu/earthwherewater.html.

43. World Health Organization, "10 Facts on Sanitation," 2011, Available at www.who.int/features/factfiles/sanitation/en/index.html.

44. R. H. Friis, *Essentials of Environmental Health,* 2007, 204.

45. V. Markham, *U.S. National Report on Population and the Environment,* 2006.

46. D. W. Kolpin et al., "Pharmaceuticals, Hormones, and Other Organic Wastewater Contaminants in U.S. Streams, 1999–2000: A National Reconnaissance," *Environmental Science & Technology* 36, no. 6 (2002): 1202–11.

47. G. Bruce et al., "Toxicological Relevance of Pharmaceuticals in Drinking Water," *Environmental Science & Technology* 44, no.14 (2010): 5619–26; J. Donn et al., "AP Probe Finds Drugs in Drinking Water," March 2010, Available at www.breitbart.com/article.php?id=D8VADOP80.

48. J. Donn et al., "AP Probe Finds Drugs in Drinking Water," 2010.

49. M. Tiemann, "Environmental Legislation: Leaking Underground Storage Tanks (USTs): Prevention and Cleanup," May 2010, Available at http://environmental-legislation.blogspot.com/2010/05/leaking-underground-storage-tanks-usts.html.

50. Agency for Toxic Substances and Disease Registry (ATSDR), "Toxic Substances Portal: Polychlorinated Biphenyls (PCBs)," Updated April 2010,

Available at www.atsdr.cdc.gov/substances/tox-substance.asp?toxid=26.

51. U.S. Environmental Protection Agency, "Pesticides: Topical and Chemical Fact Sheets: Assessing Health Risks from Pesticides," Updated September 2009, Available at www.epa.gov/pesticides/factsheets/riskassess.htm.

52. U.S. Environmental Protection Agency, *Municipal Solid Waste Generation, Recycling, and Disposal in the United States: Facts and Figures for 2009* (Washington, DC: U.S. Environmental Protection Agency, 2010), Available at www.epa.gov/epawaste/nonhaz/municipal/msw99.htm.

53. Ibid.

54. Ibid.

55. Ibid.

56. U.S. Environmental Protection Agency, "Superfund: Superfund National Accomplishments Summary, Fiscal Year 2009," Updated May 2010, Available at www.epa.gov/superfund/accomp/numbers09.html.

57. World Health Organization, "Electromagnetic Fields and Public Health: Mobile Phones," Fact Sheet no. 193, May 2010, Available at www.who.int/mediacentre/factsheets/fs193/en/; U.S. Food and Drug Administration, "Radiation-Emitting Products: Health Issues: Do Cell Phones Pose a Health Hazard?" Updated May 2010, Available at www.fda.gov/Radiation-EmittingProducts/RadiationEmittingProductsandProcedures/HomeBusinessandEntertainment/CellPhones/ucm116282.htm; D. Hoch, MedlinePlus, "Cell Phones—Do They Cause Cancer?" Updated September 2008, Available at www.nlm.nih.gov/medlineplus/ency/article/007151.htm.

58. R. Snowden, American Cancer Society, "Major Study Complicates Debate over Cell Phone Use and Cancer Risks," May 2010, Available at www.cancer.org/Cancer/news/News/major-study-complicates-debate-over-cell-phone-use-and-cancer-risk.

59. U.S. Nuclear Regulatory Commission, "Radiation Basics," 2011, Available at http://nrc.gov/about-nrc/radiation/health-effects/radiation-basics.html.

60. National Council on Radiation Protection and Measurements, "NCRP Report No. 160 Section 1 Pie Chart," Available at www.ncrponline.org/Publications/160_Pie_charts.html.

61. Nuclear Energy Institute, "World Statistics," 2011, Available at www.nei.org/resourcesandstats/nuclear_statistics/worldstatistics.

62. J. Deutch et al., *Update of the MIT 2003 Future of Nuclear Power: An Interdisciplinary MIT Study* (Cambridge, MA: Massachusetts Institute of Technology, 2009), Available at http://web.mit.edu/nuclearpower.

63. BBC News, "Japan Earthquake," 2011, Available at www.bbc.co.uk/news/world-asia-pacific-12711226.

64. Nuclear Energy Institute, "Key Issues," 2010, Available at www.nei.org/keyissues.

65. Public Citizen, "Just the Facts: A Look at the Five Fatal Flaws of Nuclear Power," 2010, Available at www.citizen.org/cmep/article_redirect.cfm?ID=13447; Friends of the Earth, "Nuclear Reactors," 2010, Available at www.foe.org/energy/nuclear-reactors.

66. American Lung Association, "State of the Air," 2011, Available at www.stateoftheair.org/2011/city-rankings.

Chapter 15

1. R. de la Fuente-Fernandez et al., "Expectation and Dopamine Release: Mechanism of the Placebo Effect in Parkinson's Disease," *Science* 293 (2001): 1164–66.

2. J. Friedman and R. Dubinsky, "The Placebo Effect," *Neurology* 71, no. 9 (2008): e25–e26; N. Diedrich and C. Goetz, "The Placebo Treatments in Neurosciences: New Insights from Clinical and Neuroimaging Studies," *Neurology* 71 (2008): 677–94.

3. American Academy of Orthopaedic Surgeons, "Information Statement: The Importance of Good Communication in the Physician-Patient Relationship," September 2005, Available at www.aaos.org/about/papers/advistmt/1017.asp.

4. MedicineNet, "Definition of Defensive Medicine," Reviewed June 2004, Available at www.medterms.com/script/main/art.asp?articlekey=33262.

5. D. Merenstein et al., "Use and Costs of Non-recommended Tests during Routine Preventive Health Exams," *American Journal of Preventive Medicine* 30, no. 6 (2006): 521–27; Thomson Reuters, "Waste in the U.S. Healthcare System Pegged at $700 Billion in Report from Thomson Reuters," October 26, 2009, Available at http://thomsonreuters.com/content/press_room/tsh/waste_US_healthcare_system.

6. N. Kwon, "Patient Rights," 2006, Available at www.emedicinehealth.com/patient_rights/article_em.htm.

7. Mayo Clinic Staff, "Complementary and Alternative Medicine: What Is It?" Mayo Clinic, October 2009, Available at www.mayoclinic.com/health/alternative-medicine/PN00001.

8. National Center for Complementary and Alternative Medicine, "The Use of Complementary and Alternative Medicine in the United States," Updated December 2008, Available at http://nccam.nih.gov/news/camstats/2007/camsurvey_fs1.htm.

9. J. Tsao, "Effectiveness of Massage Therapy for Chronic, Non-Malignant Pain: A Review," *Evidence-Based Complementary and Alternative Medicine* 4, no. 2 (2007): 165–79; National Cancer Institute, "Acupuncture: Human/Clinical Studies," 2008, Available at www.cancer.gov/cancertopics/pdq/cam/acupuncture/HealthProfessional/page6.

10. National Center for Complementary and Alternative Medicine, "The Use of Complementary and Alternative Medicine in the United States," 2008.

11. Ibid.

12. National Center for Complementary and Alternative Medicine, "What Is CAM?" NCCAM Publication no. D347, Updated November 2010, Available at http://nccam.nih.gov/health/whatiscam/.

13. National Center for Complementary and Alternative Medicine, "Ayurvedic Medicine: An Introduction," NCCAM Publication no. D287, Updated March 2011, Available at http://nccam.nih.gov/health/ayurveda/introduction.htm.

14. American Institute of Homeopathy, "Homeopathy: Efficacy and Evidence Base," 2007, Available at http://homeopathyusa.org/homeopathy-now.html; Health Alternatives Online, "Homeopathy," 2008, Available at www.healthalternativesonline.com/homeopathy.html.

15. National Center for Complementary and Alternative Medicine, "Chiropractic: An Introduction," NCCAM Publication no. D403, Modified February 2011, Available at http://nccam.nih.gov/health/chiropractic/#intro.

16. Bureau of Labor Statistics, U.S. Department of Labor, "Chiropractors," *Occupational Outlook Handbook, 2010–11 Edition,* December 2009, Available at www.bls.gov/oco/ocos071.htm.

17. J. Tsao, "Effectiveness of Massage Therapy for Chronic, Non-Malignant Pain: A Review," 2007.

18. Mayo Clinic Staff, "Massage: Get in Touch with Its Many Health Benefits," January 2010, Available at www.mayoclinic.com/health/massage/SA00082; National Center for Complementary and Alternative Medicine, "Massage Therapy," 2009, Available at http://nccam.nih.gov/health/massage.

19. National Center for Complementary and Alternative Medicine, "Massage Therapy," 2009.

20. Bureau of Labor Statistics, U.S. Department of Labor, "Massage Therapists," *Occupational Outlook Handbook, 2010–11 Edition,* 2009.

21. National Center for Complementary and Alternative Medicine, "What Is CAM?" 2010, Available at http://nccam.nih.gov/health/whatiscam; U.S. Trager Association, "The Trager Approach," 2010, Available at www.trager-us.org/trager-approach.html.

22. National Center for Complementary and Alternative Medicine, "What Is CAM?" 2010.

23. American Cancer Society, "Acupuncture," 2010, Available at www.cancer.org/docroot/ETO/content/ETO_5_3X_Acupuncture.asp.

24. National Center for Complementary and Alternative Medicine, "Acupuncture: An Introduction," NCCAM Publication no. D404, Modified March 2011, Available at http://nccam.nih.gov/health/acupuncture/introduction.htm.

25. B. Seaward, *Managing Stress,* 6th ed. (Sudbury, MA: Jones and Bartlett, 2009); D. Tosevski and M. Milovancevic, "Stressful Life Events and Physical Health," *Current Opinion in Psychiatry* 19, no. 2 (2006): 184–89.

26. J. Robins et al., "Research in Psychoneuroimmunology: Tai Chi as a Stress Management Approach for Individuals with HIV Disease," *Applied Nursing Research* 19, no. 1 (February 2006): 2–9; M. Opp et al., "Sleep and Psychoneuroimmunology," *Immunology and Allergy Clinics of North America* 29, no. 2 (May 2009): 295–307; A. Starkweather et al., "Immune Function, Pain, and Psychological Stress in Patients Undergoing Spinal Surgery," *Spine* 31, no. 18 (August 2006): E641–E647.

27. Office of Dietary Supplements, National Institutes of Health, "Dietary Supplements: Background Information," Updated July 2009, Available at http://ods.od.nih.gov/factsheets/dietarysupplements.asp.

28. U.S. Food and Drug Administration, "The Possible Dangers of Buying Medicine over the Internet," 2010, Available at www.fda.gov/ForConsumers/ConsumerUpdates/ucm048396.htm.

29. AARP and National Center for Complementary and Alternative Medicine Survey Report, Complementary and Alternative Medicine, "What People Aged 50 and Older Discuss with Their Health Care Providers," NCCAM, 2011, Available at http://nccam.nih.gov/news/camstats/2010/findings1.htm

30. National Center for Complementary and Alternative Medicine, "Kava," June 2008, Available at http://nccam.nih.gov/health/kava/ataglance.htm.

31. Mayo Clinic Staff, "Herbal Supplements: What to Know before You Buy," November 2009, Available at www.mayoclinic.com/health/herbal-supplements/SA00044.

32. Kaiser Family Foundation, "The Uninsured: A Primer: Key Facts about Americans without Health Insurance," 2010, Available at www.kff.org/uninsured/7451.cfm.

33. C. Schoen et al., "How Many Are Underinsured? Trends among U.S. Adults, 2003 and 2007," *Health Affairs* Web Exclusive (June 10, 2008): w298–w309.

34. American College Health Association, American College Health Association-National College Health Assessment Reference Group Data Report Fall 2010 (Baltimore: American College Health Association, 2011.

35. National Center for Health Statistics, *Health, United States, 2010* (Hyattsville, MD: National Center for Health Statistics, 2011), Available at www.cdc.gov/nchs/hus.htm.

36. Kaiser Family Foundation, "Total HMO Enrollment, July 2010," 2011, Available at www.statehealthfacts.org/comparemaptable .jsp?ind=348&cat=7.

37. Centers for Medicare and Medicaid Services, "NHE Fact Sheet," Modified June 29, 2010, Available at www.cms.gov/NationalHealthExpendData/ 25_NHE_Fact_Sheet.asp.

38. Centers for Medicare and Medicaid Services, "Medicare Enrollment: National Trends 1966–2009," Modified June 2011, Available at www.cms .gov/MedicareEnRpts/01_Overview.asp.

39. Centers for Medicare and Medicaid Services, "Medicaid Data Sources—General Information," Modified December 2005, Available at www.cms .gov/MedicaidDataSourcesGenInfo.

40. National Center for Health Statistics, *Health, United States, 2010,* 2011; Centers for

Medicare and Medicaid Services, "National Health Care Expenditures Projections: 2009–2019," 2009, Available at www.cms.gov/ NationalHealthExpendData/03_National HealthAccountsProjected.asp.

41. National Center for Chronic Disease Prevention and Health Promotion, "Chronic Diseases and Health Promotion," Updated July 2010, Available at www .cdc.gov/chronicdisease/overview/index.htm.

42. Ibid.

43. Bureau of Labor Statistics, U.S. Department of Labor, "Physicians and Surgeons," *Occupational Outlook Handbook, 2010–11,* Modified December 2009, Available at www.bls.gov/oco/ ocos074.htm.

44. The White House, "Health Care Reform: The Affordable Care Act," 2010, Available at www.whitehouse .gov/healthreform/healthcare-overview.

45. Right to Health Care ProCon.org, "Should All Americans Have the Right (Be Entitled) to Health Care?" Updated October 2010, Available at http:// healthcare.procon.org.

46. United Nations, "The Universal Declaration of Human Rights," 1948, Available at www.un.org/ en/documents/udhr.

47. Right to Health Care ProCon.org, "Should All Americans," 2010.

48. Environmental Protection Agency, "Medical Waste Frequent Questions," 2010, Available at www.epa.gov/wastes/nonhaz/industrial/medical/ mwfaqs.htm.

49. U.S. Food and Drug Administration, "How to Dispose of Unused Medicines," 2009, Available at www.fda.gov/ForConsumers/ConsumerUpdates/ ucm101653.htm.

50. National Conference of State Legislatures, "State Prescription Drug Return, Reuse, and Recycling Laws," 2010, Available at www.ncsl.org/default .aspx?tabid=14425.

Photo Credits

Front matter p. v top: Comstock/Getty Images; p. v bottom: STEVE LINDRIDGE/Alamy; p. vi top: Jose Luis Pelaez Inc/Blend Images/Photolibrary; p. vi bottom: Adam Borkowski/iStockphoto.com; p. vii: Adam Hart-Davis/Photo Researchers, Inc.; p. viii top: ACE STOCK LIMITED/Alamy; p. viii bottom: Comstock Images/Getty Images; p. ix top: Brian Hagiwara/Food Pix/Getty Images; p. ix bottom: Jim Esposito Photography L.L.C./Photodisc/Getty Images; p. x: Thomas Smith Photography/Alamy; p. xi top: John Giustina/Digital Vision/Getty Images; p. xi bottom: Doruk Sikman/iStockphoto.com; p. xii left: Martin Heitner/Photolibrary; p. xii right: Dave King/Dorling Kindersley; p. xiii: Willie Hill, Jr./The Image Works.

Chapter 1 Opener: Goodluz/Shutterstock.com; p. 2: Ale Ventura/Jupiterimages; p. 3: MBI/Alamy; p. 4 left to right: UK Stock Images Ltd/Alamy; webphotographeer/iStockphoto.com; Cat London/iStockphoto.com; Yeko Photo Studio/Shutterstock.com; p. 5: AP Photo/Steve Holland; p. 6: amana images inc./Alamy; p. 8: Corbis Super RF/Alamy; p. 10: Hola Images/Alamy; p. 12: manley099/iStockphoto.com; p. 13: STEVE LINDRIDGE/Alamy; p. 15: Christina Kennedy/Alamy; p. 17: Jacob Wackerhausen/iStockphoto.com; p. 18: Lisa F. Young/iStockphoto.com; p. 19 all: ZoneCreative/iStockphoto.com.

Chapter 2 Opener: Ipatov/Shutterstock.com; p. 23 left: Comstock/Thinkstock; p. 23 right: Terry Vine/Getty Images; p. 25: Exactostock/SuperStock; p. 26: Pascal Broze/AGE Fotostock; p. 28: Corbis Super RF/Alamy; p. 29: George Doyle/Stockbyte/Getty Images; p. 31 left: Keren Su/China Span/Alamy; p. 31 right: Neal & Molly Jansen/SuperStock; p. 32: Michael Valdez/iStockphoto.com; p. 33 top: Exactostock/SuperStock; p. 33 bottom: Jumpstart/Kathleen VanDernoot Pearson Foundation; p. 35: John Bell/iStockphoto.com; p. 36: Comstock/Getty Images; p. 38: Bubbles Photolibrary/Alamy; p. 39: Blend Images/SuperStock; p. 40: SIMON RAWLEY/Alamy; p. 43: ZoneCreative/iStockphoto.com.

Chapter 3 Opener: Comstock/Getty Images; p. 46: CREATISTA/Shutterstock.com; p. 47 top left: John Pendygraft/St. Petersburg Times/PSG/Newscom; p. 47 top right: Blend Images/Alamy; p. 47 bottom: Scott Griessel/iStockphoto.com; p. 49: Oliver Furrer/Alamy; p. 50: Adam Borkowski/iStockphoto.com; p. 51: Michael Krinke/iStockphoto.com; p. 52: Gladskikh Tatiana/Shutterstock.com; p. 53: Radius Images/Jupiter Images; p. 54: Radius Images/Corbis; p. 55: David Grossman/Alamy; p. 56: Imagerymajestic/Alamy; p. 58: Sam Chrysanthou/All Canada Photos/Photolibrary; p. 59: Corbis/SuperStock; p. 60: parema/iStockphoto.com; p. 61: Richard Rodvold/iStockphoto.com; p. 62: Andy Crawford/Dorling Kindersley; p. 63: John Dowland/Photoalto/Photolibrary; p. 64: Hannah Gleghorn/iStockphoto.com; p. 65: Sharon Dominick/iStockphoto.com.

Chapter 4 Opener: iofoto/Shutterstock.com; p. 68: Jose Luis Pelaez Inc/Blend Images/Photolibrary; p. 70: Royalty-Free/Masterfile; p. 72: Royalty-Free/Masterfile; p. 73: Justmeyo | Dreamstime.com; p. 74: Copyright David Young-Wolff/PhotoEdit; p. 75: Copyright Colin Young-Wolff/PhotoEdit; p. 77: Ryan McVay/Photodisc/Getty Images; p. 78: PhotoAlto/John Dowland/Getty Images; p. 80: Gaz Shirley/Kevin Perkins, PacificCoastNews/Newscom; p. 81 top: Kevin Dodge/Masterfile; p. 81 bottom: Hannibal Hanschke/dpa/picture-alliance/Newscom; p. 84: David J. Green - lifestyle themes/Alamy; p. 87 left: Westend61 GmbH/Alamy; p. 87 right: Mangostock | Dreamstime.com; p. 88: PhotoAlto/Alamy; p. 89: Banana Stock/Jupiterimages; p. 90: Allison Michael Orenstein/Photodisc/Getty Images; p. 91: Yanik Chauvin/iStockphoto.com.

Chapter 5 Opener: Somos Images/Alamy; p. 95 top: Dorling Kindersley; p. 96 left: Renn Sminkey/Pearson Science; p. 96 right: SIU BIOMED COMM Custom Medical Stock Photo/Newscom; p. 97 left: Jules Selmes and Debi Treloar/Dorling Kindersley; p. 99: Adam Hart-Davis/Photo Researchers, Inc.; p. 100: Courtesy of Johnson & Johnson; p. 101 top: Reproduced with permission of N.V. Organon, subsidiary of Merck & Co., Inc. All rights reserved. NuvaRing is a registered trademark of N.V. Organon.; p. 101 bottom: PHANIE/Photo Researchers, Inc.; p. 102: Saturn Stills/Photo Researchers, Inc.; p. 103: Maureen Spuhler/Seelevel.com/Pearson Science; p. 106: Imagesource/PhotoLibrary; p. 107: Fancy/Alamy; p. 110: Phase4Photography/Shutterstock.com; p. 111: Stockbrokerxtra Images/Photolibrary; p. 113: Lisa Spindler Photography Inc./Getty Images; p. 114: Cagri Özgür/iStockphoto.com; p. 117: Plush Studios/Getty Images; p. 118: Donna Coleman/iStockphoto.com; p. 119 top: Christoph Achenbach/iStockphoto.com; p. 119 bottom: winterling/iStockphoto.com.

Chapter 6 Opener: Kuzma/Shutterstock.com; p. 122: UpperCut Images/Alamy; p. 123 left: WENN/Newscom; p. 123 right: DAVID MCKNEW/UPI/Newscom; p. 124: UpperCut Images/Alamy; p. 125 top: Digital Vision/Alamy; p. 125 bottom: Denis Pepin/iStockphoto.com p. 127: Science Photo Library/Alamy; p. 128: Lori Sparkia/Shutterstock.com; p. 129: Image Source/Getty Images; p. 130: Courtesy of Charles Tatlock; p. 131: Banana Stock/PhotoLibrary; p. 132: RayArt Graphics/Alamy; p. 133 top: Copyright Park Street/PhotoEdit; p. 133 bottom: Karen Mower/iStockphoto.com; p. 134: Gregor Buir/Shutterstock.com; p. 135: David Hoffman Photo Library/Alamy; p. 136: Martyn Vickery/Alamy; p. 137 top: ACE STOCK LIMITED/Alamy; p. 137 bottom: Bob Cheung/Shutterstock.com; p. 138: Janine Wiedel Photolibrary/Alamy; p. 139: Image of Sport Photos/Newscom; p. 140: Design Pics/Jupiter Images; p. 141: Cultura/Alamy; p. 142: Jupiterimages/Getty Images; p. 143: TommL/iStockphoto.com.

Chapter 7 Opener: Mark Yeoman/Alamy; p. 148: Steve Gorton/Dorling Kindersley; p. 149: INSADCO Photography/Alamy; p. 151: i love images/Photolibrary; p. 152 left: CNRI/SPL; p. 152 right: Martin M. Rotker/Photo Researchers, Inc.; p. 154: vario images GmbH & Co.KG/Alamy; p. 155: Roger Lee/Superstock/Photolibrary; p. 156: Thinkstock/Comstock/Getty Images; p. 158: INSADCO Photography/Alamy; p. 159: Bubbles Photolibrary/Alamy; p. 160: image100/Alamy; p. 161: Image courtesy of Romano & Associates Inc./Oral Health America; p. 162: Biophoto Associates/Photo Researchers, Inc.; p. 163: allOver photography/Alamy; p. 164: Image Source/Alamy; p. 167: Comstock Images/Getty Images; p. 168: Fadyukhin/iStockphoto.com; p. 169: milosluz/iStockphoto.com.

Chapter 8 Opener: Brand X Pictures/Thinkstock.com; p. 172: webphotographeer/iStockphoto.com; p. 173: design56/Shutterstock.com; p. 174 all: Pearson Learning Photo Studio; p. 175: Frank Greenaway/Dorling Kindersley, Courtesy of the Natural History Museum, London; p. 176: Miflippo | Dreamstime.com; p. 179: David R. Frazier Photolibrary, Inc./Alamy; p. 180 all: Barry Gregg/Corbis; p. 181 top: Brand Pictures/AGE Fotostock; p. 181 middle: C Squared Studios/Photodisc/Getty Images; p. 181 bottom left: Barry Gregg/Corbis; p. 181 bottom right: Barry Gregg/Corbis; p. 182 all: Brand Pictures/AGE Fotostock; p. 183 all: Barry Gregg/Corbis; p. 184: Suzannah Skelton/iStockphoto.com; p. 187 all: Kristin Piljay/Pearson Science; p. 188: Ted Pink/Alamy; p. 190: Brian Hagiwara/Food Pix/Getty Images; p. 193: MorePixels; p. 194: rtyree1/iStockphoto.com; p. 196: Denise Kappa/iStockphoto.com; p. 197: alxpin/iStockphoto.com.

Chapter 9 Opener: A Green/Photolibrary; p. 201: Big Cheese Photo LLC/Alamy; p. 202: Wavebreakmediamicro | Dreamstime.com; p. 203 all: Brand X Pictures/Getty Images; p. 204: Fancy/Alamy; p. 206: Jim Esposito Photography L.L.C./Photodisc/Getty Images; p. 209: Davidcrehner | Dreamstime.com; p. 210: Luislouro | Dreamstime.com; p. 211: Asia Images Group Pte Ltd/Alamy; p. 212: Tony DiMaio iPhoto Inc./Newscom; p. 213: Howard Shooter/Dorling Kindersley; p. 214 left: Custom Medical Stock Photo/Alamy; p. 214 right: Sakala/Shutterstock.com; p. 216 left: Brand X Pictures/JupiterImages; p. 216 right: gollykim/iStockphoto.com; p. 217: Christopher LaMarca/Redux; p. 218: Moodboard/Corbis; p. 219 top: Photodisc/Thinkstock.com; p. 219 bottom: Lucas Allen White/Shutterstock.com; p. 220 top: Catherine Lane/iStockphoto.com; p. 220 bottom: Sharon Dominick/iStockphoto.com; p. 221: Angelika Schwarz/iStockphoto.com; p. 222: Kristen Johansen/iStockphoto.com; p. 223: Gustavo Andrade/iStockphoto.com.

Chapter 10 Opener: Fancy/Alamy; p. 227 left to right: Teo Lannie/Getty Images; Elena Dorfman/Pearson Science; Photodisc/Getty Images; Exactostock/SuperStock; Paul Matthew Photography/Shutterstock.com; p. 229: Philip Date/Shutterstock.com; p. 231: Andresr | Dreamstime.com; p. 232 top, left to right: Walter Cruz/MCT/Newscom; Craig Veltri/iStockphoto.com; PaulMaguire/iStockphoto.com; Tatuasha/Shutterstock.com; M.w.lao | Dreamstime.com; Graca Victoria/Shutterstock.com; Royalty-Free/Masterfile; Sandra Caldwell/Shutterstock.com; p. 232 bottom, left to right: Kirsty Pargeter/iStockphoto.com; Ali Ender Birer/iStockphoto.com; Bob Jacobson/Corbis; Ali Ender Birer/Shutterstock.com; dandanian/iStockphoto.com; p. 233 left to right: Dan Dalton/Digital Vision/Getty Images; MIXA/Getty Images; Image Source/Getty Images; p. 234 left: Creative Digital Visions/Pearson Science; p. 234 right: Karl Weatherly/Photodisc/Getty Images; p. 235: Courtesy of OSU Office of News & Communication; p. 236: Royalty-Free/Masterfile; p. 237 left to right: Blue Jean Images/Alamy; Pearson Science; Pearson Science; Courtesy of HOGGAN Health Industries, Inc.; p. 238 all: Pearson Science; p. 239: Nenad Aksic/iStockphoto.com; p. 240 top: Thomas Smith Photography/Alamy; p. 240 bottom: Pearson Science; p. 242 top: Thomas Northcut/Getty Images; p. 242 bottom: Morgan Lane Studios/iStockphoto.com; p. 243: Dennis Welsh/AGE Fotostock; p. 244: Ingram Publishing/Photolibrary; p. 245: Juice Images/Alamy; p. 246: MARK COWAN/UPI/Newscom; p. 248 top: Aleksandr Lobanov/iStockphoto.com; p. 248 middle: Pearson Science; p. 248 bottom: Elena Dorfman/Pearson Science.

Chapter 11 Opener: Haveseen | Dreamstime.com; p. 257: Irina Iglina/iStockphoto.com; p. 259: Radius Images/Alamy; p. 260: Juanmonino/iStockphoto.com; p. 261: Iofoto | Dreamstime.com; p. 263: Dorling Kindersley; p. 266: Photolibrary RF; p. 267: Dawn Poland/iStockphoto.com; p. 268: BSIP SA/Alamy; p. 269: Robert Convery/Alamy; p. 270: Kevin Winter/Getty Images; p. 272: Rick Gomez/Masterfile; p. 273 left to right: James Stevenson/Photo Researchers, Inc.; Dr. P. Marazzi/Photo Researchers, Inc.; Dr. P. Marazzi/Photo Researchers, Inc.; p. 275: David Sacks/Lifesize/Getty Images; p. 280: John Giustina/Digital Vision/Getty Images; p. 282: Scott Bauer/Photo Researchers, Inc.; p. 284: Ioana Davies/iStockphoto.com; p. 285 top: vm/iStockphoto.com; p. 285 bottom: Max Delson Martins Santos/iStockphoto.com; p. 287 mark wragg/iStockphoto.com.

Chapter 12 Opener: Sam Edwards/Alamy; p. 290: Losevsky Pavel/Alamy; p. 291: Blend Images/SuperStock; 294 Lezh/iStockphoto.com; p. 295 left to right: Dr. Gary Gaugler/Photo Researchers, Inc.; Dr. Linda M. Stannard, University of Cape Town/Photo Researchers, Inc.; Steve Gschmeissner/Photo Researchers, Inc.; Eye of Science/Photo Researchers, Inc.; Medical-on-Line/Alamy; p. 296: Sidea Revuz/Photo Researchers, Inc.; p. 298: Antagain/iStockphoto.com; p. 299: Michael Krinke/iStockphoto.com; p. 300: Gabriel Moisa/iStockphoto.com; p. 301: Doruk Sikman/iStockphoto.com; p. 302: Kevin Foy/Alamy; p. 304: Western Ophthalmic Hospital/Photo Researchers, Inc.; p. 305: Courtesy of The Centers for Disease Control and Prevention; p. 306: SPL/Photo Researchers, Inc.; p. 307: Copyright 2010 NMSB - Custom Medical Stock Photo, All Rights Reserved; p. 308: Dr. P. Marazzi/Photo Researchers, Inc.; p. 309: Eye of Science/Photo Researchers, Inc.; p. 310 top: Tomaz Levstek/iStockphoto.com; p. 310 bottom: arturbo/iStockphoto.com; p. 311 top: Simon Valentine/iStockphoto.com; p. 311 bottom: Brandon Brown/iStockphoto.com.

Chapter 13 Opener: i love images/Alamy; p. 314: Jochen Tack/Alamy; p. 315: D. Hurst/Alamy; p. 316: Dean Millar/iStockphoto.com; 317 top: Felix Mizioznikov/Shutterstock.com; 317 bottom: Thinkstock.com; p. 318: Janine Wiedel Photolibrary/Alamy; p. 320: David White/Alamy; p. 321: Copyright Bill Aron/PhotoEdit; p. 322: Peter M Fisher/Photolibrary; p. 323: Anthony Dunn/Alamy; p. 324: Charles Sturge/Alamy; p. 326: Olivier Douliery/ABACAUSA/Newscom; p. 328: Martin Heitner/Photolibrary; p. 329: Copyright Paul Conklin/PhotoEdit; p. 330 all: Kristin Piljay/Pearson Science; p. 331: Laurel Scherer/Photolibrary; p. 333: Copyright Jeff Greenberg/PhotoEdit; p. 334 all: Science Photo Library/Alamy; p. 336 top: Gerville Hall/iStockphoto.com; p. 336 bottom: Dmitry Melnikov/Shutterstock.com; p. 337 left: Eric Ferguson/iStockphoto.com; p. 337 right: Daniel Deitschel/iStockphoto.com.

Index